Plant Regulation and World Agriculture

NATO ADVANCED STUDY INSTITUTES SERIES

A series of edited volumes comprising multifaceted studies of contemporary scientific issues by some of the best scientific minds in the world, assembled in cooperation with NATO Scientific Affairs Division.

Series A: Life Sciences

Recent Volumes in this Series

Volume 15 – The Lipoprotein Molecule
edited by Hubert Peeters

Volume 16 – Amino Acids as Chemical Transmitters
edited by Frode Fonnum

Volume 17 – DNA Synthesis: Present and Future
edited by Ian Molineux and Masamichi Kohiyama

Volume 18 – Sensory Ecology: Review and Perspectives
edited by M. A. Ali

Volume 19 – Animal Learning: Survey and Analysis
M. E. Bitterman, V. M. LoLordo, J. B. Overmier, and M. E. Rashotte

Volume 20 – Antiviral Mechanisms in the Control of Neoplasia
edited by P. Chandra

Volume 21a – Chromatin Structure and Function:
Molecular and Cellular Biophysical Methods
edited by Claudio A. Nicolini

Volume 21b – Chromatin Structure and Function:
Levels of Organization and Cell Function
edited by Claudio A. Nicolini

Volume 22 – Plant Regulation and World Agriculture
edited by Tom K. Scott

Volume 23 – The Molecular Biology of Picornaviruses
edited by R. Pérez-Bercoff

Volume 24 – Humoral Immunity in Neurological Diseases
edited by D. Karcher, A. Lowenthal, and A. D. Strosberg

The series is published by an international board of publishers in conjunction with NATO Scientific Affairs Division

A	**Life Sciences**	Plenum Publishing Corporation
B	**Physics**	New York and London
C	**Mathematical and Physical Sciences**	D. Reidel Publishing Company Dordrecht and Boston
D	**Behavioral and Social Sciences**	Sijthoff International Publishing Company Leiden
E	**Applied Sciences**	Noordhoff International Publishing Leiden

Plant Regulation and World Agriculture

Edited by
Tom K. Scott
University of North Carolina
Chapel Hill, North Carolina

PLENUM PRESS • NEW YORK AND LONDON
Published in cooperation with NATO Scientific Affairs Division

Library of Congress Cataloging in Publication Data

Nato Advanced Study Institute on Plant Regulation and World Agriculture, Izmir, 1978.

Plant regulation and world agriculture.

(NATO advanced study institutes series: Series A, Life sciences; v. 22)
"Published in cooperation with NATO Scientific Affairs Division."
Includes indexes.
1. Plant regulators–Congresses. 2. Agriculture–Congresses. I. Scott, Tom K. II. North Atlantic Treaty Organization. Division of Scientific Affairs. III. Title. IV. Series.
SB128.N37 1978 631.8 79-14597

ISBN 978-1-4684-3514-6 ISBN 978-1-4684-3512-2 (eBook)
DOI 10.1007/978-1-4684-3512-2

Proceedings of a NATO Advanced Study Institute on Plant Regulation and World Agriculture, held in Izmir, Turkey, September 21–30, 1978.

Softcover reprint of the hardcover 1st edition 1979

To

YUSUF VARDAR

A pioneer in a time when

pioneering is a disappearing quality of humankind

PREFACE

By the year 2000, the most critical world problem--as things stand now--will be sustaining the human race. The quality and the availability of food will continue to be central to this issue. However, since the beginning of the final quarter of the twentieth century, few attempts have been made to organize and integrate information applying our knowledge of the regulation of plant growth to the enhancement of the world's yield of food, forage, fiber, and other useful plants. It is appropriate, therefore, to approach a solution to future human needs by combining an area of basic science with a defined and needed application of it.

The purpose of this NATO Advanced Study Institute--Plant Regulation and World Agriculture--is reflected in the content of this volume. It covers a wide range of physiological processes including photosynthesis, translocation, seed germination, source-sink relationships, water relationships, flowering, fruiting, and adaptations to stress. The identification, chemistry, and biochemistry of naturally occurring as well as known and new synthetic plant growth regulators are discussed in relation to productivity, growth retardation, and herbicidal activity. Other topics include plant breeding and genetics, tissue culture and its use in the improvement of and the increase in plant varieties, and ecological implications in agriculture. Chapter titles in bold print in the Table of Contents designate keynote presentations for the three major subtopics in Section II.

The organization of this NATO Advanced Study Institute--Plant Regulation and World Agriculture--was made possible with the collaboration and through the outstanding efforts of Dr. Johan Bruinsma (The Netherlands), Dr. A. Carl Leopold (U.S.A.), Dr. Yusuf Vardar (Turkey), Dr. A. J. Vlitos (United Kingdom), and Dr. R. Louis Wain (United Kingdom). Their encouragement and advice brought a highly complex and unusually diverse program to a successful and productive culmination. They are to be congratulated. The Scientific Affairs Division of NATO sponsored the Advanced Study Institute held in Izmir, Turkey, September 21-30, 1978. There were 68 participants representing 16 countries. A productive characteristic of this program was the combination of scientists from universities with those from industry.

The Advanced Study Institute attracted the interests of and received support from the following organizations and companies: Aegean Chamber of Industry; BASF Aktiengesellschaft; Central Treaty Organization; Chamber of Commerce (Izmir); CIBA-GEIGY Corporation; Commercial Stock Exchange (Izmir); Deutsche-Forschungesgemeinschaft; Diamond Shamrock Corporation; E. I. du Pont de Nemours & Company; FMC Corporation; R. Maag Ltd. Chemical Works; Monsanto Company; National Science Foundation; Sandoz Ltd.; Schering AG; Shell Development Company; Tate & Lyle, Limited; Turkish Scientific Organization (TUBITAK); and The University of North Carolina at Chapel Hill. I should like to thank each of them for the extra latitude that their support enabled the Conference to enjoy.

The topic of the Advanced Study Institute evolved naturally from two previous NATO Conferences pertaining to plant growth regulation held in Izmir in 1967 and 1971. Unique to this Conference, however, was a stress on recommendations and strategies which should be pursued in the future in order to insure the necessary increase in agricultural output. It follows that these recommendations and strategies should have a worldwide and long-lasting impact.

It was the uniformly held hope of the participants that there will be future meetings to sustain the momentum gained and to improve upon these suggested initiatives. In short, although this was the third meeting in the series, the participants nevertheless consider it to be a forerunner to other Conferences which might easily include a wider representation. This representation should soon include economists, lawmakers, and industrial policymakers who must now be brought closer to world food problems.

A number of very dedicated and helpful individuals made this Conference and this volume possible. Foremost amongst them is Mrs. Henrietta Brandt, who attended to virtually every detail from the very beginning to the very end of this venture. She has my special thanks. I should also like to express my sincere thanks to Ms. Suzanne Appelbaum for her expert copy-editing services; to Ms. Karen Hildebrandt for her superb typing of the entire manuscript; to Ms. Anna E. Birkner for her fine art work; and to Mrs. Betty Zouck for her help with many bibliographic problems.

Though many of us feel this volume to be a group effort, I, in the end, take full responsibility for all acts of editorial commission and omission.

Tom K. Scott
Chapel Hill, North Carolina
March 1979

CONTENTS

1

FOOD PLANTS AND PLANT HORMONES IN OUR FUTURE

Kenneth V. Thimann

University of California
Santa Cruz

"There is no profession which can be compared in importance with that of agriculture, for to it belongs the production of food for man and animals; on it depends the welfare and development of the whole human species, the riches of states, and all commerce."
Justus Liebig, 1840 (trans. J. W. Webster, 1841)

This NATO Advanced Study Institute on Plant Regulation and World Agriculture is the first conference ever aimed at drawing together the plant hormones or growth substances and the production of food. It seems that people in general have become aware only in the last few years of the real problem of food production, though some of us, via a United States National Academy of Sciences report, called this problem "pressing" back in 1966.

The problem at the world level can be put very simply. We can use the well-balanced United Nations projections for the next 20 years. During this period:

The annual growth of population in the developed countries will be *ca* 0.8%.
The annual growth of population in the undeveloped countries will be *ca* 2.5%.

Furthermore, during this period:

The annual growth of income per capita in developed countries will be 3.0%.
The annual growth of income per capita in undeveloped countries will be 3.0-3.5%.

The United Nations calculates that:

The net growth in food demand in developed countries will be 1.25%.
The net growth in food demand in undeveloped countries will be 3.5-4.0%.

During the last 20 years the annual increment in world food production has been close to 2.5%. It follows that the previous annual increment must not only be maintained, but must be increased by about 1%. The figures are worse for Africa outside of South Africa and Rhodesia, for in the 52 undeveloped countries there the food production has increased in the last seven years by only 1.3%.

Since the total world grain production is now about 1.5×10^9 tons per year, the need will be for an additional 5.2×10^7 or 52 million tons every year. Whether such an amount can be achieved depends on a large number of interacting factors, some favorable and some unfavorable.

Under unfavorable factors we note the following:

(1) As is often said, most of the potentially arable land is already under cultivation; additional lands will probably be of low productivity. We shall examine this point a little later.

(2) Town and country populations have conflicting needs. If food prices are kept low enough to keep the poor people fed then the farmer cannot earn enough to buy equipment and fertilizer. This is a problem with which many countries are wrestling.

(3) The high price of oil, which is not likely to decrease, has advanced the costs of large-scale agriculture. On a small scale recourse can be had to farm animals, but they have to be fed.[1]

(4) The continued need for high production in the major producing countries is leading to eutrophic conditions in lakes and streams. In some places it is also leading to serious soil erosion.

Under favorable factors the following are to be considered:

First, the population problem is beginning to show some improvement.

(1) The rates of growth of population are genuinely decreasing in a number of "third world" countries. There are encouraging figures from Chile, Costa Rica, Egypt, Hong-Kong, Taiwan, and Tunisia.

(2) Official information and assistance on family planning is installed and now available in China, India, and Eastern Europe; it is beginning to be available in other countries.

Second, the rate of production of food does have some elasticity.

(3) There is great room for improvement in farm practice. Rice

---

[1]In the past, the United States devoted about 100 million acres of farm land to raising feed for farm horses.

yields under experiment station conditions are about 10,000 kg/ha, while the world average is only 2,200 kg/ha. Thus with education, advice, incentive, and fertilizer, large increments are possible without additional lands.

(4) There is always the hope for scientific developments such as those discussed in this conference.

It will be a difficult task to meet the necessary production quota, and every possible scientific and technical advance will be needed. Should we all go and join production teams, as in China? Or become county agricultural agents, as in the United States and Britain? Before we answer these questions, and before we get too far into the future, let us take a brief look into the past, beginning about fifty years ago.

Modern developments in growth substance research can be said to have started with Went's demonstration that the growth substance from coleoptile tips could be worked with quantitatively. From that sprang bioassays, chemical identification, and the growth of hormone physiology. Went is now primarily interested in the ecology of deserts; I will return to that subject shortly.

In the United States the work began with the coming of Herman Dolk to Cal Tech. Dolk and I were joined there by James Bonner; then after Dolk's tragic death I took over as biologist, ably assisted by Mrs. Dolk, Charles Schneider, and two graduate students, Bonner and Folke Skoog. It was a fascinating area of research, and there was no thought of applications. Later Went joined us, and the first possible application began to appear--the induction of root formation on cuttings--first on etiolated pea stems in the dark-room, then on lemon shoots in the greenhouse, and later on most horticultural plants. This particular development came in the laboratory. But later, with the advent of other workers, there came in other places the delaying of abscission by auxins and then the use of auxins as herbicides. This last soon became an affair of ton lots. But the largest result was the general use of many kinds of substances (not only auxins) on crop plants. Agricultural chemicals became a major field of development. This was, needless to say, not wholly due to the success with auxins, but industrial chemists were turning their attention to plants and the auxins provided a strong stimulus. The whole scenario supports the view that <u>the broadest applications come eventually from advances in basic science</u>. This answers the questions above about our own most worthwhile activity, at least for some of us.

Before we get to growth substances I plan to make one more digression, this time on the subject of land. It is said that almost all arable land is already under cultivation. The United States could perhaps add 1.5% per year for a while, and Argentina could probably do the same. But what is the definition of arable land? Many hillsides are not cultivated because of difficulty with mechanized equipment and risk of erosion. Yet in western and southern Europe such slopes, and very steep ones, are used for grapes; sunny slopes along the Rhine and the Swiss lakes are covered over every inch with vineyards. If someone were to develop a food-yielding shrub that can grow in cool and temperate climates it could be planted in large areas now neglected. In warm climates olives fill this niche. In the old days, of course, such areas would be terraced as on Capri, or like rice fields in the tropics, but the human labor required would be too costly today. What is much needed, as an alternative, is a machine which makes terraces quickly and cheaply; some agricultural engineer might consider that. It would make a major contribution.

Then there are the arid lands. These generally have the highest light intensities and are therefore most desirable for agriculture. Conventional thought is that they can only be brought into cultivation by irrigation. But irrigation is expensive; it is estimated that one-half of all the energy used on irrigated farms is for water delivery. Irrigation also involves problems of salination, now serious both in California and Pakistan. It would be much better, if possible, to raise those plants that normally grow in arid lands. Legumes are usually thought to require much water, but our western deserts have two leguminous genera, *Krameria* and *Dalea*, and a program aimed at intergeneric hybrids of these with some of the common agricultural legumes might just possibly yield some very exciting plants. Ingenious plant geneticists could find this a worthwhile challenge, i.e., to breed a food-yielding, water-sparing, legume.

I am also impressed by the pineapple (*Ananas*). This plant has not only a thick cuticle and semi-succulent leaves, but--and this is its notable characteristic--it is a CAM plant. That means that its stomata are mainly open at night and gradually close during the day--a perfect adaptation to arid climates. The pineapple is, as far as I know, the only CAM plant used for food. But would it not be worthwhile to study this type of plant systematically to identify one or more that could be the basis of a breeding program? Such forms could have edible leaves, seeds, or fruits, or all of these. They could well revolutionize the agriculture of arid lands. Indeed, we do tend to adapt our agriculture to those plants that have historically always been used for food, and I think the time has come when we should now be adapting our plants, or developing new ones, to the special requirements of the present day.

A development in some ways comparable has recently begun at the University of California at Davis. Here Emanuel Epstein has selected a few out of a large number of cultivars of barley (*Hordeum*) and grown them in saline soil near the shore. As you know, barley and rape are grown in Holland in the first years of newly recovered polders when the soil is still saline. By further selection from these barley plantings Epstein has found a few which can grow and even yield seed when watered with undiluted seawater. The yields may be small, but could furnish the beginning of a major breeding program. Even one small variety of tomato, belonging to *Lycopersicum pimpinellifolium*, gave a few fruits under these unpromising conditions.

Perhaps the land suitable for agriculture is not quite so limited after all.

And while thinking about land we should not forget the ocean. Aquatic farming in ponds, particularly for carp, has been quite successful in Central Europe. But marine farming (in enclosures) is better in principle because the water is continually renewed by the tide. Why, indeed, do we traditionally have to go out into the ocean to collect our fish? Is it not more sensible to have the ocean come to us, to bring the food for our fish on marine farms? Shallow bays in Japan and Spain are already farmed in this way, especially for shellfish, and are said to produce high yields. There are many more areas worldwide that could be so used. Sewage diluted with seawater is being tried as fertilizer in one experimental enclosure at Woods Hole. With the new restrictions on fishing in territorial waters one can foresee a big future for marine farming. Besides, fish are readily digestible, high in protein, and the protein is of desirable amino acid composition.

Let us now turn to our own preoccupation, plant hormones or growth substances. In the 1975 Conference on Crop Productivity--Research Imperatives (held in Michigan) several of the research needs that this large group agreed are urgent concerned hormones. The group discussing carbon input listed "Investigate hormonal and chemical regulation in crop plants" and "Determine effect of leaf senescence on photosynthesis." Another group, covering plant development, listed "Attain a better understanding of the hormonal control of growth and development." The stress group pointed to the importance of understanding the control of stomata, a subject which now is just coming into the realm of hormones. Thus the stage is set for the field of plant hormones to make its major contribution to agriculture and horticulture. Of course this field has already given us the rooting of cuttings, the control of abscission, and the understanding, if not quite the control, of the ripening of fruit. In field-type agriculture such as concerns the big five crops (wheat, rice, corn, potatoes, and barley), however, the only contribution up to now has been the auxin-type herbicides. These ushered in the great modern development of organic weed killers of many widely different structural types. Their great diversity makes them capable of adaptation to a variety of crops and growing conditions. They are also helping to make possible the recent development of limited tillage, or even zero tillage.

There is one transfer from the laboratory which might well be worth some further study--the treatment of seed with auxin. It shortens the root length but then stimulates the emergence of additional roots. In oats the normal number of seedling roots is 5 but after auxin treatment there are 10 to 12. This increased root number can give the seedlings an early start which, if the growing season is short, can be most important. The seedling really wastes a lot of space in the field and the sooner it can spread its canopy the better. Polish workers have recently reported similarly good results by soaking tree seeds in either auxin or gibberellin. In China it is the custom to grow several crops a year on the same ground, by transplanting half-grown plants from the nursery, and in this (very labor-intensive) system any improvement in the length or number of the roots would be important. But because in the early experiments, 30 or more years ago, the results were sensitive to temperature and other conditions the matter has not been much studied. The effects may possibly be due to ethylene production caused by the auxin treatment rather than to the auxin itself, but that remains to be proved.

One aspect of plant development that is fundamental to agriculture and yet should be amenable to growth substance research is one that we seem not to know anything about. I refer to the filling of the seed. This is a strange process; it involves the steady accumulation of dry weight--sugars or amino acids, or both, depending on the plant--without corresponding accumulation of water. It is not directly dependent on photosynthesis, of course, since the ovary wall is usually quite opaque. It is hard to see how this process could be simply osmotic, since evaporation of the necessary water from the seed, enclosed in the ovary, must be minimal. The hard dry seed can be surrounded by watery tissue, as in the grape or orange. The only reasonable way it can be visualized seems to be that the activity of polymerizing systems in the growing seed must be so high that the concentration of the small molecules is kept far lower than in the surrounding tissues; in this way there would be a continuous flow or gradient of solutes from the phloem sap (even though that is relatively concentrated) to the endosperm or cotyledon cells of the seed. For an agriculture which is so heavily based on seeds it is remarkable that this problem seems not to have attracted much research interest. It is not even mentioned in the proceedings of the congress on research imperatives I just mentioned. It is not included in the list of topics eligible for support in the new extramural program of the U.S. Department of Agriculture (a list, by the way, that would have seemed more up-to-date a quarter of a century ago than it does today). Yet with the old work of Mitchell on dry matter attraction by auxin and the more recent work of Mothes and others on the amino acid-attracting action of cytokinins we do have a handle on how plant hormones influence the movement of materials, and I conclude that this is a problem to which our special fraternity might well turn its attention.

Indeed, the whole field of the mobilization and transport of organic substances in the plant is now opened up to researchers on plant hormones and artificial growth regulators. Has it not been dominated for too long by osmotic and mechanical considerations? The broad lines of phloem anatomy are understood, and the faithful aphid is spending its energies, and indeed sacrificing its life, to help understand the mechanism of phloem flow. But that hormones control directional transport and entry into cells can hardly be doubted, in the light of the considerations just mentioned. I feel that this factor will be the next in line to be drawn into the complex picture of transport within the whole plant, and the ability to control it will ultimately be critical for a successful agriculture.

A pertinent development of the last few years has been the detailed study of plant senescence. When leaves start to senesce, proteolysis begins at once, amino acids move out of the leaf by a sort of polar transport, the chloroplasts are then attacked and the pigments decolorized. Light delays but does not prevent the process. When whole plants undergo senescence the interrelations are more complex, and there is evidence for a factor or signal coming from the young fruits and slowly spreading an aging response throughout the plant body. The process can be postponed, perhaps indefinitely, by repeated defloration or removal of the newly forming fruits. The defloration of potatoes to increase the yield of tubers was described as early as 1839. Soybeans, progressively deflowered, continue growth indefinitely, and in Noodén's laboratory at Michigan they produce trees. In one strain of peas senescence is postponed indefinitely by a simple change in day-length. Since all the cytokinins that have been tested have the power to delay senescence, at least in leaves, the matter comes definitely within the purview of plant growth regulators. Indeed, in our laboratory in the last few weeks we have found other materials quite as active as cytokinins in this respect. So, senescence can be both hastened and delayed by simple treatments. The possible application of these findings is evident when we recall that many crops are harvested at a time when there are still several months of growing season remaining. At the International Agricultural Research Institute in New Delhi I saw recently some delayed-senescence cultivars of rice, which remain fully green when the grain is formed and when the ordinary varieties have yellowed. These should provide most interesting breeding material.

However, it would not be enough merely to prevent senescence, for then all that flow of amino acids out of the leaves, most of which undoubtedly goes into the fruits, would be prevented; we must be able to delay senescence and then, near the end of the growing season, to bring it on as desired. The costs of both treatments would have to be small. With such a development, some crop yields should be markedly increased. We can hope that this line of work may reach the stage of field experiments in the near future.

Another limitation on fertility is posed by the stomata. In many crop plants the stomata close during the afternoon, and this is not wholly due to loss of water, for we have found that even in leaves floating on water in continuous light the stomata still tend to close. Such closure naturally limits photosynthesis. Hence, the control of stomatal aperture in plants that are not under water stress could markedly improve yields. We know already that abscisic acid causes closure and in the last year or two it has been found (and we have confirmed) that cytokinins cause opening. Also fusicoccin, surprisingly enough, causes stomatal opening. Thus we have a strong lead toward ultimately being able to control stomatal aperture in crop plants by growth substances. Doubtless there are many situations where one would prefer to leave the control to nature (as for instance, because of complex or conflicting requirements) but there are also many where control would be desirable. Work in this area also seems to be approaching the stage of field experiment.

It has often been said that the most fundamental advance in agriculture would come if we could control flowering. Evidence for a florigen and an anthesin is still being adduced, but understanding of the true control of flowering remains elusive. Meanwhile plant hormone research has given us two partial solutions to the problem. Ethylene can bring on almost immediate flowering in a few plants. What is more, gibberellin can cause long-day plants to flower in short days. But the application of these well-established facts seems to have been pretty much limited to pineapple culture. Economics has prevented the spraying of gibberellins over vast acreages, and, besides, agricultural practices are already adapted to normal seasons, so that flowering out of season may not be as useful as it sounds.

I have a feeling, too, that flowering research may have been held back by the fierce adherence to the dogma of a universal florigen. Auxin and ethylene are universal, it is true, but zeatin seems to be limited to a few plants, and there are almost enough different gibberellins to apportion one to each family of angiosperms! Thus the flowering influence may well be multiple, i.e., a hormone accompanied by a specific set of conditions, or an interaction of hormones, and it may differ in different plants or families. I believe we could make more progress if we began to wonder what happens during a long day or a long night, i.e., if we made a simple-minded study of the physiology of vegetative and reproductive phases in a selected suitable plant, especially with modern sophisticated methods. Thus we might get away from the endless red and far-red exposures and reach some inkling of what the inception of these phases means in physiological terms.

I would like to take a moment to turn from specific topics to a couple of hopeful notes on research support and awareness. We in the United States have long been trying to push the U.S. Department of Agriculture into developing an extramural research program, that is, a system of competitively awarded grants to universities, colleges, and private research institutions to support research on subjects basic to agriculture. Normally the U.S. Department of Agriculture funds only research within its own laboratories and experiment stations, and gives partial support to work in state experiment stations. These studies are mainly those having a direct bearing on agricultural procedures, such as breeding for increased yields or for pest resistance, care of crops and fruit trees, soil conservation methods, etc. There have been few really basic research projects undertaken in this system, though we must in fairness pay tribute to the fundamental work on day-length begun by Garner and Allard, and to the work on light-sensitive seeds which led to the recognition of phytochrome, begun by Flint and Macalaster, then continued by Borthwick and Hendricks. But the tremendous program of extramural research support developed by the National Institutes of Health, which has brought out a vast volume of new discoveries in biochemistry, animal and human physiology, and pharmacology, shows what can be done with widespread support of competent researchers distributed all through our varied institutions of learning. It was for some parallel to this that our numerous resolutions and reports called, but without avail. Then rather suddenly about two years ago the principle was accepted in Congress and the Department was instructed to make plans for such a program. This spring applications were requested, and a committee is even now at work to judge these applications. The topics have been expressly limited to photosynthesis, nitrogen fixation, plant response to stress, and a few others, with no direct mention of effects of plant growth substances, yet the program does come at a time when awareness of the urgency of the food problem is growing, and I feel sure that some of the work thus financed will lead to discoveries bearing on many phases of food production. Though its future financial support is a little unclear, it is indeed a welcome development.

A step forward in the international sphere is also notable. The International Council of Scientific Unions, ICSU, or CIUS, has responded to a strong urging in last year's United Nations General Assembly by setting up a new body, an Inter-Union Commission on the Application of Science to Agriculture. It will be staffed by representatives of interested Unions with some additional experienced people. Its tasks will be fourfold: (1) to stimulate awareness of food problems among members of the ICSU family; (2) to develop a program of international studies that will help ensure the more rapid application of basic research to food production; (3) to act as a clearinghouse for suggestions for novel research into food problems; and (4) to suggest sources of funding for such work. I hope that the Proceedings of our NATO meeting will be made available to this ICSU commission, and indeed they may constitute the first direct response to its initiative.

Lastly I feel I must return, if only for a moment, to make a point related to some of the points made earlier. Let me introduce you to a young lady. Her name was Atalanta, and she was Greek, or rather, Aeolian. She was so excessively fleet of foot that she was content to remain single and to enjoy hunting, but at her father's urging she finally agreed to marry. However, she would only marry a man who could beat her in a race--a race which we can visualize as something like the 1,000 meters today. The various suitors all failed and duly paid the penalty of death. But young Milanion was given three golden apples by the goddess Aphrodite, and while he ran he quietly dropped these one after the other along the track; they were so attractive that Atalanta stooped to pick them up and so lost the race. Is it possible, I wish to ask, that if we stoop to pay so much attention to the gold of economic applications we run the risk of losing the greater race, the race toward a deeper understanding of how plants live and grow?

2

AGRICULTURAL PRODUCTION--RESEARCH IMPERATIVES FOR THE FUTURE[1]

Sylvan H. Wittwer

Michigan State University
East Lansing, MI 48824

INTRODUCTION

Many studies have assessed the potential contributions of research for the enhancement of food production and of other renewable resources. An equal number have inventoried the earth's resources of land, water, minerals, climate, etc. for absolute production capability. Recent emphasis on the "Politics of Food" suggests a strong third determinant for agricultural production potential. The tripartitions of productivity--new technologies, resource inputs, and economic incentives--must be constantly reviewed.

The emphasis in this paper relates primarily to technology inputs for enhancement of stable crop production at high levels. Dependability of supply is equally important to that of improvement of yields. The focus will be on crops. Plants provide directly,

---

[1]This paper is an extension, updating, and further amplification of five previous documents by the author: "Research Recommendations for Increasing Food, Feed, and Fiber Production in the U.S.A." (National Science Foundation, Washington, D.C., 1974); "Food Production, Technology and the Resource Base" (Science, 188:579-584, 1975); "Increased Crop Yields and Livestock Productivity," World Food Prospects and Agricultural Potential, pp. 66-135 (The Hudson Institute, New York, 1977); "Assessment of Technology in Food Production," presented at the 143rd Annual Meeting of the American Association for the Advancement of Science, Denver, Colorado, February 24, 1977; and "The Shape of Things to Come," the concluding chapter in the book Biology of Crop Production, Peter Carlson, ed., Academic Press, New York, 1978. Other resource documents included

or indirectly, up to 95% of the world's food supply. They are also our chief source of renewable resources for industrial materials.

Regulation or control of the biological processes that limit crop productivity holds top priority. Many global problems relate to failures of productivity (Table 1). There are already a number of crises in relation to the production and stability of our food supply and other renewable resources.

Reference is made, herewith, to the "next generation of agricultural research" (Wittwer, 1978b). Details as to the initiatives to be taken are listed in Table 2. Each can be characterized as mission oriented basic research for enhancement of production. They can add to, rather than diminish, resources essential to crop productivity. They are nonpolluting and without noise. They are the areas identified in recent National Academy of Sciences/National Research Council reports and elsewhere as grossly underfunded; where no nation is making any substantial research investment; where industrialized developed nations, including the United States with its vast human, financial, and natural resources, could make their greatest contributions to the agricultural development of third world nations. If the research efforts were directed toward economically important crops as test materials, the productivity and stability of output of forests, grasslands, and cropland would be greatly improved. These are three of the four biological systems which, according to Brown (1978), form the foundation of the global economic system; and they would indirectly improve the fourth, that of fisheries. Such technologies would be scale neutral and economically, socially, politically, and ecologically sound. They

---

those of the Board on Agriculture and Renewable Resources (BARR) of the National Research Council, National Academy of Sciences, "Agricultural Production Efficiency" (1975), "Enhancement of Food Production for the United States" (1975), and "Climate and Food" (1976); "World Food and Nutrition Study, The Potential Contributions of Research" (1977), National Research Council, National Academy of Sciences, A Report of the Steering Committee; Proceedings of the World Food Conference of 1976 (1977), Iowa State University Press, Ames, Iowa; The Proceedings of the International Conference, "Crop Productivity--Research Imperatives," jointly sponsored by the Michigan Agricultural Experiment Station and the Charles F. Kettering Foundation (1976); the Report of the Office of Technology Assessment (U.S. Congress) Panel on "Assessment of Alternatives for Supporting High Priority Basic Research to Enhance Food Production," the May 1975 Food Issue of Science, 188:503-651; the Food and Agriculture September 1976 issue of Scientific American, 253:31-205; and the special issue, Future of Biological N_2 Fixation, of Bioscience, 28:September 1978.

Michigan Agricultural Experiment Station Journal Article 8720.

Table 1. Global Problems Relating to Crop Productivity

Poverty	Soil erosion
Inflation	Changing climate
Malnutrition	Shortage of firewood
Unemployment	Uncertainties of energy supplies
Deforestation	Toxic chemicals in the environment
Desertification	Adequacy and dependability of food supply
Population increase	

could ease the inevitable transition we must make from nonrenewable to renewable resources.

The biological processes or phenomena that limit the stability and magnitude of crop productivity and the most efficient use of resources (land, water, fertilizer, energy, climate) include photosynthesis, biological nitrogen fixation, photorespiration, transpiration, leaf senescence, dormancy, growth rates, nutrient and water uptake, flower bud differentiation, fruit and seed set, harvest index, and resistance to chemical, biological, and environmental stresses. All are hormonal or special substance mediated.

Meanwhile, in the chemical plant regulation field, new application and assay technologies have been developed. Considerable progress has been made in identification of new active compounds. There are now 52 gibberellins (Hedden et al., 1978). Farm chemical industrial interest has intensified. In 1975, there were at least 29 major companies in the United States actively engaged in some phase of plant regulation research with the focus on major food, feed, and industrial crops. A Plant Growth Regulator Working Group has been created. Annual conferences are held and a proceedings published (Plant Growth Regulator Working Group, 1978). Favorable responses have been recorded for representatives of all the major food crops. These include the cereal grains, the seed legumes and pulses, the oil, sugar, and root crops, many tropical species, and a great variety of fruits, vegetables, and ornamentals. Equally exciting possibilities exist for forest trees and biomass production, and for other renewable resources used for industrial purposes.

Until now, there have been few reviews on the practical uses of chemical regulators and crop productivity, apart from those dealing with the acquisition of new scientific knowledge. There has been little effort to focus growth regulator studies on significant food crop species or on whole plants of economic importance. Most of the locally financed agricultural research in developing countries has been on plantation and export crops. Food crops for domestic consumption have been largely ignored. What is needed in the chemical growth regulator field is for scientists, especially in

Table 2. Next Generation of Plant Science Research

Greater photosynthetic efficiency
Improved biological nitrogen fixation
Genetic improvement and new cell fusion technologies
Greater resistance to competing biological systems
More efficiency in nutrient uptake and utilization
Reduction in losses from nitrification and denitrification
Greater resistance to environmental stresses
Identification of hormonal systems and mechanisms

developing countries, to participate personally in field research to solve food production problems, rather than to contribute to the burgeoning growth of scientific journals. Much of the information resulting from research in the plant sciences has not been brought to bear on the practical problems of crop productivity. There is yet no effective linkage between the molecular biologist and the field scientist.

AGRICULTURAL PRODUCTIVITY--A HISTORICAL PERSPECTIVE

Gains in agricultural output came almost entirely from increases in area cultivated until the midpoint of the twentieth century. Since World War II, other resource inputs (water, fertilizer, machinery, pesticides) have played a major role. Crop research strategy has been to grow two blades of grass or two ears of corn where one grew before--irrespective of resource input. Greater production efficiency measured by output was the goal. The result was plentiful food at low cost. Meanwhile, nearly all existing agricultural technologies in the United States and some other industrialized nations, heavily dependent on fossil fuels and chemicals, have evolved during an era characterized by low cost and abundant energy. Few agricultural scientists, even as of this writing, recognize the impending impact of resource constraints. The high fossil energy subsidy to American agriculture cannot continue forever. The agricultural output of the United States and many other developed nations has been closely tied to the availability of fossil fuel inputs. New varieties of crops (wheat, rice, maize, potatoes, sorghum, millet) have also been developed that are highly responsive and dependent on industrial (energy) inputs of fertilizer, pesticides, irrigation, and mechanization. Direct spinoffs of an energy intensive agriculture include increased specialization (monoculture), less resiliency, and large scale operations accompanied by a movement away from small and medium sized production units.

There is now a worldwide shift from a natural resource-based to a science-based agriculture. The emphasis is to raise output per unit resource input and release the constraints imposed by relatively inelastic supplies of land, water, fertilizer, and energy. Ruttan (1977) has pointed out that this has already occurred during the first part of the twentieth century in Japan and certain western European countries. Whereas the United States has followed a mechanical technology pathway, Japan has followed a biological one. Increasing yield technology in the United States has lagged until recently, compared to Japan and some European countries, because of the abundance and low cost of resources. It is projected now, however, that by the end of this century almost all increases in agricultural production will be a result of increases in yield (output per unit land area per unit time). New high payoff agricultural technologies for the future will be not only those which result in stable production and high yields, but are sparing of resources. They will be the ones which address and offer solutions to global problems (Table 1), increase the demand for underutilized labor resources, and put people to work more days per year and more productively. An expanded use of chemical growth regulants may fulfill some of these criteria.

Meanwhile, there are some immediate problems. The food and agricultural events of the 1960s and 1970s have been kind neither to the prophets of doom nor the optimists. Recent events have jolted all prognostications (Wortman and Cummings, 1978). There was the food crisis, drought in India and Pakistan, and crunch in grain supplies during the mid-1960s. This was followed by the optimism and potential of the green revolution. There was the United States corn blight of 1970; Soviet grain shipments in 1972; the poor, as well as good, harvests of 1973-1974; escalating food prices and shortages; a resurgence of food production in 1975 through 1978; disastrously low prices to producers in 1977; and the development of an American agricultural movement known as a Farmers' Strike. Dramatic behaviors have characterized world agricultural commodity markets. Since 1972, prices have been volatile, unstable, and unpredictable, and markets periodically peppered with nagging shortages and surpluses.

There is much current interest in exploring the biological limits of crop productivity. They have not been achieved nor defined. World grain production for the 1977-1978 crop year was an all-time record of 1,300 million metric tons. The United States has just experienced an all-time record in corn production for 1978. The global increases in yields of the major cereal crops since World War II are without precedent in agricultural history. Particularly significant have been some of the records in Japan, western Europe, Mexico, Colombia, the United States, and the Punjab state in India. Yields of wheat in northern European countries and Japan are significantly higher than in the United States. The most remarkable crop production record for all time has been in India's Punjab. A threefold increase in food grain production was achieved in ten years (1966 to 1976).

Many have estimated ultimate or maximum crop productivity. Buringh (1977) has computed productivity in grain equivalents to be forty times its present global level. Biological limits have not been achieved for the productivity of any of the major food crops. Average and world record yields are listed in Table 3. The current and potential productivity of nine major crops--maize, sugarcane, sugar beets, rice, wheat, soybeans, peas, potatoes, and cotton--are reviewed by Evans (1975), who points out that record yields to date are about one-half of the estimated maximum yields.

A careful review of parameters responsible for the ever increasing record yields of corn (Table 4) could be informative for the design of future models of crop productivity. All have occurred in the United States, and two of the most recent ones in Michigan. Other case histories are available for analysis (Hageman, 1978). The study of comparative productivity of various successful agricultural ecosystems could be most rewarding. New technologies, resource inputs, and economic incentives are the parameters which will determine future agricultural crop productivity. The combinations that work will be site and location specific.

Table 3. Average and World Record Yields

Food Crop	United States Average--1977 (metric tons/hectare)	World Record (metric tons/hectare)
Maize	5.6	22.2
Wheat	2.1	14.5
Soybeans	2.2	5.6
Sorghum	3.3	21.5
Oats	1.9	10.6
Barley	2.4	11.4
Potatoes	27.6	95.0
Cassava[1]	8.0	60.0
Rice (crop/112 days)	2.5	14.4
Sugarcane (tons/ha/yr)	50.0	250.0
Sugar beets (tons/ha/yr)	52.0	120.0

[1]Data from Colombia.

Table 4. World Record Corn Yields

Year	Yield (bu/acre)	Person	Location
1955	304	L. Ratcliff	Mississippi
1973	306	O. Montri	Michigan
1975	338	H. Warsaw	Illinois
1977	353	R. Lynn, Jr.	Michigan

1066--Theoretical maximum yield (bu/acre).

Analysis of Current Yield Plateaus

Within the very shadow of unprecedented progress for enhancement of food crop productivity has come a plateauing of yields of the major food crops of the earth. This is an ominous trend in that the number of years in which food production will need to be doubled in most developing countries to meet estimated consumption requirements ranges only from 7 to 20 years (Wortman and Cummings, 1978). Yields of wheat, maize, sorghum, soybeans, and potatoes in the United States have not increased since 1970 (Wittwer, 1978b). This is true of maize, potatoes, wheat, and cassava in Latin America. The yields of rice in India, Bangladesh, Indonesia, Nepal, Pakistan, Philippines, Sri Lanka, and Thailand were the same in 1976 as in 1970, even with a substantial input of high yielding varieties (IRRI, in press). Overall world grain (wheat) yields are beginning to plateau (Jensen, 1978). Increased production has been achieved largely by bringing more land under cultivation.

This phenomenon needs careful analysis. Possible causal factors are listed in Table 5. There are fewer options in the use of water, land, energy, fertilizer, pesticides, and for mechanization. These resources are becoming more costly, subject to more constraints, and less available. Some are nonrenewable. Meanwhile, soil erosion continues unabated nationally and globally. Topsoil continues to be lost at an enormous rate. Soil organic matter is still on the decline. There is greater soil compaction from excess and untimely tillage. Air pollution is progressively more severe. Additional land areas brought under cultivation may be less productive.

The changing composition of the earth's atmosphere and its projected effects for either enhancing or reducing crop production deserves special emphasis. Particulates and gases found therein--natural or of human origin--are absorbed by the aerial parts of plants, and if released through precipitation, may be taken up by

Table 5. Causes of Decline in Agricultural Productivity

Soil erosion--Loss of topsoil
Loss of organic matter--Soil compaction
Chemical soil residues--Air pollution
More less-productive land under cultivation
Increased pressures on productive land base
Fewer options for water, fertilizer, pesticide uses
Climate and weather fluctuations
Increased regulatory constraints
Decreased support for agricultural research

roots. Acid rainfall is common over all the United States east of the Mississippi River, localized industrial areas of the western United States, much of western Europe, and around all major cities in the world. Its impact on the productivity of agricultural crops, forests, and natural ecosystems has not been assessed. Air quality standards, thus far, have been associated with activities of people, with little attention given to renewable resources productivity (Williams, 1978). Crop losses from air pollution may be minimized by the selection and development of tolerant cultivars, modification of cultural practices, application of antioxidant chemicals and growth regulants, and modifying the nutrition of plants. The effects of the atmosphere on the biosphere, and what we do about it, will help shape the world of tomorrow.

Some would attribute the recent plateauing of crop yields to adverse and fluctuating climate and weather. Season-to-season variations, however, are far more significant than any identifiable long-term trends. There is no evidence that technology has reduced the sensitivity of grain yields to weather. On the other hand, technology may be working to insulate yields from unfavorable weather. Many of the recent advances in technology which could enhance productivity are highly dependent on use of more energy resources. The rising costs of energy relative to crop prices may be limiting the adoption of new practices that could increase yields. If this is true, then the plateauing of yields may be expected to continue. Obstacles to increased crop productivity in many nations may be more political than technological (Brown, 1978).

Regulatory and financial constraints on the use of labor, chemicals, water, and energy are increasingly costly and stifle production (Table 6).

Finally, there has been a 13-year erosion of public support for agricultural research, not only in manpower, but in new equipment and facilities. Enrollments in the colleges of agriculture in the

Table 6. Recently Imposed Regulations upon Agricultural Research and Productivity

Occupational safety and health
Human subjects requirements
Personnel relations
Union/management relationships
Affirmative action
Waste handling and disposition
Chemicals handling and disposition
Laboratory animals
Building codes, ordinances, standards
Accountability
Budget management
Freedom of information
Acts--Clean Water; Federal Insecticide, Fungicide, and Rodenticide (FIFRA); Toxic Substance; Clean Air; Rebuttable Presumption Against Registration (RPAR)

United States land grant universities have tripled in ten years with little, if any, increase in teaching faculty. Scientist years in support of agricultural research have not changed since 1966. Teaching needs had to be met. Research was the remnant left behind. Particularly disastrous has been the lack of effort on mission oriented basic research relating to the biological processes that control and limit crop productivity (Wittwer, 1978b). In 1976, scarcely $15 million total was being invested in the United States for combined research on photosynthesis, biological nitrogen fixation, and cellular approaches to plant breeding which was crop productivity related. The human resources for a much expanded effort in these three areas are available. This was indicated by over 500 proposals received in the modestly funded ($10 million) competitive grant program administered by the United States Department of Agriculture for fiscal year 1978. The manpower is available, but the financial resources are not.

RESEARCH IMPERATIVES FOR THE FUTURE

Increased Photosynthetic Efficiency and Yield Enhancement

Photosynthesis is the most important biochemical process on earth. Its improved efficiency holds the key to the future adequacy of our food supplies. The greatest unexploited resource available to the earth is sunlight. Photosynthesis is the most extraordinary mechanism ever devised. Man has specialized in and depends on the culture of sun-loving plants. Green plants, as yet, are the primary harvesters of free solar energy. They are net producers of food and energy on a renewable basis. All farm practices directed toward increased crop productivity must ultimately relate to an increased appropriation of solar energy in the plant system. Agriculture is, basically, a solar energy processing machine. It is the only industry that utilizes today's incident solar radiation, and is man's largest current user of solar energy. Yet, few studies of photosynthesis have focused on crop productivity and biomass production. The whole intent in agriculture is to collect and store solar energy as food, feed, and fiber in plant and animal products, and to do it with utmost efficiency. That efficiency, however, which averages less than 2% annually for the major food crops, is very low. For most crops, the efficiency of solar energy utilization does not exceed 1%. Many environmental pressures affect photosynthesis, and there is great diversity among plants.

There are many researchable alternatives for enhancement of photosynthesis. They include identification and control of the mechanisms that regulate and could reduce the wasteful processes of both dark and light induced (photo) respiration, mechanisms responsible for redistribution of photosynthates which, in turn, regulate yield and maximize the "harvest index"; resolution of the hormonal mechanisms and identification of growth regulators and heritable components that control flowering and leaf senescence; improvements in plant architecture and anatomy, cropping systems, planting designs, and cultural practices for better light reception; and carbon dioxide enrichment of crop atmospheres. Plant breeding research has not generally been aimed at improving the photosynthetic process. Furthermore, the relationship between photosynthesis and crop yield is complex. Photosynthetically positive mutants should be sought after. Any physiologic-genetic prolongation of the functionally active state of chloroplasts and/or delay in leaf senescence would be important for enhancement of photosynthetic productivity. The future of the world's food supply and much of the energy resides at the door of photosynthesis and subsequent partitioning of the products of photosynthesis into the harvested parts. The simplicity of the approach belies its credibility among the many options for support of new solar energy producing and conserving technologies. Even with the high fossil energy inputs consumed in the culture of major agronomic crops, the ratio of food energy produced to that consumed is greater than one, and ranges from two to five for major cereal grains. The energy output exceeds the input by a factor of two to five.

Enhancement of crop productivity for increasing biological solar energy conversion in the future is a topic of much discussion. A plethora of reports have appeared. Next to hydropower, biomass is now the largest source of commercial solar energy in the United States and many other nations. On a global scale, net photosynthesis "produces" about ten times the world's annual use of energy. The problem is one of collection. The biomass resource could increase dramatically with more efficient photosynthetic conversion of solar energy. The sources of biomass now available for conversion to energy, however, represent only about 2% of the current fossil energy consumption. Expectations of large increases in energy from energy farming in the United States are not realistic. The constraints on the use of land and water resources are too great. Nevertheless, the development of photobiological energy conversion systems has long term implications for the production of energy, food, and industrial materials in the tropics and countries with large amounts of sunshine. Many efforts are under way to identify food crops and management practices for energy production. Some crops receiving special attention are sugarcane, sorghum, and cassava (Da Silva et al., 1978).

There are special opportunities for yield enhancement by chemical regulants with managed forest tree plantings, plantation crops, and food crops. Great interest currently exists in hybrid poplars and other inherently vigorous species as pulpwood sources and for energy conversion. Among the potential growth factors are chemical regulants, specifically the gibberellins, which, over twenty years ago, gave demonstrable increases in tree growth and productivity. The use of diverse sugarcane ripeners for enhancement of sugar production in Hawaiian sugar plantations is now standard practice. Increases in sugar yield of over 10% are achieved. An almost equal increase has been realized with gibberellin. The oleoresin ("pitch") yield of conifers has been greatly increased in remote areas with such materials as paraquat. Ethylene generating compounds ("Ethrel," "Ethad") have greatly improved the flow of latex in the commercial production of rubber trees. Gibberellins have induced important species of conifers to flower in 4 to 6 years, compared with the natural sequence of 10-20 years to flower, and another 20 years to produce significant quantities of seed. The treatment of young guayule plants with 2-(3,4-dichlorophenoxy)-triethylene markedly stimulates the accumulation of natural rubber in the stems and roots. This could make the desert shrub of North America a viable domestic source of hydrocarbons, including rubber (Yokoyama et al., 1977). It would also bring into production millions of acres of desert land now only marginally useful.

Most of the irrigated rice, the number one food crop of the earth, is sown in nursery beds and then hand transplanted in the field. Transplanted rice is more productive than that sown broadcast. Millions of plants are grown in small areas. Greater ease of transplanting could likely be enhanced by treatment of seedlings with appropriate growth regulators that would produce stronger and more uniform plants.

The pattern of crop canopies and plant architecture can be dramatically changed with growth regulators. This has been achieved with many fruit trees, soybeans, and some cereal grains. Better light receiving systems are formed and, with some cereal grains, lodging is prevented and yields are increased.

Considerable progress has occurred in the identification of new biologically active compounds, both synthetic and natural, which directly enhance plant growth. Tricontanol has opened a new dimension for higher alcohols. Foliar sprayings in milligram quantities per hectare or in spray concentrations ranging from 1 ppm to 1 ppb have significantly increased the yields of field grown crops and stimulated the growth of rice plants in the dark. Field results showing yield enhancements now confirm those in growth chambers and the greenhouse (Ries et al., 1978).

Biological Nitrogen Fixation

Chemically fixed nitrogen is a nonrenewable resource. It is also the largest single and most costly industrial input into agricultural productivity. Up to 35% of the total productive capacity of all crops is now accredited to this single input. Almost one-third of all fossil energy now used in agricultural production goes to chemical nitrogen fertilizer synthesis.

The global use of chemically fixed nitrogen fertilizer for crop production has grown precipitously. In 1905, 400,000 metric tons were produced. This increased to 3.5 million tons in 1950, and to an output of 40 million tons in 1974. The estimate for 1978 is 50 million tons. Meanwhile, the contribution of biologically fixed nitrogen, estimated at 150-175 million tons annually, has not changed.

The United States is the world's largest consumer of nitrogen fertilizer. Over 10 million metric tons--almost one-fourth of the world's total--are applied to crops annually. Half goes to a single crop--maize. The average annual investment for nitrogen fertilizer for corn alone is $1 billion. It is $1.5 billion for all grain crops. The total for all crops approximates $2 billion.

Natural gas is the primary fuel (95%) used to produce anhydrous ammonia. It requires 30 cubic feet of natural gas to produce one pound of nitrogen. The current and projected natural gas dependency of chemically fixed nitrogen fertilizer remains as one of the most flagrant violations of good economics, use of a nonrenewable resource, and threatens a possible environmental disaster. It is inconceivable for us to continue to go this route.

The alternative is research directed toward enhancing biological nitrogen fixation. The many possible research frontiers and the inadequacy of current funding levels have been thoroughly documented by numerous National Research Council/National Academy of Science reports, assessments by several federal agencies, the United States Congress, national and international conferences and symposia, and the September 1978 issue of BioScience. The opportunities lie in the establishment of rhizobial technology centers. A return to research in farming systems specifically relating to cropping systems, making more extensive use of legume green manure and winter cover crops, forage legumes, and possible intercropping of legumes with non-legumes, have been suggested. A third initiative lies in genetic engineering for improvement of both host and microorganism. Symbiotic relationships now exist for legumes, the actinomycete-nodulated angiosperms, and in the Anabenae-Azolla combinations that enrich rice paddies. These relationships need to be optimized. Finally, there should be an effort toward improving the biological nitrogen fixation associations with grasses, cereal grains, and non-legumes. One of the most remarkable opportunities resides with forage legumes (alfalfa, clovers). Their capacity for N_2 fixation exceeds that of the seed legumes (soybeans, field beans, peas, lentils, peanuts) by a factor of two. Biologically fixed nitrogen is slow release nitrogen. Losses from nitrification and denitrification which now approximate 50-75% of the fertilizer nitrogen could be reduced by 50%.

Further research breakthroughs in biological nitrogen fixation that will be important for enhancement of agricultural productivity will be hastened if active linkages are now created between scientists engaged in basic fundamental research in the laboratory and those in mission-oriented, applied, and problem-solving areas under field conditions. There is a unique opportunity with research on biological nitrogen fixation to apply science to problems in agriculture and contribute mightily to the enhancement of food and fiber production. The economic, resource, and environmental stakes are too high to do otherwise (Wittwer, 1978a).

Abiotic nitrogen fixation, utilizing renewable energy resources, must also remain an option. One possibility is the production of ammonia in solar cells utilizing nitrogen gas, water, and catalysts. Zero energy inputs into nitrogen fixation, with appropriate catalysts, is another. A nitrogen fixation generator for farm use, which will appropriate the renewable energy resources of wind, waterfalls, or sunlight, is being designed (Treharne et al., 1978).

Genetic Improvement

The genetic resources of the earth for crop improvement are enormous. A resume of accessions, assembled from the latest annual reports of the several International Agricultural Research Centers, shows 40,000 for rice, 26,000 for wheat, 12,000 for maize, over 14,000 for grain sorghum, and 5,000 for pearl millet. There were over 12,000 accessions for potatoes in 1976, and over 2,000 for cassava. Chick-peas show a figure of near 11,000, plus 47 wild species. There are 5,530 accessions for pigeon peas, and 3,000 each for peanuts and field beans. The ultimate goal, however, is not fulfilled in the collection and preservation of genetic resources, but in their utilization. These plant genetic resources now being assembled will truly shape the future for world crop productivity.

The standard techniques of selection, based on phenotypic expression, controlled hybridization, and more recently, selection for better nutritional qualities, have given us super strains of rice, wheat, maize, sorghum, millet, some legumes, and many new fruits and vegetables. The process is relatively simple for cereal grains, the seed legumes, forages, and many vegetables. Those that are vegetatively propagated (potatoes, sweet potatoes, cassava, fruit trees), however, pose a special problem. There is now an effort to freeze meristems in liquid nitrogen for the preservation of genetic stocks of vegetatively propagated food crops. The challenge will then be to initiate regrowth, utilizing appropriate metabolites, growth regulants, and culture media.

An equally exciting area for the future is that of genetically altering crops for greater climatic adaptability, and thus getting higher yields from soils which are infertile, too acid, toxic, or saline for varieties now in use. No wheat varieties are yet suitable for the lowland tropics, and there are at least 100 million acres not suited for present rice paddies. Vast land areas of the earth, including those in the United States, are either not utilized, or are underutilized for economically important crop production. It has been suggested that crop (biomass) production is limited more by nutritional incompatibility of the plant with its environment than the inefficiency of the photosynthetic process (Brown, 1978).

The report of Epstein and Norlyn (1977) is a classic. Marketable yields have been obtained in California with a salt-tolerant research line of barley irrigated with water from the Pacific Ocean. Barley grown with seawater was found satisfactory as a feed, and yields were appreciable. The genetic approach to saline crop production has been proven with barley, and is applicable to other crops. Considerable progress has been made with the tomato. This development could be the shape of things to come in genetically opening a vast new water resource for crop production, one that was heretofore not accessible. Few regulatory constraints would likely be imposed on this new technology. Genetically controlled plant nutrition will surely play a key role in the future of crop production.

Genetic resources will continue to be utilized for improvement of the nutritional (biological) value of food crops. Cereals still dominate the diets of most people. Progress in genetically raising the levels of protein and critically deficient amino acids with cereal grains has been singular. Rice, wheat, and barley selections have been identified with higher protein levels. Both the biological value and the level of the protein of maize have been enhanced using the opaque-2-recessive gene, and, more recently, in maize of normal background. There is no cheaper, better, or quicker way to solve the protein needs of people in most agriculturally developing nations than to improve the cereals they eat. Combining the high productivity of certain cereal crops (maize, sorghum, millet) with the superior protein quality and "noble" grain characteristics of others (wheat, rice) remains, however, as a major challenge for plant scientists. The solution can be approached both genetically and chemically.

"Genetic engineering" has emerged as a series of events to cover new techniques of cell culture, protoplast fusion, and plasmid modification and transfer. An entire volume has recently been devoted to "Genetic Engineering for Nitrogen Fixation" (Hollaender, 1977). Significant advances have occurred in defining techniques for isolating protoplasts (plant cells without walls), their fusion, and providing cultures, with appropriate growth regulants, for rapid regeneration into new plants. With protoplast culture has come haploid production. New freeze-storage techniques and the establishment of gene banks of plant cells, as well as for meristems, will be a means of preserving rare and useful genetic materials. These new cellular approaches to plant breeding, sometimes described as somatic cell genetics, could become a major avenue for broad corsses--building new species with greater yield, resistance to biological and environmental stresses and to toxins, and for improved nutritional quality. Protoplast fusion offers hope of tapping genetic material not now available because of other sterility barriers between genera and species. Transformations and regeneration of parasexual hybrids from fixed protoplasts could revolutionize agricultural crop productivity. The ability to produce material, however, that can be readily introgressed into established plant breeding programs remains a major challenge.

The potential wealth of new crops as resources for food, feed, energy, fiber, and for industrial uses has often been emphasized. Wild plants also offer a genetic resource that is virtually unexplored. Many underexploited crops have received the attention of the Commission of International Relations of the United States Academy of Sciences National Research Council. As many as 36 are mentioned in a single report. There is the winged bean of the tropics and leucaena as a forage legume. Guayule and jojoba are desert shrubs, both of which have great value as producers of renewable resources that are important--both strategically and industrially. The productivity of hybrid napier grass as a forage crop for the tropics could revolutionize livestock production, as it is now doing in the Gujarat State of India.

Efficiency in Nutrient Uptake

It has been estimated that only 50% of the nitrogen and less than 35% of the phosphorus and potassium applied as fertilizer in the United States are recovered by crops. The recovery of fertilizer nitrogen in the rice paddies of the tropics is 25-35%. The rest is lost to the environment. Denitrification loses nitrogen to the atmosphere. Nitrification encourages losses in the soil from leaching. Nitrification is also a prerequisite to losses from denitrification. Food production and crop productivity could be greatly improved if these enormous losses, particularly in the warm soils of the tropics, could be even partially reduced. The single factor, recently identified, as responsible for no increase in rice yields on Asian farms is the low level of nitrogen fertilizer available.

A worldwide annual loss of 12-15 million tons of nitrogen fertilizer can be ascribed to denitrification alone. Losses from nitrification are equally as great. Nitrification inhibitors, both natural and synthetic, applied with ammonia or urea, are effective deterrents to leaching and atmospheric losses of nitrogen. The result could be a significant reduction in fertilizer cost and usage. Nonrenewable resources would be preserved. Crop productivity would be increased, and a potential environmental hazard reduced (Bremner and Blackmer, 1978).

Denitrification occurs only under anaerobic soil conditions. This may be alleviated by reduced nitrification, soil compaction, improved drainage, use of soil improving crops, and careful attention to irrigation procedures. Research emphasis on reduction of losses of nitrogen fertilizer applied to crops should hold priority equal to that for devising means of nitrogen fixation utilizing renewable, rather than nonrenewable, resources.

The facilitation of nutrient uptake by microorganisms (fungi) in symbiotic associations with the roots of higher plants is emerging as one of the most exciting frontiers for enhancement of crop production. The efficiency of plant roots in absorption of nutrients from the soil can be improved. Mycorrhizae, particularly the endomycorrhizae and the subgroup referred to as vesicular-arbuscular, may result in large increases in the uptake of phosphorus and other poorly mobile nutrients. Almost all crops respond. Vesicular-arbuscular mycorrhizae can be viewed as fungal extensions of roots. They help roots absorb fertilizer and can stimulate growth and nitrogen fixation by legumes, especially in phosphorus deficient soils.

There are superior strains of mycorrhizae, and crops can be inoculated with them. Mycorrhizae fungi have been reported to increase significantly the yields of cereal grains and many vegetable crops. The profound effects of these fungi have only recently been appreciated. They facilitate nutrient uptake by changing the amounts, concentrations, and properties of minerals available to plants both in forestry and in agriculture. The potential is not only for a substantial increase in conventional crop production, with conservation of nonrenewable resources, but to expand the land base so that plants can be grown in areas which now have an unfavorable climate and nonproductive soils. Equally fascinating is the microbiology of aerial plant surfaces and the role of phyllosphere microorganisms in plant mineral nutrition.

Foliar applications of fertilizer have long been declared the most efficient method of fertilizer placement. Technology of application, however, is still lacking. Future yield barriers may be broken by utilizing the absorptive capacity of leaves, as well as the roots, for applying nutrients at crucial stages of development. Great hope was expressed for nutrient foliar sprays following results on soybeans in 1975. Extensive experimental foliar spraying of nutrients in all the major soybean producing areas in the United States during 1976 and 1977 for yield enhancement has not, however, confirmed the outstanding results achieved in 1975.

There are other possibilities for increasing crop productivity and, simultaneously, reducing fertilizer loss. The gradient mulch system for growing tomatoes in Florida is one. It is a high-level, low-cost concept utilizing and maintaining a nonvariable root environment; achieved by a plastic mulch, a constant water table, and precise fertilizer placement.

Resistance to Competing Biological Systems

Field losses from pests (insects, diseases, weeds, nematodes, rodents) for the world's major food crops approximate 35%. Regional losses vary from 25-29% for Europe, Oceania, and North America to 42-43% for Africa and Asia (Table 7). All major crops suffer losses before harvest that exceed 20%. Chemical pesticides have played a dominant role in the control of pests, and will continue to do so in the near future. Approximately 1.4 billion pounds of synthetic organic pesticides were produced worldwide in 1976. The United States expended $1.8 billion for pesticides in 1975. Chemical pesticides have accounted for 20% of the increase in farm output during the past 25-30 years, during which time production has doubled. Since World War II, there has been an ever increasing dependence on pesticides. Historians will likely refer to the latter half of the twentieth century as the "organic pesticide era." Meanwhile, reliance on this single line of defense has introduced

Table 7. Crop Losses to Pests

Region	% Loss
North America	29
South America	33
Europe	25
Africa	42
Asia	43
Oceania	28
USSR and China	30

problems of pesticide resistance, destruction of natural enemies, outbreaks of secondary pests, reductions in pollinators, potential environmental, livestock, and human health problems, rising economic costs, and increasing regulatory constraints. Regulatory constraints and costs relating thereto in the use of pesticides have multiplied exponentially (Table 6).

Future alternative strategies for integrated pest control, as now being developed by teams of scientists, if implemented, will likely result in the use of more pesticides in agriculturally developing nations, and less in the more developed (Glass and Thurston, 1978). For small farm peasant agriculture, it is not a future option; it is an immediate urgency. The intent of the projected widely used systems approach in pest management will be to reduce costs for pest control, impose less of an environmental insult, create greater production dependability, and increase yields. This will come through the use of natural enemies and parasites, identification and creation of genetically resistant varieties, improved cultural practices, environmental monitoring, and more timely and efficient use of chemicals. Whereas the possibility may exist for some agriculturally developing nations to bypass the fossil fuel age, it is not likely for the chemical pesticide era. One of the big steps in the next ten or twenty years will be real time management of agricultural systems, including pests. In an era of few stable resources, we must develop integrated pest control measures.

Allelopathy

Considerable evidence has now accumulated to implicate secondary plant metabolites as defensive agents in plant-to-plant relationships. Allelopathy is a widespread phenomenon among crop plants. Studies of allelopathy in crop plants have revealed toxic compounds in asparagus and sorghum roots and shoots and in cucumber fruits and seeds. Residues of sorghum plants and sudan grass have provided excellent control of annual grass weeds in both the greenhouse and field. Production of common purslane and smooth crabgrass is greatly reduced by both living sorghums and their residues. The use of allelopathic cover crops in conservation tillage crop production is being pursued.

Crops or crop residues with weed suppressing ability have the potential to reduce dependence on synthetic herbicides and to reduce the number of viable weed propagules. Considerable reductions in cost and energy inputs may be realized. The discovery of natural toxins could lead to synthesis of analogs with better efficacy and safety (Putnam and Duke, 1978).

There has been, until now, a constant battle between man, the scientist, and nature in achieving disease resistance in high yielding plants. Resistance has an average half life of only five years. One of the inevitable consequences of modern agriculture appears to be that the most widely adapted of the improved crop varieties are highly vulnerable to new strains of plant diseases. The southern corn leaf blight that destroyed a substantial part of the United States crop in 1970 was one example. Another was downy mildew, which afflicted hybrid pearl millet in the late 1960s. Traditional plant breeding methods have resulted in new varieties in which disease resistance is specific and dependent upon a single gene.

A possible alternative approach is the "multiline" concept. It is being pursued with new rust-resistant wheats. A multiline variety is created mechanically. Seeds of several lines that are similar in appearance and genetic makeup, but which have different genes for resistance to rust, are mixed together. This concept, if proven, could shape the future. Immunity would be lasting, and resistance would be permanent and achieved at low cost.

Resistance to Environmental Stresses

Environmental stresses, alone or in combination, constitute the primary limiting factor(s) for increasing and expanding the production of many, if not most, of the world's crops. Those that limit crop productivity include drought, cold, heat, salt, toxic ions, and air pollutants. Plants, unlike people, livestock, and other animals, are immobile. They are fixed by location. Environmental adaptability, thus, becomes preeminent. Any means of increasing the resistance of plants to high and low temperatures, drought and water stress, to adverse soil conditions, and other environmental hazards, holds great promise for enhancement of the amount of food, as well as the dependability of the supply. Through the use of short season, early planted, single-cross maize hybrids, commercial production in the United States has moved 500 miles further north during the past fifty years. Winter wheat production has been extended northward by 200 miles. Hybrid sorghum and millets are moving into hot-dry areas, not heretofore adapted for cereal grain production. The new synthetic species, triticale, has resistance to aluminum toxicity. Thus, millions of acres of previously nonproductive land can be opened for food cropping. Characteristic of the new seeds (rice and wheat) of the "green revolution" are varieties that are day-neutral and will produce grain at any latitude. There are also genetic strains of rice, wheat, and barley having greater resistance to both cold and alkalinity. This, coupled with earlier maturity, has made possible a "two paddy system" in South Korea where heretofore only one crop of grain per year could be grown. Potato varieties have been identified in the high Andes with moderate frost resistance and cold hardiness.

Plants can be made more "climate-proof" by genetic improvement and by appropriate soil, water, and pest management. The use of weather and climatic information in the selection of crop varieties for a particular climatic setting, the strategic planning of the size, the type, and operation of an irrigation system, or alternative strategies in pest management can reduce the adverse effects of climate and weather on crop productivity.

Controlled environment agriculture can greatly increase food crop productivity and the dependability of supply. By far, the most extensive means of modifying the environment is irrigation. Food production suffers from some degree of water deficiency over the entire globe. Currently, there are more than 100 million hectares of the land surface of the earth under irrigation for crop production. Irrigated cropland constitutes about 15% of the total under cultivation. The higher productivity of irrigated land, however, results in 30% of the world's food. Egypt's agriculture is entirely dependent on irrigation. There are 6.5 million acres that support 40 million people. The Nile River is now a closed system.

Looking to the future, India, Sri Lanka, the Soviet Union, and Bangladesh expect to double the amount of irrigated land, and they have the renewable water resources to do it. This will not only increase the productivity of a given crop, but will enable year around production. It will require vast capital inputs. Irrigation will also greatly increase food security, through greater dependability of supply and with less vulnerability to climatic and weather variables. Largely through irrigation, new seeds, and fertilizer, China has doubled the yields of the major food grains in two decades, despite recurring droughts. "Drip" or "trickle" irrigation referred to as the "blue revolution" offers great potential for water, energy, soil, and fertilizer conservation. It puts the water where the roots are, and alleviates some problems of alkalinity.

The most intensive food producing systems on earth are those where crops are grown in greenhouses or under the protection of other structures. This offers the ultimate in stable production at high levels. The chief constraint of fully controlled-environment agriculture is that it demands a maximum in capital, management, and resource inputs. It is high technology and resource intensive. Nevertheless, great agricultural production potential exists. Hydroponic culture facilitates control of both the top and root environments. The latest developments in hydroponics have occurred in northern Europe with the nutrient film technique. This is the most sophisticated technology yet conceived for improvement and control of crop production in greenhouses. It takes full advantage of maximizing control of the total environment and optimizing the uptake of both water and nutrients by plant roots.

CONCLUSIONS

Our immediate challenge is to enhance yields and improve the dependability of production of the food, feed, and industrial crops of the world. Future plant growth regulator research should be restructured to permit a multidisciplinary approach to the regulation of the basic biological processes that control productivity of the major crops. There is an urgent need for a chemical to enhance the productivity of soybeans and other legumes. The corn plant offers another challenge; as do rice, wheat, sugar beets, and sorghum. Root crops and tubers should receive special attention.

Root and tuber responses to growth regulators, as well as the behavior of aerial plant parts, should be evaluated. Thus far, observations have been confined largely to above-ground plant parts. Studies of effects on root growth are few and incomplete. A knowledge of the responses of roots to plant growth regulators when applied repeatedly, in combination, and with variations in the carbon dioxide and oxygen levels in the atmosphere, should give some exciting and useful results.

There are new technologies for application and bioassay of growth regulators. Ultra low volume (ULV) and aerial spraying permit coverage of vast areas with a minimum of water carried and energy expended. These approaches are important in treatment of forest lands and major food and pasture crops; and in the application of chemicals that counteract the effects of air pollutants (serious consideration is being given to the development of the latter). The nutrient film technique in hydroponic greenhouse culture enables complete control of not only the top, but the root environment of plants. It also offers a means for uniform application, and for simultaneously observing and measuring growth regulator effects on both roots and tops. Drip irrigation of field crops offers similar possibilities.

All effects possible with chemical regulators may eventually be duplicated genetically. Meanwhile, these regulators offer an immediate and very practical solution to many food production problems. It is likely that a useful role can be found for all crops, for all biological processes, and for all developmental stages.

Thirty-five years after the publication of Missouri Research Bulletin 371, "Growth Hormone Production During Sexual Reproduction of Higher Plants" (Wittwer, 1943), the mysteries of the growth of the corn plant still intrigue me. It is the most important crop we grow in America. It is the world's third most important food crop. Millions depend on it for sustenance. There are two major periods of accelerated plant growth that are hormone related. One follows the development of the microgametophytes preparatory to the shedding of pollen. The second follows gametic union and the early development of the kernels. Tremendous quantities of growth promoting substances are found in fresh corn pollen and immature corn kernels at the milk stage. There is still no good inventory of the growth substances in these reproductive structures whose appearance parallels precisely the remarkable upsurges in growth. Their true nature remains obscure.

Finally, history may record many achievements for the twentieth century, but I am optimistic enough to believe that we will see, through the great potential for enhancement of food production, the dread scourge of famine eliminated from the face of the earth.

REFERENCES

Bremner, J. M., and Blackmer, A. M., 1978, Nitrous oxide: Emission from soils during nitrification of fertilizer nitrogen, Science, 199:295-296.

Brown, J. C., 1978, Genetic improvement of nutrient uptake in plants, BioScience 28:(in press).

Brown, L. R., 1978, "The Global Economic Prospect: New Sources of Economic Stress," Worldwatch Paper 20, Washington, D.C.

Buringh, P., 1977, Food production potential of the world, World Development, 5:477-485.

Da Silva, J. G., Serra, G. E., Moreira, J. R., Concalves, J. C., and Goldemberg, J. 1978, Energy balance for ethyl alcohol production from crops, Science, 201:903-906.

Epstein, E., and Norlyn, J. D., 1977, Seawater-based crop production: A feasibility study, Science, 197:249-251.

Evans, L. T., ed., 1975, "Crop Physiology," Cambridge Univ. Press, Cambridge.

Glass, E. H., and Thurston, H. D., 1978, Traditional and modern crop protection in perspective, BioScience, 28:109-115.
Hageman, R. H., 1978, in: "Proceedings Fourth Annual Meeting Plant Growth Regulator Working Group," E. F. Sullivan, Great Western Sugar Co., Longmont, Colo.
Hedden, P., MacMillan, J., and Phinney, B. O., 1978, The metabolism of the gibberellins, Ann. Rev. Plant Physiol., 29:149-192.
Hollaender, A., ed., 1977, "Genetic Engineering for Nitrogen Fixation," Plenum Press, New York.
International Rice Research Institute, in press, Los Banõs, The Philippines, 1978.
Jensen, M. F., 1978, Limits to growth in world food production, Science, 201:317-320.
Plant Growth Regulator Working Group, 1978, "Proceedings Fourth Annual Meeting Plant Growth Regulator Working Group," E. F. Sullivan, Great Western Sugar Co., Longmont, Colo.
Putnam, A. R., and Duke, W. B., 1978, The role of allelopathy in agroecosystems, Ann. Rev. Phytopathology, 16:431-451.
Ries, S. K., Richman, T. L., and Wert, V. F., 1978, Growth and yield of crops treated with tricontanol, Jour. Amer. Soc. Hort. Sci., 103:361-364.
Ruttan, V. W., 1977, Induced innovation and research resource allocation, Food Policy, 2:196-216.
Treharne, R. W., Moles, D. R., Bruce, M. R., and McKribben, C. K., 1978, "A Nitrogen Fertilizer Generator for Farm Use," Technical Note 1, Charles F. Kettering Foundation Research Laboratories, Yellow Springs, Ohio.
Williams, W. T., 1978, "Effects on Plants of Sulfur Pollutants from Coal Combustion," Citizens for a Better Environment Report 7866, San Francisco.
Wittwer, S. H., 1943, "Growth Hormone Production During Sexual Reproduction of Higher Plants," Missouri Research Bulletin 371.
Wittwer, S. H., 1978a, Nitrogen fixation and agricultural productivity, BioScience, 28:555.
Wittwer, S. H., 1978b, The next generation of agricultural research, Science, 199:375.
Wortman, S., Cummings, R. W., Jr., 1978, "To Feed This World: The Challenge and the Strategy," John Hopkins Univ. Press, Baltimore.
Yokoyama, H., Hayman, E. P., Hsu, W. J., and Poling, S. M., 1977, Chemical bioinduction of rubber in guayule plant, Science, 197:1076-1078.

3

ROOT HORMONES AND OVERGROUND DEVELOPMENT

Johan Bruinsma

Agricultural University
Wageningen, The Netherlands

AGRICULTURE AND ROOT HORMONES

Many cultural measures in crop production are exerted through the soil. Soil cultivation, fertilization, drainage, and irrigation affect root growth initially and subsequently the development of the overground plant parts. That plants develop into harmonious organisms, with balanced proportions between their various organs, is mainly due to correlative interactions between these organs. Well-developing shoots allow the root system to develop accordingly and vice versa. This is not just a matter of adequate supply of nutrients. Of course, roots need to be supplied with photosynthetic assimilates from the leaves, such as sucrose and vitamins and sometimes amino acids; and the leaves, in turn, feed water, minerals, and amino acids into the shoot. But this is not the whole story. The various correlative effects between organs are mediated by hormonal substances that, by definition, are produced at a particular site and affect one or more developmental processes at another site after translocation. They are the "calines" suggested by Went (1938), produced by one organ and evoking the growth of another plant part. We shall be concerned with what Went called "caulocalines," root-produced hormonal substances influencing the growth and development of such overground parts as stems, leaves, buds, flowers, and fruits. To these organs they convey effects of soil humidity, aeration, fertilization, man-made chemicals, root nodules, etc. In this way, root hormones play an important role as a link in the chain between cultural measures of the grower and overground crop growth.

NATURE OF THE HORMONES INVOLVED

Which hormones are involved as messengers from root to shoot? Representatives of all known classes of phytohormones have been detected in root extracts: auxins, gibberellins, cytokinins, and abscisins have all been demonstrated to occur in root extracts, while roots are also known sites of biosynthesis of ethylene (e.g., see Torrey, 1976). Because all phytohormones can be circulated through the whole plant via the phloem and xylem vessels, their occurrence in root extracts gives hardly any information about their site of synthesis, unless different areas of roots are analyzed separately. The occurrence of relatively high concentrations of indoleacetic and abscisic acids in root caps, for example, indicates their local synthesis. Also the occurrence of phytohormones in roots grown in cultures in vitro is highly indicative for local synthesis of auxin and gibberellin (Torrey, 1976).

Hormones acting as messengers from root to shoot should occur in the xylem sap exuded from the cut stem of a decapitated plant. Again, all four groups of hormones have been detected in the root exudate. However, the main flow of auxin is from shoot to root. Shoot apices, leaves, flowers, and developing seeds are the main sites of auxin synthesis. From these organs in the top of the plant, auxin is translocated downward into the root system. Within the roots, auxin is predominantly transported acropetally, and on its way to the root tip it is strongly inactivated by conjugation and oxidation. This implies a direction of auxin from over- to underground plant parts rather than the reverse.

Likewise, abscisins are formed predominantly in mature leaves (Zeevaart, 1977), also in response to changes in such a soil factor as water supply. Like auxins, abscisins in roots are mainly involved in root development itself: straight and tropistic growth, as well as initiation of laterals. However, in some cases such inhibiting substances as abscisins do play the role of messengers from the roots as will be seen later.

This is certainly the case with gibberellins, although their biosynthesis is by no means restricted to roots or even unambiguously demonstrated to occur in roots. Gibberellins are produced by shoot tips, leaves, flowers, and seeds, but also in isolated root systems and decapitated plants. They have frequently been shown to occur in bleeding sap, especially under conditions of root aeration and with sprouting trees in the spring. This occurrence is diminished by the addition of growth retardants to the roots (e.g., see Reid and Carr, 1967). Roots may convert inactive gibberellins from shoots into active ones (Crozier and Reid, 1971), but also incorporate radioactivity from mevalonic acid into kaurene (Sitton et al., 1967), so that Torrey (1976) rightly concludes: "That roots serve as the source of gibberellins which move in the xylem sap to the shoot and there elicit effects seems established beyond doubt."

The best candidates for root-produced messengers are the cytokinins. Their production in overground parts, such as developing seeds (Hahn et al., 1974), leaves (Wareing et al., 1977), and cotyledons (Uheda and Kuraishi, 1977), has been surmised but the evidence is very inconclusive (e.g., see Krechting et al., 1978). There are indications that overground parts may synthesize cytokinins under special conditions, for instance at a high level of mineral nutrition (Wareing et al., 1977). Moreover, the occurrence in aerial parts of their glucosides (Hoad et al., 1977) indicates that in these parts cytokinins are metabolized rather than synthesized (Wareing et al., 1977). Admittedly, their biosynthesis from adenosine phosphate(s) and mevalonic acid has not been explicitly demonstrated in root tips either. But their occurrence in high concentrations in root tips, nodules, and exudate, dependent on the activity of root tips under different environmental conditions, strongly suggests them to be the main messengers transferring information about these conditions to the overground parts.

This article will not deal with effects of root hormones on root and tuber growth which indirectly also affect overground development. It will rather be confined to the direct effects of root-produced cytokinins, gibberellins, and possibly substances which inhibit the growth and development of the aerial plant parts.

ROOT HORMONES AND SHOOT GROWTH

The first indication that root-produced cytokinins may act as messengers of changed soil conditions to the plant shoot was found by Itai and Vaadia (1965). They observed that the root exudate of sunflower plants suffering from water stress contained less cytokinin than the bleeding sap of well-watered plants. They suggested that the drought-induced changes of the leaves are connected with the decreased hormonal supply from the roots. The opposite treatment, waterlogging, induces similar effects owing to lack of oxygen. Waterlogging of tomato roots decreases the gibberellin content of roots, bleeding sap, and stems, as well as the growth of the shoot (Reid and Crozier, 1971). They found that shoot growth could be restored by gibberellin application, but that it also slightly recovered of its own after three to four days, probably due to gibberellin production by newly formed adventitious roots. Other symptoms of these waterlogged tomato plants besides growth reduction could be combatted with exogenous cytokinin rather than gibberellin. Such effects as chlorophyll breakdown, epinasty of petioles, and appearance of adventitious roots, which can be ascribed to auxin or auxin-induced ethylene, were successfully suppressed by benzyladenine (Railton and Reid, 1973).

Effects caused by changes in soil temperature can also be transmitted by these hormones, probably in cooperation with abscisins. The root exudate of decapitated maize plants normally contains three cytokinins, four gibberellins, and four growth-inhibiting substances (Atkin et al., 1973). At the optimum root temperature for shoot growth, 33°C, the inhibitor content in the xylem sap was at a minimum. At lower root temperatures the inhibitor content slightly increased and the supply of cytokinins and gibberellins strongly decreased. This suggests a relationship between soil temperature and shoot growth by means of the hormonal composition of the sap supply from the roots. Similarly, Itai et al. (1973) found that a short heat stress to the roots of bean and tobacco of 2 min at 46-47°C reduced shoot growth and was accompanied by a decreased cytokinin content and increased abscisic acid content of the root exudate.

The sprouting of Douglas fir in spring is retarded when the soil temperature remains low. Shoot growth can then be improved by a spray with gibberellic acid. At increasing soil temperature gibberellins appear in the xylem sap about a week prior to bud growth (Lavender et al., 1973). Jones and Lacey (1968) collected xylem sap of flowering apple and pear trees and found gibberellin activities compatible with those required for shoot growth.

Also, effects of mineral nutrition can be mediated to the shoot via the hormonal composition of the transpiration stream. The mediation of phosphorus nutrition by cytokinins in flower formation will be dealt with later. Nitrogen deficiency reduces the growth and longevity of shoots. This has generally been ascribed to shortage of such nitrogen-containing substrates as amino acids. However, Wagner and Michael (1969), who found a sharp decrease of cytokinin level in the xylem sap of nitrogen-deficient sunflower plants, suggested that the reduction in growth and longevity of the shoot may be caused by a hormonal rather than nutritional deficiency.

Thus we come to two interesting problems of sprout physiology: senescence and apical dominance.

ROOT HORMONES AND APICAL DOMINANCE

The phenomenon of apical dominance has alternately been looked upon as a matter of lack of nutrients in lateral buds and as one of presence of an inhibitor of lateral bud growth. After the discovery of auxin as a correlative regulator with the ability to replace the apex in repressing the growth of lateral buds, the old view was disregarded. The new theory held that these buds fail to grow because the apex exclusively attracted the substances required for growth. The further observation that cytokinin applied to a lateral bud of, for example, Alaska pea, counteracts the inhibitory effect of the apex and allows the bud to grow, corroborated the theory of correlative inhibition.

Gregory and Veale (1957), when studying apical dominance in oil and linen flax, unexpectedly hit upon the old theory when they found that apical dominance in flax could be diminished by ample nitrogen nutrition. Later work (e.g., Phillips, 1968), however, showed that the lateral buds were not in need of nutrients but of another factor required for growth. Among the accumulating evidence that this factor must be root-produced hormone the data obtained by Chang and Goodin (1974) are particularly convincing (Fig. 1). They demonstrated that the outgrowth of lateral buds of decapitated Alaska pea seedlings is inhibited by excision of the roots, but can largely be restored by the addition of root hormones to the basal cut. They further indicated, by the application of radioactive cytokinin, that this substance moves toward sites of auxin activity. Apical dominance can, therefore, be largely looked upon as a morphogenetic phenomenon regulated by hormones from the two extremities of the plant: auxin from the shoot apex and especially cytokinins from the root tips. These cytokinins, the production of

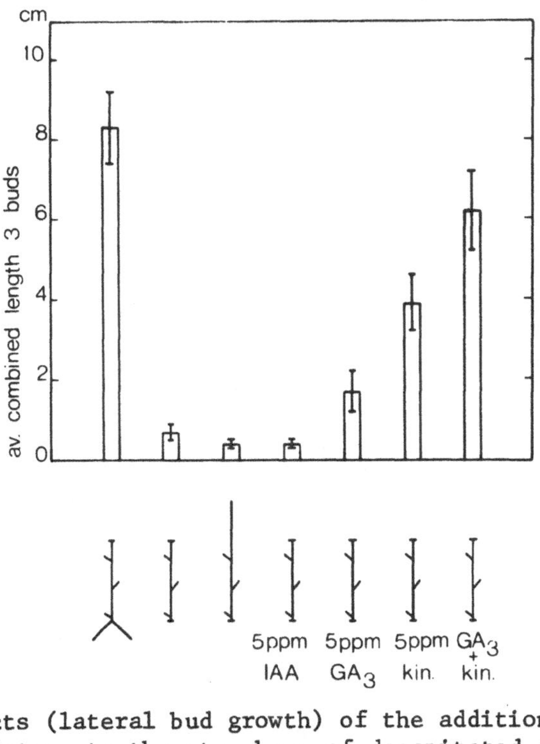

Fig. 1. Effects (lateral bud growth) of the addition of growth regulators to the stem base of decapitated and derooted *Pisum sativum* seedlings (after Chang and Goodin, 1974).

which depends on soil conditions (for example, the amount of fertilization), are required for bud growth but attracted to the shoot apex by the activity of auxin at that site. This main relationship may further be influenced by other hormonal substances. For instance, the shape of tomato plants is controlled by a balance between cytokinin, auxin, and abscisin that, as an inhibitor, reduces lateral sprout formation (Tucker, 1976).

ROOT HORMONES IN SENESCENCE AND JUVENILITY

Root-produced hormones influence the growth and shape of the overground plant by their regulation of cell division and elongation. Moreover, they can affect the longevity of aerial plant parts by regulating their senescence, also in response to soil conditions.

This effect was one of the earliest known actions of cytokinins. As early as 1964, Engelbrecht reported that the aging of an excised leaf can be halted and reversed by adventitious root formation on the petiole. Also, a cytokinin solution sucked through the petiole could delay the aging process. This cytokinin effect has frequently been confirmed and the (re)activation of cell metabolism and postponement of senescence in leaves and fruits are well established. For example, root pruning of dwarf pea seedlings caused reduced photosynthesis and advanced senescence of leaves (MacDavid et al., 1973). Addition of cytokinin compensated these effects and promoted the retention of assimilates in the shoot. Cytokinins generally increase the resistance of plants to such stress conditions as cold, heat, drought, and salt, probably because the stability of cell membranes is also improved when anabolic processes are promoted. Cytokinins counteract the closing effect of abscisic acid on stomatal aperture, so that a cytokinin-containing transpiration stream induces stomata to open, also to the advantage of photosynthetic assimilation.

A related phenomenon is the juvenility of shoots carrying adventitious roots, but here gibberellins rather than cytokinins play a role. Ivy, *Hedera helix*, has creeping shoots with many adventitious roots which are juvenile and flowering occurs only on the short, rootless, erect shoots. Also leaf shape and phyllotaxy differ between juvenile and mature shoots. Adult shoots can be reverted to the juvenile phase by treatment with gibberellin. Both this induced rejuvenation and the spontaneous rejuvenation in weak light can be counteracted by abscisic acid and growth retardants (Rogler and Hackett, 1975a,b). The hypothesis that the juvenility of shoots in the proximity of roots is promoted by root-produced gibberellins is corroborated by the observation with black currant (*Ribes nigrum*) that the occurrence of aerial roots at mature internodes rejuvenates the shoots. In mature shoots, gibberellins are normally not detectable, in contrast with roots, and gibberellic acid inhibits flowering in black currant (Schwabe and Al-Doori, 1973).

ROOT HORMONES AND FLOWER INDUCTION

The phenomenon of juvenility brings us to reproductive development. In studying hormonal regulation of flowering, one has to distinguish between the induction of the reproductive stage and the morphogenetic realization of flowering. Hormones may exert opposite effects in these two processes. Gibberellins, for instance, induce the reproductive stage in rosetted plants that require long days or vernalization for stem elongation. However, the inhibiting effect of gibberellins in actual flower development of already reproductive plants explains such phenomena in fruit growing as biennial bearing and increased fruitfulness by reduction of shoot growth. With biennial bearing it is the gibberellin production of the developing seeds which prevents simultaneous flower development for the next season, and the gibberellins produced by growing shoots exert a similar effect.

Roots influence flowering differently, not only because of the difference between flower induction and realization, but also because gibberellins and cytokinins may act in opposite ways and, moreover, their action may differ in different plant species.

That root conditions can greatly affect flowering is shown in Fig. 2, derived from experiments of Wellensiek (1968) on flower induction with the long-day plant _Silene armeria_. Otherwise exposure of the roots to a soil temperature of 35°C for three weeks induces the reproductive stage under short days at 20°C. Wellensiek assumes a hormone connected with flowering to be produced by the roots at 35°C. Also, chilling temperatures can provoke roots to produce such a hormone as Wellensiek (1962) demonstrated for the "root vernalization" of _Lunaria biennis_ root cuttings. The site of vernalization is probably dividing cells in the root tips. The nature of this root-produced hormone involved in the induction of flowering of rosetted plants may well be gibberellin-like. However, recent evidence obtained by Bernier (1976) indicates that cytokinins may also play a role in flower induction. In the short-day plant _Xanthium strumarium_, root-produced cytokinin seems to inhibit flower induction (Henson and Wareing, 1977). One short day induces flowering and lowers the cytokinin supply from the roots, unless the long night is interrupted. This interesting observation indicates that day-length perceiving leaves are able to transmit a signal to the roots to induce suppression of cytokinin synthesis.

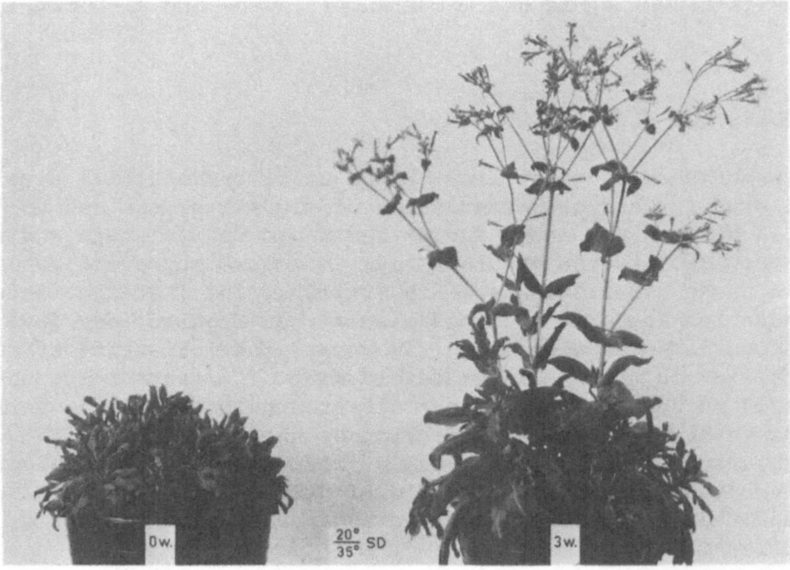

Fig. 2. Flowering of Silene armeria under short days at 20°C air temperature and 35°C soil temperature, shown at right. At left a control plant at 20°C soil temperature.

ROOT HORMONES AND FLOWER DEVELOPMENT

In the realization of flower formation roots exert opposing effects. Often flowering and fruit production are promoted by reducing root growth. Root pruning promotes flowering in lilac, an effect that can be replaced by the application of growth retardants. Also, a weak parent stock of fruit trees or incompatible grafting of trees considerably increases fruit and seed yields and here, too, growth retardants act in a similar way. However, the conclusion that such negative effects of roots on fruitfulness can wholly be ascribed to their production of gibberellin is premature. In vine, the addition of the growth retardant chlormequat to the soil greatly improves flower formation and fruit set, and increases the cytokinin activity of the bleeding sap (Skene, 1968).

Cytokinins are known to promote flower morphogenesis, not only in vine where flower primordia of cuttings with insufficient roots often shrivel away unless cytokinin is supplied (Mullins, 1967). Many flowers require cytokinin for their development in vitro culture. We grow flower primordia on liquid media of known compositions and usually find that the addition of, for instance, 10^{-6} M benzyladenine is essential, for example, in Begonia (Berghoef and Bruinsma, in press). In earlier experiments with the spider flower, Cleome sp., we found that the occurrence of pistil abortion in developing flowers was caused by the attraction of the sap stream by the rapidly growing fruits underneath the flower buds (de Jong and Bruinsma, 1974a). Culture of flower buds in vitro demonstrated cytokinin to be the factor essential for pistil development (de Jong and Bruinsma, 1974b). It is depletion in the sap stream of cytokinins produced by the root tips which causes pistil abortion in the flower buds at the other extreme end of the plant (de Jong and Bruinsma, 1974c). Recent observations on sex expression in hemp plants point in the same direction (Chailakhyan and Khryanin, 1978). If the roots are removed from hemp plants the percentage of female flowering is reduced from 80-90% to 10-20%. However, the addition of 15 ppm benzyladenine during 28 hours to these derooted plants increases the percentage of female flowering to 81% again.

At the Long Ashton Research Station, the promotive action of root-produced cytokinins on flower formation is the core of the theory on fruitfulness of pome trees (Luckwill, 1970). The hypothesis, based on the gradual drop in cytokinin activity of xylem sap during the growing season, holds that flower formation depends on the relative rates at which cytokinins from the roots and gibberellins from the shoot tip decrease. If the cytokinin content is still sufficiently high when shoot growth ends, then the cytokinin: gibberellin ratio allows flower buds to develop. If this ratio becomes too low, which is always the case when fruits with their gibberellin-producing seeds develop, then flower differentiation fails to occur.

Nitrogen fertilization plays a role in the antagonism between shoot growth and flower formation in pome trees, with ammonium nitrogen, particularly, favoring flower morphogenesis (Grasmanis and Edwards, 1974). We found a sudden increase in the zeatin content of the xylem sap of starved apple trees only one day after nitrogen fertilization, and a larger one after ammonium than upon nitrate application (Bubán et al., 1978). Similarly, the cytokinin activity of the bleeding sap of phosphorus-deficient tomato plants increased upon phosphate nutrition. Both the addition of phosphate and that of kinetin to the nutrient solution increased the rate and amount of flower formation (Menary and van Staden, 1976). This indicates the possibility of removing adverse effects of such soil conditions as mineral deficiencies by the application of plant growth regulators that can replace root-produced hormones.

ROOT HORMONES AND FRUIT DEVELOPMENT

Finally, from the onset of reproductive development the overground organs mutually compete for the root-produced hormones. The already mentioned pistil abortion in <u>Cleome</u> flowers in the presence of growing fruits underneath the flower buds is an example of such a competition. This competition occurs particularly between fruits and leaves. It can be changed by reducing the numbers of fruits or leaves and this may influence the cytokinin content of these organs considerably. In tomato, reduction of the foliage to one-third increased the cytokinin content of the fruits seventeenfold (Varga and Bruinsma, 1974). On the other hand, removal of grape berries markedly enhanced the cytokinin content of the grape leaves which, in turn, inactivated the excess of zeatin and its riboside from the xylem by glucosidation (Hoad et al., 1977). The ripening of fruits can be retarded by hormones obtained from the root exudate. As with senescence of vegetative organs, both gibberellins and cytokinins delay the ripening process, for example, in tomato fruits (Dostal and Leopold, 1967; Varga and Bruinsma, 1974).

CONCLUSION

Hormones produced by the roots and supplied to the overground plant parts via the xylem sap can be translocated into the phloem and circulated throughout the shoot system. They transmit information from the environment, mainly about soil conditions, but even about such influences as the day-length regime. In this way they play an important role as intermediate factors in the chain from agricultural measures to overground growth and development by regulating the amount and rate of shoot growth and branching, of flower and fruit production, as well as the longevity of the crop. A better understanding of the production, distribution, mode of action, and metabolism of these intermediate factors may contribute to a quantitatively and qualitatively improved crop production. The recent availability of exact and rapid methods for hormone determination enables the study of changes in hormonal composition of the root exudate of, for instance, plants with and without root nodules or mycorrhizae, and of C_4 plants subjected to varying degrees of drought and salinity. The application of growth-regulating substances with a similar action as the natural root-produced hormones may be an alternative for energy-consuming growing measures in the production of food and fiber crops.

REFERENCES

Atkin, R. K., Barton, G. E., and Robinson, D. K., 1973, Effect of root-growing temperature on growth substances in xylem exudate of Zea mays, J. Exp. Bot., 24:475-487.

Berghoef, J., and Bruinsma, J., 1978, Flower development in Begonia franconis, Z. Pflanzenphysiol., in press.

Bernier, G., 1976, La nature complexe du stimulus floral des facteurs de floraison, in: "Etudes de Biologie Végétale. Hommage au Professeur P. Chouard," R. Jacques, ed., Paris.

Bubán, T., Varga, A., Tromp, J., Knegt, E., and Bruinsma, J., 1978, Effects of ammonium and nitrate nutrition on the levels of

zeatin and amino nitrogen in xylem sap of apple rootstocks, Z. Pflanzenphysiol., in press.
Chailakhyan, M. K., and Khryanin, V. N., 1978, The role of roots in sex expression in hemp plants, Planta, 138:185-188.
Chang, W. C., and Goodin, J. R., 1974, The role of root system in lateral bud growth of pea (Pisum sativum L., var. Alaska), Bot. Bull. Acad. Sinica, 15:112-122.
Crozier, A., and Reid, D. M., 1971, Do roots synthesize gibberellins?, Can. J. Bot., 49:967-975.
Dostal, H. C., and Leopold, A. C., 1967, Gibberellin delays ripening of tomatoes, Science, 158:1579-1580.
Engelbrecht, R., 1964, Ueber Kinetinwirkungen bei intakten Blättern von Nicotiana rustica, Flora Allg. Bot. Z., 154:57-69.
Grasmanis, V. O., and Edwards, G. E., 1974, Promotion of flower initiation in apple trees by short exposure to the ammonium ion, Aust. J. Plant Physiol., 1:99-105.
Gregory, F. G., and Veale, J. A., 1957, A reassessment of the problem of apical dominance, Symp. Soc. Exp. Biol., 11:1-20.
Hahn, H. R. de Zacks, and Kende, H., 1974, Cytokinin formation in pea seeds, Naturwiss., 61:170.
Henson, I. E., and Wareing, P. F., 1977, Cytokinins in Xanthium strumarium L.: Some aspects of the photoperiodic control of endogenous levels, New Physiol., 78:35-45.
Hoad, G. V., Loveys, B., and Skene, K. G. M., 1977, The effect of fruit removal on cytokinins and gibberellin-like substances in grape leaves, Planta, 136:25-30.
Itai, C., and Vaadia, Y., 1965, Kinetin-like activity in root exudate of water-stressed sunflower plants, Physiol. Plant., 18:941-944.
Itai, C., Ben-Zioni, A., and Ordin, L., 1973, Correlative changes in endogenous hormone levels and shoot growth induced by short heat treatments to the root, Physiol. Plant., 29:355-360.
Jones, O. P., and Lacey, H. J., 1968, Gibberellin-like substances in the transpiration stream of apple and pear trees, J. Exp. Bot., 19:526-531.
Jong, A. W. de, and Bruinsma, J., 1974a, Pistil development in Cleome flowers. I. Effects of nutrients and of the presence of leaves and fruits on female abortion in Cleome spinoza Jacq., Z. Pflanzenphysiol., 72:220-226.
Jong, A. W. de, and Bruinsma, J., 1974b, Pistil development in Cleome flowers. III. Effects of growth-regulating substances on flower buds of Cleome iberidella Welw. ex Oliv grown in vitro, Z. Pflanzenphysiol., 73:142-151.
Jong, A. W. de, and Bruinsma, J., 1974c, Pistil development in Cleome flowers. IV. Effects of growth-regulating substances on female abortion in Cleome spinoza Jacq., Z. Pflanzenphysiol., 73:152-159.
Krechting, H. C. J. M., Varga, A., and Bruinsma, J., 1978, Absence of cytokinin biosynthesis in pea seeds developing in vitro, Z. Pflanzenphysiol., 87:91-93.

Lavender, D. P., Sweet, G. B., Zaerr, J. B., and Hermann, R. K., 1973, Spring shoot growth in Douglas fir may be initiated by gibberellins exported from the roots, Science, 182:838-839.
Luckwill, L. C., 1970, The control of growth and fruitfulness of apple trees, in: "Physiology of Tree Crops," L. C. Luckwill and C. V. Cutting, eds., Academic Press, London, New York.
MacDavid, C. R., Sagar, G. R., and Marshall, C., 1973, The effect of root pruning and 6-benzylaminopurine on the chlorophyll content, $^{14}CO_2$, fixation and the shoot/root ratio in seedlings of Pisum sativum L., New Phytol., 72:465-470.
Menary, R. C., and van Staden, J., 1976, Effect of phosphorus nutrition and cytokinins on flowering in the tomato, Lycopersicon esculentum Mill., Aust. J. Plant Physiol., 3: 201-205.
Mullins, M. G., 1967, Morphogenetic effects of roots and of some synthetic cytokinins in Vitis vinifera L., J. Exp. Bot., 18: 206-214.
Phillips, D. J., 1968, Nitrogen, phosphorus, and potassium distribution in relation to apical dominance in dwarf bean Phaseolus vulgaris c.v. Canadian Wonder, J. Exp. Biol., 19:617-627.
Railton, I. D., and Reid, D. M., 1973, Effects of benzyladenine on the growth of waterlogged tomato plants, Planta, 111:261-266.
Reid, D. M., and Carr, D. J., 1967, Effect of a dwarfing compound, CCC, on the production and export of gibberellin-like substances by root systems, Planta, 73:1-11.
Reid, D. M., and Crozier, A., 1971, Effects of waterlogging on the gibberellin content and growth of tomato plants, J. Exp. Bot., 22:39-48.
Rogler, C. E., and Hackett, W. P., 1975a, Phase change in Hedera helix: Induction of the mature to juvenile phase change by gibberellin A_3. Physiol. Plant., 34:141-147.
Rogler, C. E., and Hackett, W. P., 1975b, Phase change in Hedera helix: Stabilization of the mature form with abscisic acid and growth retardants, Physiol. Plant., 34:148-152.
Schwabe, W. W., and Al-Doori, A. H., 1973, Analysis of a juvenile-like condition affecting flowering in the black currant (Ribes nigrum), J. Exp. Bot., 24:969-981.
Sitton, D., Richmond, A., and Vaadia, Y., 1967, On the synthesis of gibberellins in roots, Phytochem., 6:1101-1105.
Skene, K. G. M., 1968, Increases in the levels of cytokinins in bleeding sap of Vitis vinifera L. after CCC treatment, Science, 159:1477-1478.
Torrey, J. G., 1976, Root hormones and plant growth, Ann. Rev. Plant Physiol., 27:435-459.
Tucker, D. J., 1976, Endogenous growth regulators in relation to side shoot development in the tomato, New Phytol., 77:561-568.
Uheda, E., and Kuraishi, S., 1977, Increase of cytokinin activity in detached etiolated cotyledons of squash after illumination, Plant & Cell Physiol., 18:481-483.

Varga, A., and Bruinsma, J., 1974, The growth and ripening of tomato fruits at different levels of endogenous cytokinins, J. Hort. Sci., 49:135-142.

Wagner, H., and Michael, G., 1969, Cytokininbildung in Wurzeln von Sonnenblumenbei unterschiedlicher Stickstoffernährung und Chlorophenicol-Zusatz, Naturwiss., 56:379.

Wareing, P. F., Horgan, R., Henson, I. E., and Davis, W., 1977, Cytokinin relations in the whole plant, in: "Plant Growth Regulation," P. E. Pilet, ed., Springer-Verlag, Berlin, New York.

Wellensiek, S. J., 1962, Dividing cells as the locus for vernalization, Nature, 195:307-308.

Wellensiek, S. J., 1968, Floral induction through the roots of Silene armeria, R. Acta Bot. Neerl., 17:5-8.

Went, F. W., 1938, Specific factors other than auxin affecting growth and root formation, Plant Physiol., 13:55-80.

Zeevaart, J. A. D., 1977, Sites of abscisic acid synthesis and metabolism in Ricinus communis, Plant Physiol., 59:788-791.

4

THE ROLE OF HORMONES IN PROMOTING AND DEVELOPING GROWTH TO SELECT NEW VARIETIES IN STERILE CULTURE

C. Nitsch and M. Godard

Génétique et Physiologie du Développement des Plantes
Centre National de la Recherche Scientifique
Gif-sur-Yvette, France

INTRODUCTION: THE AIM OF IN VITRO CULTURE FOR HAPLOID PRODUCTION

In most plant breeding programs, the possibility of having haploids would allow for more rapid progress. Several procedures for obtaining haploid and homozygous diploid (named "homodiploid") plants have been described in the literature (Nitzsche and Wenzel, 1977). The use of the in vitro culture technique has proved to be very advantageous in several respects:

(1) The number of haploid plants obtained may be essentially unlimited when the technique is properly adapted to the species. Thus it allows maximum combination possibilities of the genomes.

(2) In vitro culture is a means to rescue tissues that for various reasons would not grow in nature, therefore making available genotypic combinations which have never been or will never be obtained by normal sexual crosses. For example, when reduction at the meiotic cell level produces a nonviable pollen grain, such pollen grains may be rescued by in vitro culture and may eventually grow into plants showing characters normally unseen in nature. In this regard, it may be noted that "spontaneous mutations" have been observed in plants originating from pollen cultures in a larger number than normally. Therefore, new characters are made available which breeders may judiciously use in their breeding programs.

(3) Starting from pollen alone, that is to say the male gametophyte, gives the possibility of studying in a simple system the cytoplasmic effect on a cross. This method can be contrasted with the somatic hybridization technique (Vasil, see Chapter 5), where the new plant has an enriched cytoplasm resulting from the

fusion of cytoplasm from the two parents (Gleba, 1978). The pollen plant has the cytoplasmic inheritance reduced to a minimum, less than in a regular cross since the plant obtained originated from only one cell, namely the vegetative pollen cell, with a small cytoplasm rather than one resulting from the fusion of the sperm nucleus with the female zygotic cell. It also allows a new approach for studying the maternal effect. Starting from a plant with cytoplasmic inheritance reduced to a minimum allows the breeder to follow any single effect of cytoplasmic inheritance.

(4) Another main advantage of the in vitro culture technique is that it allows the scientist to follow the growth and development of the plant in conditions where it is possible, at any time, to observe, modify, or stop its development. For fundamental research in morphology and biochemistry, this is indeed a very important point, especially since it pertains to the entire period from uninucleate cell level (i.e., from the microspore) to the complete plant.

(5) The last but a still very important point is that this tissue culture method is probably the fastest way to obtain homodiploid plants, although not necessarily the cheapest. To date, in all successful cases less than six months have been needed to achieve the goal of obtaining haploid or homodiploid plants starting from a hybrid.

GROWTH SUBSTANCES AND THE PRODUCTION OF PLANTS ORIGINATED FROM POLLEN CELLS

It is now possible, for several families, to produce plants by culturing the pollen in vitro. This is done either while the pollen is still enclosed in the anther or as a free cell suspension.

The mechanism of "androgenesis," namely the development of a pollen cell into a plant without going through the fertilization process, is the result of two aberrations in the normal pollen ontogenesis:

First, it is necessary to either prevent the formation of the generative cell or to stop it from its normal sexual development.

Second, it is necessary to enhance vegetative cell division instead of its normal sexual way (Fig. 1).

From the work reported in the literature, several points seem to be of special importance in gearing the metabolism and the development of the pollen away from its normal maturation. The goal is twofold:

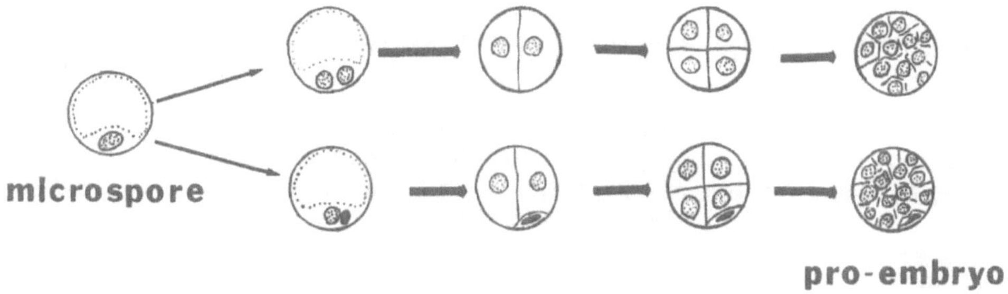

Fig. 1. Routes toward androgenesis.

First, to modify the pollen development, namely to force it toward androgenesis. The time when this occurs is called the induction period. The plant has to be conditioned to trigger off cell division in the vegetative pollen cell.

The second goal is to direct the vegetative growth toward embryogenesis by preventing the rupture of the exine too early. In many cases the second goal is not fully reached--high auxin concentration promotes cell division in a manner which does not allow the cell to be kept confined in the exine. The tissue becomes undifferentiated and grows as a callus. A third goal is therefore necessary: the regeneration of a plant from the callus with all that that implies.

Several important steps are necessary for successful results with in vitro culture for haploid production.

(1) The plant material from which the pollen is taken has to be kept in optimum growth conditions. Not only is good fertile soil required, but also the quality of light as well as its intensity must be taken into consideration. This has proved to be particularly important for cereal crops. The best results in cereals have been obtained from field grown plants. No artificial lighting seems to equal sunlight for the viability of the cereal pollen, and *Zea mays* and *Pennisetum* are the most sensitive to it. It should also be noted that any pesticide and especially systemic chemical treatment are extremely harmful for the further growth of the pollen.

(2) The state of pollen development when the flower is taken off the plant is another crucial point. Before starting any culture, one has to select flowers having pollen at the stage of the first mitosis. This means, depending on the variety, either just before mitosis as in the case of maize (Anonymous, 1975), when the microspore nucleus is migrating to the side of the grain, or at the end of mitosis, as for *Nicotiana sylvestris*, when the generative nucleus is

present but before the reproductive cell is fully differentiated. In all cases it should always be before starch has accumulated in the pollen grain.

Insuring a good selection of the pollen at the right stage requires first determining the relationship between flower bud development and pollen development. For this, careful cytological analysis is necessary. Feulgen staining technique is widely used and allows a clear observation of the two types of nuclei, the vegetative nucleus being light pink and the generative nucleus being smaller, denser, and darker in color.

(3) Preconditioning of the donor plant increases the induction frequency. Preconditioning can be done either by giving a physical stress to the pollen at the time of mitosis or by giving a chemical treatment to the very young flower in vivo.

(a) A temperature shock, given to the flower itself or to the anthers as soon as they are placed in culture, increased the number of plants produced.

Low temperature shock, between 3-12°C depending on the species, multiplies three- to fourfold the number of plants. The cold shock given to the pollen:

- Increases the viability of the pollen and the synchrony of the cells.

- Modified the mitosis axis which, instead of resulting in asymmetrical division, gives rise to an equal division of the microspore cell into two "androgenetic cells."

- Favors the start of a new developmental pathway, namely toward vegetative growth, by slowing down the existing metabolism for the pathway leading to sexual maturation.

- Induces supplementary divisions of the vegetative cell, even after an asymmetrical first division.

A high temperature shock, between 32-38°C, seems to be effective in the Brassica (Keller and Armstrong, 1978).

(b) A hormonal treatment given to the flower in vivo rather than in vitro allows the plant to prevent harmful effects of the high auxin concentration which in some species, especially cereals, appears necessary to trigger off cell division.

- If put in the culture medium, 2,4-dichlorophenoxyacetic acid (2,4-D) at a concentration ranging from 2 to 10 mg/l will induce cell division of the microspore but also produce dedifferentiation of the cells. The pollen therefore develops as a callus which will have to be transferred to a bud differentiating medium.

- By feeding the flower still attached to the plant with the solution of growth substances (Fig. 2), we have been able to induce divisions of the vegetative cell without destroying its embryogenic ability; in other words, the daughter cells are still enclosed in the exine (Fig. 3).

(4) Induction of pollen originated plants can be achieved several ways depending on the species.

(a) The simplest way is that for Datura innoxia or Nicotiana tabacum, sylvestris, or otophora when no growth substances are required. The important factor here is the stage of the pollen at the time it is placed in culture. At that time the cold shock is enough to achieve the induction toward embryogenesis (Fig. 4).

(b) Other species require an induction by auxin in addition to the physical stress given to the pollen.

As in the case of Nicotiana alata, numerous plants are obtained by adding to the culture medium 2, 3, 5, 6-tetrachlorobenzoic acid (2, 3, 5, 6-T) at a concentration of 0.1 mg/l. The pollen develops into an embryo (Fig. 5) and then into a plant which can be grown in a pot after ten weeks from the start of the culture.

(c) Other species which have been successful require a stronger auxin such as naphthalene acetic acid (NAA) or 2,4-D for inducing division of the microspore. It is the case for all cereals. In such instances, the auxin induces a dedifferentiating process and the growth of a callus originating from the pollen. It is therefore necessary to induce bud formation from the callus. A medium containing indoleacetic acid (IAA) and a cytokinin is necessary. Most cereals respond positively and produce plants (Kuo et al., 1977; Picard and De Buyser, 1973).

However, in other species and especially for fruit trees, it has not yet been possible to induce bud differentiation from haploid callus of pollen origin (Fig. 6). In order to overcome this difficulty we have applied the 2,4-D in vivo in the manner described in item 3. The tissue is therefore still connected to the regulatory system of the whole plant, thus preventing the disorganization that occurs at the cellular level when the cells are devoid of correlation.

Another disadvantage of callus is that plants regenerated from anther derived callus may be originating from more than one pollen cell and thus be chimeric. Others may be derived from somatic tissue

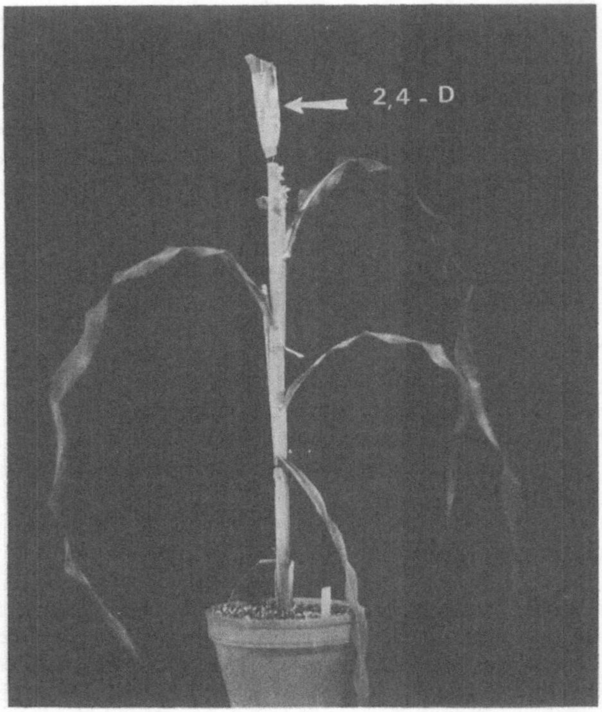

Fig. 2. In vivo preconditioning of the donor plant. The corn male inflorescence still enclosed in the leaf blade is placed inside plastic tubing which is tightly fastened at the base to the stem. Aqueous solution of 2,4-D + BAP + GA at 2 mg/l of each in 2% dimethylsulfoxide is poured into the plastic tubing at the end of the day (6:00 pm), after which the plant is kept in its normal growing condition for three more days. At the end of the three days, the anthers are taken out and placed in sterile culture.

either entirely or in part, nuclear fusion thus giving rise to heterozygous chromosomes (D'Amato, 1977).

(5) The effect of growth substances on embryo development. It is the task of the scientist to adapt the cell-division promoting effect of the growth substances to prevent dedifferentiation of the cell.

Production of plants from pollen origin is a rather complex event if one wants to preserve the genetic character of the starting cell, namely the microspore. From what has been discussed previously, we realize that the most promising way to obtain haploid or

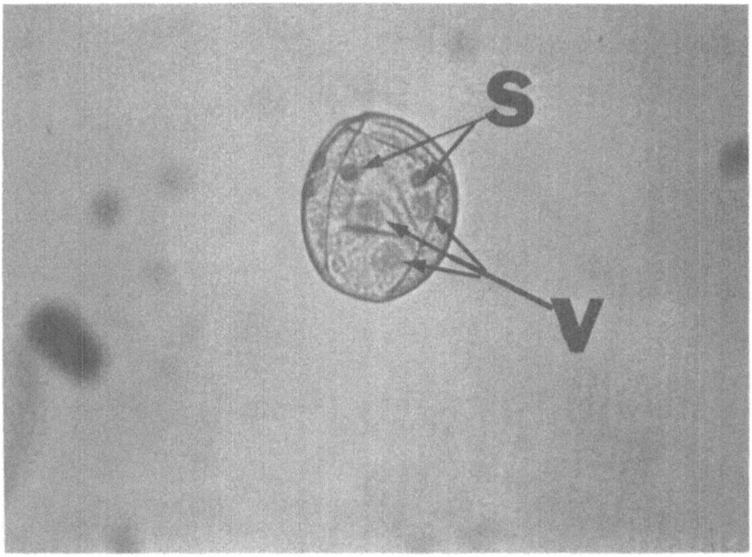

Fig. 3. Pollen of the plant treated as in Fig. 2 after 5 days in vitro culture on medium without 2,4-D but with IAA 0.3 mg/l added (Feulgen staining). S = 2 small dense sperm nuclei and V = 3 pale vegetative nuclei.

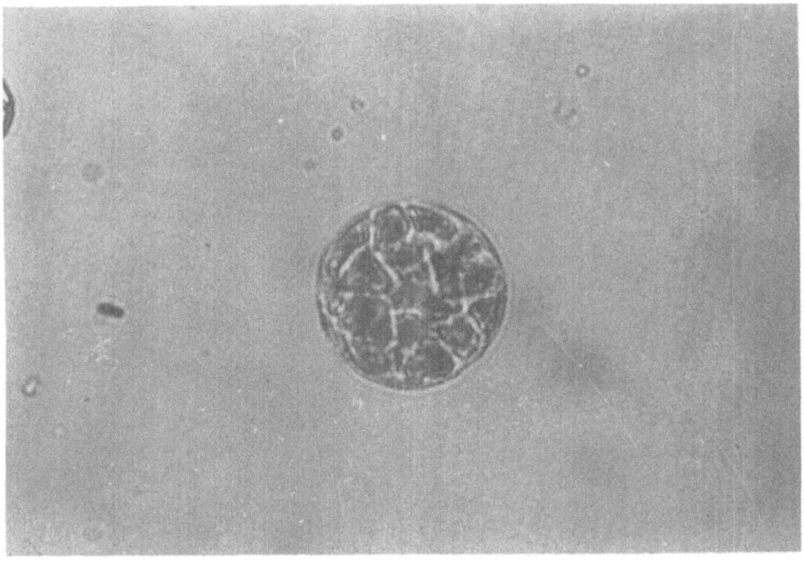

Fig. 4. Pro-embryo of N. sylvestris still enclosed in the exine induced by a cold shock (7°C) alone. No growth substances were added in the medium (Feulgen staining).

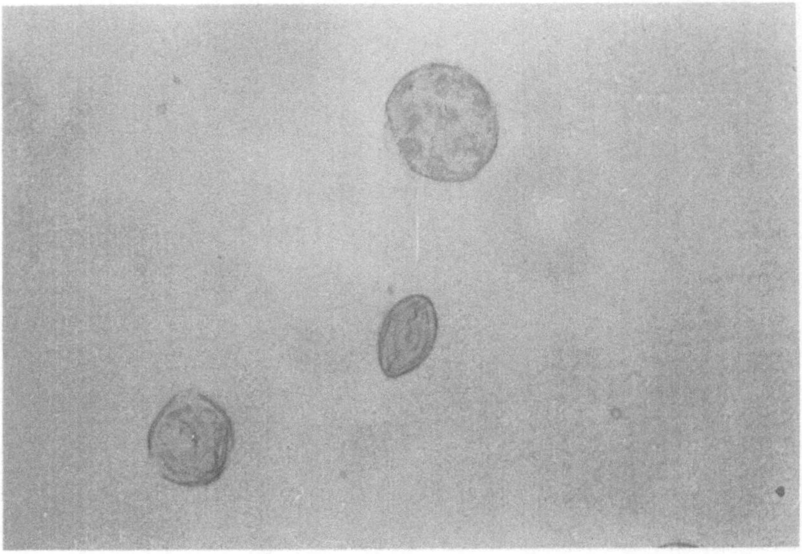

Fig. 5. Pro-embryo of N. alata still enclosed in the exine induced by a cold shock (7°C) plus the presence of 2, 3, 5, 6-T at 0.1 mg/l in the medium (Feulgen staining).

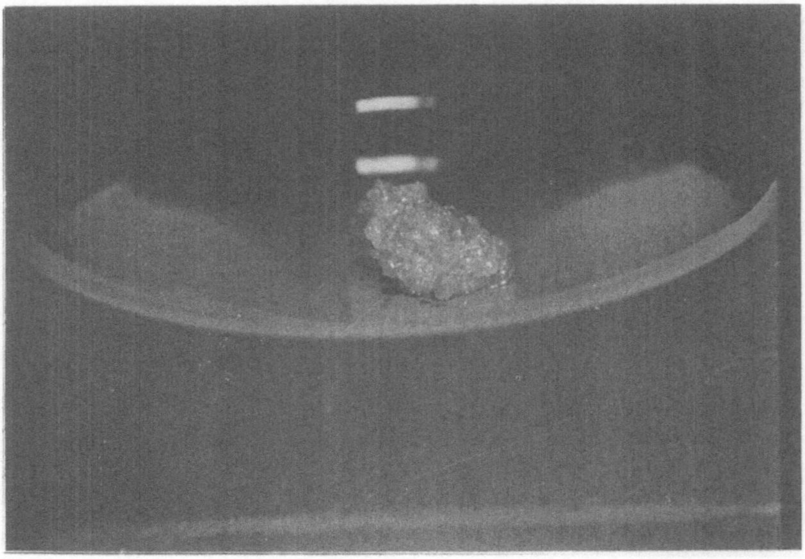

Fig. 6. Haploid callus originating from anther culture of "Golden Delicious" apple after one month in culture on 2,4-D 0.3 mg/l.

homodiploid plants is to prevent dedifferentiation of the cells from occurring at any time.

To achieve such a goal, it is necessary to think in terms of a change in nutritional requirements during development from the one microspore cell to the multicellular polarized embryo.

The induction period is the time of cell division when the cells are enclosed in the exine, and during this time some growth substances may be required in the culture medium. Once the pro-embryo is formed and becomes polarized the exine breaks open (Fig. 7). Thereafter the requirement for the growth of the young embryo is different; amino acids become more important in the medium than any growth substances although the latter may still be necessary in low amounts.

Since the metabolism of the plant is very different from one species to another, it is advisable to study the requirement for embryo development in each case in order to adapt the medium used to the species in culture. Following this idea, we have analyzed the variation of amino acids during the growth of the embryos of Datura and Nicotiana. Only glutamine and serine have attracted our attention since they increased and then decreased during the growth phase. Thus it is possible there is both production as well as utilization

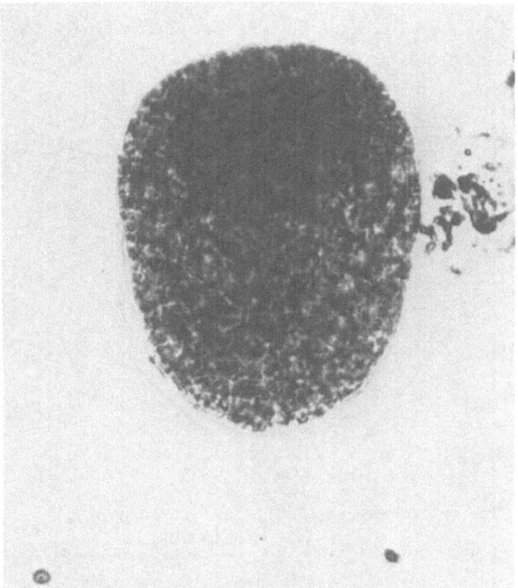

Fig. 7. Embryo of N. sylvestris after one week in culture emerging from the exine.

of these two amino acids (Fig. 8). In cereals (in this case corn and millet), the analysis showed the same profile for glutamine again as well as proline (unlike Datura and Nicotiana).

Contrary to what has been found for the Solanaceae, where the growth of the young embryo is inhibited by growth substances, in millet the presence of auxin and, most important, gibberellin is beneficial.

Very young zygotic embryos of millet taken out four days after fertilization can only be grown to plants if IAA at 0.1 mg/l and gibberellic acid (GA) at 1 mg/l are added to the culture medium enriched by glutamine (3×10^{-3} M) and proline (3×10^{-4} M). The addition of a cytokinin may be beneficial when used at very low concentration (0.01 mg/l); at higher concentration it will inhibit root growth thus preventing the evolution of the embryo to plant.

Indeed this new development is not directly related to haploid production. However, we think that it is noteworthy since it is a valuable tool for plant breeders. This technique shortens the cycle of one generation by three to four weeks. Moreover, the in vitro culture conditions may allow the rescue of embryos which would not otherwise develop. In any case results of a study on embryo development can be a valuable guideline for future work in this area.

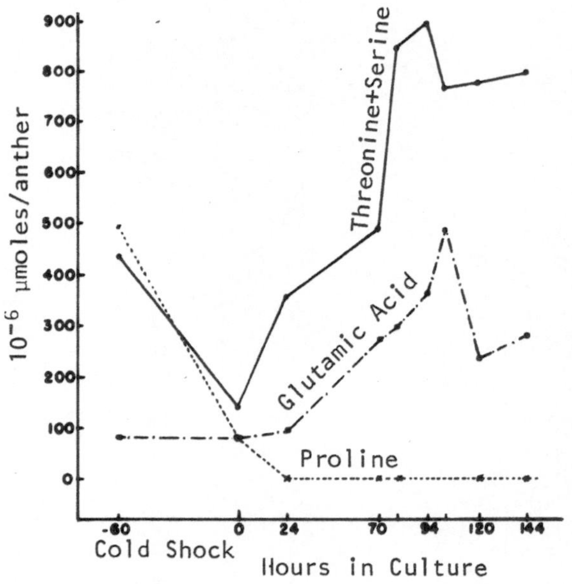

Fig. 8. Evolution of amino acid concentration during embryo development.

THE USE OF POLLEN-ORIGINATED PLANTS FOR AGRICULTURE

Out of numerous haploid plants obtained in vitro culture, the potential offered to the breeder is large but the work of making the right selection is still to be done.

The haploid production technique described above has the main advantage of bringing out on the palette of plant breeders a wider range of variability in pure lines and in a much shorter time than when using the conventional method for obtaining pure lines. It is then the breeder's task to judiciously pick out the right combinations to obtain the most desirable plant (Dore, 1974; Thevenin and Dore, 1976).

The first step, however, is to find the right way to double the chromosome number of the haploid plant without losing homozygosity.

Depending on the species, different procedures may be used:

(1) The colchicine treatment, which has been known for a number of years, is one of them. Its success varies with the plant varieties and the quality of the chemical used.

(2) In many instances, spontaneous diploidization occurs during the induction process. The two nuclei formed at the first mitosis of the microspore fuse to form one nucleus with 2n chromosomes which indeed are homozygous.

In our work with Datura and Nicotiana we could observe the occurrence of such an event (Figs. 9 and 10) and in a day-by-day observation of the development of the embryo starting at the microspore we have seen that the nuclear fusion event is enhanced by the cold shock given to the flower at the time of the first pollen mitosis.

The results obtained on cereals (Picard and De Buyser, 1975; Anonymous, 1974, 1976) indicate chromosome doubling occurs spontaneously in large numbers.

(3) Growth as a callus, originating either from the pollen directly or from the stem of a haploid plant, also results in chromosome doubling (Nitsch et al., 1969) in regenerated plants. This phenomenon, called "endomitosis," occurs very frequently during in vitro culture when the tissue is kept in an undifferentiated state, namely in a callus kind of growth. The occurrence varies depending on the species but also on the culture medium used as well as the time in culture.

(a) Many examples from the literature indicate the degree of response to endomitosis in relation to the species.

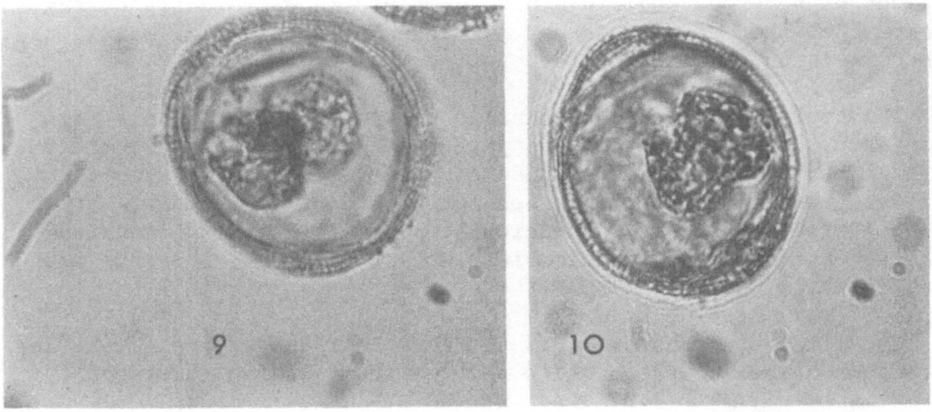

Figs. 9-10. Nuclear fusion observed in D. innoxia following induction toward androgenesis by cold shock (3°C) (Feulgen staining).

(b) The auxin and the cytokinin used for callus formation and bud regeneration influence the degree of polyploidization (Nitsch, 1973). From the different auxins commonly used in the culture medium to induce callus proliferation, IAA at a concentration ranging from 10^{-6} M to 10^{-5} M promotes 100% polyploidization on N. sylvestris. For the cytokinin necessary in the bud regenerating medium, B.A.P. is the most effective, followed by kinetin. Zeatin appears less effective.

(c) The time during which the tissue is kept in the callus state has important consequences.

The degree of polyploidization increases with increasing time in culture as callus. However in our study on the progeny of the diploid plants obtained via endomitosis, we have observed that as the time in culture in a callus form increases, the degree of homozygosity in the progeny decreases. As an example, with N. sylvestris we have examined one hundred diploid plants regenerated after endomitosis by having placed in culture a piece of stem of the haploid plant. When the callus is kept growing for 20 days only, 85 of the one hundred diploid plants are homozygous. If the callus is kept 40 days, only 62 of the one hundred diploid plants regenerated are homozygous.

It is therefore important to note that during the in vitro culture for chromosome doubling of the haploid plants, chromosomal aberrations may be introduced in the genome. This may be a cause of heterozygosity in the offspring of pollen-originated plants.

CONCLUSION

So far, the successes achieved with in vitro culture for haploid production have not been very numerous. They are, however, increasing in number as time goes by. The positive and very important results recently obtained in China and Japan on cereal crops should encourage research workers to become active in the area of those crops (Hu Han et al., 1978; Niizeki, 1977). The legume family does not appear to have been as successful, although this may be due to the fact that not as many scientists have been working on the production of haploid plants in leguminosae.

Several varieties of tobacco, wheat, and rice obtained by the pollen culture method of selection are already cultivated in a wide area in China. Field tests have shown an increase in yield of the new varieties compared to the parents ranging from 10-30% as well as increases in quality and resistance to disease of up to 15%.

Noteworthy is the observation that in several cases, the pollen-derived plants obtained by anther culture are superior to both parents and also to their hybrid. These first results are encouraging for the development of in vitro culture technique, despite the few necessary precautions, as a tool which will speed up new advances in agriculture.

REFERENCES

D'Amato, F., 1977, Cytogenetics of differentiation in tissue and cell cultures, in: "Applied and Fundamental Aspects of Plant Cell, Tissue and Organ Culture," J. Reinert and Y. P. S. Bajaj, eds., Springer-Verlag, Berlin, Heidelberg, New York.

Anonymous, 302 Research Group, Rice Research Laboratory, 1976, New rice varieties "Hua Yu I" and "Hua Yu II" developed from anther culture, Acta Genetica Sinica, 3:19-25.

Anonymous, 401 Research Group, 1975, Primary study on induction of pollen plants of Zea maize, Acta Genetica Sinica, 2:138-143.

Anonymous, 2nd Division, 3rd Laboratory Institute of Genetics--Academia Sinica, 1974, Investigation on the induction and genetic expression of rice plants, Scientia Sinica, 17:209-226.

Dore, C., 1974, Production de plantes homozygotes mâles et femelles à partir d'anthères d'asperge, cultivées in vitro, C. R. Acad. Sci., 278D:2135-2138.

Gleba, Y. Y., 1978, Non-chromosomal inheritance in higher plants as studied by somatic cell hybridization, in: "Fourth Annual College of Biological Sciences Colloquium, Ohio State Univ. Press, Columbus (in press).

Hu Han, Hsi Tze-ying, Tseng Chun-Chih, Ouyang Tsun-wen, and Ching Chien-Kang, 1978, Anther cultures, principles and application to crop plants in China, in: "Proceedings of the IVth

International Plant Cell and Tissue Culture Congress," Calgary, Canada (in press).

Keller, W. A., and Armstrong, K. C., 1978, High frequency production of microspore derived plants from *Brassica napus* anther cultures, *Z. Pflanzenzütchtg.*, 80:100-108.

Kuo Ming-Kwang, Cheng Wan-Chen, Hwaing Ta-nian, Hwang Jiao-Shang, and Kuan Yue-Lan, 1977, The culture of pollen grains of wheat, rice and tobacco *in vitro*, *Acta Genetica Sinica*, 4:333-340.

Niizeki, M., 1977, Haploid, polyploid and anueploid plants from cultured anthers and calluses in species of *Nicotiana* and forage crops, *Jour. Fac. Agr. Hokkaido Univ.*, 58:343-466.

Nitsch, C., 1973, Transformations génétiques obtenues au moyen de cultures in vitro, *in*: "Comptes Rendus du 96ème Congrès Societé Savantes Toulouse 1971," Vol. IV.

Nitsch, J.P., Nitsch, C., and Hamon, S., 1969, Production de *Nicotiana* diploïdes à partir de cals haploïdes cultivés *in vitro*, *C. R. Acad. Sci.*, 269D:1275-1278.

Nitzsche, W., and Wenzel, G., 1977, Advances in plant breeding, *in*: "Fortschritte der Pflanzenzüchtung," 8th ed., Paul Parey, Berlin and Hamburg.

Picard, E., and De Buyser, J., 1973, Obtention de plantes haploïdes de *Triticum aestivum* L. à partir de culture d'anthères *in vitro*, *C. R. Acad. Sci.*, 277D:1463-1466.

Picard, E., and De Buyser, J., 1975, Nouveaux résultats concernant la culture d'anthères *in vitro* de blé tendre, *C. R. Acad. Sci.*, 281D:127-130.

Thevenin, L., and Dore, C., 1976, L'amélioration de l'asperge et son atout majeur, la culture *in vitro*, *Ann. Amélior. Plantes*, 26:655-674.

5

SOMATIC HYBRIDIZATION AND GENETIC MANIPULATION IN PLANTS

Indra K. Vasil, Vimla Vasil, Derek W. R. White, and
Howard R. Berg

University of Florida
Gainesville, Florida

INTRODUCTION

Following the discovery of cytokinins and their role in plant development (Skoog and Miller, 1957), and the demonstration of the totipotency of plant cells (Vasil and Hildebrandt, 1965; Vasil and Vasil, 1972), plant regeneration has been achieved in vitro from a wide variety of plant species (Murashige, 1974; Vasil et al., 1978). Although plant regeneration from the most important groups of crop plants, namely the cereals and the legumes, still remains a serious problem, the ability to rapidly clone plants through tissue culture techniques fulfills an important prerequisite for the utilization of the novel methods of somatic hybridization and genetic manipulation of plants. These cloning procedures ensure that any changes effected through somatic hybridization or other parasexual methods in the information content of plant cells can be perpetuated without necessarily going through the sexual cycle where they might very well be eliminated.

There has recently been an extensive discussion of the potential of genetic manipulation of plants through tissue culture techniques (Ledoux, 1975; Markham et al., 1975; Dudits et al., 1976b; Vasil, 1976; Barz et al., 1977; Beers and Bassett, 1977; Kleinhofs and Behki, 1977; and Rubenstein et al., 1977). Most of this interest has centered on the following:

(1) Production of haploid and/or homozygous plants or tissues and their use in mutagenesis, mutant selection, and hybridization. Plants obtained from such cultures have resulted in the introduction of improved cultivars of rice and tobacco in Japan and the Peoples Republic of China. This technique appears to have the best prospect

for utilization in crop improvement in the near future (Vasil and Nitsch; 1975; Nitzsche and Wenzel, 1977; Nitsch, see Chapter 4).

(2) Isolation and culture of plant protoplasts, and production of somatic hybrids following induced fusion of protoplasts.

(3) Transplantation of organelles, and the fusion of enucleated protoplasts with nucleated protoplasts for the production of cytoplasmic hybrids (cybrids).

(4) Genetic engineering for nitrogen fixation (Hollaender et al., 1977), and forced association of nitrogen fixing bacteria with non-legume tissue cultures (Vasil et al., 1977).

(5) Genetic transformation of plants through DNA uptake, etc. (Ledoux, 1975; Kleinhofs and Behki, 1977; Vasil et al., 1978).

The following discussion is limited to only those aspects of the above in which some experimental work is currently being carried out in the senior author's laboratory.

PLANT PROTOPLASTS IN SOMATIC HYBRIDIZATION AND GENETIC MANIPULATION

Much of the interest in modern protoplast research can be attributed to two recent reports: Power et al. (1970) described a method for the induced fusion of protoplasts, and Carlson et al. (1972) reported the formation of the first somatic plant hybrids by fusing protoplasts of two species of Nicotiana. The enzymatic removal of the cell wall from the plant cell not only provides an opportunity to fuse protoplasts of unrelated species, but also permits a variety of novel experimental procedures--such as the introduction of cell organelles, microorganisms, foreign genetic materials, etc.--that can be used to obtain new gene recombinations or to produce genetically modified cells and/or plants that cannot otherwise be obtained by normal sexual means.

ISOLATION AND CULTURE OF PROTOPLASTS

Mechanical isolation of protoplasts, in very limited numbers, was successfully demonstrated toward the end of the last century (Klercker, 1892), but enzymatic removal of the plant cell wall to yield comparatively large numbers of viable protoplasts was first reported by Cocking in 1960. Since then, largely owing to the potential of the system and easy availability of potent commercial preparations of cell wall degrading enzymes, techniques have been developed for the isolation of large and homogeneous populations of protoplasts from a variety of plant cells, tissues, and organs (Cocking, 1972; Gamborg and Wetter, 1975; Vasil, 1976). In most cases protoplasts are prepared by exposing plant cells or tissues to fairly crude preparations of cellulases and pectinases, which can be used either simultaneously or sequentially. The most suitable sources of protoplasts have proven to be leaf tissues (mesophyll cells) and plant cells grown in suspension. With the loss of the cell wall, the protoplast loses protection against osmotic swelling, and thus it is critical that proper osmoticum be maintained during the isolation procedure and the early stages of culture. This is accomplished by preparing the enzyme solutions in mannitol and/or various sugars as somatic agents.

Protoplasts must be removed rapidly from enzyme solutions after the cell walls have been completely digested. This is achieved by filtration and/or centrifugation, and repeated washing by fresh nutrient media. The cleanest protoplast preparations, almost completely devoid of any cellular debris, are obtained when the protoplasts are floated during centrifugation in sucrose solutions. The washed protoplasts are suspended in various nutrient media (Gamborg and Wetter, 1975; Gamborg et al., 1976; Vasil, 1976, 1977), and cultured either in suspension (Eriksson and Jonasson, 1969; Vasil and Vasil, 1974), liquid droplets (Kao et al., 1971; Gleba, 1978), or mixed with a soft agar nutrient medium and plated (Nagata and Takebe, 1971). A very complex nutrient medium has been developed by Kao and Michayluk (1975) which even supports the growth of single isolated protoplasts.

Synthesis and deposition of cellulosic microfibrils appears to start within minutes after the removal of the protoplasts from enzyme solutions (Williamson et al., 1977), and the protoplasts lose their perfectly spherical shape as the new wall is deposited. Within 2-7 days following culture, the first mitotic division takes place resulting in the formation of two cells, and within 1-3 weeks multicellular colonies are formed. These can be subcultured as callus tissues or placed in liquid media to obtain suspension cultures.

Although regeneration of cell walls and sustained cell divisions have been obtained in protoplasts of a wide variety of plants (Gamborg, 1977; Vasil et al., 1978), the culture of cereal protoplasts has proven to be extremely difficult (Vasil and Vasil, 1974; Potrykus et al., 1976; Kinnersley et al., 1978). Some success has been achieved in the culture of rice (Deka and Sen, 1976), corn (Potrykus et al., 1977), and pearl millet protoplasts (Vasil and Vasil, 1978). We have recently isolated protoplasts from suspension cultures of pearl millet (*Pennisetum americanum*), and plated them in a soft-agar overlay on nutrient agar. A large number of protoplasts (15-20% plating efficiency) not only regenerate cell walls, but continue to divide to form cell colonies (Figs. 1-5). These colonies, when isolated and cultured on fresh nutrient media, give rise to continuing callus tissue cultures (Fig. 6). The success in pearl millet was

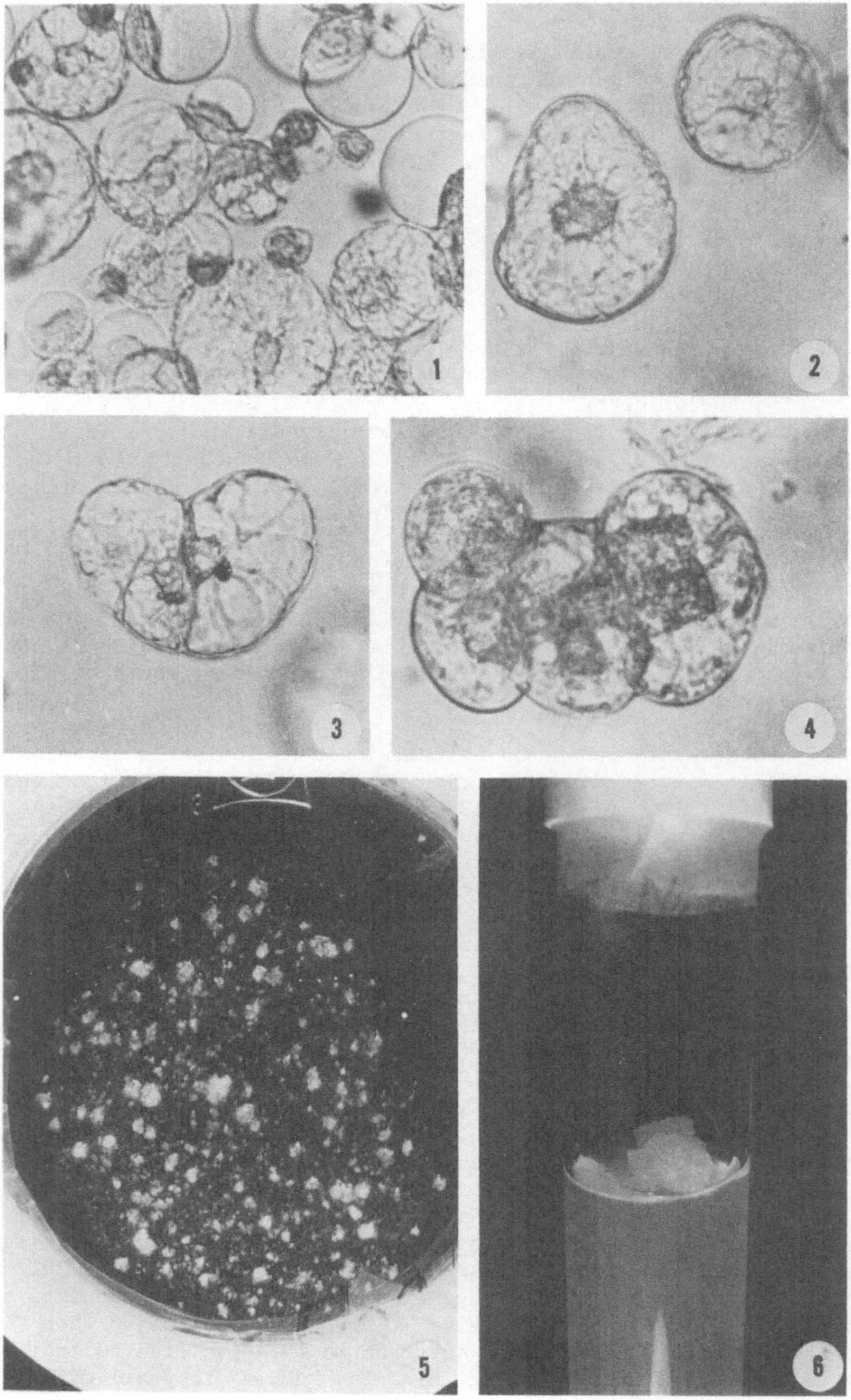
1
2
3
4
5
6

made possible by the use of a rapidly proliferating cell suspension culture, extended incubation of cells in enzyme solutions at low temperatures, isolation of clean protoplast preparations by floatation on sucrose, and by the use of a modified nutrient medium.

Like other somatic--and some reproductive--plant cells (Vasil and Vasil, 1972; Vasil and Nitsch, 1975), protoplasts are also totipotent, and under suitable nutritional and hormonal conditions will give rise to normal plants. A perusal of the species listed in Table 1 clearly shows that it includes largely model plant systems like Datura, Daucus, Nicotiana, and Petunia, and that plant regeneration from cereals and legumes has not been achieved so far. The only important food crop listed is potato. If somatic hybridization and genetic manipulation is to play any important role in crop improvement in the future, it is necessary that vigorous attempts be made to achieve plant regeneration from protoplasts of important crop plants--primarily cereals and legumes--which represent a major portion of man's food resources. In several species of legumes cell colonies have been obtained from protoplasts, but all attempts to induce shoot or plant morphogenesis in such cultures have failed.

Somatic Hybridization

Sodium-nitrate induced fusion of enzymatically isolated protoplasts was first reported by Power et al. (1970). Later it was shown that sodium nitrate at best produces fusion at low frequencies, and is generally useful for protoplasts derived from meristematic tissues only, such as root tips. A search for more effective fusogenic treatments led to the discovery by Keller and Melchers (1973) that incubation of mixed protoplasts at high temperatures (37°) in media containing high concentrations of Ca^{++} in a highly akaline environment (pH 10.5) led to fusion frequencies of 25% or more. At about the same time it was demonstrated that polyethylene glycol (PEG) causes tight agglutination of protoplasts, followed by the fusion of their membranes (Constabel and Kao, 1974; Kao and Michayluk, 1974; Wallin et al., 1974). The most effective fusion of protoplasts is obtained by treatment with PEG followed by elution with a medium containing high amounts of Ca^{++} at pH 10.5 (Kao, 1977). PEG-induced fusion is completely nonspecific, and very high fusion frequencies can be obtained. It can be readily applied to both inter- and intraspecific fusions. PEG induces fusion of plant protoplasts with animal cells (Dudits et al., 1976c; Jones et al., 1976;

Figs. 1-6. Culture of pearl millet protoplasts. Fig. 1. Protoplasts after 24 hr in liquid nutrient medium. Figs. 2-5. Cell wall formation, cell division, and colony formation in protoplasts plated on agar nutrient medium. Fig. 6. Protoplast-derived callus tissue.

Table 1. List of Species in Which Plants Have Been Regenerated from Cultured Protoplasts

Species	Reference
Asparagus officinalis	Bui Dang Ha and Mackenzie, 1973
Atropa belladonna	Gosch et al., 1975
Brassica napus	Kartha et al., 1974
Brassica napus (haploid)	Thomas et al., 1976
Bromus inermis	Kao et al., 1973
Datura metel (haploid and diploid)	Schieder, 1977
Datura meteloides (haploid and diploid)	Schieder, 1977
Datura innoxia (haploid and diploid)	Schieder, 1975
Daucus carota	Grambow et al., 1972; Dudits et al., 1976a
Nicotiana alata (haploid)	Bourgin and Missonier, 1973
Nicotiana debneyi	H. H. Smith (personal communication)
Nicotiana langsdorffii	H. H. Smith (personal communication)
Nicotiana otophora	Banks and Evans, 1976
Nicotiana sylvestris	Bourgin et al., 1976; Nagy and Maliga, 1976; Banks and Evans, 1976
Nicotiana sylvestris x N. otophora (F_1 hybrid)	Banks and Evans, 1976
Nicotiana tabacum	Takebe et al., 1971; Nagata and Takebe, 1971
Nicotiana tabacum (haploid)	Ohyama and Nitsch, 1972

Table 1 cont'd.

Species	Reference
Nicotiana tabacum x _N. otophora_ (F_1 hybrid)	Banks and Evans, 1976
Petunia axillaris	Power et al., 1976a
Petunia hybrida	Durand et al., 1973; Frearson et al., 1973; Vasil and Vasil, 1974
Petunia hybrida (haploid)	Binding and Nehls, 1974
Petunia hybrida x _P. parodii_ (hybrid)	Power et al., 1976b
Petunia inflata	Power et al., 1976a
Petunia parodii	Hayward and Power, 1975
Petunia parviflora	Sink and Power, 1977
Petunia violacea	Power et al., 1976a
Ranunculus sceleratus	Dorion et al., 1975
Solanum dulcamara	Binding and Nehls, 1977
Solanum tuberosum	Shepard and Totten, 1977

Willis et al., 1977), and has also been found to be useful for the fusion of animal cells without the aid of Sendai virus (Pontecorvo, 1975; Davidson and Gerald, 1977; Wacker and Kaul, 1977).

A variety of fusion products may be formed when protoplasts of two different species, identified as A and B, are given a fusion treatment: AA, AAA, BB, BBB, AAB, ABB, AB . . . , and unfused A and B protoplasts. Under normal conditions of fusion, heterokaryotic fusions are apparently quite common, as indicated by reports of 35-50% heterokaryotic fusions (Kao and Michayluk, 1974; Vasil et al., 1975). Nuclear fusion does not necessarily follow protoplast fusion, and true hybrid cell formation is, therefore, not too common.

Even the formation of true hybrid cells following protoplast fusion does not assure the recovery of hybrid tissues and plants, as the unfused protoplasts of both the parental species, as well as the products of homokaryotic fusions, grow vigorously to dilute or eliminate the few true hybrid cells which may be present in the population. Recovery of hybrid cells growing on normal media under nonselective conditions is highly unlikely. Therefore, selective nutrient media that would not only favor but will preferentially allow the growth of only the hybrid cells must be used to isolate hybrid cell colonies. Such media have been successfully and elegantly employed in isolating and growing animal somatic cell hybrids (Davidson and de la Cruz, 1974; Ringertz and Savage, 1976). Unfortunately, very little information is available to develop effective selective media for plant cells. The few cases where some selective methods are available have indeed been used successfully to produce somatic hybrid plants (Table 2).

The first reported somatic hybrid plants were produced by fusing mesophyll protoplasts of *Nicotiana glauca* with those of *N. langsdorffii* (Carlson et al., 1972). Fusion was achieved by treatment with sodium nitrate. Protoplasts of both species were reported to regenerate a cell wall and occasionally go through one division cycle, but were never observed to form a callus. Protoplasts isolated from a sexually produced amphiploid hybrid also behaved similarly, but about 0.01% of these protoplasts eventually gave rise to a mass of cells. This difference in the growth characteristics of the protoplasts from the two parental species and protoplasts of the hybrid plant, which allowed the growth of only the hybrid cells, was used as the first selection screen. The regenerated calli were later transferred to a medium containing no hormones. This provided an additional and powerful selection for the elimination of parental tissues, which are known not to be able to grow in vitro in the absence of exogenously supplied hormones, while the hybrid tissues continued to grow, as they do not require any added hormones for growth. Hybrid plants regenerated from such selected calli were identical to sexual amphiploids, and had a 2n chromosome number of 42 (24 from *N. glauca* and 18 from *N. langsdorffii*).

Smith et al. (1976) also produced somatic hybrids of *N. glauca* (G) and *N. langsdorffii* (L), but they used the PEG fusion procedure and a complex nutrient medium. They also employed the two-step selection screen used by Carlson et al. (1972), and reported that although both the parental and the hybrid protoplasts grew in their nutrient medium, the hybrid colonies developed more rapidly. More significantly, none of the somatic hybrid plants isolated by Smith et al. (1976) showed 42 chromosomes. The 2n chromosome number in these plants varied from 56 to 64, which probably resulted from triple fusions (LL+G = 60 or L+GG = 66) and some degree of aneuploidy introduced during callus formation and plant regeneration.

Table 2. Somatic Hybrids Have Been Produced in the Following Plants Through Protoplast Fusion

1. Datura innoxia + D. innoxia (Schieder, 1977).

2. Daucus carota + D. capillifolius (Dudits et al., 1977).

3. Nicotiana glauca + N. langsdorffii (Carlson et al., 1972; Smith et al., 1976).

4. Nicotiana sylvestris + N. knightiana (Maliga et al., 1977).

5. Nicotiana tabacum + N. sylvestris (Melchers, 1977)

6. Nicotiana tabacum + N. tabacum (Melchers and Labib, 1974; Gleba et al., 1975; Glimelius et al., 1978).

7. Petunia hybrida + P. parodii (Power et al., 1976b).

8. Datura innoxia + D. discolor (Schieder, 1978).

9. Datura innoxia + D. stramonium (Schieder, 1978).

Sexual hybrids are known in all of the above combinations, except in 4, 8, and 9 which are presumably sexually incompatible.

The experiments of Carlson et al. (1972) and Smith et al. (1976) adequately demonstrated the feasibility of somatic hybridization by protoplast fusion. It must be pointed out here that no hybrids could have been isolated from these experiments without the prior knowledge of the auxin autotrophic nature of the sexually produced hybrids. It is unlikely, therefore, that such a system can be widely or usefully employed for somatic hybridization.

Melchers and Labib (1974) fused protoplasts isolated from two anther-derived chlorophyll-deficient and light-sensitive mutants of Nicotiana tabacum. Taking advantage of the genetic complementation of the two recessive genes in the fusion products, somatic hybrid plants were regenerated showing normal green leaves and resistance to high light intensities. Gleba et al. (1975) obtained normal green plants of tobacco following fusion of protoplasts derived from a nuclear and a plastome mutant of tobacco. Chlorophyll-deficient mutants have also been used recently to obtain somatic hybrids of Nicotiana tabacum + N. sylvestris (Melchers, 1977) and Datura innoxia + D. innoxia (Schieder, 1977). Unless unexpected difficulties are faced in complementation of genes controlling chlorophyll deficiency in hybrid cells of unrelated species, this system could be widely applied for the selection of somatic hybrids.

A complementation-selection system based on the differential growth characteristics and sensitivity to actinomycin D was used by Power et al. (1976b) to obtain somatic hybrids of Petunia hybrida + P. parodii.

Glimelius et al. (1978) have used nitrate reductase-deficient (NR-deficient) mutants of Nicotiana tabacum to select somatic hybrids following protoplast fusion. The NR-deficient mutants are complete auxotrophs, and do not grow on a minimal medium containing nitrate as sole nitrogen source (Muller and Grafe, 1978). The NR deficiency is a recessive genetic character, found to be complementing in the somatic hybrids, which show NR activity and are able to utilize nitrate (Glimelius et al., 1978). The NR-deficient cell lines used in these experiments are probably the first completely auxotrophic cell lines reported in higher plants, and clearly provide a very powerful and efficient system for the preferential selection of hybrid cells from mixed populations which result after protoplast fusion.

As stated earlier, an ideal selection system should be able to effectively eliminate the parental cell types and yet support the growth of hybrid cells. We have attempted intraspecific somatic hybridization of Nicotiana sylvestris by isolating and using two variant cell lines which are resistant to amino acid analogues, 5-methyl-tryptophan (5MT) and S-2-aminoethyl-L-cysteine (AEC), respectively (White and Vasil, unpublished). This selection system is based on the assumption that the resistance to the analogues is a dominant characteristic. Growth of wild type N. sylvestris cells in suspension culture is completely inhibited by 10 μg/ml AEC or 5MT. Spontaneous resistant cell lines were selected which were able to grow normally without inhibition in 200 μg/ml AEC (AEC^R) and 30 μg/ml 5MT ($5MT^R$) (Figs. 7,8). Both the cell lines retained resistance after cloning by protoplast culture, and differed from each other in morphological characteristics. The $5MT^R$ cell colonies are dull white in color and grow predominantly as chains of cells, while the AEC^R colonies are yellow in color and grow in tight clumps. These characteristics permitted morphological differentiation of the cell types in mixed populations. In order to enhance the chance of survival of any hybrid protoplasts resistant to both the analogues, the fused protoplasts were allowed to grow to cell colonies of about 50 cells before any selection was applied. Screening of 10^4 mixed (1:1) AEC^R and $5MT^R$ protoplasts on 200 μg/ml AEC + 30 μg/ml 5MT (control), after 45-60 days initial culture in the absence of the two analogues, did not produce any calli capable of growth. AEC^R and $5MT^R$ cells were observed in close association in such mixed cultures, but none of these survived, eliminating the possibility of any cross feeding. AEC^R and $5MT^R$ protoplasts (1:1) were fused with

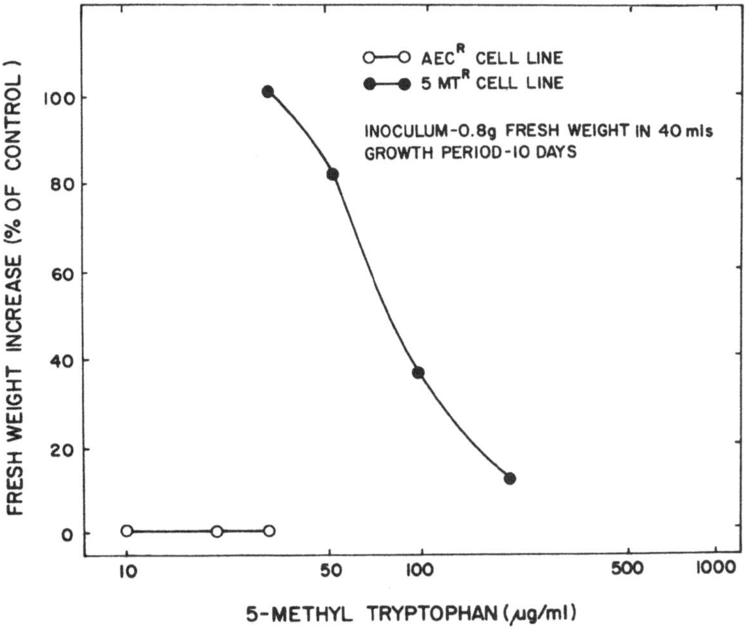

Fig. 7. Growth of AEC^R and $5MT^R$ cell lines in 5-methyl tryptophan.

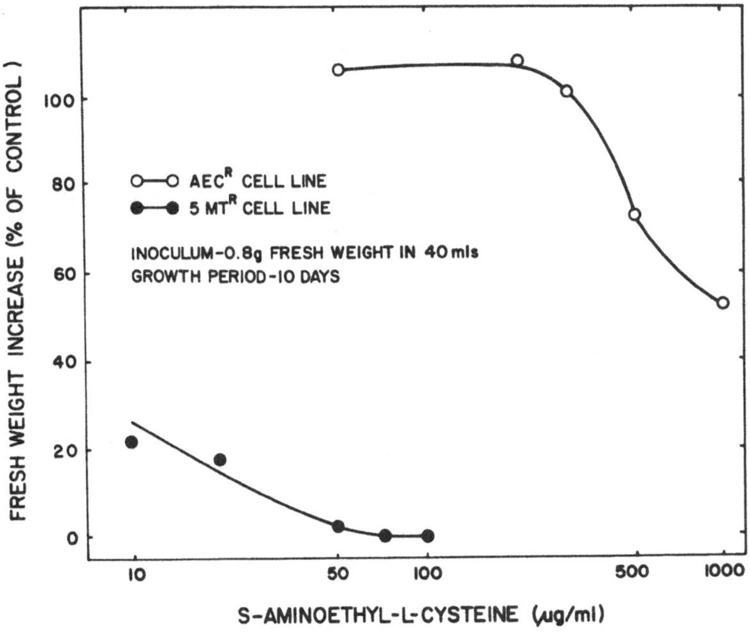

Fig. 8. Growth of AEC^R and $5MT^R$ cell lines in S-2-aminoethyl-L-cysteine.

the aid of polyethylene glycol and cultured on a normal medium for 35 days prior to screening for double amino acid analogue resistance. From 656 calli screened, 6 have been isolated which are capable of rapid growth in the presence of both the analogues (Table 3). These presumptive $AEC^R + 5MT^R$ cell hybrids are being tested to compare their degree of resistance with parental cell lines.

Strong evidence is now available of the random elimination of chromosomes of one of the parental species from heterokaryons as well as true hybrid cells during cell division. This is particularly true in intergeneric somatic hybrid cells (Kao, 1977; Binding and Nehls, 1978). One of the finest examples of chromosome elimination in somatic hybrid cells of plants comes from the elegant work of Kao (1977), who fused protoplasts derived from the suspension culture of soybean with the mesophyll protoplasts of *Nicotiana glauca*. The morphologically identifiable fusion products were mechanically isolated and cultured in about 25 µl of a highly complex nutrient medium. Cytological analyses of hybrid calli showed that although no obvious change took place in the structure or number of soybean chromosomes, only a few chromosomes of *N. glauca* were retained. These were structurally modified owing to the breaking and sticking together of chromosome pieces. No organogenesis or regeneration of plants occurred in the hybrid tissues. It is unlikely that normal organogenesis will take place in hybrid tissues containing entire genomes of very widely separated plant species. Stabilization of a few or of only parts of chromosomes in somatic hybrid tissues would probably not seriously interfere in regeneration phenomena. Such cell lines will also be of much use in chromosome mapping of higher plants.

Gleba and Hoffmann (1978) mechanically isolated and cultured fusion products of *Arabidopsis thaliana* + *Brassica campestris* protoplasts in microdroplets. Cytological examination of the cell lines after about 30 cell generations (6-7 months of culture) showed that specific chromosomes of both the parents were still retained in the hybrid cells, and their activities were confirmed by isozyme analyses. Loss or retention of chromosomes, therefore, may depend on specific characteristics of the parental species used in somatic hybridization.

Mechanical isolation of fusion products has been successfully used in some cases where suitable morphological markers are present. Thus, Kao (1977) and Gleba and Hoffmann (1978) isolated chloroplast-containing mesophyll protoplasts from the leaves of one parent and fused these with protoplasts from suspension cultures of a second parent. Culture of such isolated single fusion products can be carried out in microquantities of nutrient media for continued growth and formation of hybrid tissues.

Table 3. Fusion and Control Experiments with AEC^R and $5MT^R$ Protoplasts on 200 μg/ml AEC + 30 μg/ml 5MT Selection

Source of Protoplasts	Period of Culture Prior to Selection (days)	Number of Colonies Screened	Number of Colonies Growing After Transfer to 200 μg/ml AEC + 30 μg/ml 5MT
Mixture of AEC^R and $5MT^R$ Protoplasts (control)	60	5×10^3	0
Mixture of AEC^R and $5MT^R$ Protoplasts (control)	45	10^4	0
Fused AEC^R + $5MT^R$ Protoplasts	35	656	6*

*Presumptive hybrid calli.

As is evident from the above discussion, auxotrophic mutants, or cell lines resistant/sensitive to drugs, etc., have so far not been widely used in plant somatic hybridization experiments. The work with nitrate reductase-deficient mutants has demonstrated how useful such mutants can be in the selection of somatic hybrid cells. Much more work needs to be done, therefore, to isolate auxotrophic and other mutant or variant cells lines from important crop plants so that suitable selection systems can be developed.

PLANT TISSUE CULTURES AND NITROGEN FIXATION

One of the most important factors limiting the yield of important agronomic crops is the availability of fixed nitrogen. In view of the high energy cost and price of synthetic nitrogen fertilizers, it will be advantageous to develop alternative sources of fixed nitrogen (Hardy and Havelka, 1975; Newton and Nyman, 1976; Vasil, 1976; Evans and Barber, 1977; Hollaender et al., 1977). The principal biological source of fixed nitrogen is the very specific symbiotic association of *Rhizobium* with legumes. Attempts are being made, therefore, to overcome the specificity of *Rhizobium*-legume associations so that highly effective strains of the bacterium can be used to nodulate desirable legumes, as well as to confer on non-legumes the ability to form symbiotic associations with Rhizobium and other nitrogen fixing bacteria.

Plant tissue cultures derived from legumes as well as non-legumes have been shown to induce nitrogenase activity in Rhizobium (Child and LaRue, 1974; Child, 1975; Scowcroft and Gibson, 1975), and are being increasingly used in a variety of experiments to engineer associations of nitrogen fixing bacteria with non-legume plant species: (1) Fusion of legume and non-legume protoplasts, and the possible regeneration of hybrid plants that will have the ability to associate with Rhizobium. (2) Forced association of nitrogen fixing bacteria with non-legume tissue cultures, and possible regeneration of plants. (3) Fusion of bacteroid-containing legume root nodule protoplasts with non-legume protoplasts. (4) Induced transfer of nitrogen fixing bacteria into protoplasts. (5) Transfer of nif-genes, through plasmids or DNA, from bacteria to non-legumes. These experimental approaches are adequately discussed elsewhere (Vasil et al., 1977, 1978).

Some recent studies have shown nitrogenase activity in microorganisms associated with the roots of some forage grasses and cereals (Dobereiner and Day, 1976; Nelson et al., 1976). The potential of a nitrogen fixing association between the free-living bacterium Spirillum (Azospirillum) and higher plants has received considerable attention (Barber et al., 1976; Day et al., 1975; Dobereiner and Day, 1976; von Bulow and Dobereiner, 1975; Albrecht et al., 1977). We have attempted to force an association of Azospirillum brasilense SP7 with tissue cultures of sugarcane (V. Vasil, R. H. Berg, I. K. Vasil, D. A. Zuberer, and D. H. Hubbell, unpublished). Sugarcane callus tissues, growing on a nitrogen-free or low nitrogen nutrient medium, were inoculated by placing one drop (2×10^8 cells/ml) of a washed bacterial suspension on the surface of the callus tissue. Measurements of acetylene reduction activity showed that inoculated callus cultures support a population of Azospirillum that is actively fixing nitrogen, while the controls show no acetylene reduction activity. Since the young and actively growing sugarcane callus cultures contain little or no intercellular air space, the bacterial growth is limited to the surface layers of the callus. With age the tissue develops substantial intercellular spaces, and these are progressively occupied by the bacteria which are embedded in a capsular slime formed as a result of plant-bacterial interaction. The bacteria principally grow in the intercellular space system of the callus or on its surface, and there is no evidence of any intracellular growth of the bacteria (Figs. 9,10). Large numbers of bacteria are seen adjacent to normal, healthy cells. We have maintained sugarcane callus cultures inoculated with A. brasilense for about 18 months, and have recently regenerated plantlets from such associated cultures. This material is currently being examined to determine if the bacteria are also present in the tissues of the regenerated plants. These experiments indicate a certain degree of

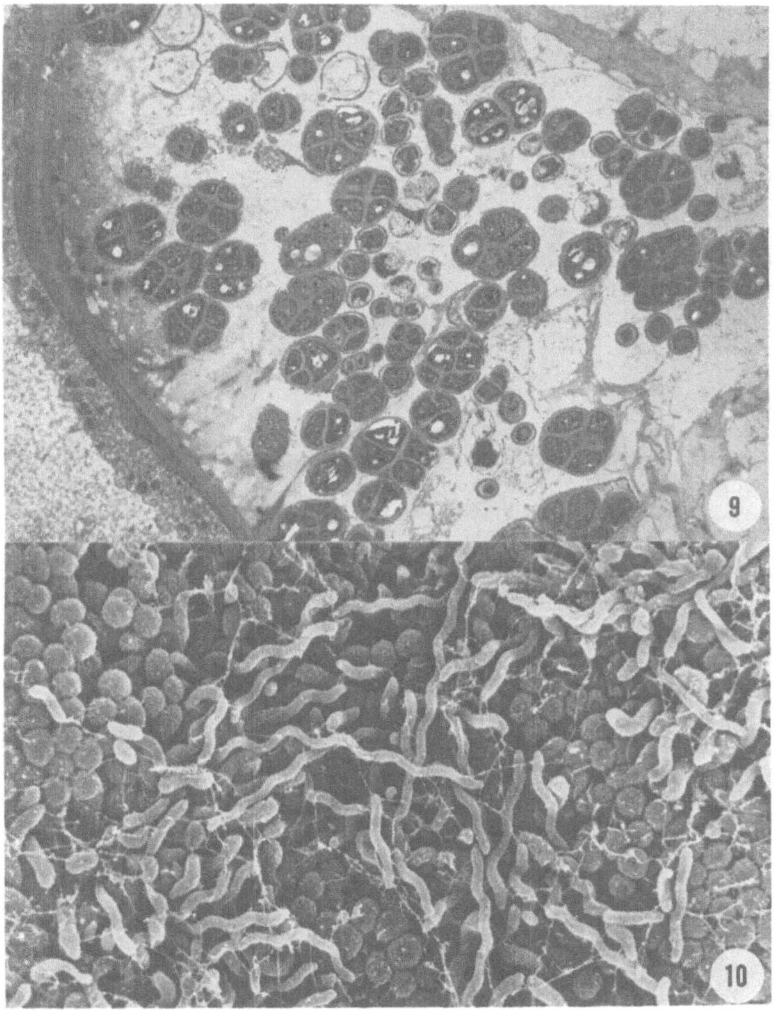

Figs. 9-10. Associated cultures of sugarcane callus tissue and *Azospirillum brasilense*. Fig. 9. Transmission electron micrograph of bacterial growth in the intercellular space system. Note healthy sugarcane cell adjacent to encapsulated forms of bacteria. X4,500. Fig. 10. Scanning electron micrograph of rod-shaped and encapsulated forms of bacteria growing on the surface of sugarcane callus tissue. X3,600.

compatibility between the sugarcane callus tissues and *Azospirillum*. Further work needs to be carried out to establish the nature of the association.

It is hoped that this brief discussion of some of the more recent and important work adequately demonstrates the potential of plant protoplast and cell culture techniques in somatic hybridization and genetic manipulation of plants. Utilization of these techniques in the improvement of important crop plants, contrary to some overly optimistic views, is certainly not imminent. The full realization of the potential of these novel techniques depends on our ability to overcome the serious difficulties currently faced in the culture and regeneration of plants from protoplasts of cereals and legumes, and to isolate and characterize true mutant cell lines which can be used to develop procedures for selecting hybrid cells from mixed populations following protoplast fusion.

ACKNOWLEDGMENTS

The preparation of this review was supported by funds from the Graduate School and the Agricultural Experiment Station, University of Florida, and grants from the National Science Foundation (INT76-17525) and the U.S. Agency for International Development (931-1004A).

REFERENCES

Albrecht, S. L., Okon, Y., and Burris, R. H., 1977, Effects of light and temperature on the association between Zea mays and Spirillum lipoferum, Pl. Physiol., 60:528-531.

Banks, M. S., and Evans, P. K., 1976, A comparison of the isolation and culture of mesophyll protoplasts from several Nicotiana species and their hybrids, Pl. Sci. Let., 7:409-416.

Barber, L. E., Tjepkema, J. D., Russell, S. A., and Evans, H. J., 1976, Acetylene reduction (nitrogen fixation) associated with corn inoculated with Spirillum, Appl. Environ. Microbiol., 32:108-113.

Barz, W., Reinhard, E., and Zenk, M. H., eds., 1977, "Plant Tissue Culture and Its Bio-technological Applications," Springer-Verlag, New York.

Beers, R. F., Jr., and Bassett, E. G., eds., 1977, "Recombinant Molecules: Impact on Science and Society," Xth Miles International Symposium, Raven Press, New York.

Binding, H., and Nehls, R., 1974, Regeneration von haploiden and diploiden Pflanzen aus Protoplasten von Petunia hybrida L. Regeneration of haploid and diploid plants from protoplasts of Petunia hybrida L., Z. Pflanzenphysiol., 74:327-356.

Binding, H., and Nehls, R., 1977, Regeneration of isolated protoplasts to plants in Solanum dulcamara L., Z. Pflanzenphysiol., 85: 279-280.

Binding, H., and Nehls, R., 1978, Molec. Gen. Genet., in press (personal communication).

Bourgin, J. P., and Missonier, C., 1973, Culture de protoplastes de mésophylle de Nicotiana alata Link et Otto haploide. Culture of haploid mesophyll protoplasts from Nicotiana alata, Z. Pflanzenphysiol., 87:55-64.

Bourgin, J. P., Missonier, C., and Chupeau, Y., 1976, Cytophysiologie végétale--Culture de protoplastes de mésophylle de Nicotiana sylvestris spegazzini et comes haploide et diploide, C. R. Acad. Sci. (Paris), 282D:1853-1856.

Bui Dang Ha, D., and Mackenzie, I. A., 1973, The division of protoplasts from Asparagus officinalis L., and their growth and differentiation, Protoplasma, 78:215-221.

Carlson, P. S., Smith, H. H., and Dearing, R. D., 1972, Parasexual interspecific plant hybridization (Nicotiana/leaf mesophyll/ plant tissue culture/genetics/selective media), Proc. Nat. Acad. Sci. USA, 69:2292-2294.

Child, J. J., 1975, Nitrogen fixation by a Rhizobium sp. in association with non-leguminous plant cell culture, Nature (London), 253:350-351.

Child, J. J., and LaRue, T. A., 1974, A simple technique for the establishment of nitrogenase in soybean callus culture, Pl. Physiol. 53:88-90.

Cocking, E. C., 1960, A method for the isolation of plant protoplasts and vacuoles, Nature (London), 187:927-923.

Cocking, E. C., 1972, Plant cell protoplasts--Isolation and development, Ann. Rev. Pl. Physiol., 23:29-50.

Constabel, F., and Kao, K. N., 1974, Agglutination and fusion of plant protoplasts by polyethylene glycol, Canad. J. Bot., 52:1603-1606.

Davidson, R. L., and de la Cruz, F. F., eds., 1974, "Somatic Cell Hybridization," Raven Press, New York.

Davidson, R. L., and Gerald, P. S., 1977, Induction of mammalian somatic cell hybridization in polyethylene glycol, in: "Methods in Cell Biology," D. M. Prescott, ed., Academic Press, New York, 15:329-338.

Day, J. M., Neves, M. C. P., and Dobereiner, J., 1975, Nitrogenase activity on the roots of tropical forage grasses, Soil Biol. Biochem., 7:107-112.

Deka, P. C., and Sen, S. K., 1976, Differentiation in calli originated from isolated protoplasts of rice (Oryza sativa L.) through plating technique, Molec. Gen. Genet., 145:239-243.

Dobereiner, J., and Day, J. M., 1976, Associative symbioses in tropical grasses: Characterization of microorganisms and dinitrogen-fixing sites, in: "Proceedings of the International Symposium on Nitrogen Fixation," W. E. Newton and C. J. Newman, eds., Washington Univ. Press, Pullman, 2:518-538.

Dorion, N., Chupeau, Y., and Bourgin, J. P., 1975, Isolation, culture and regeneration into plants of Ranunculus scelerata L. leaf protoplasts, Pl. Sci. Let., 5:325-331.

Dudits, D., Kao, K. N., Constabel, F., and Gamborg, O. L., 1976a, Embryogenesis and formation of tetraploid and hexaploid plants from carrot protoplasts, Canad. J. Bot., 54:1063-1067.
Dudits, D., Farkas, G. L., and Maliga, P., eds., 1976b, "Cell Genetics in Higher Plants," Akademiai Kiado, Budapest.
Dudits, D., Hadlaczky, G., Levi, E., Fejer, O., Haydu, Z., and Lazar, G., 1977, Somatic hybridization of Daucus carota and D. capillifolius by protoplast fusion, Theoret. Appl. Genet., 51:127-132.
Dudits, D., Rasho, I., Hadlaczky, G., and Lima-de-Faria, A., 1976c, Fusion of human cells with carrot protoplasts induced by polyethylene glycol, Hereditas, 82:121-124.
Durand, J., Potrykus, I., and Donn, G., 1973, Plantes issues de protoplastes de Petunia, Z. Pflanzenphysiol., 69:26-34.
Eriksson, T., and Jonasson, K., 1969, Nuclear division in isolated protoplasts from cells of high plants grown in vitro, Planta (Berlin), 89:85-89.
Evans, H. J., and Barber, L. E., 1977, Biological nitrogen fixation for food and fiber production, Science, 197:332-339.
Frearson, E. M., Power, J. B., and Cocking, E. C., 1973, The isolation, culture and regeneration of Petunia leaf protoplasts, Dev. Biol., 33:130-137.
Gamborg, O. L., 1977, Somatic cell hybridization by protoplast fusion and morphogenesis, in: "Plant Tissue Culture and Its Bio-technological Application," W. Barz, E. Reinhard, and M. H. Zenk, eds., Springer-Verlag, New York.
Gamborg, O. L., Murashige, T., Thorpe, T. A., and Vasil, I. K., 1976, Plant tissue culture media, In Vitro, 12:473-478.
Gamborg, O. L., and Wetter, L. R., eds., 1975, "Plant Tissue Culture Methods," National Research Council of Canada, Ottawa.
Gleba, Y. Y., 1978, Microdroplet culture: Tobacco plants from single mesophyll protoplasts, Naturwiss., 65:158.
Gleba, Y. Y., Butenko, R. G., and Sytnik, K. M., 1975, Fusion of protoplasts and parasexual hybridization in Nicotiana tabacum L., Dokl. Akad. Nauk. S.S.S.R., 221:1196-1198.
Gleba, Y. Y., and Hoffmann, F., 1978, in: "Proceedings of the IVth International Plant Tissue and Cell Culture Congress, Calgary, Canada" (personal communication).
Glimelius, K., Eriksson, T., Grafe, R., and Muller, A. J., 1978, Somatic hybridization of nitrate reductase-deficient mutants of Nicotiana tabacum by protoplast fusion, Physiol. Plant., 44:273-277.
Gosch, G., Bajaj, Y. P. S., and Reinert, J., 1975, Isolation, culture and induction of embryogenesis in protoplasts from cell-suspensions of Atropa belladonna, Protoplasma, 86:405-410.
Grambow, H. J., Kao, K. N., Miller, R. A., and Gamborg, O. L., 1972, Cell division and plant development from protoplasts of carrot cell suspension centers, Planta (Berlin), 103:348-355.
Hardy, R. W. F., and Havelka, U. D., 1975, Nitrogen fixation research: A key to world food, Science, 188:633-643.

Hayward, C., and Power, J. B., 1975, Plant production from leaf protoplasts of Petunia parodii, Pl. Sci. Let., 4:407-410.

Hollaender, A., Burris, R. H., Day, P. R., Hardy, R. W. F., Helinski, D. R., Lamborg, M. R., Owens, L., and Valentine, R. C., eds., 1977, "Genetic Engineering for Nitrogen Fixation," Plenum Press, New York.

Jones, C. W., Mastrangelo, I. A., Smith, H. H., Liu, H. Z., and Meck, R. A., 1976, Interkingdom fusion between human (HeLa) cells and tobacco hybrid (ggLL) protoplasts, Science, 193:401-403.

Kao, K. N., 1977, Chromosomal behaviour in somatic hybrids of soybean--Nicotiana glauca, Molec. Gen. Genet., 150:225-230.

Kao, K. N., Gamborg, O. L., Michayluk, M. R., Keller, W. A., and Miller, R. A., 1973, The effects of sugars and inorganic salts on cell regeneration and sustained division in plant protoplasts, in: "Protoplastes et fusion de cellules somatiques végétales," J. Tempe, ed., C.N.R.S. (Paris), 212:207-213.

Kao, K. N., Gamborg, O. L., Miller, R. A., and Keller, W. A., 1971, Cell divisions in cells regenerated from protoplasts of soybean and Haplopappus gracilis, Nature, New Biol., 232:124.

Kao, K. N., and Michayluk, M. R., 1974, A method for high-frequency intergeneric fusion of plant protoplasts, Planta (Berlin), 115: 355-367.

Kao, K. N., and Michayluk, M. R., 1975, Nutritional requirements for growth of Vica hajastana cells and protoplasts at a very low population density in liquid media, Planta (Berlin), 126: 105-110.

Kartha, K. K., Michayluk, M. R., Kao, K. N., and Gamborg, O. L., 1974, Callus formation and plant regeneration from mesophyll protoplasts of rape plants (Brassica napus L. cv. Zephyr), Pl. Sci. Let., 3:265-271.

Keller, W. A., and Melchers, G., 1973, The effect of high pH and calcium on tobacco leaf protoplast fusion, Z. Naturforsch., 28B:737-741.

Kinnersley, A. M., Racusen, R. H., and Galston, A. W., 1978, A comparison of regenerated cell walls in tobacco and cereal protoplasts, Planta (Berlin), 139:155-158.

Kleinhofs, A., and Behki, R., 1977, Prospects for plant genome modification by nonconventional methods, Ann. Rev. Genet., 11:79-101.

Klercker, J. A., 1892, Eine Methode zur Isolinung lebender Protoplasten, Oefvers Vet. Akad. (Stockholm), 9:463-471.

Ledoux, L., ed., 1975, "Genetic Manipulations with Plant Material," Plenum Press, New York.

Maliga, P., Lazar, G., Joo, F., Nagy, A. H., and Menczel, L., 1977, Restoration of morphogenic potential in Nicotiana by somatic hybridisation, Molec. Gen. Genet., 157:291-296.

Markham, R., Davies, D. R., Hopwood, D. A., Horne, R. W., eds., 1975, "Modifications of the Information Content of Plant Cells," North-Holland, Amsterdam.

Melchers, G., 1977, Microbial techniques in somatic hybridization by fusion of protoplasts, in: "International Cell Biology 1976-1977," B. R. Brinkley and K. R. Porter, eds., Rockefeller Univ. Press, New York.

Melchers, G., and Labid, G., 1974, Somatic hybridisation of plants by fusion of protoplasts. I. Selection of light resistant hybrids of "haploid" light sensitive varieties of tobacco, Molec. Gen. Genet., 135:277-294.

Muller, A. J., and Grafe, R., 1978, Isolation and characterization of cell line of Nicotiana tabacum lacking nitrate reductase, Molec. Gen. Genet., 161:67-76.

Murashige, T., 1974, Plant propagation through tissue cultures, Ann. Rev. Pl. Physiol., 25:135-166.

Nagata, T., and Takebe, I., 1971, Plating of isolated tobacco mesophyll protoplasts on agar medium, Planta (Berlin), 99: 12-20.

Nagy, J. I., and Maliga, P., 1976, Callus induction and plant regeneration from mesophyll protoplasts of Nicotiana sylvestris, Z. Pflanzenphysiol., 78:453-455.

Nelson, A. D., Barber, L. E., Tjepkema, J., Russell, S. A., Powelson, R., Evans, H. J., and Seidler, R. J., 1976, Nitrogen fixation associated with grasses in Oregon, Canad. J. Microbiol., 22:523-530.

Newton, W. E., and Nyman, C. J., eds., 1976, "Proceedings of the International Symposium on Nitrogen Fixation," Vols. 1 and 2, Washington Univ. Press, Pullman.

Nitzsche, W., and Wenzel, G., 1977, Haploids in plant breeding, Fortsch. Pflanzenzuchtg., Suppl., 8:1-101.

Ohyama, K., and Nitsch, J. P., 1972, Flowering haploid plants obtained from protoplasts of tobacco leaves, Pl. Cell Physiol., 13:229-236.

Pontecorvo, G., 1975, Production of mammalian somatic cell hybrids by means of polyethylene glycol treatment, Som. Cell Genet., 1:397-400.

Potrykus, I., Harms, C. T., and Lorz, H., 1976, Problems in culturing cereal protoplasts, in: "Cell Genetics in Higher Plants," D. Dudits, G. L. Farkas, and P. Maliga, eds., Akademiai Kiado, Budapest.

Potrykus, I., Harms, C. T., Lorz, H., and Thomas, E., 1977, Callus formation for stem protoplasts of corn (Zea mays L.), Molec. Gen. Genet., 156:347-350.

Power, J. B., Cummins, S. E., and Cocking, E. C., 1970, Fusion of isolated plant protoplasts, Nature (London), 225:1016-1018.

Power, J. B., Frearson, E. M., George, D., Evans, P. K., Berry, S. F., Hayward, C., and Cocking, E. C., 1976a, The isolation, culture and regeneration of leaf protoplasts in the genus Petunia, Pl. Sci. Let., 7:51-56.

Power, J. B., Frearson, E. M., Hayward, C., George, D., Evans, P. K., Berry, S. F., and Cocking, E. C., 1976b, Somatic hybridisation of Petunia hybrida and P. parodii, Nature (London), 263:500-502.
Ringertz, N. R., and Savage, R. E., 1976, "Cell Hybrids," Academic Press, New York.
Rubenstein, I., Phillips, R. L., Green, C. E., and Desnick, R., eds., 1977, "Molecular Genetic Modification of Eucaryotes," Academic Press, New York.
Schieder, O., 1975, Regeneration von haploiden und diploiden Datura innoxia Mill. Mesophyll-Protoplasten zu Pflanzen, Z. Pflanzenphysiol., 76:462-466.
Schieder, O., 1977, Hybridisation experiments with protoplasts from chlorophyll-deficient mutants of some Solanaceous species, Planta (Berlin), 137:253-257.
Schieder, O., 1978, Somatic hybrids of Datura innoxia Mill. + Datura discolor Bern, L. and of Datura innoxia Mill. + Datura stramonium L. var. tatula L. I. Selection and characterisation, Molec. Gen. Genet., 162:113-119.
Scowcroft, W. R., and Gibson, A. H., 1975, Nitrogen fixation by Rhizobium associated with tobacco and cowpea cell cultures, Nature (London), 253:351-352.
Shepard, J. F., and Totten, R. E., 1977, Mesophyll cell protoplasts of potato isolation, proliferation and plant rejuvenation, Pl. Physiol., 60:313-316.
Sink, K. C., and Power, J. B., 1977, The isolation, culture and regeneration of leaf protoplasts of Petunia parviflora Juss., Pl. Sci. Let., 10:335-340.
Skoog, F., and Miller, C. O., 1957, Chemical regulation of growth and organ formation in plant tissues cultured in vitro, Symp. Soc. Exp. Biol., 11:118-131.
Smith, H. H., Kao, K. N., and Combatti, N. C., 1976, Interspecific hybridization by protoplast fusion in Nicotiana: Confirmation and extension, J. Hered., 67:123-128.
Takebe, I., Labib, G., and Melchers, G., 1971, Regeneration of whole plants from isolated mesophyll protoplasts of tobacco, Naturwiss., 58:318-320.
Thomas, E., Hoffmann, F., Potrykus, I., and Wenzel, G., 1976, Protoplast regeneration and stem embryogenesis of haploid androgenetic rape, Molec. Gen. Genet., 145:245-247.
Vasil, I. K., 1976, The progress, problems and prospects of plant protoplast research, Adv. Agron., 28:119-160.
Vasil, I. K., 1977, Nutrient requirements of plant tissues in culture for growth and differentiation, in: "Handbook Series in Nutrition and Food," M. Rechcigl, Jr., ed., Vol. 1, Sec. D., CRC Press, Cleveland, Ohio.
Vasil, I. K., Ahuja, M. R., and Vasil, V., 1978, Plant tissue cultures in genetics and plant breeding or some alternatives to sex in plants through plant tissue cultures, Adv. Genet., 20: (in press).

Vasil, I. K., and Nitsch, C., 1975, Experimental production of pollen haploids and their uses, Z. Pflanzenphysiol., 76:191-212.
Vasil, I. K., and Vasil, V., 1972, Totipotency and embryogenesis in plant cell and tissue cultures, In Vitro, 8:117-127.
Vasil, I. K., Vasil, V., and Hubbell, D. H., 1977, Engineered plant cell or fungal association with bacteria that fix nitrogen, in: "Genetic Engineering for Nitrogen Fixation," A. Hollaender et al., eds., Plenum Press, New York.
Vasil, I. K., Vasil, V., Sutton, W. D., and Giles, K. L., 1975, Protoplasts as tools for the genetic modification of plants, in: "Proceedings IV International Symposium on Yeast and Other Protoplasts," Univ. of Nottingham, England.
Vasil, V., and Hildebrandt, A. C., 1965, Differentiation of tobacco plants from single, isolated cells in microcultures, Science, 150:889-892.
Vasil, V., and Vasil, I. K., 1974, Regeneration of tobacco and Petunia plants from protoplasts and culture of corn protoplasts, In Vitro, 10:83-96.
Vasil, V., and Vasil, I. K., 1978, Isolation and culture of cereal protoplasts. I. Callus formation from pearl millet Pennisetum americanum protoplasts, Z. Pflanzenphysiol., in press.
von Bulow, J. F. W., and Dobereiner, J., 1975, Potential for nitrogen fixation in maize genotypes in Brazil (grass-bacteria associations/Spirillum lipoferum/acetylene reduction), Proc. Nat. Acad. Sci. USA, 72:2389-2393.
Wacker, A., and Kaul, S., 1977, Polyäthelenglykol-induzierte Fusion von Saugetierzellen mit Cytoplasten in Suspension, Naturwiss., 64:146.
Wallin, A., Glimelius, K., and Eriksson, T., 1974, The induction of aggregation and fusion of Daucus carota protoplasts by polyethylene glycol, Z. Pflanzenphysiol., 74:64-80.
Williamson, F. A., Fowke, L. C., Weber, G., Constabel, F., and Gamborg, O. L., 1977, Microfibril deposition on cultured protoplasts of Vichia hajastana, Protoplasma, 91:213-219.
Willis, G. E., Hartmann, J. X., and de Lamater, E. D., 1977, Electron microscopic study of plant-animal cell fusion, Protoplasma, 91:1-14.

6

GENETIC HERBICIDE RESISTANCE: PROJECTIONS ON APPEARANCE IN WEEDS AND BREEDING FOR IT IN CROPS

J. Gressel

Weizmann Institute of Science
Rehovot, Israel

INTRODUCTION

With the worldwide energy crisis, herbicides have come into greater use and importance as they afford a less energy expensive form of weed control than tractor drawn implements. The use of herbicides often affords an additional advantage in many areas as a factor in saving irrigation water; they reduce competition from weeds. Thus, it becomes increasingly important to know if the weed/herbicide relationship will follow in the footsteps of all other pest/pesticide relationships vis à vis appearance of resistance.

As a case in point it should be remembered that in the mid-forties and fifties antibiotics, chlorinated hydrocarbon insecticides, dicoumarol rodenticides, many new fungicides, as well as the MCPA and 2,4-D type herbicides were all introduced. Except for the herbicides, genetically resistant biotypes were selected in species that were susceptible to each pesticide, severely limiting each pesticide's usefulness. By 1957, resistance to insecticides was a well known phenomenon (see Newman, 1957). At that time Harper (1957) warned that there would be selection for herbicide resistance. Agriculturalists were told to rotate herbicides to prevent the appearance of resistant strains (Abel, 1954). Not all farmers listened. There are large areas where economics have encouraged monoculture, e.g., of grain with continuous deployment of a single herbicide 2,4-D. In some areas a single crop and a single herbicide have been used repeatedly for more than 25 years.

In the past few years reports of isolated field appearances of complete herbicide resistance have appeared. All the cases reported were due to two S-triazine herbicides that have been in use for a much shorter period and to a lesser extent than the phenoxy herbicides. So that we may plan how to use herbicides judiciously, it is imperative to know at what rate resistance will appear, to which herbicides, and why. This might help us in better choosing herbicides for integrated weed control systems. The economics of introducing new herbicides, despite the need and market, make it highly unlikely that our arsenal of effective compounds will enlarge very much. Unless there are regulatory changes in licensing procedures, the number of new compounds that will become available for "minor" crops will also diminish even more. We must then learn to "live with" the compounds available to the best of our ability.

For the past few years we have been cogitating over the factors which might be delaying the appearance of herbicide resistance, especially by studying the literature on weed biology, antibiotic and insecticide resistances, as well as reports on the appearance of plant resistance to other toxic compounds, e.g., heavy metals. From this we have developed a picture, described below, of the factors governing the appearance of resistance. After remarking on the nature of herbicide resistance, we shall consider the various factors affecting the appearance of such resistance: mutation, selection pressure, fitness, and the particular "plasticity" of weed growth and especially the large bank of dormant weed seeds in the soil.

The discussion will be devoted to the appearance of resistance in species that were heretofore susceptible. In this article, we shall not consider well known changes of weed populations due to changes in agronomic procedures including the use of herbicides for species which are naturally insensitive, as discussed by Harper (1957, 1960), Baker (1974), and Holm et al. (1977). We have been able to integrate these factors into a simple (i.e., algebraic) equation. Using "plug in" data from analogous situations and "guesstimations" we used the equation to generate graphs which allow us to weigh the relative importance of each factor. We believe that these models help us in understanding what has happened, as well as what may happen and how we can influence what will happen. Some of our conclusions presented later in this article are conspicuously different from those proposed in weed control tests of yesteryear.

We also believe that these models suggest better strategies for selecting for herbicide resistant strains of crops. These strategies will be discussed.

ARE THERE GENES FOR RESISTANCE IN WEED POPULATIONS?

Resistance[1] to phytotoxic compounds such as herbicides can occur at many levels. Selective permeation, for example, can occur at various levels, e.g., uptake into the root, through the cuticle, or uptake into target organelles. Prevention of toxicity by lack of translocation is also known, especially in the root endodermis. Selectivity can be based on the differential ability to detoxify a compound enzymatically. Phenological modes of resistance occur, for example, by germination after the normal time of application of contact herbicides or after degradation of mildly persistent herbicides. Thus the modes of selective resistance are quite varied, making it all the more surprising that there have been few reports of genetic resistance to herbicides.

A few cases are known where resistant genes seem not to be a part of the genetic framework of an organism. Unlike many other bacteria, streptococci are still controlled by penicillin. They seem to lack both the gene for resistance and the ability to take up a plasmid conferring resistance. Bordeaux mixture is still used to control many fungi even after about a century of use. No weed has acquired resistance to a hoe (yet dandelions have been selected that are lawn mower "resistant," i.e., very dwarf strains). These cases are rare exceptions. Cases of selected resistance in genomes thought to be evolution proof have occurred. Gonococcus, which like streptococcus was controlled by penicillin, has recently become immune. Among the list of fungi becoming resistant to fungicides, we find a single report of resistance to the venerable Bordeaux mixture (Ogawa et al., 1977). Considering that many herbicides are selective, killing one plant but not another, and that the modes of action of species selectively span from biochemical detoxification to morphological barriers, we should expect the existence of a small frequency of resistant biotypes to be present in nature. The resistance genes would be available within the population waiting for selection. Their frequency is another matter. The gene for DDT resistance has not been expressed in the African strain of the yellow fever mosquito, but is easily selected for the Asian and American strains which interbreed with it (Inwang et al., 1967). This means that DDT can still be effectively used for yellow fever control in Africa, but not elsewhere.

---

[1]Resistance is herein defined as being completely tolerant to a concentration of herbicide that kills the "wild" type. Lesser degrees of tolerance are noted as tolerance of differential tolerance. This definition conforms to that of the United Nations Food and Agriculture Organization (FAO) Working Party on Pesticide Resistance (Anonymous, 1967).

With herbicides, we now have some data on the appearance of tolerance and resistance (Appendix 1), along with some genetic information. Siduron tolerance in Hordeum is inherited by three dominant genes (Schooler et al., 1972). Atrazine tolerance in Linum is quantitatively inherited (Comstock and Andersen, 1968) and in maize is controlled by a single recessive nuclear gene (Grogan et al., 1963), but in Brassica campestris the same trait is maternally inherited in the chloroplast (Souza-Machado et al., 1978), which probably controls the structure of a plastid lamellar protein which binds atrazine (Arntzen, 1978).

Recently, a highly picloram-tolerant, possibly resistant strain of Nicotiana was selected. The tolerance was due to a single dominant nuclear gene with a frequency of $\sim 10^{-5}$ (Chaleff and Parsons, 1978).

Thus it would be very hard to predict the frequency of resistants to any given herbicide in an untreated weed population. This would depend on the number of genes for resistance, dominance, and the ploidy of the plant involved. From analogous situations we can predict that it would be between $<10^{-10}$ and 10^{-5}.

From all the above it seems reasonable to assume that genetic resistance is feasible, at least with most weed species and most herbicides.

HAVE HERBICIDES BEEN USED LONG ENOUGH FOR RESISTANCE TO APPEAR?

The frequency of herbicide resistance in diploid plants and insecticide resistance in insects should be the same. We can with validity ask if sufficient generations of selection have gone by for resistance to be apparent. If DDT is analogous to 2,4-D and flies to plants, the answer is yes. Within the first year of DDT use, resistance was reported from Italy to Denmark (cf. Newman, 1957). This occurred in fewer generations than the number of years 2,4-D has been used continually in some areas. Thus, it is not a question of number of generations per se; it must be more a question of enrichment for resistance per generation. 2,4-D and DDT exert different pressures on their pests, and plants have some properties quite different from flies, which when compounded, strongly affect the rate of evolution of resistance. These factors governing the rate of enrichment of resistance will be discussed in the following sections.

SELECTION PRESSURE (RATE OF KILL) OF HERBICIDES

It is empirically observable that the greater the kill rate of a pesticide, the more rapidly the enrichment for resistant strains, unless 100% kill is achieved. There have been interesting reports on pasture revegetation on toxic mine tailings. Bradshaw's group found a selection for ecotypes of various species that are resistant to much higher levels of copper, zinc, and lead than allow survival of normal ecotypes. The frequency of such types in the normal population is low and yet it only takes a few seasons for such areas to become revegetated by the resistant strains (Antonovics, 1971; Antonovics and Bradshaw, 1970; McNeilly, 1968).

There is a basic difference between the field phytotoxicities of heavy metals and herbicides: the degree of selection pressure, i.e., the percent kill achieved by the phytotoxic compound. Heavy metals are not degraded nor do they leach rapidly from the soil, a quite different situation from most herbicides. Most herbicides are applied at rates which give 90-95% kill. Higher kill rates still leave escapees but often kill the crops. At 90% kill without intervening factors there would be a tenfold yearly enrichment of resistants in the population. This in itself is different from the other pesticides which are used at higher kill rates. If the initial frequency of resistance is 10^{-10}, in 10 years of repeated treatment the resistants would totally "inherit the earth." This has not quite happened. If we measure "kill" in a biological manner and not an agronomic one, we will see that the effective pressure may actually be lower. For these purposes, kill should not be measured as the percentage of plants remaining after treatment but as the weed seed yield at the end of the year compared to the untreated situation. If we kill 90% of the weed plants the weed seed yield will not be 10%. The 10% of plants remaining will somewhat "expand to fill the space available" as suggested by Parkinson's Law, putting out much more seed per plant. From the work of Harper (1960) and Isenee et al. (1973) (see also Fig. 1 in Gressel and Segel, 1978) we know that "Parkinsonian" plasticity exists. It will increase both the resistant and the susceptible weed seed populations of the soil, possibly to different extents as will be discussed later.

Many herbicides are ineffective and disappear shortly after application. This rapid loss was once thought to be "bad." It allows late germination and growth of the weed species, which in economic agricultural situations is not always detrimental to the crops. This late germination allows much herbicide susceptible seed to be added to the soil, especially in areas with longer growing seasons. There the weeds can expand considerably after the crop is cut. In addition susceptible weed seed carried in by wind, water, and animals contributes to lowering effective kill. Using the seed criterion, the effective kill may be lowered to a rate estimated to be 60-80% with ephemeral herbicides, although precise seed counts have not been reported as far as we can ascertain. From the above we can conclude that when the effective selection pressure is high, plants resistant to the toxic pressure can rapidly "evolve." This, we will see, is part of the reason that resistance has probably appeared to S-triazines and not the phenoxy herbicides. The triazines have higher kill rates and greater persistence.

FITNESS: THE COST OF SELECTION

Despite his being an avowed communist, the great geneticist Haldane (e.g., 1960) sounded like the epitome of a capitalist when discussing selection. He stated that all selection has a genetic "cost" which is "charged" against "fitness." Fitness in our case is best defined as the ability of a resistant strain to compete with the sensitive wild type of the same species under nonselective conditions, i.e., without herbicide. The decreased fitness can be at any one of many levels of plant growth; it can be at the level of germination, establishment, growth, ability to be "plastic" upon thinning, or the number of seeds produced per plant. Overall fitness is a compounded fitness from each stage of growth and would be measured empirically as the relative number of seed produced per unit area of the resistant vs. the wild type when the two are in mixed culture under conditions where there is no selection pressure. Decreased fitness of pesticide resistants has been shown in antibiotic resistant bacteria, fungicide resistant molds, and insecticide resistant insects. A few cases have also been reported with plants: When the heavy metal tolerant genotypes discussed above were interseeded with the wild type plants on a normal nonselective soil, the metal tolerant type genetically "disappeared" back toward its normal frequency. The tolerant type was less fit to compete with the wild type (McNeilly, 1968). There have been similar findings with resistant weeds. S-triazine resistant *Chenopodium* germinated 2-3 days after the sensitive wild type (Bandeen and McLaren, 1976). That this can have a strong competitive disadvantage has been discussed previously (Gressel and Holm, 1964). Conard and Radosevich (1979) have measured an overall resistant *Amaranthus*, *Chenopodium*, and *Senecio*. Resistant plants were about half as fit (i.e., had half the seed yield per unit area) as wild type plants in nonselective competitive situations, both in terms of heavy metal resistance (McNeilly, 1968) and atrazine resistance (calculated from Conard and Radosevich, 1979). This large differential in fitness is part of the reason that when the usage of a particular pesticide is stopped, susceptibility slowly reappears, as will be seen later.

An important consideration with herbicides is that there is the possibility of having differential fitness play an important role in delaying the appearance of resistance even in the season in which the herbicide is used. There can be a considerable part of the growing season in which the herbicide is not present. With rapidly degraded herbicides, this nonselective competitive period predominates and may be most of the growing season. With some highly persistent herbicides, there is little or no time for this competitive period, and differential fitness will be unimportant. Thus susceptible weed seeds germinating after a pesticide disappears not only decrease the effective selection pressure, they also are more fit to compete with resistant seeds.

THE SOIL BANK OF DORMANT WEED SEEDS

That weed seeds which undergo asynchronous germination may severely decrease the effective selection pressure of an ephemeral herbicide and compete better because of fitness was discussed above. This asynchrony is not just over one growing season, but over many. Unlike crop seed, dormant weed seeds usually germinate over a period of years (e.g., Roberts and Dawkins, 1967). This property of weeds is unique to the plant kingdom and can be a major factor in delaying the appearance of resistance. The more fit susceptible seed keep germinating, partially diluting out the enrichment of resistant seeds from each previous year.

THE INTERPLAY BETWEEN THE PARAMETERS

A series of mathematical considerations were used to try to construct a model describing the appearance of resistance (Gressel and Segel, 1978). Using values from some of the analogous situations, we tried to ascertain if we should have expected or when to expect the appearance of resistance and under what conditions. A series of mathematical considerations, simplifications, and estimations (16 equations) culminated rather simply as:

$$N_n = N_o(1 + \frac{f\alpha}{\bar{n}})^n.$$

The proportion of resistants of a given species in the nth year of continued treatment of a given herbicide (N_n) equals the proportion in the field prior to herbicide treatment (N_o) times the factor in parentheses to the power of n, the number of years of treatment. N_o itself is a function of the frequency of natural mutation to the resistant biotype and the fitness of such a biotype, i.e., $N_o = \mu \cdot f$ where μ is the frequency of natural mutation to the resistant biotype and f is the overall fitness of the resistant compared to the susceptible. The factor in parentheses governs the rate of increase of resistance and is composed of the following: The overall fitness (f) which in the known cases for herbicide and heavy metal resistance is about 0.5. The selection pressure (α) is defined as the proportion of remaining susceptibles. Thus, if no resistants are killed and 95% of susceptibles are killed, $\alpha = 1/0.05 = 20$; in the case of heavy metal resistance α will approach infinity because of the extremely high kill. If we use seed set to measure selection pressure and guess that effectual kill is 50% then α will be lowered to $1/0.5 = 2.0$. All this is divided by the average lifespan of the soil seed bank of the species ($\bar{n}$). If we were dealing with crops which germinate immediately, then $\bar{n} = 1$ year. With most weed species $\bar{n}$ would be between 2 and 5. Because of $\bar{n}$ being in the denominator it depresses the rate at which resistance will increase. Upon looking at the possible numbers that can be inserted into the equation, we can see empirically that in most cases the low effectual selection pressure has the greatest effect on reducing the rate of appearance of herbicide resistance. The fitness differential would be a less important modifier and the seed bank would be a major modifier. This is even more apparent when we use the equation to generate lines from different scenarios of kill, average seedbank lifespan, and fitness (Fig. 1). We have arbitrarily started in year zero from a field frequency of something less than 10^{-10}, e.g., where resistance is inherited by a single recessive gene in a diploid weed with a resistant biotype mutation frequency of 10^{-10}. The field frequency is lower because of fitness. If we have any other initial field frequency, it is possible to move the frequency scale in Fig. 1 to fit the case, or use the right hand scale. From the slopes it is clear that we should be enriching yearly for herbicide resistance. If we follow the slopes we see that it will take many years to reach a frequency of resistants that will be noticeable, i.e., more than the 5-10% that remain anyway after a treatment (Fig. 1). Thus we will not realize that we are enriching for herbicide resistance until it is upon us. This rate of enrichment is not easy to measure, even in laboratory experiments.

The right hand scale of Fig. 1 shows that when the selection pressure is lowered, or when average seed bank longevity is longer, the lesser fitness of resistants will have a greater effect. At the low effective selection pressures of the less persistent herbicides, fitness exerts its greatest effect. Under these circumstances, differential fitness will also have its greatest mathematical effect of depressing the rate of appearance of resistance.

Various groups of scientists tried isolating resistant biotypes in experimental field trials with no success until very recently (Holliday and Putwain, 1977). It was possible though to isolate partial tolerants; e.g., Holliday and Putwain (1974), Devine et al. (1975), and Faulkner (1976). A typical case would be 90% kill of the normal strain and 50% kill of the partially tolerant strain. The selection pressure for such a situation is lower than with resistance, i.e., $\alpha = 0.5/0.1 = 5$. Thus the rate of increase of partial tolerance to herbicides should be rather slow, in seeming contradiction to the large number of reports on finding such biotypes (Appendix 1). In any genetic framework of resistance, it is expected that there will be many more individuals partially

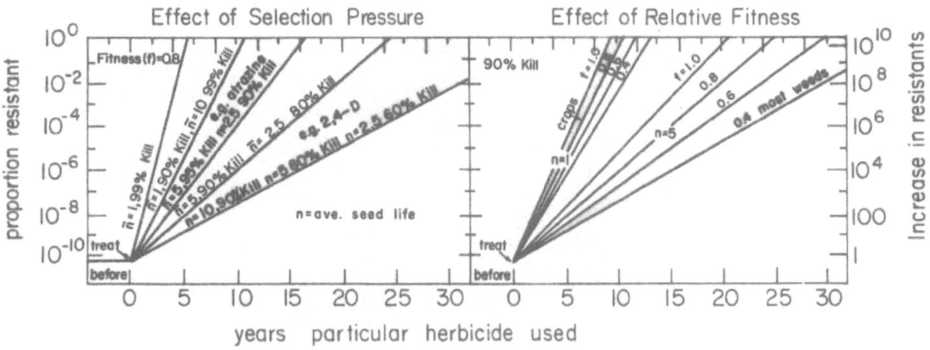

Fig. 1. The effects of various combinations of selection pressure, average soil seedbank longevity ($\bar{n}$), and fitness (f) on the rates of enrichment of herbicide resistance. Resistance would only become apparent in the field when there are more than 20% resistant plants. The scale on the right indicates the increase in resistance from any unknown initial frequency of resistants in the population, whereas the scale on the left starts from an expected frequency of a recessive monogene. (Modified from Gressel, 1978.)

tolerant than those resistant. In the model equation, this can be summarized as: Though α is lower with tolerants, N_o, the frequency of tolerants before spraying, is probably a few orders of magnitude higher than N_o for resistants.

What are we then to expect as a result of this mathematical modeling? In the left hand scale of Fig. 1 we see that in most agronomic cases we would expect resistance to occur after more than twenty years of annual spraying of the same compound and in many cases more than thirty years of spraying. Only with high selection pressures would resistance appear within ten years. This has occurred so far with only one group of herbicides, the S-triazines. S-triazines have a longer soil persistence than most herbicides (Burnside and Schultz, 1978) and are widely used. In one of the cases where resistance was found, two applications were made per year (Bandeen and McLaren, 1976). We must carefully note that S-triazine resistance has been noted in various places in the world (Fig. 2). There is a strong possibility that these are not the only places where resistance to triazine has appeared and the reports are probably a function of (at least) two factors; in those areas S-triazines are in great use and there are leading groups of weed scientists at nearby institutions. Seed and gene flow are not expected to be the important disseminators of the newly appeared resistance. It is more likely that local selection and enrichment of resistance will cause a continued popping up of the problem.

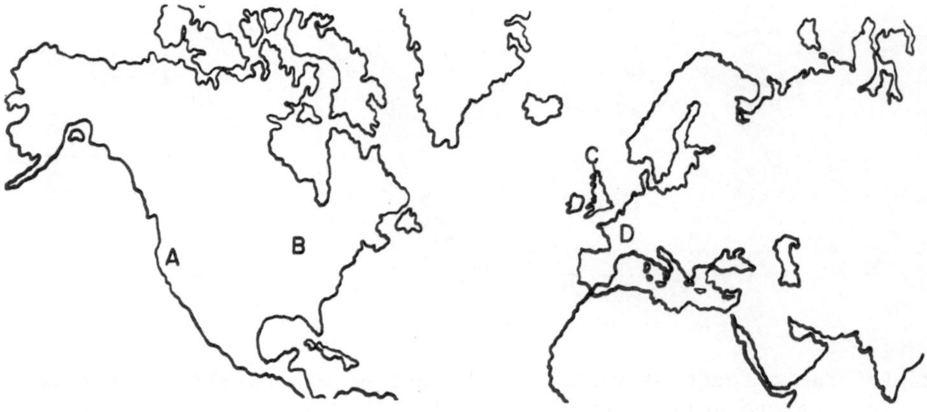

Fig. 2. The first appearances of resistance of field weeds to persistent S-triazine herbicides.
Point A--Western Washington, USA, 1968-1972; resistances of Senecio vulgaris, Amaranthus retroflexus, and Chenopodium album to atrazine. The Senecio was isolated in a nursery with an 8-year history of two atrazine applications per year and then 2 years with atrazine and simazine (Ryan, 1970; Anonymous, 1974).
Point B--Ontario, Canada, 1976; resistances in Chenopodium album in field where atrazine was used for 10 years in maize (Bandeen and McLaren, 1976). More recently Brassica campestris and Ambrosia artemisiifolia resistant to atrazine were found (Souza-Machado et al., 1978).
Point C--England; Senecio vulgaris resistant to simazine was isolated from an orchard population receiving 6 years simazine and one generation of experimental selection with simazine (Holliday and Putwain, 1977).
Point D--Montpellier, France; Echinochloa crusgalli and Setaria viridis partially tolerant (an increase from 5-30% viability) to 5 kg/ha atrazine after 9 annual treatments in vineyards (Grignac, 1975).

Thus, we may expect more and more reports of resistance to persistent herbicides over the next few years.

Senecio achieved S-triazine resistance at two locations (Fig. 2). It has a genetic limitation that in theory says this species should be slow to evolve; it is an inbreeder. Either the theory is wrong or the S-triazines indeed have a very high selection pressure. As Senecio is easily controlled by other herbicides which have been in use for longer periods, it can be presumed that selection pressure was an overriding feature in the selection for resistance.

One lesson from these mathematical games is that it would be wise, if feasible, to consider curtailing use of the high soil persistent, high selection pressure herbicides. Possibly, instead of searching for persistent formulations, the opposite should be sought. This will help prevent furthering the appearance of herbicide resistance in a twofold manner--by reducing the magnitude of selection pressure within the equation and by having a longer period of the season in which the differential fitness can be effective. The fitness differential, as detailed above, is only effective in the absence of the herbicide. If the use of persistent S-triazines is not replaced by less persistent S-triazines or other herbicides, we may soon get such widespread resistances. This will severely deplete the farmers' effective herbicide arsenal of an important group of compounds and the manufacturers of a market for all S-triazine herbicides.

It is necessary to reconsider one of the old concepts from the weed control texts which "pushed" the importance of high selection pressure. This concept has been stated as follows: "Hence herbicide applications aimed at control but not elimination are especially dangerous" (Harper, 1957). There has never been total elimination of a pest with pesticides exept in a minuscule number of cases. It must thus be decided which level of selection pressure, i.e., control, is desirable. More and more practitioners and theoreticians using pesticides, from antibiotics through insecticides, have come to the conclusion that to prevent resistance and help the patient or crop it is best to control the pest just to the level where the desired individuals can compete naturally. We should be most wary, as we have already found out in the field, of the persistent herbicides which are meant to bring about "total kill." Close to total kill may give us totally diminished returns in the not too long run, as resistance will appear more rapidly. The same wariness should be turned to the efforts to achieve slow release formulations of less persistent herbicides. There are some crops where such high persistence makes sense; those with an open type vegetation which cannot compete with weeds long into the season. The use of high persistence herbicides has caused other problems. A prime example was described by Burnside and Schultz (1978): Maize and sorghum which had to be used as fodder or plowed under because of drought in a large geographic area. The presence of residual atrazine in the soil precluded planting winter wheat in the same year.

Another problem is cross-resistance; the *Chenopodium*, *Amaranthus*, and *Senecio* with atrazine or simazine resistance were found to be resistant to all other S-triazines tested (Radosevich and Appleby, 1973; Bandeen and McLaren, 1976). This cross-resistance is quite worrisome as it means that once resistance has appeared, it is too late to switch to less persistent S-triazines. The S-triazine cross-resistance is disturbing, but we may be luckier with herbicides than farmers were with insecticides. As the various S-triazines seem to have similar modes of action, the cross-resistance between them would be expected. In insects there are selected cross-resistances to metabolically unrelated insecticides; when one appeared, all appeared. The weeds developing resistance to triazines remained susceptible to most other herbicides (cf. Jensen et al., 1977).

Long ago Abel (1954) advised that herbicides be rotated like crops. Will this prevent or delay the appearance of resistance? A similar question is what happens when we stop spraying with a herbicide? This situation is depicted in Fig. 3 where the rate of increase was calculated from the model equation, but the rate of decay of resistance was calculated on a yearly basis because of complications imposed by the soil seed bank. From the equation we see that the rate of increase in resistance is affected by the selection pressure and slightly decreased by fitness. When herbicide usage is topped, i.e., there is no longer selection pressure (α=1), the rate of disappearance of resistance is due only to fitness. This rate will be much less than the rate of increase obtained with a herbicide.

When we resume herbicide treatment with the same herbicide, we initially induce a more rapid increase which later parallels the original rate of increase (Fig. 3). Thus, if we rotate herbicides of differing groups which are not cross-resistant, we will considerably delay resistance. For example, if it would take 25 years of repeated use to attain field resistance to a given herbicide, it will take 75 years to achieve resistance if the herbicide is used every third year in rotation.

HERBICIDE MIXTURES: THEIR EFFECTS ON SELECTION

It is becoming more fashionable to use herbicide mixtures. When this is done, there is simultaneous selection for resistance to each of the herbicides in each of the susceptible weed species. This happens because each herbicide in the mixture is added to kill different weed species. These mixture groupings may be divided into two types; those where a full rate of each herbicide is used and the weed spectrum killed by each is exclusive; and those where the rates used are less than would be used alone, with the weed spectrum killed by each overlapping. The first case is easier to analyze within the model. We are just increasing the number of years in which each herbicide is used and thus achieve a greater enrichment for resistance in the weeds that each herbicide controls. Care must be taken in considering the long run necessity to do this vs. the added control one gets from the additional herbicide.

The second situation with subnormal application rates and overlapping spectra is harder to analyze within the models. Some complex mathematical models have already been suggested to help ascertain if

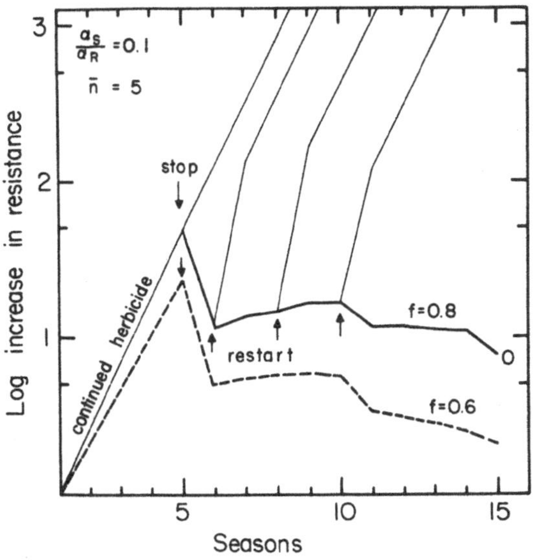

Fig. 3. The effect of stopping and restarting herbicide treatment. The ratio of resistant seeds deposited in year n to those deposited in reference year 1 is plotted, giving slopes similar to that in Fig. 1. Continual herbicide application is shown with fitnesses of 0.8 and 0.6. The lines show the decline in resistance expected when treatment is topped after year 5 (↓) and the reappearance of resistance when herbicide treatment is restarted after years 1, 3, and 5 (↑). These graphs are drawn for the case where 90% of the susceptibles are destroyed by the herbicide and none of the resistants, and where the average seed longevity is five years (reproduced from Gressel and Segel, 1978).

components of such mixtures have additive effects or synergic effects (Morse, 1978). Thus, it is not yet clear whether the lower dosages will effect a much lower selection pressure (α) for each herbicide and considerably delay appearance of resistance, possibly overweighing the effect of using the herbicide more often in a rotation. If there is a true synergy, there also exists the possibility that only plants genetically resistant to >1 herbicides will survive; this in theory will have an enormous delaying effect on the appearance of resistance. Roughly it could potentially square the number of years until resistance becomes apparent, if two herbicides are used.

HERBICIDE ROTATION AND DISCONTINUATION

When resistance is reached and the particular herbicide is no longer useful, the loss of resistance will be the same as depicted in

Fig. 3 for a stoppage part way to full resistance. There will be a slow loss of resistance but a rapid resurgence if the particular herbicide or any of its metabolic relatives are used. This is very similar to what has occurred with insects: There it has been postulated that fitness of the resistant strains increases due to interbreeding with the wild type. Thus, if we return to the long-term doomsday picture painted for the high selection pressure herbicides, we see that if resistance does become widespread, loss of the whole group of similar compounds may essentially become irrevocable, even years after use was stopped.

GERMINATION STIMULATORS AND HERBICIDE RESISTANCE

It is necessary to reassess another suggestion in the "theoretical" weed control literature. Many have suggested and looked for ways to force uniform, synchronous germination of weed seeds. This might be called the "shaving cream" strategy: "get them up so we can mow them down." If the "mowing" is done mechanically or by frost this should have little effect on the appearance of herbicide resistant weeds. If the "mowing" is to be done with a herbicide used as part of the normal herbicide rotation it may be contra-indicated. The induced germination will strongly increase the effective selection pressure of the herbicide on the species, and will only advance the time when resistance appears. In the mathematical terms of the model it means that the average span of existence in the seedbank will become $\bar{n} = 1$, with all the implications of achieving $\bar{n} = 1$ seen in Fig. 1.

HERBICIDE PROTECTANTS AND HERBICIDE RESISTANCE

There is an increasing interest in compounds which protect crops from the action of a herbicide that would otherwise be toxic. These compounds have been termed "safeners," "protectants," or (with inaccurate semantics) "antidotes," and are used to treat crops before, or along with, the herbicide application. One such compound, a diallyl diacetamide, is already marketed in combination with a thiocarbamate herbicide and others are at various stages of development. The compounds will thus broaden the utilization of some herbicides with the expected implications; there will be enrichment for resistance to those herbicides. If they are highly persistent and already used with other crops in the rotation this can obviously be detrimental in the not too long run. If the herbicides to be used have a low effective selection pressure, they will pose a far lesser problem, especially if they are to replace high persistence herbicides.

SELECTION FOR HERBICIDE RESISTANCE IN CROPS

The number of selective herbicides available is both finite and small, especially when compared to the number of crops. All too often there is not a good match between a crop, the weeds attacking it, and an economical selective herbicide. The expense of developing new herbicides seems almost prohibitive but the costs of obtaining permission to use a known and used herbicide on other crops are not nearly as large. For these reasons it would be useful to select for herbicide resistant strains in many crops. Differential tolerance to pesticides has been noted in crops as well as in weeds (Appendix 1) and is often a factor in choosing varieties for use with some herbicides. Karim and Bradshaw (1968) have noted "there is no good reason why the improvement of herbicide resistance of crop plants should not be undertaken." Because of the slowness of enrichment for herbicide resistance imposed by the fitness and selection pressure, one may arrive at the opposite conclusion. With crops the problem of "fitness" should be marginal; crop species have been so heavily selected for, for so long, they already are quite naturally "unfit" except in the highly artificial "cultural" environments where they are grown. Anyway they are not usually grown in mixed intraspecific combinations. Thus, herbicide resistance should hardly decrease this lack of fitness in a crop species, in its crop environment. Conversely, the homozygosity of crops may pose a problem if we can extrapolate from insects; there was a relative ineffectiveness of selection for insecticide resistance within inbred lines (cf. Crow, 1960). This would be especially severe where resistance is a multigenic quantitative effect.

It is a greater problem to find ways of exerting sufficient selection pressure to obtain resistance, and this is probably the reason for the fact that there seems to be but one report of successful selection for herbicide tolerance in a crop (Faulkner, 1976). The pasture grass *Lolium temulentum* is somewhat tolerant to treatments with paraquat. Faulkner took a population that had already undergone repeated paraquat treatment over several years and then performed recurrent selection (J. F. Faulkner, personal communication, 1978). He thus achieved sufficient resistance such that subnormal rates of paraquat can be used to severely inhibit other unwanted species within a pasture while allowing the *Lolium* to expand (Faulkner, 1976). This could be done despite the low level of multigenic hereditability of the paraquat tolerance (Faulkner, 1974a). The differences in susceptibility seem not to be at the level of uptake, translocation, distribution, or metabolism of paraquat (Harvey et al., 1978) but to activities of enzymes which may detoxify the toxic products of paraquat action (Harper and Harvey, 1978). It should be easier to select resistance for the more persistent herbicides, but there are pervading agronomic and ecological reasons (described above) not to consider this type of compound. Even with high selection pressures, no loss of fitness, and no seedbank, it will still take a long time (Fig. 1) and large populations of plants to test over substantial areas of field to select for complete resistance in a sensitive crop. If even 99% kill could be used and 10^{12} plants are sprayed, you are left with seed from 10^{10} plants to test the following season, clearly a prohibitive amount. There are pervading reasons to consider the use of in vitro cell culture systems to select for resistance. They have been used with a modicum of success for studies of pesticide metabolism (cf. reviews by Sandermann et al., 1977 and Gressel et al., 1978), toxicity, and screening (cf. review by Gressel et al., 1978). In a series of studies we have shown that cell cultures are not homogeneously affected by herbicides as might be presumed, but if judicious use is made of systems, cell cultures do mirror plants in their response to herbicides (cf. Gressel et al., 1978). There are a variety of reasons to prefer the use of cell cultures over field selection or classical genetic means with whole plants. The selection pressure which we can impose in the field can rarely be made to exceed 90-95% kill; the vast majority of plants remaining are "escapees." Increasing the dose rate in the field hardly increases kill of susceptible plants but may be lethal to the few truly resistant plants among the escapees. The possibility of greater uniformity of application to cells in culture should vastly reduce the number of "escapees." Another advantage of cultures is that if we start out with a given variety in culture, upon regeneration of plants we should return (in theory) to that same variety. If we select for a resistant cell line, we should still be able to return to that same variety. If the resistant gene(s) was/were recessive, then no additional genetic crossing should be necessary. If resistance is dominant then a few crosses are needed to check for homozygosity. Multigenic inheritance would cause considerable additional work under <u>any</u> method of selection. With good reason it is fashionable to want to select for mutants in haploid cultures; the frequency of monogenic recessive mutants is squared compared to diploids. Using haploid <u>Nicotiana sylvestris</u> suspensions, a strain resistant to 1 mM, 2,4-D was isolated (Zenk, 1974). As appealing as haploids may be, for the purpose of crop selection they are undesirable since upon regeneration you would get a homozygous plant quite unlike the parent variety, necessitating a great amount of "classical" breeding to transfer the desirable genes. The usefulness of mutagens to increase the frequency of resistant mutations can also be questioned. There is a strong possibility that many resulting resistants will have received more than one "hit" and will have other undesirable features. Mutagenesis was used only in one case (Aviv and Galun, 1977), reflecting either lack of efficacy or conservatism on the part of other researchers. There is good reason to believe that herbicide resistance can be selected for using diploid cell cultures, and the first evidence for this is just arriving (see Appendix 1). An example of a typical case is presented in Fig. 4. Here we see the possibility of isolating a strain of cells from carrot lines which

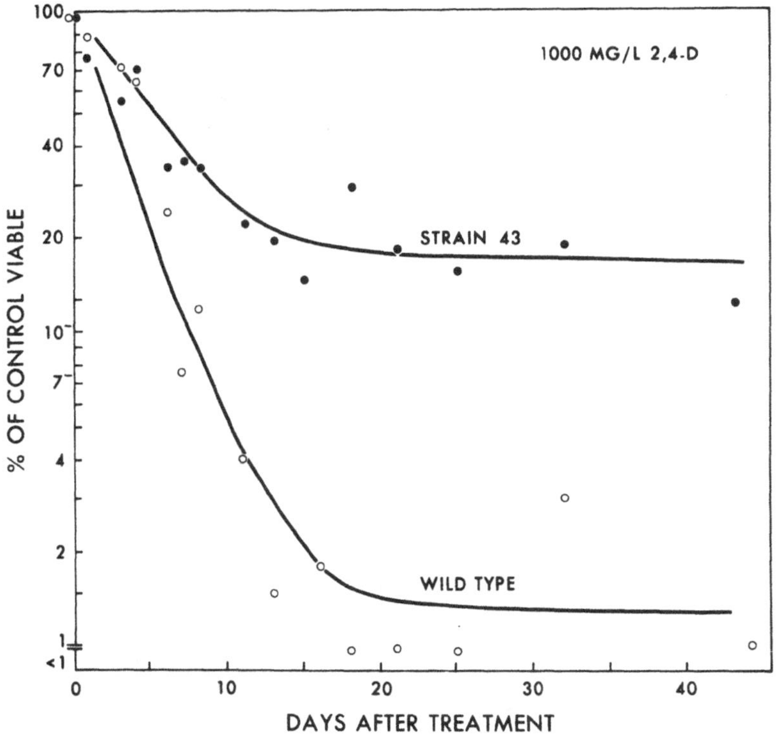

Fig. 4. The isolation of a herbicide tolerant strain of carrot by cell culture techniques; viability following a supralethal dose of 2,4-D. Calli of Daucus carota were isolated from roots and subcultured on solid media, and later suspended in liquid media. Suspension cultures were treated for 3 hours with 4 X 10^{-3}M, 2,4,D, rinsed with fresh medium, and then plated on solid medium. The few resulting calli were separately suspended and the suspension cultures retreated with 2,4-D, rinsed, and plated. The data in this figure show the viability of the wild type and of one resistant strain in suspension culture following four treatments, rinses, and resuspension in liquid medium. Viability was checked with fluorescein diacetate according to Widholm (1972). The drawbacks of this staining procedure are described in Zilkah and Gressel (1978). These data are from an unpublished experimental series by J. Gressel and N. Cohen.

could partially withstand a dose 100 times greater than the wild type. This type strain, to be useful, must be regenerated into plants, and seedlings developing from seeds of selfed plants must also be resistant. Other groups have achieved a modicum of success with diploid cultures: atrazine resistant soybean suspensions (Zenk, 1974) and carboxin (a fungicide) resistant tobacco calli (really a haploid of an amphidiploid) (Polacco and Polacco, 1977). Further, partial toleration has been observed in clones of suspensions exposed to phenoxy herbicides (Oswald et al., 1977), and tobacco calli are partially tolerant to amitrole (Barg and Umiel, 1977). Finally tobacco protoplasts are somewhat tolerant to propham (Aviv and Galun, 1977). To our knowledge most of these cases have not been successfully carried through a sexual cycle. Carboxin resistance has been carried through seeds to calli, though it is not clear if the seedlings had enhanced carboxin resistance (Polacco, personal communication). The full circle of isolation of herbicide resistance using cell cultures and regeneration of resistant plants has been achieved by Chaleff and Parsons (1978). They isolated picloram resistant tobacco cells and the resistance carried through to seedlings from seed of regenerated plants. The segregation of selfed plants was indicative of a single dominant gene which they estimated as having a frequency of about 10^{-5} in the _Nicotiana_ cell line they used.

Whereas brute selection without haploidization or mutagens may be considered by users of cell culture techniques to be "unsophisticated," there are sophisticated methods that should be of value. It may be well worth considering using methods of somatic hybridization by protoplast fusion, especially when the desired trait cannot be transferred because of incompatibility or when it is cytoplasmic. In the latter case all the necessary backcrosses are precluded. A possible case in point might well be the case of plastid inherited atrazine resistance in _Brassica campestris_ noted by Souza-Machado et al. (1978). It is conceivable that this cytoplasmic genome may be transferred to various _Brassica_ crops without deleterious effects, conferring S-triazine resistance upon them. Other potential uses of protoplast fusion for crop improvement have been well reviewed by Galun and Aviv (1978).

Care must be taken in choosing the species and the correct "multi-homogeneous" cell type for selection of resistants. There are many more species in culture than can be reproducibly regenerated into reproducing plants. More work on propagation from cells will be needed. At the cell level, the use of white calli for isolating resistance to a herbicide known to act primarily (i.e., at its lowest inhibitory concentration) on photosynthesis would seem misconceived. Equally misconceived would be to try to use cell cultures to isolate mutants to herbicides whose known mechanism of selectivity is based on a morphological barrier. Considering the possibilities for genetic drift occurring in cultures it might be wise to use recently isolated cells if we wish to return to our original variety. Still, there is great potential in using cell cultures for isolating genetically resistant varieties, a technique requiring far less effort and cost than selecting for resistance in the field.

REFERENCES

Abel, A. L., 1954, The rotation of weed killers, in: "Proceedings of the 2nd British Weed Control Conference," British Weed Control Council.
Anonymous, 1967, Report of the First Session of the FAO Working Party of Experts on Resistance of Pests to Pesticides, FAO Public PL/1965/18.
Anonymous, 1974, Weeds Today, 5:14.
Antonovics, J., 1971, The effects of a heterogeneous environment on the genetics of natural populations, Amer. Sci., 59:593-599.
Antonovics, J., and Bradshaw, A. D., 1970, Evolution in closely adjacent plant populations. VIII. Clinal patterns at a mine boundary, Heredity, 25:349-362.
Arntzen, C. J., 1978, in: "Proceedings 18th Meeting Weed Science Society of America Abstracts," No. 164, p. 75.
Aviv, D., and Galun, E., 1977, Isolation of tobacco protoplasts in the presence of isopropyl N-phenylcarbamate and their culture and regeneration into plants, Z. Pflanzenphysiol., 83:267-273.
Baker, H. G., 1974, The evolution of weeds, Ann. Rev. Ecol. Systemat., 5:1-24.
Bandeen, J. D., and McLaren, R. D., 1976, Resistance of Chenopodium album to triazine herbicides, Can. J. Plant Sci., 56:411-412.
Barg, R., and Umiel, N., 1977, Development of tobacco seedlings callus cultures in the presence of amitrole, Z. Pflanzenphysiol., 83:437-447.
Burnside, O. C., and Schultz, M. E., 1978, Soil persistence of herbicide for corn, sorghum, and soybeans during the year of application, Weed Sci., 26:108-115.
Chaleff, R. S., and Parsons, M. F., 1978, Direct selection in vitro for herbicide-resistant mutants of Nicotiana tabacum, Proc. Natl. Acad. Sci., USA, 75:5104-5107.
Comstock, V. E., and Andersen, R. N., 1968, An inheritance study of tolerance to atrazine in the cross of flax (Linum usitatissimum L.), Crop Sci., 8:508-509.
Conard, S. G., and Radosevich, S. R., 1979, J. Ecol., in press.
Costa, J., and Appleby, A. P., 1976, Response of two yellow nutsedge varieties to three herbicides, Weed Sci., 24:54-58.
Crow, J. F., 1960, Genetics of insecticide resistance: General considerations, in: "Research Progress on Insect Resistance," Misc. Public. Entom. Soc. Amer., 2:69-74.
Devine, T. E., Seaney, R. R., Linscott, D. L., Hagin, R. D., and Brace, N., 1975, Results of breeding for tolerance to 2,4-D in birdseed trefoil, Crop Sci., 15:721-724.
Ellis, M., and Kay, Q. O. N., 1975, Genetic variation in herbicide resistance in scentless mayweed (Tripleurospermum indorum (L.)

Schultz Bip.). III. Selection for increased resistance to ioxynil 4-chloro-2-methylphenoxyacetic acid and simazine, Weed Res., 15:327-333.

Faulkner, J. S., 1974a, Heritability of paraquat tolerance in Lolium perenne L., Euphytica, 23:281-288.

Faulkner, J. S., 1974b, The effect of dalapon on thirty-five cultivars of Lolium perenne, Weed Res., 14:405-413.

Faulkner, J. S., 1976, A paraquat resistant variety of Lolium perenne under field conditions, in: "Proceedings of the 1976 British Crop Protection Conference," Weeds, Vol. 2, British Crop Protection Council.

Fryer, J. D., and Evans, S. A., eds., 1968, "Weed Control Handbook, Vol. 1, Principles," 5th ed., Blackwell Scientific, Oxford.

Galun, E., and Aviv, D., 1978, Newsletter; Intl. Assoc. Plant Tissue Culture, No. 25, pp. 2-5.

Gressel, J., 1978, Outlook in Agric., in press.

Gressel, J., and Holm, L. G., 1964, Chemical inhibition of crop germination by weed seeds and the nature of inhibition by Abutilon theophrasti, Weed Res., 4:44-53.

Gressel, J., and Segel, L. A., 1978, J. Theor. Biol., in press.

Gressel, J., Zilkah, A., and Ezra, G., 1978, in: "Proceedings of the Fourth International Plant Tissue Culture Congress," T. A. Thorpe, ed., Univ. of Calgary Press, Calgary.

Grignac, P., 1974, Selection of a biotype of annual grass (Poa annus L.) resistant to metoxuron by repetition of herbicide treatments, C.R. Acad. Agric. (France), 60:401-408.

Grignac, P., 1975, Status and Control of Grassweeds in Europe, in: "Proceedings of European Weed Research Society Symposium."

Grogan, C. O., Eastin, E. F., and Palmer, R. D., 1963, Inheritance of susceptability of a line of maize to simazine and atrazine, Crop Sci., 3:451.

Haldane, J. B. S., 1960, More precise expressions for: The cost of natural selection, J. Genet., 57:351-360.

Harper, D. B., and Harvey, B. M. R., 1978, Plant Cell Envir., in press.

Harper, J. L., 1957, Outlook in Agric., 1:197.

Harper, J. L., 1960, in: "The Biology of Weeds," J. L. Harper, ed., Blackwell Scientific, Oxford.

Harvey, B. M. R., Muldoon, J., and Harper, D. B., 1978, Plant Cell Envir., in press.

Hayes, R. M., and Wax, L. M., 1975, Differential intraspecific responses of soybean cultivars to bentazon, Weed Sci., 23:516-521.

Holliday, R. J., and Putwain, P. D., 1974, Variation in the susceptability to simazine in three species of annual weeds, in: "Proceedings of the 12th British Weed Control Conference, British Weed Control Council.

Holliday, R. J., and Putwain, P. D., 1977, Evolution of resistance to simazine in Senecio vulgaris L., Weed Res., 17:291-296.

Holm, L. G., and Pluckett, D. L., Pancho, J. K., and Hershberger, J. P., 1977, "The World's Worst Weeds: Distribution and Biology," Univ. of Hawaii Press, Honolulu.
Hunter, J. H., and Smith, L. W., 1972, Environment and herbicide effects on Canada thistle ecotypes, Weed Sci., 20:163-167.
Inwang, E. E., Khan, M. A. Q., and Brown, A. W. A., 1967, DDT-resistance in West African and Asian strains of Aedes aegypti L., Bull. Wld. Hlth. Org., 36:409-421.
Isenee, A. R., Shaw, W. C., Genter, W. A., Swanson, C. R., Turner, B. C., and Woolson, E. A., 1973, Revegetation following massive application of selected herbicides, Weed Sci., 21:409-412.
Jensen, K. I. N., Bandeen, J. D., and Souza-Machado, V., 1977, Studies on the differential tolerance of two lamb's-quarters selections to triazine herbicides, Can. J. Plant Sci., 57: 1169-1178.
Karim, A., and Bradshaw, A. D., 1968, Genetic variation in simazine resistance in wheat, rape and mustard, Weed Res., 8:283-291.
Kochba, J., Spiegel-Roy, P., and Saad, S., 1978, Mutations in vegetatively propagated plants, IAEA Bull., in press.
McNeilly, T., 1968, Closely adjacent plant populations. III. Agrostis tenuis on a small copper mine, Heredity, 23:99-108.
Miles, C. D., 1976, Selection of diquat resistance photosynthesis mutants from maize, Plant Physiol., 57:284-285.
Miller, F. R., and Bovey, R. W., 1969, Tolerance of Sorghum bicolor (L.) Moench. to several herbicides, Agron. J., 61:282-285.
Morse, P. M., 1978, Some comments on the assessment of joint action in herbicide mixtures, Weed Sci., 26:58-71.
Nalewaja, J. D., and Bothun, R. E., 1969, Response of flax to post-emergence herbicides, Crop Sci., 9:160-162.
Narsaiah, D. B., and Harvey, R. G., 1977, Differential responses of corn inbreds and hybrids to alachlor, Crop Sci., 17:657-659.
Newman, J. F., 1957, Resistance to insecticides, Outlook in Agric., 1:235-239.
Ogawa, J. M., Gilpatrick, J. D., and Chiarappa, L., 1977, FAO Plant Protection Bull., 25:97.
Oliver, L. R., and Schrieber, M. M., 1971, Differential selectivity of herbicides on six Setaria taxa, Weed Sci., 19:428-431.
Osgood, R. V., Romanowski, R. R., and Hilton, H. W., 1972, Differential tolerance of Hawaiian sugarcane cultivars to diuron, Weed Sci., 20:537-539.
Oswald, T. H., Smith, A. E., and Phillips, D. V., 1977, Herbicide tolerance developed in cell suspension cultures of perennial white cloves, Can. J. Bot., 55:1351.
Polacco, J. C., and Polacco, M. L., 1977, Producing and selecting valuable mutation in plant cell culture, a tobacco mutant resistant to carboxin, Ann. N.Y. Acad. Sci., 287:385-400.
Radosevich, S. R., and Appleby, A. P., 1973, Relative susceptability of two common groundsel (Senecio vulgaris L.) biotypes to six s-triazines, Agron. J., 65:553-555.

Roberts, H. A., and Dawkins, P. A., 1967, Effect of cultivation on the numbers of viable weed seeds in soil, Weed Res., 7:290-301.
Roché, Jr., B. F., and Musik, T. J., 1964, Ecological and physiological study of Enchinochloa crusgalli (L.) Beauv. and the response of its biotypes to sodium 2,2-dichlorophospionate, Agron. J., 56:155-160.
Rochecouste, E., 1962, Studies on the biotypes of Cynodon dactylon (L.) Pers. II. Growth response to trichloroacetic and 2,2-dichloropropionic acids, Weed Res., 2:136-145.
Ryan, G. F., 1970, Resistance of common groundsel to simazine and atrazine, Weed Sci., 18:614-616.
Sandermann, H., Diesperger, H., and Scheel, D., 1977, Metabolism of xenobiotics by plant cell cultures, in: "Plant Tissue Culture and Its Bio-technological Application," W. Barz, E. Reinhard, and M. H. Zenk, eds., Springer-Verlag, Berlin, Heidelberg, New York.
Schooler, A. B., Bell, A. R., and Nalewaja, J. D., 1972, Inheritance of siduron tolerance in foxtail barley, Weed Sci., 20:167-169.
Sexsmith, J. J., 1964, Morphological and herbicide susceptability difference among strains of hoary cress, Weed Sci., 12:19-22.
Souza-Machado, V., Bandeen, J. D., Stephenson, G. R., and Lavigne, P., 1978, Can. J. Plant Sci., in press.
Wedderspoon, I. M., and Burt, G. W., 1974, Growth and development of three johnson grass selections, Weed Sci., 22:319-322.
Whitehead, C. W., and Switzer, C. M., 1963, The differential response of strains of wild carrot to 2,4-D and related herbicides, Can. J. Plant Sci., 43:255-262.
Whitworth, J. W., 1964, The reaction of strains of field birdseed to 2,4-D, Weeds, 12:57-58.
Widholm, J. M., 1972, The use of fluorescein diacetate and phenosafranine for determining viability of cultured plant cells, Stain Tech., 47:189-194.
Zenk, M. H., 1974, Haploids in physiological and biochemical research, in: "Haploids in Higher Plants: Advances and Potentials," K. J. Kasha, ed., Univ. of Guelph, Guelph, Canada.
Zilkah, S., and Gressel, J., 1978, Differential inhibition by dikegulac of dividing and stationary cells in in vitro cultures, Planta, 42:281-285.

Appendix 1. Appearance of Genetic Tolerance and Resistance to Herbicides

Herbicide[1]	Species	Type of Tolerance[2]	Notes	Reference[3]
PHENOLS	None reported			
BENZONITRILES				
ioxynil	*Tripleurospermum inodorum*	diff. tolerance	Found with natural variations	1
THIOCARBONYLS	None reported			
QUATERNARY AMMONIUMS				
paraquat	*Lolium perenne*	diff. tolerance	Selected from strain differences	2
diquat	*Zea mays*	resistant	Artifically selected albino	3
PHENOXY ACIDS				
MCPA	*Tripleurospermum inodorum*	diff. tolerance	Found with natural variation	1
	Linum usitatissimum	diff. tolerance	Varietal differences	4
2,4-D	*Cardaria chalapensis*	diff. tolerance	Strain differences in nature	5
	Citrus sinensis	diff. tolerance	Selected in callus cultures	6
	Cirsium arvense	diff. tolerance	Clonal ecotypes	7
	Convolvulus arvensis	diff. tolerance	Clonal differences	8
	Cyperus esculentus	diff. tolerance	Varietal differences	9
	Daucus carota (wild)	diff. tolerance	Biotype variations	10
	Daucus carota (cultivated)	resistant	Selected in cell cultures	11
	Lotus corniculatus	diff. tolerance	Repeated field selection	12
	Nicotiana sylvestris	resistant	Selection in haploid tissue cultures	13
	Saccharum L.	diff. tolerance	Clonal differences	14
	Trifolium repens	diff. tolerance	Selected in cell cultures, resistant to other phenotypes	15
BENZOIC ACIDS				
TBA	*Cardaria chalepensis*	diff. tolerance	Strain differences in nature	5
dicamba	*Cirsium arvense*	diff. tolerance	Clone ecotypes	7

Appendix 1. (con't)

Herbicide[1]	Species	Type of Tolerance[2]	Notes	Reference[3]
HALOGENATED ALIPHATICS				
dalapon	Cynodon dactylon	diff. tolerance	Biotype variation	16
	Echinochloa crusgalli	diff. tolerance	Biotype differences	17
	Saccharum L.	diff. tolerance	Clonal variations	14
	Setaria	diff. tolerance		18
	Sorghum halapense	diff. tolerance	Ecotype variations	19
	Lolium perenne	diff. tolerance	Cultivar variations	35
TCA	Cynodon dactylon	diff. tolerance	Biotype differences	16
CARBAMATES AND THIOCARBAMATES				
propham	Nicotiana tabacum	diff. tolerance	Selected in isolated protoplasts	20
AMIDES				
propachlor	Sorghum bicolor	diff. tolerance	Found among 40 varieties	21
alachlor	Zea mays	diff. tolerance	Found in inbred lines and hybrids	22
UREAS				
diuron	Saccharum L. cvs.	diff. tolerance	Clonal types	14
linuron and norea	Sorghum bicolor	diff. tolerance	Found among 40 varieties	21
siduron	Hordeum jubatum	diff. tolerance	Biotype differences controlled by three dominant genes	23
metoxuron	Poa annua	diff. tolerance	Artificially selected	24
DIAZINES				
bentazon	Glycine max	diff. tolerance		25
TRIAZINES (note: species tolerant to one S-triazine are usually tolerant to others)				
simazine	Brassica napa	diff. tolerance	Varietal responses	26
	Capsella bursa pastoris	diff. tolerance	Response related to number of repeated treatments	27 27
	Chenopodium album	diff. tolerance	Response related to number of repeated treatments	27
	Senecio vulgaris	diff. tolerance	Response related to number of repeated treatments	27
	Sinapis alba	diff. tolerance	Varietal difference	26
	Tripleurospermum inodorum	diff. tolerance	Wide natural variation	1
	Triticum aestivum	diff. tolerance	Varietal difference	26

Appendix 1. (con't)

Herbicide[1]	Species	Type of Tolerance[2]	Notes	Reference[3]
atrazine	Amaranthus retroflexus	resistant	Field strains	28
	Ambrosia artemisiifolia	resistant	Field	29
	Brassica campestris	resistant	Field	29
	Chenopodium album	resistant	10 year repeated treatment in maize	30
	Cyperus esculentus	diff. tolerance	Varietal differences	9
	Echinochloa crusgalli	diff. tolerance	5 repeated treatments	31
	Glycine max	resistant	Selected in cell cultures	13
	Linum usitatissimum	diff. tolerance	Quantitatively inherited	32
	Senecio vulgaris	resistant	10 years repeated treatment in nursery	33
	Setaria sp.	diff. tolerance	In repeatedly sprayed vineyard (31)	18,31
propazine	Sorghum bicolor	diff. tolerance	Among 40 varieties	21
MISCELLANEOUS				
amitrole	Cirsium arvense	diff. tolerance	Clonal ecotypes	7
picloram	Nicotiana tabacum	resistant	Selected in cell cultures	34

[1]Common names of herbicides according to Weed Science Society of America or British Standards Institute. The groupings used in Fryer and Evans, 1968 are used in this table.

[2]Resistance is complete tolerance to a herbicide rate normally used. Anything less is differential tolerance (Anonymous, 1967). In some cases this was hard to determine from the published data.

[3]References: 1. Ellis and Kay (1975) 2. Faulkner (1976) 3. Miles (1976) 4. Nalewaja and Bothun (1969) 5. Sexsmith (1964) 6. Kochba et al. (1978) 7. cf. Hunter and Smith (1972) 8. Whitworth (1964) 9. Costa and Appleby (1976) 10. Whitehead and Switzer (1963) 11. Gressel and Cohen, unpub. (see Fig. 4) 12. Devine et al. (1975) 13. Zenk (1974) 14. cf. Osgood et al. (1972) 15. Oswald et al. (1977) 16. Rochecouste (1962) 17. Roché and Musik (1964) 18. Oliver and Schrieber (1971) 19. Wedderspoon and Burt (1974) 20. Aviv and Galun (1977) 21. Miller and Bovey (1969) 22. Narsaiah and Harvey (1977) 23. Schooler et al. (1972) 24. Grignac (1974) 25. cf. Hayes and Wax (1975) 26. Karim and Bradshaw (1968) 27. Holliday and Putwain (1977) 28. Anonymous (1974) 29. cf. Souza-Machado et al. (1978) 30. Bandeen and McLaren (1976) 31. Grignac (1975) 32. Comstock and Andersen (1968) 33. Ryan (1970) 34. Chaleff and Parsons (1978) 35. Faulkner (1974b).

7

THE PROBLEM OF PLANT BREEDERS

G. M. Simpson, R. C. Durley, T. Kannangara, and D. G. Stout

University of Saskatchewan
Saskatoon, Saskatchewan, Canada

The art of plant breeding, particularly successful in the last one hundred years, but nevertheless several thousand years old, relies essentially on the identification of superior traits in individuals. These individuals are either removed from the general population and multiplied to constitute a new population with superior attributes or crossed to other plants to combine specific characteristics which are desirable from an agronomic or utilization perspective.

Perhaps the two most important practical difficulties associated with improving any specific crop species are the identification of selection indexes and the long time-scale to select or recombine desirable indexes.

For example, in the self-pollinated crops such as rice, wheat, barley, oats, and rye the production of a superior new variety with any one of the characteristics of higher yield, disease resistance, more efficient morphology, earliness of flowering, or resistance to lodging is likely to take anywhere from 12 to 15 years (Table 1). Parents with desirable characteristics are first crossed and combinations of desirable traits are recovered in the homozygous form by selection through about fifteen generations (Briggs and Knowles, 1967). Backcrossing can speed up the process for some traits. The guesswork that underpins plant breeding is aptly described by one plant breeder:

"Without the perceptivity born of thorough knowledge of the crop, it is doubtful whether the visual evaluation necessary in the early generations of a pedigree program can be successful in identifying the infrequent valuable types that most hybrid

Table 1. The Numbers of Generations and Plants Selected in the Pedigree Method of Breeding[1]

	Number Grown		Number Selected	
	Plants	Lines	Plants	Lines
F_1	50		50	
F_2	5,000		250	
F_3		250	125	50
F_4		125	90	40
F_5		90	80	35
F_6		80		15
F_7		15		4
F_{8-10}		4		1
F_{11-12}		1		1

[1]After Briggs and Knowles, 1967.

combinations are capable of producing by segregation. . . . Conditions necessary for the expression of the genetic characteristics must be present" (Allard, 1960).

Hybrids, from cross- or self-pollinated crops, generally require identification of specific traits in the homozygous parents. Most frequently yield characteristics which when combined confer hybrid vigor on the first generation heterozygote. The increased vigor declines rapidly in the general population in successive generations; an example is corn.

In cross-pollinated species, such as most forage crops which would include many grasses and legumes, there is also great difficulty in identifying desirable parameters and also in fixing them permanently as a superior population. The time-scale for producing a new cultivar can be of the same order as for self-pollinated species but is often as long as twenty years. The main method is to devise a selection grid of characteristics for a specific environment such as high leaf area and dry matter, disease resistance, prolonged seasonal growth, high protein for animal feed, etc. The key index or "sieve" is ultimately the

Table 2. Minimum Sampling Numbers to Identify a Spectrum of Hormone Changes in Leaves of Drought-Stressed *Sorghum bicolor*

Identification Step		Total Number of Samples
3 leaf positions (young, intermediate, old)		3
3 positions along a single leaf		9
3 replications		27
2 cultivars		54
Control versus stress environment		108
3 arbitrary stages of the life cycle		316
4 hormones (a cytokinin, auxin, abscisin, and gibberellin)		1,264
Diurnal study (2-hour intervals)	Minimum	288
	Maximum	15,168

gravimetric balance to select high yield. Desirable parents are allowed to cross-fertilize in a polycross block and the bulked progeny constitute the new "mixed" variety. Such a variety will lose the superior traits through outcrossing from wind and insect pollination. There is thus a need for continuous release of new selections to maintain a steady level of improved forage production.

The central practical problem for plant breeders using any of the above approaches is the technique of sieving out the one, dozen, or fifty plants, with desirable traits, from the tens or hundreds of thousands of individuals that constitute the population. With the exception of final yield of grain, the attribute measured in the plant which is used as the selection index must be a measurement that does not destroy the plant. This would prevent seed production and thus the establishment of the next generation. The half-seed technique used for selecting superior oil-producing genotypes in rapeseed (Downey and Harvey, 1963; Harvey and Downey, 1963) is a nice example of selection early in the life cycle without preventing normal growth and seed production of each generation.

Because of the practical difficulties of using selection indexes, the single main tool of the plant breeder has been the gravimetric balance to measure yield, either of grain or forage. Probably the second selection tool has been the artificial disease epidemic to select disease resistance. Despite considerable improvement in the last twenty-five years of our physiological knowledge about the contribution of plant architecture to superior yield, plant breeders have not been able to adopt indexes such as high leaf area index, high net assimilation rates, or vertically oriented leaves in cereals as selection criteria because the techniques of measurement

Table 3. Plant and Environment Parameters Correlated with Changes in Hormones of Sorghum bicolor

Plant Measurements	Environment Measurements
Leaf characters	Temperature
- area and length	Relative humidity
- water content	Soil moisture potential
- water potential (ψw)	Applied soil moisture
- osmotic potential (ψs)	Net radiation
- pressure potential (ψp)	Pan evaporation
- ionic conductivity	CO_2 exchange
- stomatal density	
- diffusive resistance	
- leaf temperature	
- senescence:	
area	
chlorophyll content	
Plant height and weight	
Grain yield	
Inflorescence length	
Anther development	

are too time-consuming and expensive on a field scale. In practical terms it is still much easier for a plant breeder to select higher yielding plants at random from a population by measuring only the yield of grain than to measure and combine desirable physiological traits which could produce a photosynthetically more effective plant.

The extreme difficulty in plant breeding is reached in selecting for such important, but general, attributes as "cold resistance" or "drought resistance." A physiological description of drought resistance (Levitt, 1972) will include the notions of drought avoidance and drought tolerance. Avoidance can be achieved variously by increased root growth, earlier maturation, premature reduction in leaf area by leaf senescence, or reduced evapotranspiration through leaf-rolling and stomatal closure (Stout and Simpson, 1978). On the other hand tolerance of drought stress may be effected by osmoregulation, differentiation, and development of plasmatic resistance (Kaul and Crowle, 1971; Stout et al., 1978). Our current understanding of cold resistance can be described in similar terms as drought resistance (Burke et al., 1976); e.g., avoidance of ice crystal formation, with its associated dehydration and physical damage, and tolerance to dehydration. Salinity resistance has similar attributes of avoidance and tolerance (Flowers et al., 1977; Levitt, 1972).

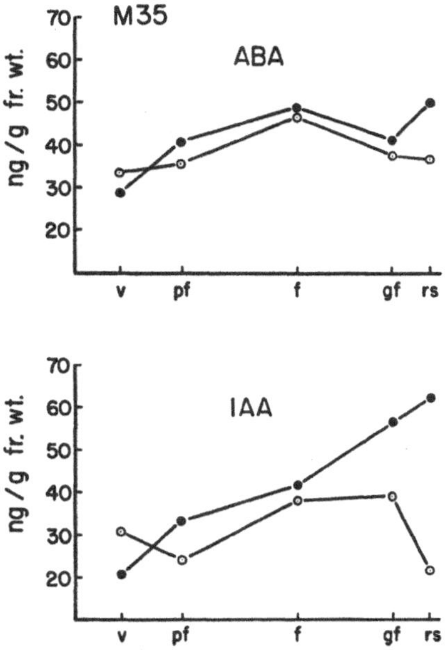

Fig. 1. Levels of abscisic acid (ABA) and 3-indoleacetic acid (IAA) during the life cycle of a sorghum cultivar (M35). 0-0 = control; x-x = drought stressed. Phases of growth: v - vegetative, pf - preflowering, f - flowering, gf - grain filling, rs - recovery from stress following irrigation.

In the case of cold, salinity, and drought resistance there is a complex of attributes in the plant that confers both productivity potential and survival at various stages of the life cycle. Seen from both a physiological and genetic perspective crop yield is the result of a complex series of events involving the interaction of a specific genotype with a specific environment. Unfortunately, while a single measurement of weight at the termination of the life cycle can signify yield, there are no single or even simple indexes which will signify drought or cold resistance. Ideally, a plant breeder needs some simple mechanical, electronic, or chemical instrument that can be taken as a "magic box" into the field, held over a plant (preferably at the seedling stage or earlier), and which then gives a signal to accept or reject the plant for each of the desirable attributes to be incorporated into a new cultivar.

Both physiological and genetic understanding of drought and cold resistance in crop plants suggests that it is improbable that any single parameter can predict, say, drought tolerance, in a particular genotype. Nevertheless, for practical reasons, it is desirable to have as small a number of indexes as possible which collectively constitute the plant breeder's sieve. In our laboratory we have been

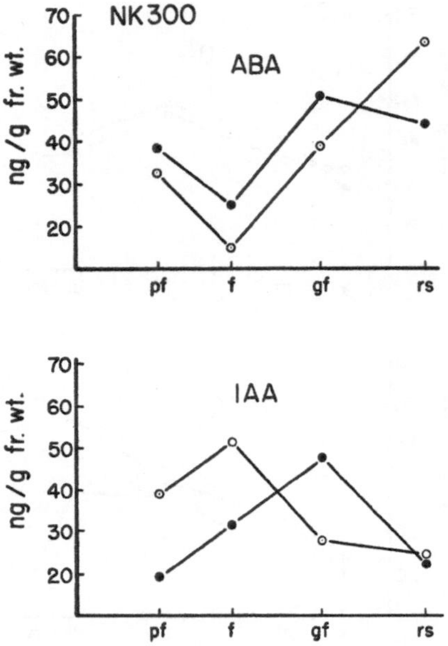

Fig. 2. Levels of abscisic acid (ABA) and 3-indoleacetic acid (IAA) during the life cycle of a sorghum cultivar (NK300). 0-0 = control; x-x = drought stressed. Phases of growth: v - vegetative, pf - preflowering, f - flowering, gf-grain filling, rs - recovery from stress following irrigation.

approaching the problem of selection for drought resistance in Sorghum bicolor by investigating the possibility of using a spectrum of endogenous plant hormones as the predictor of genotypic response to drought stress.

From the outset of this study we have been faced with certain stringent objectives to ensure that the analytical procedures developed are consistent with the basic requirements of a practical plant breeding program where large populations of plants are grown in field conditions. Examples of these restrictions are:

(1) Hormone analysis must be made on a part of a single plant, without destroying seed production.

(2) The method must be simple enough to use on hundreds of individual plants in a short time span.

(3) The analytical procedures should be suited for automation under the supervision of technicians who do not need high levels of technical training.

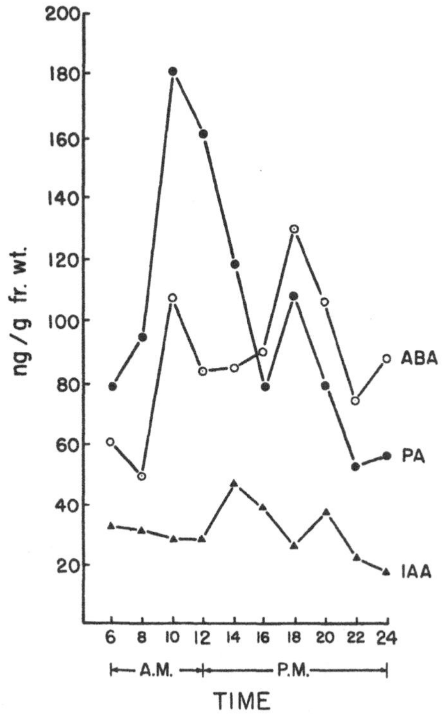

Fig. 3. Diurnal fluctuations in the leaves of sorghum of three endogenous hormones, abscisic acid (ABA), phaseic acid (PA), and 3-indoleacetic acid (IAA).

(4) The analytical procedures should permit adequate replication at all levels.

(5) Instrumentation should be inexpensive and suitable for use, without special environmental precautions, in the tropical or temperate zone and easy to maintain.

(6) The analytical procedure should be capable of resolving all the known endogenously occurring plant growth regulators in nano or picogram levels ideally from a single tissue extract.

The reasoning behind choosing a hormone spectrum as an index included the belief that the known plant growth regulators, such as the families of auxins, gibberellins, cytokinins, and abscisins, all play a role as triggers of certain growth processes and therefore should reflect any growth changes following environmental stress. Adaptation to drought stress by such processes as, for example, differentiation, osmoregulation, senescence, or stomatal movement

Table 4. Summary of Dry Weight Reduction During Purification of Hormone Extracts

IAA/ABA	Weight	Cytokinins	Weight
Tissue – Fresh	5 g	Tissue – Fresh	50 g
Tissue – Dry	1 g	Tissue – Dry	10 g
After PVP (ammonium salt)	110 mg	After cellulose phosphate cation exchange	350 mg
After Bondapak C_{18} HPLC	4 mg ↓	After Bondapak C_{18} HPLC	8 mg ↓
Analysis on 10 μm diameter silica	--	Analysis on octyl-silica	5 μm

should be reflected as changes in composition and quantity of hormones in the tissue.

Because of the current difficulties of assaying hormones in less than "pooled tissue" levels (it is impossible yet to measure hormones in single cells), we chose young actively growing leaves as the primary tissue for our investigation. The magnitude of the task of searching for the optimal conditions of analysis with new untried techniques which must be verified in the initial stages by the older, more cumbersome methods using chemical, physical, and bioassay techniques can be illustrated by a simple example (Table 2).

It becomes immediately apparent that in the interests of reducing extracts and increasing the range of hormones the technique of hormone identification should be able to identify all the known hormones from a single tissue extract. Because of the significant differences in chemical properties of the family of cytokinins from the group of substances included in the auxins, gibberellins, and abscisins the prospects for identification from less than two tissue extracts are not high at present.

Our approach to this particular problem has been to concentrate on a single instrument, the high performance liquid chromatograph (HPLC) as the basic tool for identifying the naturally occurring hormones (Durley et al., 1978; Kannangara et al., 1978). At the same time we have attempted to simplify the extraction procedures so that tissue samples are less than 50 g fresh weight but in

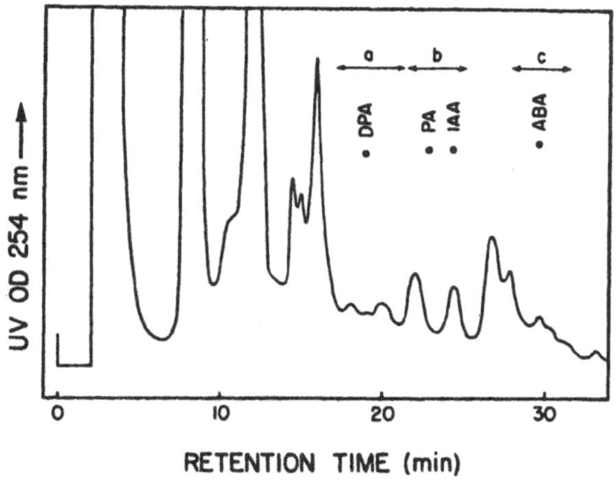

Fig. 4. Purification of abscisin/auxin extract from sorghum leaves by HPLC on Bondapak/C_{18} poracil B. Conditions: 56 cm X 2.1 mm i.d. column gradiently eluted (linearly) at 1 ml/min for 40 min starting with water (adjusted to pH 4.0 with acetic acid)/methanol (90:10) and ending with water/methanol (30:70).

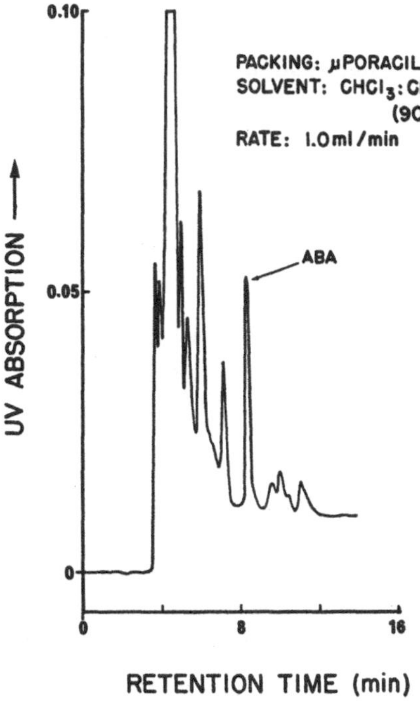

Fig. 5. Analysis of abscisic acid (ABA) in an extract of sorghum leaves.

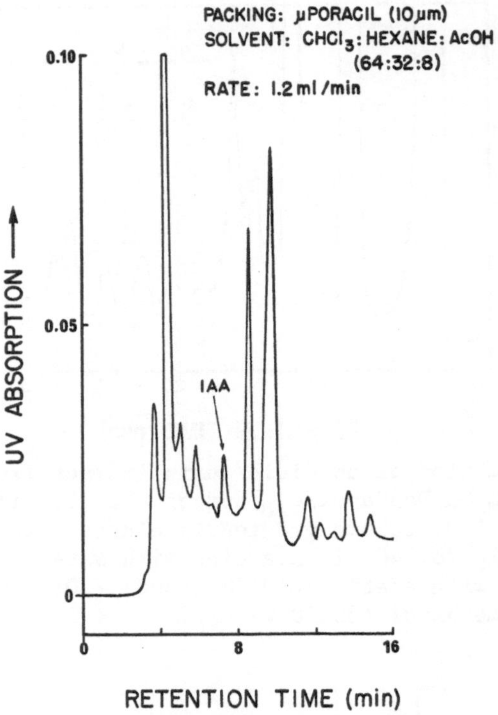

Fig. 6. Analysis of 3-indoleacetic acid (IAA) in an extract of sorghum leaves.

amounts containing sufficient hormone to stay above the limit of the UV detector of the instrument. The sensitivity of our current methods is: 1-2 ng for abscisins, 3-6 ng for auxins, and 4-6 ng for cytokinins.

The general objectives of our group of two chemists, three physiologists, and two technicians has been first to develop the analytical procedures for the hormones. These should be fast, accurate, and highly efficient. Second, we have attempted to make an inventory of representatives of the four groups of hormones (auxins, cytokinins, gibberellins, and abscisins) which can be found in sorghum leaves at various stages of the life cycle. We have compared two cultivars of sorghum grown under drought-stressed and normal conditions. Third, we have measured a number of growth and water relations parameters in the sorghum plants together with environmental descriptors both over the life cycle of the plant and coincident with the times of assay for hormones (Table 3). The ultimate objective is to test whether the hormone spectrum can be of any predictive value in selecting characters which will enhance

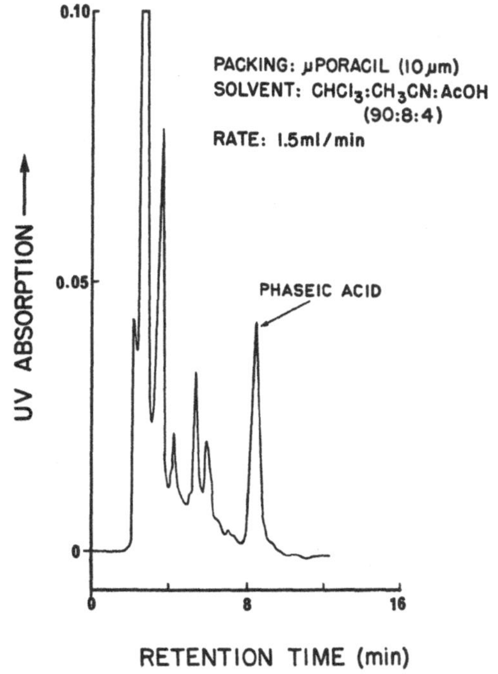

Fig. 7. Analysis of phaseic acid (PA) in an extract of sorghum leaves.

drought avoidance or tolerance which together can be defined as drought resistance.

The sorghum plants for analysis are grown essentially under field conditions in undisturbed soil. Graduated drought stress has been achieved routinely by erecting a rainout shelter (an old greenhouse) over the field site to keep off rainfall. Plants are watered by flood irrigation in compartments of soil separated by deep cement walls. Stress is achieved by withholding graded amounts of water. Saskatoon is in a prairie semiarid zone with high light intensities and temperatures in the summer months. It is thus easy to induce high levels of stress in plants.

We have just completed the second of two growth cycles in the rainout shelter. The data for growth and water relations parameters are complete but it will take some months to complete the analysis of hormones. Nevertheless, at this stage there are good indications that the two cultivars we have been using as test plants (NK300 and M35) not only show different growth responses to drought stress (Stout et al., 1978; Stout and Simpson, 1978) but also show different patterns of hormones at similar growth stages and in

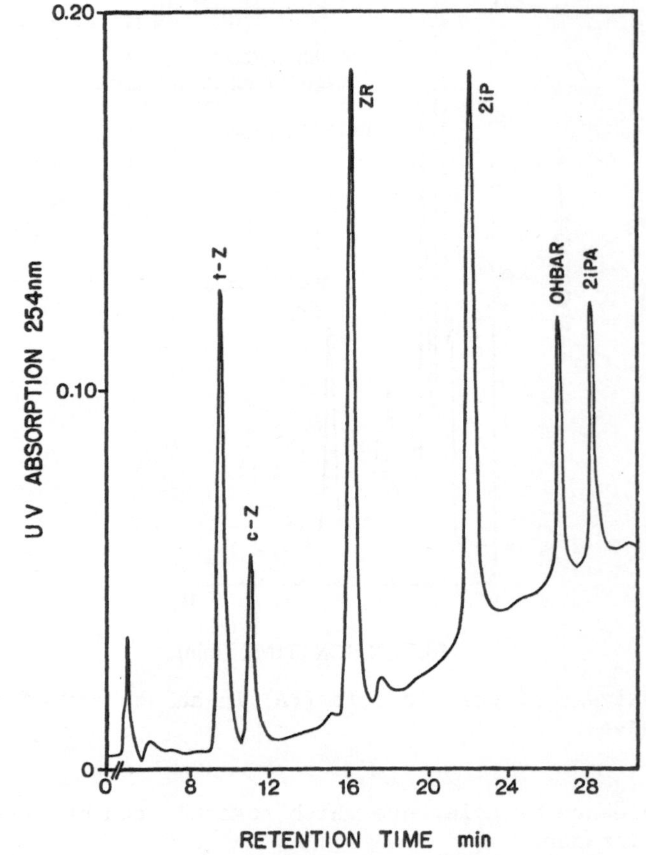

Fig. 8. HPLC chromatogram of authentic samples of trans-zeatin (t-Z), cis-zeatin (c-Z), zeatin riboside (ZR), 2iP - isopentenyladenine, 2iPA - isopentenyl adenine riboside, OHBR - orthohydroxy benxylaminopurine riboside.

response to drought stress. This can be illustrated by reference to 3-indoleacetic acid (IAA) and abscisic acid (ABA).

At flowering time M35 has double the level of ABA found in NK300, whether stressed or unstressed (Figs. 1 and 2). In the case of IAA drought stress reduced the level by one-half in NK300 but there was little change in M35. NK300 is the type of plant that responds to stress by senescing leaves and accelerating its life cycle whereas M35 tends to quiesce and resume growth if moisture becomes available again. The balance between IAA and ABA in M35 remains stable under stress with a concomitant increase in the levels throughout most of the life cycle. Rewatering and recovery after stress (RS) evoked an increase in both ABA and IAA.

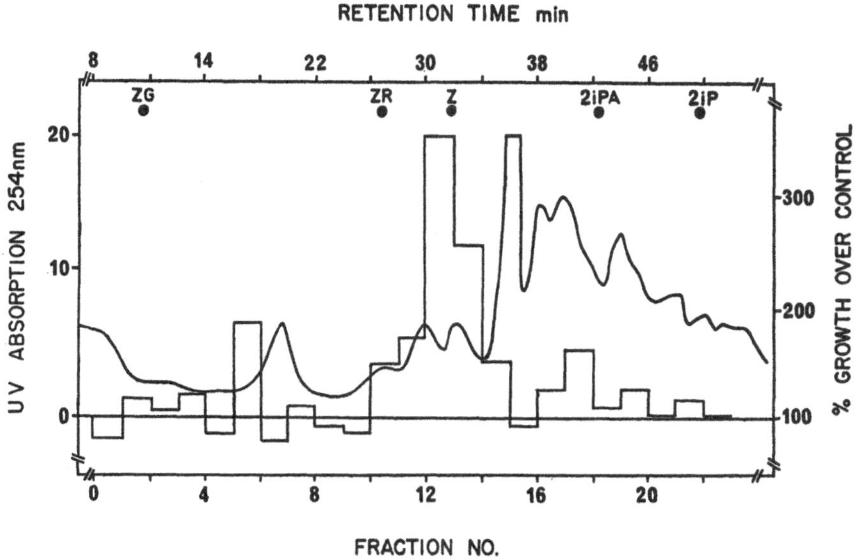

Fig. 9. Elution of a partially purified extract for cytokinins through a 56 X 0.65 cm i.d. Bondapak C_{18}/poracil B column. Biological activity and UV trace superimposed. Elution conditions: linear gradient at 1 ml per min for one hr starting with water (0.2 N acetic acid)/methanol (90:10) and ending with 100% methanol.

On the other hand, in NK300 whenever IAA went up ABA went down and vice versa. On rewatering stressed plants of NK300 both IAA and ABA declined and so did growth. The difference in hormone levels between stressed and nonstressed plants was more marked in NK300.

From these preliminary results we are optimistic that the basic requirement for beginning a selection program, namely the demonstration of significantly different qualitative and/or quantitative differences between genotypes in a general population of sorghum, is present if a spectrum of endogenous hormones is used as a selection index. It remains for us to complete a sound inventory of the kinds and amounts of hormones present in the two cultivars which we are examining closely and then to limit the choice of hormones which constitutes a good "fingerprint" of drought resistance potential. Before moving our analysis to a larger number of genotypes we are attempting to refine the sampling and analytical procedures by such steps as:

(a) Optimizing leaf tissue selection for both leaf position on the plant and position of a sample on an individual leaf.

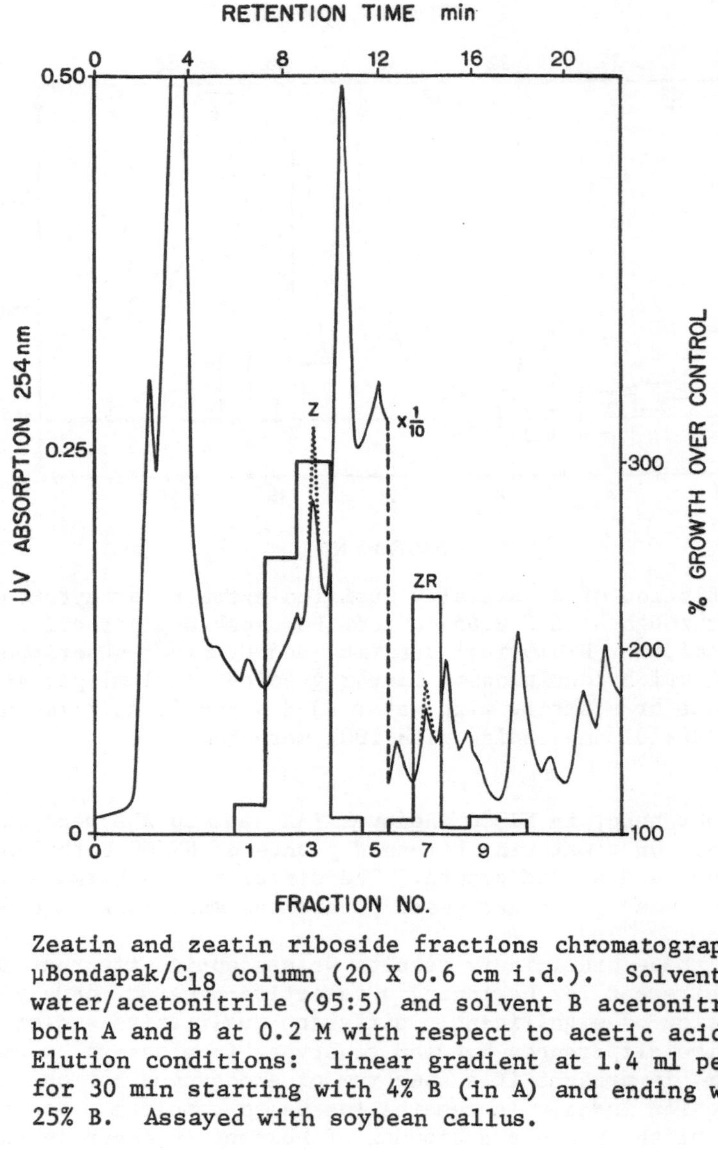

Fig. 10. Zeatin and zeatin riboside fractions chromatographed on a μBondapak/C_{18} column (20 X 0.6 cm i.d.). Solvent A was water/acetonitrile (95:5) and solvent B acetonitrile, both A and B at 0.2 M with respect to acetic acid. Elution conditions: linear gradient at 1.4 ml per min for 30 min starting with 4% B (in A) and ending with 25% B. Assayed with soybean callus.

(b) Optimizing the daily sampling time since we have found considerable diurnal fluctuations in some hormones (Fig. 3).

(c) Improving the preliminary purifications to remove background dry weight of the sample before the use of the final analytical microcolumn. Compared to tissues conventionally assayed for hormones such as fruits and buds of various species, the leaves of sorghum have relatively low amounts of hormones. Also in the later

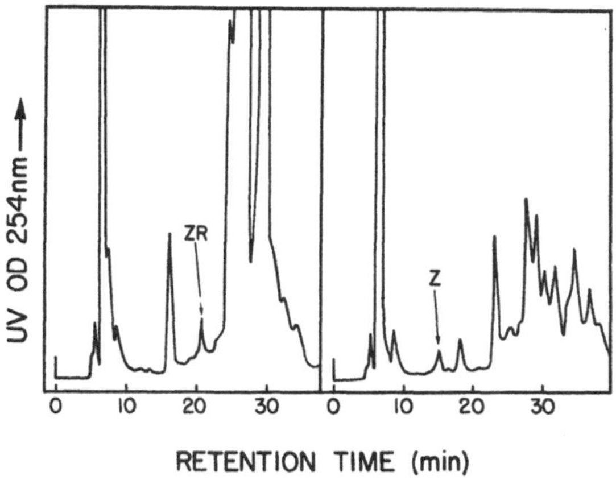

Fig. 11. Analysis of cytokinins zeatin and zeatin riboside purified from sorghum leaves on a 25 cm X 4 mm i.d. μBondapak/C_{18} column. Solvent A = water/acetonitrile and solvent B = acetonitrile, both solvents 0.2 M with respect to acetic acid. Elution conditions: linear gradient at 1.4 ml/min for 40 min starting with 4% B (in A) and ending with 25% B.

stages of the life cycle there is a considerable build-up of compounds which create extraneous background dry weight that can markedly decrease the sensitivity of microcolumns.

(d) Automating sample processing and recording for the HPLC. We also are currently adopting a fluorescence detector which will increase the sensitivity of detection of IAA tenfold.

A brief summary of the purification and analysis techniques we have adopted for abscisins, auxins, and cytokinins indicates the enormous scale change from the original tissue to the final identification of the individual hormone. The scale change is epitomized both by the proverbial needle in the haystack analogy and the interesting parallel problem of a plant breeder finding a single plant in a huge population!

In general, purification of extracts involves two stages. The first is designed to reduce dry weight and is therefore highly efficient but low in performance. The second involves a high performance resolution to select specific hormones. As examples (Table 4):

Stage 1. For IAA/ABA--the hormone extracts are chromatographed as ammonium salts on a short polyvinyl pyrrolidone (PVP) column which is eluted with water containing an antioxidant.

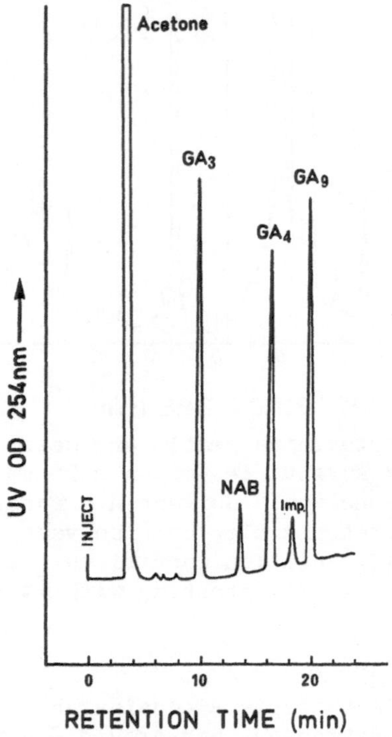

Fig. 12. Gibberellin naphthacyl esters chromatographed by HPLC on a 25 cm X 4 mm i.d. μBondapak/C_{18} column. Solvent A = water/acetonitrile (90:10) and solvent B = acetonitrile. Elution conditions: linear gradient at 1.5 ml/min for 20 min starting with 30% B (in A) and ending with 80% B. Polar (GA_3), intermediate (GA_4), and nonpolar (GA_9) gibberellins in order of appearance from the column.

For cytokinins--acidic tissue extracts are chromatographed on cellulose phosphate cation exchange columns (ammonium form). After removal of acidic and neutral substances the cytokinins are eluted with dilute ammonia.

Stage 2. All extracts are further purified by HPLC on an octadecyl-silica reverse phase column using acidified methanol water gradient elution. The desired hormones are collected according to their elution profile.

Final analysis for IAA/ABA is by HPLC on a 10 μm diameter silica; for cytokinins by HPLC on 5 μm diameter octyl-silica. Chromatograms for IAA/ABA are illustrated in Figs. 4-7. Cytokinins are seen in Figs. 8-11. We have not finalized our technique for the gibberellins, which are currently being assayed for with the dwarf rice assay. Our most promising method is to make the naphthacyl esters so that the gibberellins can be detected by ultraviolet absorption (Fig. 12). The free acids do not absorb UV sufficiently for detection with current HPLC detectors.

Clearly we still have some distance to go before we can give the plant breeder a magic box to be used in the field. Nevertheless we may be able to provide him with the magic box in a laboratory. With the rapid changes taking place in the HPLC field such as better detectors, microprocessors for automation, better columns, and other refinements coupled with constant improvement in extraction technique we are optimistic that our approach will be refined to the point where it can be used routinely in a plant breeding program. To this end we will probably be moving our system to the International Crop Research Institute for the Semi-arid Tropics (ICRISAT) in Ibadan, Nigeria in the near future so that we can work more closely with sorghum breeders with large programs and under more realistic practical conditions.

ACKNOWLEDGMENTS

The authors are grateful for the substantial financial support to this program by the International Development Research Centre, Ottawa, Canada, and for technical assistance from D. Firth, D. Flotre, L. Armstrong, and J. Montgomery.

REFERENCES

Allard, R. W., 1960, "Principles of Plant Breeding," John Wiley and Sons, New York.

Briggs, F. N., and Knowles, P. F., 1967, "Introduction to Plant Breeding," Reinhold, New York.

Burke, M. J., Gusta, L. V., Quamme, H. A., Weiser, C. J., and Li, P. H., 1976, Freezing and injury in plants, Ann. Rev. Plant Physiol., 27:507-528.

Downey, R. K., and Harvey, B. L., 1963, Methods of breeding for oil quality in rape, Can. J. Plant Sci., 43:271-275.

Durley, R. C., Kannangara, T., and Simpson, G. M., 1978, Analysis of abscisins and 3-indolylacetic acid in leaves of *Sorghum bicolor* by high performance chromatography, Can. J. Bot., 56: 157-161.

Flowers, T. J., Troke, P. F., and Yeo, A. R., 1977, The mechanism of salt tolerance in halophytes, Ann. Rev. Plant Physiol., 28:89-121.

Harvey, B. L., and Downey, R. K., 1963, The inheritance of erucic acid content in rapeseed (*Brassica napus*), Can. J. Plant Sci., 44:104-111.

Kannangara, T., Durley, R. C., and Simpson, G. M., 1978, High performance liquid chromatographic analysis of cytokinins in *Sorghum bicolor* L. Moench leaves, *Physiol. Plant.*, 44:295-299.

Kaul, R., and Crowle, W. L., 1971, Relations between water status, leaf temperature, stomatal aperture, and productivity of some wheat varieties, *Z. Pflanzenzuchtg.*, 65:233-243.

Levitt, J., 1972, "Responses of Plants to Environmental Stresses," Academic Press, New York.

Stout, D. G., Kannangara, T., and Simpson, G. M., 1978, Drought resistance of *Sorghum bicolor*. 2. Water stress effects on growth, *Can. J. Plant Sci.*, 58:225-233.

Stout, D. G., and Simpson, G. M., 1978, Drought resistance of *Sorghum bicolor*. 1. Drought avoidance mechanisms related to leaf water status, *Can. J. Plant Sci.*, 58:213-224.

8

TEMPERATURE RESPONSES AND YIELD IN TEMPERATE CROPS

P. F. Wareing

Department of Botany and Microbiology
University College of Wales
Penglais, Aberystwyth, Dyfed, U.K.

INTRODUCTION

Assuming that mineral nutrients and water supply are not limiting, crop yield depends upon: (1) the photosynthetic rate, (2) the amount of solar radiation intercepted and utilized in photosynthesis over the growing period, and (3) the proportion of total dry matter constituting the harvested part of the plant (harvest index). Under field conditions there is nothing the farmer can do about the major external factors affecting the photosynthetic rate, viz., the input of solar radiation, the CO_2 supply, and temperature, and the main prospects for increasing total dry matter production lie in improving the photosynthetic rate and/or the efficiency of light interception by selection and breeding.

Considerable attention has been devoted to the possibility of increasing yield by breeding for higher photosynthetic rates, but while this possibility should not be neglected, the prospects of substantially increasing yield in this way do not seem to be very promising in the short term (Evans, 1975). Indeed, comparison of wild and cultivated forms of crop species suggests that domestication and breeding have had little effect on photosynthetic rate and that yield has been increased mainly by improvements in the harvest index (Evans, 1975).

Watson (1952) was the first to point out that the slow development of an adequate leaf canopy (leaf area index) by spring-sown arable crops, such as sugar beet and potatoes, results in inefficient interception and utilization of solar radiation during the early part of the growing season and that dry matter production and crop yield could be increased by the earlier development of an adequate leaf area index (L). Since Watson's pioneering work, a number of studies have clearly established the direct relation between the amount of solar radiation intercepted by a crop and its yield (Biscoe and Gallagher, 1977; Monteith, 1977).

This loss of potential dry matter products in the spring is accentuated by the fact that in many temperate regions there is a pronounced lag between the time at which light conditions improve sufficiently in the spring to support active photosynthesis and the date at which the average temperature rises sufficiently to allow active crop growth. In lowland Britain, this time lag is frequently of the order of 3-4 weeks, but at higher altitudes it may amount to 6-8 weeks. Consequently, low temperature generally constitutes the major factor limiting plant growth, even during late spring. Moreover, the situation is further exacerbated by the fact that temperature minima for photosynthesis are frequently lower than for growth (Monteith and Elston, 1971). Hence crop growth in the spring is frequently limited, not by the rate of production of assimilates in photosynthesis, but by their rate of utilization in growth; i.e., under cool conditions, such as occur in the spring, dry matter production may be "sink limited" rather than "source limited" (Warren Wilson, 1966). Moreover, this situation applies not only to arable crops but also to permanent grassland, where dry matter production is limited less by inefficient light interception than in spring-sown arable crops, and in which the leaves constitute the harvested part of the crop.

Several courses of action are open to promote the earlier development of an adequate leaf area index in arable crops. Thus, autumn sowing allows earlier development of a leaf canopy in areas where this is practicable, as has been shown for autumn- and spring-sown wheat (Watson et al., 1963). Autumn-sown wheat achieved a maximum leaf area index (L) markedly earlier than spring-sown plants and the yield was 20% greater. Similarly, autumn-sown kale achieved an adequate value of L earlier than spring-sown plants and resulted in a greater yield of dry matter at harvest (Warne, 1961). With sugar beet, autumn sowing is not possible because the winter chilling results in "bolting" (flowering) of the plants in the spring. However, the yield of roots of sugar beet seedlings raised in a greenhouse for 5 weeks and subsequently planted out-of-doors was markedly greater than that of plants sown directly in the field (Scott and Bremner, 1966).

GENETIC VARIATION IN TEMPERATURE REQUIREMENTS FOR LEAF GROWTH

Another approach to the problem of developing an adequate leaf canopy earlier in the spring, one that has so far received little attention, is to breed cultivars which show higher growth rates at cool temperatures. That there are marked differences between species in their temperature requirements for growth is a matter of common observation. Thus, herbaceous species of the "pre-vernal" phase of woodlands may commence active growth some 6-8 weeks before the average temperature rises sufficiently for bud growth in tree species.

On the other hand the extent of intraspecific variation with respect to temperature/growth relations has been very little studied. It has been shown, however, that there are marked differences between Mediterranean and Scandinavian races of certain grass species, such as Dactylis glomerata, Lolium perenne, and Festuca arundinaceae in their temperature responses (Cooper, 1964; Eagles, 1967). Mediterranean races are adapted to growing during cool, moist conditions in the winter and tend to become dormant during the hot, dry summer. It is found, accordingly, that they have lower temperature minima for growth than Scandinavian races, which become semi-dormant during the winter and do not commence growth until late in the spring. Genetical variation in growth responses to temperature have recently been shown also for Festuca rubra (Ollerenshaw et al., 1976).

Until recently, little attention has been given to the design of controlled environment facilities providing a range of temperature conditions, but the development of a temperature-gradient "tunnel," providing a linear temperature gradient and adequate light intensities to support photosynthesis, now renders it possible to determine the temperature responses of seedlings with considerable accuracy (Mason, 1976). Using such facilities we have recently carried out detailed studies with young seedlings of several grass species, including D. glomerata and L. perenne (Elias, Mason, and Wareing, unpublished). These studies have shown that there are, indeed, significant differences in the temperature responses of grass populations of different geographical origin. In general, Mediterranean populations of D. glomerata show lower temperature minima for growth and less steep growth response curves to rising temperature than do races from Scandinavia. Some populations from high altitudes show response curves similar to those from Scandinavia. Between these two extremes there is a wide range of intermediate types of response, shown by races from various European regions, but it is not yet possible to correlate clearly these responses of various populations to the climatic conditions prevailing in their regions of origin. Similar, though less extreme, variation is seen in various races of L. perenne.

These response curves were obtained over an experimental period of 10-14 days with young seedlings at the two-leaf stage. In order to ascertain how far the temperature responses of young seedlings are correlated with those of mature plants of the same populations growing under field conditions, further experiments were carried out to determine the differences in relative growth rates of seedlings of various populations under controlled environment conditions at 6°C compared to differences in the growth of adult plants of the same populations under field conditions between November and March. It was found that there was indeed a high correlation between the relative growth rates of young seedlings at 6°C and those of mature plants of the same populations growing out-of-doors during winter.

These findings would seem to have two important implications for the breeding of grasses for earlier spring growth: first, the occurrence of intraspecific genetic variation with respect to growth responses to temperature has been clearly demonstrated; second, it was shown that the responses of young seedlings give a fairly reliable indication as to how the adult plants will respond under field conditions, so that it becomes possible to screen large numbers of seedlings at a very young stage.

Studies were also carried out on intraspecific variation with respect to the temperature requirements for germination in various grass species, using thermo-gradient bars (Thompson, 1970). The results demonstrated a considerable variation in the minimum temperatures for germination, the minima ranging from below 5°C to over 10°C among populations of diverse origins. Extensive intraspecific variation in the temperature requirement for germination has been demonstrated for a wide range of species (Thompson, 1973). Although such differences in germination/temperature relations are probably of little importance in perennial crop species such as pasture grasses, they could be of greater importance in spring-sown arable crops, where more rapid emergence after sowing could assist in the earlier development of the leaf canopy.

The occurrence of considerable intraspecific genetic variation in growth responses to temperature seems to be clearly indicated by the foregoing observations, and therefore there would seem to be good prospects that earlier spring growth could be attained by breeding. Strangely, this possibility has received relatively little attention by plant breeders hitherto, but there are probably several reasons for this omission. First, in general, biochemical and physiological processes conform to the Arrhenius equation relating to the effects of temperature on chemical reactions, and hence inevitably growth and metabolism must proceed more slowly at cool temperatures, so that attempts to improve the rates of growth under these conditions by breeding would appear to be in conflict with physico-chemical "laws." However, this argument is probably too simplistic and does not allow sufficiently for the complexity and adaptability of living systems, since although the constituent partial processes will follow the Arrhenius equation, other factors such as phase-transition in membranes (discussed below) are involved.

Second, it is not unreasonable to assume that adaptation to cool conditions would involve large numbers of genes and hence that improvement by breeding would be a long and difficult process.

However, it is also possible to envisage that overall rates of growth and metabolism might be limited by the rates of a few key processes, such as respiration or hormone biosynthesis, in which case the possibility of improvement by breeding may not be so intractable as has commonly been assumed. However, there is very little information on these matters and it is clear that we need a much better understanding of the biochemical basis of differences in temperature responses.

PHOTOSYNTHESIS AND RESPIRATION UNDER COLD CONDITIONS

As stated earlier, there is evidence that the overall rate of dry matter production in the early spring is frequently "sink limited" rather than "source limited"; i.e., that it is the rate of utilization of assimilates in growth rather than the rate of their production by photosynthesis which is limiting at that time. However, there is no doubt that under the short days and cloudy conditions frequently prevailing in early spring, photosynthesis could become limiting if growth activity at this time were increased by breeding. Hence in breeding programs it would be necessary to keep "sink activity" and "source activity" in balance.

The possibility that photosynthesis may limit active growth in the early spring is suggested by the fact that many woodland and other very early species, such as *Ficaria verna*, *Endymion non-scripta*, and *Galanthus nivalis*, have well-developed storage organs (root tubers, corms, or bulbs). Such species are therefore not dependent solely upon current photosynthesis in the early spring, but are able to develop an adequate leaf surface at the expense of reserve substances while light conditions are still poor. Presumably, the expenditure of such reserves on photosynthetic tissue is a sound strategy which pays "dividends" in the form of new assimilates as soon as light conditions become sufficiently favorable. It would seem that this strategy cannot be effectively exploited with crops grown from seed, except possibly in large-seeded species such as beans and peas, but the reserves present in potato "seed" tubers allows the possibility of rapidly developing an adequate leaf cover, independently of current photosynthesis.

For annual crops grown from seed and for perennial crop species lacking storage organs, high photosynthetic activity at cool temperatures could be an advantage in varieties which have been selected for early growth. The evidence for inter- and intraspecific variation in photosynthetic rate in relation to temperature has been discussed by Pisek (1973). It has been shown that if specific differences in photosynthetic rate are eliminated by equating the highest value for each species as 100, the photosynthesis/temperature curves for a wide range of species are very similar in the optima and maxima temperatures, but there is some variation in the responses at lower temperatures. The arctic and subalpine species Oxyria digyna achieves half its maximum photosynthetic rate at 0°C and at 10 k lux; the maximum rate is achieved at 7°C. Races of Picea abies and Pinus cembra from high altitudes in the alps also show active photosynthesis at low temperatures. Oxyria digyna and the subalpine species Ranuculus glacialis have the lowest compensation temperatures among the species studied followed by the central European bulbous species Leucojum vernum, which flowers in the early spring when frosts are still frequent. Thus there is good evidence that some species from arctic or subalpine regions are adapted to conduct active photosynthesis at low temperatures.

On the other hand, several studies have shown intraspecific variation in dark respiration rates, forms adapted to cold conditions having higher rates than those from warmer regions. Thus, plants of arctic populations of O. digyna have higher respiration rates than southern alpine populations (Mooney and Billings, 1961) and similar differences have been reported for Polygonatum bistortoides (Mooney, 1963). Populations of Festuca rubra showing active growth at cool temperatures have also been reported to have higher dark respiration rates than populations adapted to warmer conditions (Stewart and Ollerenshaw, in press).

It was suggested above that at cool temperatures the overall growth rate may be limited by the rate of certain key processes. Clearly the overall respiration rate constitutes such a key process, and the finding that ability to grow at cool temperatures is associated with a high respiration rate is not surprising, since presumably this reflects a high overall metabolic rate at low temperatures which would clearly be essential for active growth under these conditions. Growth involves the synthesis of major cell constituents, including DNA, RNA, proteins, lipids, and cell wall polysaccharides, and hence is dependent upon an adequate supply of free energy in the form of ATP or reduced pyridine nucleotides, so that any genetical variation affecting energy supply at low temperature could influence growth rate under these conditions. However, whether the observed higher respiration rates of plants able to grow at cool temperatures are the cause or the result of the higher growth rates is not known.

GROWTH SUBSTANCES AND TEMPERATURE RESPONSES

There is now overwhelming evidence for the involvement of growth substances in all aspects of plant growth, and where the levels of a specific growth substance are limiting, that substance can be regarded as "controlling" a particular growth process. In these circumstances the effect of temperature on the growth process may reflect primarily an effect on growth substance levels. The steady-state levels of a given growth substance will be determined by its rate of "turnover," i.e., by the balance between its rates of biosynthesis and inactivation, and both these processes will be sensitive to temperature. There are no well-established instances in which the effects of temperature on growth rate can be clearly related to effects on endogenous growth substance levels, but it has been suggested that the effects of root temperature on shoot growth may involve endogenous growth substances. There have been many reports that the growth rate of the shoot is reduced when the temperature of the roots is lowered relative to the air temperature at which the shoots are maintained. Since there is evidence that cytokinins are transported from roots to shoots in the transpiration stream, and that leaf growth is promoted by cytokinins, it has been suggested that the reduced rate of leaf growth observed when roots are maintained at lower temperatures may be due to a reduced rate of supply of cytokinins from the roots. This hypothesis was investigated by Atkin et al. (1973), who showed that when the roots of maize plants were maintained at 8°C the levels of cytokinins and gibberellins present in the xylem sap were markedly lower than in plants in which the roots were maintained at 28°C.

Since the shoot apical meristems of grasses are close to the soil surface, it is difficult to maintain them at clearly defined temperatures and the apparent effect of soil temperature on shoot growth in grasses is partly due to direct effects on the temperature of the apical meristems (Watts, 1972; Peacock, 1975). However, this problem does not arise with tomato plants, in which the root and shoot apices can be maintained at different temperatures without difficulty. In experiments in which the roots were maintained at 7°C and the shoots at 22°C, the flux of cytokinin and gibberellin activities in the xylem sap were markedly lower than in plants in which both roots and shoots were maintained at 22°C (Menhenett and Wareing, 1975). Moreover, the growth of the leaves and stems of plants with roots maintained at 7°C was significantly increased by the application of gibberellic acid (GA_3), but not by the cytokinin benzyladenine (BA).

In similar experiments with two contrasting populations of the grass *Dactylis glomerata*, low soil temperature resulted in markedly lower endogenous gibberellin levels in the shoots, but cytokinin levels were actually somewhat *higher* than in plants with roots maintained at a higher temperature (Menhenett and Wareing, 1976). Moreover, the adverse effects of low soil temperature on leaf growth in *D. glomerata* could be overcome by application of exogenous GA_3 but not by BA.

These results suggest that the effects of low root temperatures on leaf growth may result from reduced levels of gibberellins rather than of cytokinins. It is known that gibberellins may be produced in both roots and shoots (Jones and Phillips, 1966; Reid and Carr,

1967), but there is no evidence that shoots are dependent upon the roots for the supply of gibberellins.

EARLY GROWTH IN RELATION TO CHILLING INJURY AND FROST DAMAGE

If earlier growth can be achieved by breeding it will increase the liability of crops to two types of damage by low temperatures, viz., chilling injury and freezing injury. As is well known, a number of tropical and subtropical species are injured by cool temperatures (below 10-12°C) which are well above freezing temperatures. Studies on such chilling injury have revealed that an "Arrhenius plot" for various enzyme systems of such species shows a discontinuity at the critical temperatures at which chilling injury can be observed, and since certain of these enzyme systems, e.g., that for succinate oxidation (Lyons and Raison, 1970), are associated with cell membranes, it has been suggested that the membranes undergo a transition from the liquid crystal to the gel structure at the critical temperature (Lyons, 1973). There is evidence that there is a higher proportion of saturated fatty acids in the lipids of chilling-sensitive than of chilling-resistant species, suggesting that the adaptation of a species to cool temperatures may involve changes in the composition of the lipids of the cell membranes.

These membrane effects seem likely to be important in the acclimatization of subtropical species, such as maize, cucurbits, and certain species of legumes, to more temperate regions, where sowing frequently has to be delayed until May. If more rapid emergence and early growth could be achieved from earlier sowings, without increasing chilling injury, considerably increased yields could be expected from the improved light interception at that stage of the growing season.

The achievement, by breeding, of earlier growth in temperate crops, including grasses, would increase the liability to damage by spring frosts. It is well established that, in general, growing tissues are less freezing-resistant than dormant tissues as is illustrated by the greater freezing sensitivity of growing plants of D. glomerata of Mediterranean origin than of semidormant plants of Scandinavian origin. However, some species, such as rye or early woodland species, show a considerable degree of freezing resistance even in the active phase of growth, so that breeding for the capacity for early growth combined with a degree of freezing resistance in crop species may prove to be difficult but is apparently not a physiological impossibility.

However, even if an adequate degree of freezing resistance cannot be achieved in early growing cultivars in the short term, it should be possible to arrive at a compromise solution by breeding for forms in which adequate degrees of earliness and freezing resistance are developed in relation to the declining risks of freezing injury as the spring progresses.

SUMMARY

The slow development of an adequate leaf canopy by spring-sown annual crops results in inefficient interception and utilization of solar radiation during the early part of the growing season and total dry matter production and crop yield could be increased by the earlier development of an adequate leaf area index. In many species the temperature minimum for photosynthesis is lower than for growth, so that low temperature frequently constitutes the major factor limiting crop growth in the spring. Hence dry matter production could be increased if it were possible to breed cultivars with higher rates of leaf growth at cool temperatures.

Experiments with several species of pasture grasses have shown that there is considerable genetic variation between populations of different geographic origin in their temperature requirements for growth. Moreover, the temperature responses of young seedlings of a given population are highly correlated with the performance of older plants of the populations under field conditions during the winter.

Hence, there appears to be considerable intraspecific genetic variation in growth responses to temperature in these grasses and if similar variation occurs in other crop species there would seem to be good prospects that earlier spring growth could be achieved by breeding.

The advantages in attaining earlier leaf growth would be enhanced if higher photosynthetic rates at cool temperatures could also be achieved. Studies on arctic and alpine species indicate that several such species show relatively high photosynthetic rates at low temperatures. On the other hand, these species also have a high dark respiration rate, indicative of a high metabolic rate at cool temperatures.

Root temperature has a marked effect on shoot growth in some species and this effect may be mediated through effects on the supply of endogenous growth substances from the roots to the shoots.

The achievement, by breeding, of earlier growth will increase the risks of damage from chilling injury and freezing injury, and breeding strategies will be required which aim at combining early growth with adequate resistance to such injury.

REFERENCES

Atkin, R. K., Barton, G. E., and Robinson, D. K., 1973, Effect of root-growing temperature on growth substances in xylem exudate of Zea mays, J. Exp. Bot., 24:475-487.

Biscoe, P. V., and Gallagher, J. N., 1977, Weather, dry matter production and yield, in: "Environmental Effects on Crop Physiology," J. J. Landsberg and C. V. Cutting, eds., Academic Press, London.

Cooper, J. P., 1964, Climatic variation in forage grasses. I. Leaf development in climatic races of Lolium and Dactylis, J. App. Ecol., 1:45-61.

Eagles, C. F., 1967, The effect of temperature in vegetative growth in climatic races of Dactylis glomerata in controlled environments, Ann. Bot. N.S., 31:31-39.

Evans, L. T., 1975, in: "Crop Physiology," L. T. Evans, ed., Cambridge Univ. Press, London.

Jones, R. L., and Phillips, I. D. J., 1966, Organs of gibberellin synthesis in light-grown sunflower plants, Plant Physiol., 41:1381-1386.

Lyons, J. M., 1973, Chilling injury in plants, Ann. Rev. Plant Physiol., 24:445-466.

Lyons, J. M., and Raison, J. K., 1970, Oxidative activity of mitochondria isolated from plant tissues sensitive and resistant to chilling injury, Plant Physiol., 45:386-389.

Mason, G., 1976, An improved temperature-gradient tunnel for use at low temperature, Ann. Bot., 40:381-384.

Menhenett, R., and Wareing, P. F., 1975, Possible involvement of growth substances in the response of tomato plants (Lycopersicon esculentum Mill.) to different soil temperatures, J. Hort. Sci., 50:381-397.

Menhenett, R., and Wareing, P. F., 1976, Effects of soil temperature on the growth and hormone content of Dactylis glomerata L. (cocksfoot) in controlled environments, J. Exp. Bot., 27:1259-1267.

Monteith, J. L., 1977, Climate and the efficiency of crop production in Britain, Phil. Trans. R. Soc. Lond. B., 281:277-294.

Monteith, J. L., and Elston, J. F., 1971, Microclimatology and crop production, in: "Potential Crop Production," P. F. Wareing and J. P. Cooper, eds., Heinemann Educational Books, London.

Mooney, H. A., 1963, Physiological ecology of coastal, subalpine and alpine populations of Polygonum bistortoides, Ecology, 44:812-816.

Mooney, H. A., and Billings, W. D., 1961, Comparative physiological ecology of arctic and alpine populations of Oxyria digyna, Ecol. Monogr., 31:1-29.

Ollerenshaw, J. H., Stewart, W. S., Gallimore, J., and Baker, R. H., 1976, Low temperature growth in grasses from Northern latitudes, J. Agric. Sci. Camb., 87:237-239.

Peacock, J. M., 1975, Temperature and leaf growth in Lolium perenne. II. The site of temperature perception, J. App. Ecol., 12: 115-123.

Pisek, A., 1973, Effect of temperature on metabolic processes, in: "Temperature and Life," H. Precht, J. Christophersen, H. Hensel, and W. Larcher, eds., Springer Verlag, Berlin.

Reid, D. M., and Carr, D. J., 1967, Effects of a dwarfing compound, CCC, on the production and export of gibberellin-like substances by root systems, Plants (Berl.), 73:1-11.

Scott, R. K., and Bremner, P. M., 1966, The effects of growth, development and yield of sugar beet of extension of the growth period by transplantation, J. Agric. Sci. Camb., 66:279-388.

Stewart, W. S., and Ollerenshaw, J. H., in press, Intra-specific variation in rates of dark respiration and of photosynthesis at low positive temperatures in Festuca rubra L., in: Proceedings XIIIth International Grassland Congress, Leipzig, 1977.

Thompson, P. A., 1970, Characterisation of the germination responses to temperature of species and ecotypes, Nature, Lond., 225: 827-831.

Thompson, P. A., 1973, Geographical adaptation of seeds, in: "Seed Ecology," W. Heydecker, ed., Butterworths, London.

Warne, L. G. G., 1961, Potential productivity of marrow stem and thousand-headed kale, Nature, Lond., 192:579.

Warren Wilson, J., 1966, An analysis of plant growth and its control in arctic environments, Ann. Bot., 30:383-402.

Watson, D. J., 1952, The physiological basis of variation yield, Adv. Agron., 4:101-145.

Watson, D. J., Thorne, G. N., and French, G. A. W., 1963. Analysis of growth and yield of winter and spring wheats, Ann. Bot., 27:1-22.

Watts, W. R., 1972, Leaf extension in Zea mays. II. Leaf extension in response to independent variation of the temperature of the apical meristem, of the air around the leaves, and of the root zone, J. Exp. Bot., 23:713-721.

9

SINK-SOURCE RELATIONSHIPS IN FRUIT TREES

Fritz Lenz

Institut für Obstbau und Gemüsebau
Der Universität Bonn
Bonn, Federal Republic of Germany

ABSTRACT

Investigations of the effects of fruit (mainly citrus) on growth, flower formation, water consumption, nutrient uptake, photosynthesis, and respiration of plants are reviewed. The main emphasis is on photosynthetic efficiency of leaves as affected and perhaps regulated by fruit.

INTRODUCTION

Developing fruit have considerable effects on the growth of other plant organs. With increasing fruit load, growth of roots, shoots, and leaves is reduced (lit. Leonard, 1962). Moreover, flower formation can be inhibited. This leads to irregular yields in perennial fruit crops, a phenomenon which in horticulture is defined as "alternate bearing." To gain a better understanding of the physiological reasons for "alternate bearing," the effects of fruit load on such growth reactions as water consumption, nutrient uptake, photosynthesis, and respiration were investigated in citrus.

For these experiments plants were grown from cuttings in glasshouses. The plants were cultivated in sand and supplied with modified Hoagland solution. The crop load was regulated by flower removal at an early stage of development (Lenz, 1967).

Flower Formation

Flower formation can be strongly inhibited by fruit load as demonstrated in an experiment with Citrus madurensis cuttings bearing different numbers of fruit (Table 1). This effect may be due to the reduction of shoot and bud numbers, low carbohydrate concentrations (Lenz and Küntzel, 1974), or direct hormonal inhibition by the fruit as suggested by Guttridge (1962). Gibberellins deriving from the fruit could inhibit flower formation in apples (Luckwill, 1970). Also for citrus it has been shown that flower formation can be strongly inhibited by applications of gibberellins (Monselise and Halevy, 1964; Moss, 1970; Moss and Bellamy, 1972), indicating that hormonal regulation of flower formation by the fruit similar to that which takes place in apples could occur here. On the other hand flower inhibiting gibberellins could also derive from the roots; strong root growth brought about by optimal root temperatures halted the flower formation in citrus as shown in Table 2. Inhibition of flower formation by fruit was even stronger in Citrus sinensis both in "seedy" and "seedless" varieties. Even with high levels of nutrient supply flower inhibition remained strong in branches with growing fruit attached.

Water Consumption

Experiments with Citrus madurensis have shown that fruiting plants have higher transpiration rates and more water consumption per kg of dry matter formed than nonfruiting ones. An example is shown in Table 3. Water consumption per kg of leaf dry matter increased considerably with increasing fruit load. Similar results have been found for apples (Hansen, 1971a).

Nutrient Uptake

Not only water uptake but also nutrient uptake can be strongly affected by the fruit load. For apples this was demonstrated by Hansen (1971b) and for citrus by Lenz and Döring (1979). Leaves from fruit bearing plants contained a higher percentage of nitrogen, calcium, and boron, but a lower percentage of potassium than those from defruited plants. Per unit root dry matter considerably more N, P, K, Ca, and B were taken up by fruiting as compared to nonfruiting plants. High portions of the total nitrogen, phosphorus, and potassium taken up can be found in the fruits.

Dry Matter Distribution

In experiments with fruiting and nonfruiting C. madurensis plants it became obvious (Lenz, 1974) that, as in apples (Maggs,

Table 1. Effects of Fruit Load on Flower Production in Citrus madurensis Plants Grown from Cuttings

	Fruit Numbers/Plant						
	0	10	20	30	40	50	LSD ($P<0.05$)
Number of flowers produced	64.8	7.2	2.2	0.0	0.0	0.0	5.9

1963; Hansen, 1971a), increasing fruit load strongly reduced the dry matter of roots, shoots, and leaves. Total dry matter of the plants was similar, however. An example of this is shown in Fig. 1 in C. madurensis. At high fruit loads (80 fruits/plant) more than 50% of plant dry matter was in the fruits. This indicates that these organs obviously compete successfully with vegetative parts of the plants for photosynthetic products. This capacity seems to be of general occurrence (see Wardlaw, 1968; Bünemann and Grassia, 1973). As shown for eggplants (Claussen, 1976), dry matter formation in roots, leaves, and shoots is strongly inhibited when fruits have the highest growth rates. At this stage 92-95% of assimilates produced were accumulated in the fruits.

Despite reduced leaf area, fruiting plants produced under favorable growing conditions (light saturation, optimal water and nutrient supply, and root temperatures) more total dry matter than nonfruiting ones (Cary, 1970; Hansen, 1971a). This indicates that higher photosynthetic efficiencies of leaves in fruiting plants, if not in the fruit themselves, contribute substantially to dry matter production.

With citrus (Lenz, 1967), it was demonstrated that fruits at all developmental stages evolve more CO_2 than they could gain by light driven processes. They are therefore dependent on assimilates from the leaves for growth. Fruit photosynthesis might serve to limit CO_2 losses, however, and some of the CO_2 evolved from the internal fruit tissue can be refixed (Kriedemann, 1968; Laval-Martin et al., 1977).

In the experiments with fruiting and nonfruiting plants it became apparent that the dry matter production per unit leaf area, i.e., the photosynthetic efficiency of leaves, increased with higher fruit load. Similar results were found for other fruit crops, e. g. apples (Maggs, 1963; Avery, 1969, Hansen, 1971a) and strawberries (Lenz and Bünemann, 1967). There is, however, an upper limit to this photosynthetic response and in some species such as Coffea arabica and citrus "over-cropping" has been described (lit. Leonard, 1962; Smith, 1976). This condition results in total inhibition of

Table 2. Effect of Root Temperature on the Flower Formation in *Citrus madurensis* Plants Grown from Cuttings

Root Temperature	Experiment I	Experiment II
12°C	42	35
20°C	17	9
28°C	0	0
36°C	0	0
LSD $P<0.05$	6.3	7.1

vegetative growth and premature senescence of leaves with an attendant reduction in rates of CO_2 fixation. Impaired root growth or nutritional stress under heavy crop loads can be important factors in such a decline.

Photosynthetic and Dark Respiration Rates

In apples (Hansen, 1970) as well as in citrus (Lenz and Daunicht, 1971), it could be shown that the photosynthetic rates of leaves in fruiting plants are higher than in nonfruiting ones. This was particularly pronounced at low root temperatures. Fruit effects on photosynthesis could be intensified by raising the temperature of the developing organ. Regardless of uncertainties about the mechanism of this physiological coupling between leaf and fruit, the photosynthetic response in adjacent leaves is unmistakable. When fruits on *C. madurensis* were held at 32°C (other aerial organs at 20°C) leaf photosynthesis was increased by 40% over the rate previously observed at 20°C.

Similarly root growth can enhance photosynthetic rates in citrus leaves. Activating root growth by raising root temperatures increased photosynthetic rates (Lenz, 1974). The fruit effect on photosynthetic rates was most pronounced during time of intensive fruit growth. Flowers and small or mature fruits had no effect on photosynthetic rates of plants with and without fruits (Claussen, 1977). So far all the available data on citrus indicate that dark respiration in fruiting and nonfruiting plants is similar (Lenz and Daunicht, 1971).

Self-Shading and Photosynthesis

Plants without fruits often produce more shoots and leaves, so that self-shading within the leaf canopy becomes more accentuated in

Table 3. Water Consumption/kg Leaf Dry Matter as Affected by Fruit Load (Citrus madurensis Lour.)

Fruit Number/Plant		
0	50	100
370	570	1,030

the absence of a crop. This alteration in microclimate could then limit photosynthesis due to reduced light intensity, especially in plants like strawberry with rosette leaves. The different degrees of self-shading of leaves in fruiting and nonfruiting plants could be an explanation for different peak photosynthetic rates. In the experiments with citrus, however, self-shading was avoided. Despite this leaves of fruiting plants produced more dry matter, i.e., they had higher photosynthetic rates. Also, measurements at light saturation in single leaves of apples showed higher photosynthetic rates as the result of fruit load (Kazarjan et al., 1965; Hansen, 1967).

REGULATORY MECHANISMS

When considering how leaf photosynthesis might be coupled to fruit growth and development the question is whether the photosynthetic rate depends on current "demand" for assimilate or whether a more direct form of regulation is involved. So far it appears that photosynthetic efficiency of leaves in fruiting and nonfruiting plants is probably regulated by several mechanisms.

Hormonal Influences

Since fruits can have relatively high concentrations of phytohormones (Crane, 1969; Luckwill, 1970; Nitsch, 1970), it has been assumed that hormones deriving from the fruits perhaps regulate photosynthetic rates by directly activating RudP-carboxylase (Wareing, 1968).

Some experiments have shown that auxins, cytokinins, and gibberellins can stimulate photosynthetic rates of leaves (lit. Kull, 1972). The amount and activity of RudP-carboxylase in leaves could be enhanced by gibberellins (Treharne and Stoddart, 1970; Broughton et al., 1970; Huber and Sankhla, 1973). Tamas et al. (1972) showed that indoleactetic acid (IAA) can increase photosynthesis of chloroplasts by enhancement of photophosphorylation. Furthermore Hoad et al. (1977), using grapevines, found that changes in gibberellin and cytokinin levels do occur when sink strength

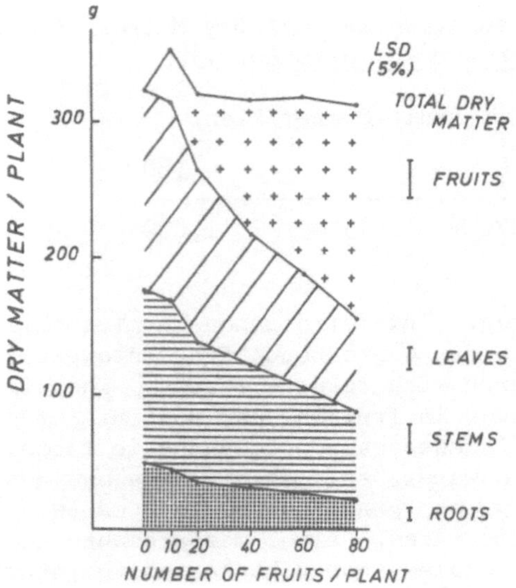

Fig. 1. Effect of fruit numbers on the total dry matter/plant and on the dry matter distribution at the stage of fruit maturity.

varies and that the rate of photosynthesis alters as a result of the observed changes in hormone levels.

Inhibitors of plant growth such as abscisic acid (ABA) and phaseic acid can also be involved in such source-sink feedback effects as shown by Kriedemann et al. (1976).

Investigations with C. madurensis revealed that leaves of fruiting plants had a 70% increase in specific activity of RudP-carboxylase (Tung et al., 1973).

It remains, however, to be seen whether phytohormones do in fact migrate from "sink" to "source" and so fulfill regulating functions on the photosynthetic enzymes. On the other hand, assimilate turnover and transport could be affected by phytohormones (Bidwell, 1973; Bidwell and Chiu-Kwong Quong, 1975), thus regulating photosynthesis. It has been indicated that hormones can stimulate transport from "source" to "sink" by increasing the metabolic activity of fruits (Booth et al., 1962) or by affecting the transport mechanisms (Davies and Wareing, 1965; Mullins, 1970). This last possibility is supported by hormonal effects on the formation of transport tissues, sieve-tube loading and unloading, as well as longitudinal transfer within the sieve-tubes (Patrick, 1976). For example, IAA not only alters permeability of membranes (Polevoi and Salamatova, 1974) but also can promote differentiation of phloem tissue (Sachs, 1975).

Finally, photosynthesis can be influenced to some degree by both stomatal and internal restrictions on CO_2 movement from the air around the leaf to photosynthetic sites within the leaf. Hormonal effects can be expressed at both locations (Loveys and Kriedemann, 1974).

Assimilate Concentration

Fruits not only affect photosynthetic rates but also assimilate concentrations in the leaves. Plants bearing fruit have lower assimilate concentrations in the leaves than nonfruiting ones (Hoffmann, 1973; Lenz and Küntzel, 1974; Quast, 1975). The probability of causal connections between photosynthetic rates and leaf assimilate concentrations has therefore been suggested (lit. Heales and Incoll, 1968). This theory is based on the assumption that an increase in concentration, particularly of sucrose, fructose, and glucose, causes the decline of photosynthetic rates by end-product inhibition of enzyme activity. Perhaps an accelerated transfer of these carbohydrates from leaves to fruits could be a main reason for higher photosynthetic rates in fruiting as compared to nonfruiting plants. Claussen (1975), in extensive investigations on photosynthetic rates and leaf contents of alcohol soluble sugars of *Solanum melongena*, showed that sucrose, fructose, and glucose in concentrations occurring in leaves do not affect photosynthetic enzymes or photosynthetic rates. Similar results for other plants were reported by Bucke et al. (1966); Bowes and Ogren (1972); Buchanan and Schürmann (1973). The possibility cannot be excluded, however, that other metabolites may have negative feedback effect on photosynthetic enzymes. For example, accumulation of 6-P-gluconate or fructose-1,6-diphosphate could strongly inhibit RudP-carboxylase activity (lit. Kelly and Latzko, 1976; Kluge, 1977) and ribulose-5-phosphate can regulate activity of RudP-carboxylase within a very small concentration range. This way fine regulation of photosynthesis would be possible.

Furthermore, an accumulation of starch in the chloroplasts could be associated with reduced rates of photosynthesis. Hoffmann's (1973) examination of chloroplasts from leaves of nonfruiting eggplants does reveal severe disruption of chloroplast fine structure compared to the situation for fruiting plants, and it seems quite remarkable that such plastids are still capable of sustaining further photosynthesis and starch accretion. Deterioration in both photochemical and biochemical properties of such plastids (Wildman, 1967) would be expected.

Although starch does not seem to be involved directly in all metabolism it appears possible that coupling of chloroplast enzymes to starch could cause reduction of their activity as well as changes of their substrate affinity and specificity as assumed for starch-synthetase (lit. Meisel, 1974). Moreover starch binds Mg ions and thus changes in Mg concentrations and pH values occur in the stroma. As Mg-ions have importance for the regulation of enzyme activities, their binding onto starch could have a regulating effect on photosynthesis (Wishnick and Lane, 1970; Klemme and Jacobi, 1974). In spite of the above, Claussen (1975), after numerous investigations of leaves in fruiting and nonfruiting eggplants, found that starch effects on photosynthesis, if they occurred at all, would be very small.

Photorespiration

An accumulation of intermediates of the Calvin cycle, in particular of ribulose-5-phosphate and ribulose-1,5-diphosphate, could increase photorespiration and thus affect photosynthetic efficiency (Zelitsch, 1975). In fact several experiments with C. madurensis have shown that nonfruiting plants have higher photorespiration rates than fruiting ones (Lenz, 1979a).

Gaseous Diffusive Resistance

As has been shown in apples (Hansen, 1971c), vine (Loveys and Kriedemann, 1974), and soybeans (Lenz and Williams, 1973; Woodward and Rawson, 1976), leaves of fruiting plants often have lower gaseous diffusive resistances than those of nonfruiting ones. In soybeans stomates of leaves in fruiting plants remain open wider and longer during the light period (Lenz and Williams, 1973). That such stomatal reactions could be hormonally controlled has been suggested by Loveys and Kriedemann (1974). They found close relationships between stomatal resistance of leaves and the abscisic acid and phaseic acid contents. Also, of course, differences in assimilate concentration in the leaves of fruiting and nonfruiting plants could be reasons for the different stomatal behavior. Possibly by accumulation of assimilates found mainly in leaves of nonfruiting plants, other resistances along the CO_2 diffusion pathways (cell walls, membranes, and cytoplasm) could affect CO_2 concentrations of the intercellular spaces and in this way stomata movement.

If by accumulation of metabolites, photorespiration is increased, rising CO_2 concentrations in the intercellular spaces can be expected. Since stomata react sensitively toward intercellular CO_2 levels (Raschke, 1976), closure of stomata must be assumed to occur. In fact in recent investigations in fruiting and nonfruiting citrus plants using a continuously recording diffusive porometer (Block and Sterzelmeier, 1978), it was found (Lenz, 1979b) that stomata of leaves in nonfruiting plants opened after the beginning of the light period. Possibly due to accumulation of intercellular CO_2, however, they partly closed and after oscillatory movement remained nearly closed for the rest of the light period. In contrast leaves of fruiting plants with lower photorespiration rates and probably intensified CO_2 uptake by chloroplasts may have had lower intercellular CO_2 concentrations. Therefore, stomata opened at the beginning of the light period and remained open until darkness even during prolonged light periods.

CONCLUSION

Developing fruits, which are often the main "sink" of the plant during the vegetation period, can considerably affect growth reactions such as water consumption and nutrient uptake. A strong reduction of root growth in a heavy bearing fruit tree can be compensated by intensified water and nutrient uptake by the remaining roots. Since the plants could be hampered by not reaching enough water and nutrients with a smaller root system it appears to be important to supply sufficient water and nutrients to the heavy cropping plants in the "on year." Numerous investigations have shown that the photosynthetic efficiency of leaves in trees can be increased by fruits. Possibly the rate of photosynthesis can be regulated by the fruit through several mechanisms, some of which were discussed in this paper. Further detailed studies on these mechanisms could bring valuable information about possible means to reduce or to improve photosynthetic efficiencies of fruit trees.

REFERENCES

Avery, D. J., 1969, Comparisons of fruiting and deblossomed maiden apple trees and of non-fruiting trees on a dwarfing and an invigorating rootstock, New Phytol., 68:323-336.

Bidwell, R. G. S., 1973, A possible mechanism for the control of photoassimilate translocation, in: "Transactions 3rd Symposium on Accumulation and Translocation of Regulators in Plant Organisms," Warsaw, 3:17-30.

Bidwell, R. G. S., and Chiu Kwong Quong, E., 1975, Indoleacetic acid effect on the distribution of photosynthetically fixed carbon in the bean plant, Biochem. Physiol. Pflanzen, 168:361-370.

Block, F. R., and Sterzelmeier, K., 1978, Kontinuierliche Messung der Blatttranspiration mit Hilfe eines neuen elektronischen Gasfeuchtemessgerätes, Gartenbauwiss., 43:142-144.

Booth, A., Moorby, J., Davies, C. R., Jones, H., and Wareing, P. F., 1962, Effects of indolyl-3-acetic acid on the movement of nutrients within plants, Nature (London), 194:204-205.

Bowes, G., and Ogren, W. L., 1972, Oxygen inhibition and other properties of soybean ribulose-1,5-diphosphate carboxylase, J. Biol. Chem., 217:2171-2176.

Broughton, W. J., Hellmuth, E. O., and Yeung, D., 1970, Role of glucose in development of the gibberellin response in peas, Biochim. Biophys. Acta, 222:491.

Buchanan, B. B., and Schürmann, P., 1973, Regulation of ribulose-1,5-diphosphate carboxylase in the photosynthetic assimilation of carbon dioxide, J. Biol. Chem., 248:4956-4964.

Bucke, C. D., Walker, D. A., and Baldry, S. W., 1966, Some effects of sugars and sugar phosphates on carbon dioxide fixation by isolated chloroplasts, Biochem. J., 101:636-641.

Bünemann, G., and Grassia, A., 1973, Growth and mineral distribution in grafted tomato/potato plants according to sink number, Scientia Horticulturae, 1:13-24.

Cary, P. R., 1970, Growth, yield and fruit composition of "Washington Navel" orange cuttings as affected by root temperature, nutrient supply and crop load, Hort. Res., 10:20-33.

Claussen, W., 1975, Untersuchungen über den Einfluss der Frucht auf die Netto-Photosyntheseraten und den Saccharose- und Stärkestoffwechsel der Blätter und Wurzeln von Auberginen (Solanum melongena L.), Diss. Fachbereich Internat. Agrarentwicklung der T. U. Berlin.

Claussen, W., 1976, Einfluss der Frucht auf die Trockensubstanzverteilung in der Aubergine (Solanum melongena L.), Gartenbauwiss., 41:236-239.

Claussen, W., 1977, Einfluss der Frucht auf Netto-Assimilationsleistung und Netto-Photosyntheseraten der Aubergine (Solanum melongena L.), Gartenbauwiss., 42:61-65.

Crane, J. C., 1969, The role of hormones in fruit set and development, HortScience, 4:108-111.

Davies, C. R., and Wareing, P. F., 1965, Auxin directed transport of radiophosphorus in stems, Planta, 65:139-156.

Guttridge, C. G., 1962, Inhibition of fruit bud formation in apple with gibberellic acid, Nature (London), 196:1008.

Hansen, P., 1967, ^{14}C-studies on apple trees. VI. The influence of the fruit on the photosynthesis of the leaves, and the relative photosynthetic yields of fruits and leaves, Physiol. Plant., 20:382-391.

Hansen, P., 1971a, The effect of cropping on the distribution of growth in apple trees, Tidssk. Planteavl., 75:119-127.

Hansen, P., 1971b, The effects of cropping on uptake, contents, and distributions of nutrients in apple trees, in: Report No. 983, State Research Station, Blangstedgaard, Germany.

Hansen, P., 1971c, The effect of fruiting upon transpiration rate and stomatal opening in apple leaves, Physiol. Plant., 24:181-183.

Hoad, G. V., Loveys, B. R., and Skene, K. G. M., 1977, The effect of fruit-removal of cytokinins and gibberellin-like substances in grape leaves, Planta, 136:25-30.

Hoffmann, E., 1973, Der Einfluss der Fruchte auf die Photosyntheseraten und die Assimilatverteilung bei fruchttragenden und nichtfruchttragenden Auberginen und Erdbeerpflanzen, Diss. T. U. Berlin.

Huber, W., and Sankhla, N., 1973, Effect of gibberellic acid on the activities of photosynthetic enzymes and $^{14}CO_2$-fixation products in leaves of Pennisetum typhoides seedlings, Z. Pflanzenphysiol., 71:275-280.
Kazarjan, M. O., Balagezjan, N. K., and Karapetjan, K. A., 1965, Effect of fruits on the physiological activity of apple leaves (Russ.), Fiziol. Rast., 12:313-319, Ref. Landw. Zbb. (1966), 10:3116.
Kelly, G. J., and Latzko, E., 1976, Regulatory aspects of photosynthetic carbon metabolism, Ann. Rev. Plant. Physiol., 27: 181-205.
Klemme, B., and Jacobi, G., 1974, Der Einfluss von Stärke auf die Aktivität der Pyrophosphatase aus isolierten Chloroplasten, Planta, 120:155-162.
Kluge, M., 1977, Regulation of carbon dioxide fixation in plants, in: "Integration of Activity in the Higher Plant," D. H. Jennings, ed., Cambridge Univ. Press, Cambridge.
Kriedemann, P. E., 1968, Observations on gas exchange in the developing Sultana berry, Aust. J. Biol. Sci., 21:907-916.
Kriedemann, P. E., Loveys, B. R., Possingham, J. V., and Satoh, M., 1976, Sink effects on stomatal physiology and photosynthesis, in: "Transport and Transfer Processes in Plants," I. Wardlaw and J. B. Passioura, eds., Academic Press, New York.
Kull, U., 1972, Wirkungen von Wuchsstoffen auf Speicherung und Stoffwechsel in vegetativen Pflanzenteilen (unter besonderer Berücksichtigung des Kohlenhydrathaushaltes), Ser. Bot. Studien Bd., 19, VEB Gustav Fischer Verlag, Jena.
Laval-Martin, D., Farinean, J., and Diamond, J., 1977, Light versus dark carbon metabolism in cherry tomato fruits. I. Occurrence of photosynthesis. Study of the intermediates, Plant Physiol., 60:872-876.
Lenz, F., 1967, Relationship between the vegetative and reproductive growth of Washington Navel orange cuttings (Citrus sinensis L. Osbeck), J. Hort. Sci., 42:31-39.
Lenz, F., 1974, Fruit effects on formation and distribution of photosynthetic assimilates, Proceedings Nineteenth International Horticultural Congress, Warsaw.
Lenz, F., 1979a, Fruit effects on photosynthesis and respiration, in: "Photosynthesis and Plant Development," H. Clysters, R. Marcelle, and M. van Pouche, eds., Dr. W. Junk, The Hague, in press.
Lenz, F., 1979b, Photosynthesis and respiration of Citrus as dependent upon fruit load, Proceedings Third International Citrus Symposium, Sydney, Australia, in press.
Lenz, F., and Bünemann, G., 1967, Beziehungen zwischen dem vegetativen und reproductiven Wachstum in Erdbeeren (Var. Senga Sengana), Gartenbauwiss., 32:227-236.
Lenz, F., and Daunicht, H. J., 1971, Einfluss von Wurzel und Frucht auf die Photosynthese bei Citrus, Angew. Bot., 35:11-20.

Lenz, F., and Döring, H., 1979, Nutrient uptake and nutrient distribution in Citrus as affected by fruit load, Z. f. Pflanzenernähr. u. Bodenk., in press.
Lenz, F., and Küntzel, U., 1974, Carbohydrate content of citrus leaves as affected by fruit load, Gartenbauwiss., 39:99-101.
Lenz, F., and Williams, C. N., 1973, Effect of fruit removal on net assimilation and gaseous diffusive resistance of soybean leaves, Angew. Bot., 47:57-63.
Leonard, E. R., 1962, Interrelation of vegetative and reproductive growth with special reference to indeterminate plants, Bot. Rev., 28:253-410.
Loveys, B. R., and Kriedemann, P. E., 1974, Internal control of stomatal physiology and photosynthesis. I. Stomatal regulation and associated changes in endogenous levels of abscisic and phaseic acids, Austr. J. Plant Physiol., 1:407-415.
Luckwill, L. C., 1970, The control of growth and fruitfulness of apple trees, in: "The Physiology of Tree Crops," L. C. Luckwill and C. V. Cutting, eds., Academic Press, London, New York.
Maggs, D. H., 1963, The reduction in growth of apple trees brought about by fruiting, J. Hort. Sci., 38:85-94.
Meisel, P., 1974, "Die Biosynthese der Stärke. Handbuch der Stärke VI-4," Paul Parey, Berlin and Hamburg.
Monselise, S. P., and Halevy, A. H., 1964, Chemical inhibition and promotion of citrus flower bud induction, Proc. Amer. Soc. Hort. Sci., 84:141-146.
Moss, G. I., 1970, Chemical control of flower development in sweet orange (Citrus sinensis), Austr. J. Agric. Res., 21:233-242.
Moss, G. I., and Bellamy, J., 1972, The use of gibberellic acid to control flowering of sweet orange (Citrus sinensis L. Osbeck), Acta Horticulturae, No. 34:207-213.
Mullins, M. G., 1970, Hormone-directed transport of assimilates in decapitated internodes of Phaseolus vulgaris L., Ann. Bot., 34:897-909.
Neales, T. F., and Incoll, L. D., 1968, The control of leaf photosynthesis rate by the level of assimilate concentration in the leaf: A review of the hypothesis, Bot. Rev., 34:107-125.
Nitsch, J. P., 1970, Hormonal factors in growth and development, in: "The Biochemistry of Fruits and Their Products," Vol. 1, A. C. Hulme, ed., Academic Press, London, New York.
Patrick, J. W., 1976, Hormone-directed transport of metabolites, in: "Transport and Transfer Processes in Plants," I. F. Wardlaw and J. B. Passioura, eds., Academic Press, New York.
Polevoi, V. V., and Salamatova, T. S., 1974, The mechanism of auxin action on membrane transport of hydrogen ions, trans. from Fiziol. Rast., 22:519-526.
Quast, P., 1975, Gibberellinbestimmung in Verbindung mit Kohlendydratgehalten und Trockensubstanzverteilung bei Solanaceen, Diss. T. U. Berlin.

Raschke, K., 1976, Transfer of ions and products of photosynthesis to guard cells, in: "Transport and Transfer Processes in Plants," I. F. Wardlaw and J. B. Passioura, eds., Academic Press, New York.

Sachs, T., 1975, The induction of transport channels by auxin, Planta, 127:201-206.

Smith, P. F., 1976, Collapse of "Mucott" tangerine trees, J. Amer. Hort. Sci., 101:23-25.

Tamas, I. A., Atkins, B. D., Ware, S. M., and Bidwell, R. G. S., 1972, Indoleacetic acid stimulation of phosphorylation and bicarbonate fixation by chloroplast preparation in light, Can. J. Bot., 50:1523-1527.

Treharne, K. J., and Stoddart, J. L., 1970, Effects of gibberellin and cytokinins on the activity of photosynthetic enzyme and plastid ribosomal RNA synthesis in Phaseolus vulgaris L., Nature (London), 228:129-131.

Tung, H. F., Broughton, W. J., and Lenz, F., 1973, Effects of fruit on ribulose diphosphate carboxylase activity in Citrus madurensis leaves, Experientia, 29:271.

Wardlaw, I. F., 1968, The control and pattern of movement of carbohydrates in plants, Bot. Rev., 34:79-105.

Wareing, P. F., 1968, The physiology of the whole tree, Ann. Rep. East Malling Res. Stn., 1967 (Kent), A51:55-68.

Wildman, S. G., 1967, The organization of grana-containing chloroplasts in relation to location of some enzymatic systems concerned with photosynthesis, protein synthesis, and ribonucleic acid synthesis, in: "Biochemistry of Chloroplasts," Vol. 2, T. W. Goodwin, ed., Academic Press, London and New York.

Wishnick, M., and Lane, M. D., 1970, The interaction of metal ions with ribulose-1,5-diphosphate carboxylase from spinach, J. Biol. Chem., 245:4939-4947.

Woodward, R. G., and Rawson, H. W., 1976, Photosynthesis and transpiration in dicotyledonous plants. II. Expanding and senescing leaves of soybean, Austr. J. Plant Physiol., 3: 257-267.

Zelitsch, J., 1975, Improving the efficiency of photosynthesis, Science, 188:626-633.

10

POTENTIAL FOR REGULATION OF PLANT GROWTH AND DEVELOPMENT

R. L. Wain

Wye College
University of London
England

A plant, unlike an animal, has to grow and survive and yet remain in the same place throughout its life. Furthermore, it is exposed to attack by pests and diseases, competition from weeds, and may be subjected to various forms of environmental stress. In man's attempts to help crop plants achieve their full potential, methods have been developed to control pests, diseases, and weeds; the plant breeder has produced improved varieties; and better performance is sometimes achieved by manipulating the crop by such devices as grafting and pruning. Better yields can be ensured by a balanced fertilizer program and unsuitable soil conditions can be improved by drainage or irrigation. Except in special situations, however, such as in glasshouses, it is not possible to control the weather--the main environmental factor which affects plant growth and development.

Basically, plant growth depends upon a wide range of diverse chemical reactions some of which are greatly influenced by temperature, water regime, and the like. In addition, through its chemistry a plant possesses built-in defense mechanisms which can operate to retard the effects of water stress, disease-causing fungi, or other potentially harmful influences.

The discovery that hormones synthesized within the plant play a vital role in controlling its growth processes has proved to be of great agricultural importance. Although great credit must be given to plant physiologists for their early pioneering work, it was not until 1934 when Kögl et al. (1934) discovered indole-3-acetic acid (IAA) as a plant growth hormone that rapid developments took place. At the present time we recognize auxins, gibberellins, cytokinins, and ethylene as hormones which operate together with growth inhibitors such as abscisic acid and xanthoxin in the complex of physiologically active chemicals which control and modify the growth of plants.

Studies on chemical structure in relation to activity have led to the discovery of a range of synthetic plant growth-regulating substances, and the consequences of this, particularly in the auxin field, have led to important developments in agriculture. Some of the effects which result from treatment can be achieved as a permanent feature by plant breeding; the responses which a growth substance can produce, however, can be obtained shortly after application and, furthermore, can be adjusted by varying the amount of chemical applied.

When a plant is treated with one of its own hormones the effect is usually not long lasting because the plant can remove excessive quantities of the chemical by degrading the molecule or by conjugating it with other substances; in doing so it uses the same mechanisms by which it controls endogenous hormone levels in its normal growth processes. Synthetic auxins in general have a longer survival rate in the plant than IAA because they are not so readily degraded or conjugated. Their uses, for example, in promoting rooting of cuttings and fruit setting and in achieving selective weed control are well known.

Gibberellins, on the other hand, have found fewer commercial uses. Although they can be much more effective than auxins in promoting elongation growth when applied to the growing plant, the yield benefits arising from this treatment, e.g., of pasture, are only marginal.

Cytokinins differ from auxins and gibberellins in that their main effect is concerned with promoting cell division. Most of the known cytokinins are derivatives of adenine, a purine derivative which is a component of nucleic acids present in the cell nucleus. A number of other cytokinins not related to adenine have recently been discovered, some of which are also highly active in promoting cell division. One of these compounds is 6-benzyloxypurine which in the sterile agar tobacco pith test causes the growing callus to undergo morphological differentiation to form plantlets (Wilcox and Wain, 1976).

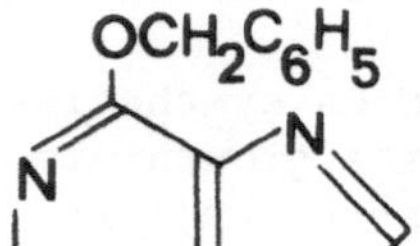

6-benzyloxypurine

Although cytokinins have so far achieved little commercial importance, their future potential in the field of tissue culture seems to be considerable. Research on derivatives of other purines and pyrimidines could be rewarding, for example, in providing easy methods for propagating difficult species. Other exciting possibilities could arise from studies now being carried out in this writer's laboratory and elsewhere on chemicals which might act as competitive antagonists to cytokinins.

One other compound which is recognized to be a growth hormone is the simple unsaturated gaseous hydrocarbon ethylene, C_2H_4. Ethylene can exert profound physiological effects; it is evolved by certain plants and especially by ripening fruits. It can promote abscission of both fruit and leaves and it also exerts detrimental effects on the growth of roots. The development of gas chromatographic techniques has greatly stimulated research on the role played by ethylene in the hormonal control of plant growth. Much of the experimental work involves the estimation of ethylene liberated by plants or plant organs followed by attempts to interpret the results in physiological terms. This interpretation, however, is very difficult because what is measured is extracellular ethylene whereas the physiological activity arises only from that present within the cells; indeed, it could well be that the same amount of intracellular ethylene is present in situations where the amount evolved is widely different. In considering the mode of action of ethylene, it would seem that the unsaturated character of the molecule and its small molecular size are of vital importance because the higher olefines are much less active and the corresponding paraffin, ethane, is inactive. A compound which breaks down to ethylene following application to plant tissues in ethephon, 2-chloroethylphosphonic acid. One striking effect it produces is to stimulate the flow of rubber latex when applied to rubber trees on a band of smoothed bark below the tapping cut. Here it is not affecting rubber biosynthesis but is preventing the plugging of the vessels through which the latex is conducted to the cut surface. Much research has been carried out, with some success, in trying to find other compounds which, like ethephon, can yield ethylene. No real breakthroughs have been made, however.

Other ways of controlling growth processes could be developed by treating the plant with a compound which hinders ethylene biosynthesis; progress made in this direction will be considered later in this report.

No important commercial uses have so far been found for the two hormone inhibitors abscisic acid and xanthoxin. One reason for this would appear to be that their physical properties are such that having been applied to the plant they do not readily move to the centers within cells from which they could exert their physiological effects. This limitation in physical properties could be of wider significance;

for example, let us just suppose that flowering is controlled by a "flowering hormone" and that to produce its effect the chemical builds up at appropriate centers within the plant. It is then quite conceivable that such a compound could be isolated from plant tissues as a stable pure substance yet never recognized as a flowering hormone because, following application, it can never find its way to its site of action.

Abscisic acid occurs in a wide range of plant tissues. Physiological studies have shown that it can inhibit the activity of auxins, gibberellins, and cytokinins. Studies in our laboratory (Wright, 1969; Wright and Hiron, 1969) have shown that abscisic acid operates in defending certain plants against effects of physiological stress. For example, when water is withheld from a tomato plant for three days the plant responds by producing up to fifty times the normal level of abscisic acid in its leaves. The effect of this is twofold--first, the resulting inhibition of growth hormone activity stops the plant from growing and energy is thereby conserved; second, closure of the leaf stomata is induced (Jones and Mansfield, 1970) and water loss by transpiration is cut down. By two mechanisms therefore, the buildup of endogenous abscisic acid provides the plant with a better chance of survival during the drought period. A challenge for research is to devise a means whereby this abscisic acid present within the tissues of a wilting crop can be removed when heavy rainfall alleviates the stress situation. As it is, although water may be abundant, retardation of crop growth is prolonged until normal hormone activity within the plant has been restored.

We have compared the capacity of a Mexican drought-resistant maize variety, "Latente," with two others which are not drought resistant (Larqué-Saavedra and Wain, 1974). It was found that when subjected to standard water stress conditions "Latente" produced much more abscisic acid than the other two varieties, again indicating the important role played by this inhibitor in plants subjected to drought. A similar finding was obtained with sorghum varieties (Larqué-Saavedra and Wain, 1976).

The abscisic acid defense mechanism which protects the plant when it is subjected to water stress also operates under conditions of waterlogging (Hiron and Wright, 1973). These findings make it not unreasonable to expect that a plant also has the capacity to protect itself when it is subjected to wounding. Earlier findings that beans can produce a wound hormone (traumatic acid) have never been substantiated but a chemical defense of this sort is possible and warrants further investigation.

Let us now consider what other research in the field of plant growth regulators might be of benefit to agriculture. Obviously there are possibilities for further developments in the various areas where plant growth substances are already producing successful results. Such progress will come from the discovery of new active chemicals, either through screening programs, research on structure activity relationships, or research on metabolic reactions, such as when inactive chemicals supplied to the plant become enzymically converted within the tissues to active growth regulators.

It is perhaps surprising that after some forty years of research very few auxins are used commercially for promoting rooting of cuttings. Although indoleacetic and butyric acids and 1-naphthylacetic acid give satisfactory results with many species, there are others which do not respond and it would seem that the wide range of known synthetic auxins ought to be examined with these species. It is becoming increasingly recognized, however, that whereas treatment with a single hormone might fail, a mixture of hormones could produce the desired effect. This applied, for example, with fruit-setting sprays on apple trees where an application of auxin, gibberellin, and cytokinin together is necessary to get good fruit setting and increased yield.

Growth retardant chemicals are now widely used in agriculture. The sturdy short-stemmed plants which arise from their use can give higher yields and withstand unfavorable weather conditions better than untreated plants. Most commercial growth retardants are synthetic chemicals and there is no doubt that more will be discovered. Some operate as "antigibberellins," thereby restricting cell elongation. A new type of retardant, however, is 3,5-dichlorophenoxyacetic acid (3,5-D) which, itself inactive as an auxin, appears to act as an antiauxin (Wain and Wightman, 1957) and as a dwarfing compound in certain plants (Smith and Moshin, 1970; Taylor and Wain, 1978). A wide range of quaternary ammonium, phosphonium, and sulphonium salts have been synthesized and examined as retardants in our laboratory and some of them are highly active (Knight et al., 1969; Chamberlain et al., 1976).

We are also following another approach to the discovery of growth retardant chemicals. In this work we have examined extracts of seedlings of genetic dwarf wheat varieties including some of those developed by Borlaug in Mexico which were important in bringing about the so-called "green revolution." When the extracts are fractionated by counter current distribution procedures and the separate fractions are sprayed onto tall wheat seedlings, one of these fractions causes marked inhibition of growth. Further work has shown that a natural growth inhibitor is responsible and it has now been isolated. The compound appears to be completely unrelated to any known growth inhibitor and when this natural growth retardant is chemically identified it should stimulate much fundamental and agricultural research.

The most important agricultural use of plant growth substances to date has been as selective herbicides. The selectivity of known compounds, such as 2,4-D and MCPA, has been extended by converting them to inactive derivatives from which the herbicidal growth regulator becomes released by enzyme action only within susceptible plants. This concept of differential lethal synthesis has been exploited successfully in our laboratory and some of the γ-phenoxybutyric acids (e.g., MCPB and 2,4-DB) arising from this work are used in world agriculture (Wain, 1955a,b). Another route to selective herbicidal activity of this kind depends upon the presence or absence of a specific amine oxidase within the plant. Thus 2,4-dichlorophenoxyethylamine becomes converted to 2,4-D only when the appropriate oxidase is present in the tissues (Nash et al., 1968). There is no doubt that many more enzymic reactions remain to be exploited in the search for new selective herbicides.

Considering the tremendous progress made in the field of antibiotics it is surprising that studies on allelopathy have been so unrewarding. Yet nature being what it is one would expect higher plants to produce chemicals which repress their competitors. Identifying such compounds could provide leads to the discovery of new selective herbicides. Again, weed seeds such as the notorious wild oat can remain dormant for many years in the soil. If the germination inhibitors which operate could be identified and chemicals which react with them discovered, this would provide a means of getting all the seeds to germinate at the same time. The whole population of seedlings could then be destroyed by cultural methods or with herbicides. Some progress is now being made in these directions.

We have so far been mainly considering chemicals which exert effects on the growth of whole plants. What about that vital part of the plant which is not normally seen--the roots growing in the soil? Research on hormones in relation to root growth has so far not been extensive and indeed it is only recently that IAA has been unequivocally shown to operate in roots. In some of our experiments we have demonstrated that root growth is restricted on exposure to light, that the light receptor is the root cap, and that with some species only a short flash of light is enough to produce an inhibitory effect (Wilkins et al., 1974; Wilkins and Wain, 1975; Wilkins et al., 1973).

A development in this area of research came unexpectedly when we were examining the biological activity of 3,5-diiodo-4-hydroxybenzoic acid (DIHB), a compound closely related to ioxynil, a selective herbicide discovered in our laboratory (Wain, 1963). When cress or rice seedlings were grown in a normal culture solution, roots exposed to light were found to grow to only one-third the length of those growing in the dark. However, this inhibitory effect was completely removed when DIHB was present in the solution at only 10^{-5}M (Wain et al., 1968). Thus, DIHB removes the constraint on root growth which is imposed by exposure to light. Unfortunately, roots in the soil are in the dark so the beneficial response to DIHB cannot be exploited. However, other constraints on the growth of roots can operate in the field, such as mechanical impedence, and when this occurs DIHB has been shown to have a beneficial effect (Wilkins et al., 1976).

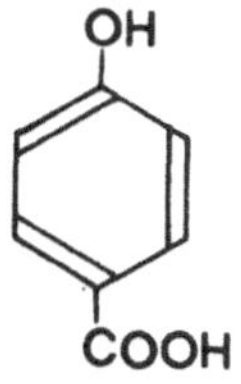

DIHB

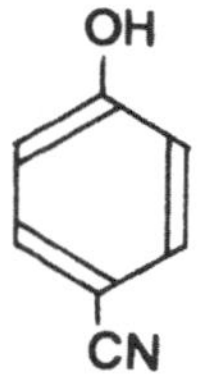

Ioxynil

Similar useful responses have been found in waterlogged and saline soils following treatment with DIHB; the agricultural implications of all these findings are now being intensively studied.

Present indications are that DIHB exerts its effect by preventing the biosynthesis of ethylene, a compound which exerts detrimental effects on the growth of roots (Robert et al., 1975). The mode of action of DIHB, however, is complex and not fully understood.

Our work on the chemical basis of plant disease resistance has provided other leads to research on plant growth substances. The approach adopted is based on the fact that most plants and their root systems are completely resistant to most of the fungal pathogens to which they are continuously exposed during their growth. Potatoes, for example, although susceptible to potato blight, are completely immune to apple scab, cereal rusts, and so on. Thus, throughout the plant kingdom, resistance is the rule rather than the exception and there is now much evidence that such resistance may be associated with the presence of defensive chemicals present within the plant. Our research within this field has recently been reviewed (Wain, 1977) and only one aspect need concern us here.

Chromatographic separation of antifungal compounds from the leaves of a species of tobacco (Nicotiana glutinosa) revealed the presence of "sclareol"--a mixture of two diterpenes, sclareol and 13-epi-sclareol. "Sclareol" proved to be a powerful fungicide and applications of only 100 ppm to beans or wheat plants gave almost complete protection against rust diseases (Bailey et al., 1975). With other fungi, e.g., Alternaria longipes, the fungicidal action of "sclareol" appears to operate in a most unusual way. Spore germination is not affected but the normally long free growing hyphae are branched and distorted and are incapable of initiating an infection. Thus, although not toxic to these fungi, "sclareol" affects the growth and morphology of the fungi hyphae. This effect, which has also been observed with griseofulvin (Brian, 1949), is in some ways similar to that produced by auxins when they are applied to higher plants. Do these compounds provide a lead to an understanding of the hormonal control of fungal growth? And do such compounds indicate a new approach to fungal disease control? More research in these fields is clearly needed.

Space does not permit discussion of other areas of research on plant regulators which might be of benefit to agriculture. Chemicals which inhibit photorespiration and thereby improve photosynthetic efficiency are being actively sought. Again, a chemical which diverts photosynthetic energy to those parts of the plant that are to be harvested, as for example from vegetative growth to roots and tubers, could make a big impact on food production.

Everything considered, there is no doubt that known plant growth regulators, and other such compounds which await discovery, will have an increasing role to play in agriculture. Further research on the biological properties and uses of these unique organic molecules is clearly warranted and should be very rewarding.

REFERENCES

Bailey, J. A., Carter, G. A., Burden, R. S., and Wain, R. L., 1975, Control of rust diseases by diterpenes from Nicotiana glutinosa, Nature (London), 255:328-329.

Brian, P. W., 1949, Studies on the biological activity of griseofulvin, Ann. Bot., 13:59-77.

Chamberlain, V. K., Chamberlain, K., and Wain, R. L., 1976, Studies on plant growth-regulating substances. XXXIX. The plant growth-retarding properties of certain quaternary ammonium halides, Ann. Appl. Biol., 82:589-596.

Hiron, R. W. P., and Wright, S. T. C., 1973, The role of endogenous abscisic acid in the response of plants to stress, J. Exp. Bot., 24:769-780.

Jones, R. J., and Mansfield, T. A., 1970, Suppression of stomatic opening in leaves treated with abscisic acid, J. Exp. Bot., 21:714-719.

Knight, B. E. A., Taylor, H. F., and Wain, R. L., 1969, Studies on plant growth-regulating substances. XXIX. The plant growth-retarding properties of certain ammonium, phosphorium and sulphonium halides, Ann. Appl. Biol., 63:211-223.

Kögl, F., Haagen-Smit, A. J., and Erxleben, H., 1934, Über ein neues Auxin ("Heteroauxin") aus Harn. XI. Mitteilung über pflanzenliche Wachstumstoffe, Z. physiol. Chemie, 228:90-103.

Larqué-Saavedra, A., and Wain, R. L., 1974, Abscisic acid levels in relation to drought tolerance in varieties of Zea mays L., Nature (London), 251:716-717.

Larqué-Saavedra, A., and Wain, R. L., 1976, Studies on plant growth-regulating substances. XLII. Abscisic acid as a genetic character related to drought tolerance, Ann. Appl. Biol., 83: 291-297.

Nash, R. J., Smith, T. A., and Wain, R. L., 1968, Studies on plant growth-regulating substances. XXVII. The growth-regulating activity and metabolism of 2,4-dichlorophenoxyethylamine and related compounds in higher plants, Ann. Appl. Biol., 61:481-494.

Robert, M. L., Taylor, H. F., and Wain, R. L., 1975, Ethylene production by cress roots and excised cress root segments and its inhibition by 3,5-diiodo-4-hydroxybenzoic acid, Planta, 126:273-284.

Smith, M. S., and Moshin, M., 1970, 3,5 dichlorophenoxyacetic acid as a growth retardant, Ann. Appl. Biol., 66:233-238.

Taylor, H. F., and Wain, R. L., 1978, Studies on plant growth-regulating substances. LII. Growth retardation by 3,5 dichlorophenoxyethylamine and 3,5 dichlorophenoxybutyric acid arising from their conversion to 3,5 dichlorophenoxyacetic acid from tomato plants, Ann. Appl. Biol., 89:271-275.

Wain, R. L., 1955a, A new approach to selective weed controls, Ann. Appl. Biol., 42:151-157.

Wain, R. L., 1955b, Herbicidal selectivity through specific action of plants on compounds applied, J. Agric. Food Chem., 3:128-130.

Wain, R. L., 1963, 3:5-dihalogeno-4-hydroxybenzonitriles as herbicides, Nature (London), 200:28.

Wain, R. L., Taylor, H. F., Intarakosit, P., and Shannon, T. G. D., 1968, Halogen derivatives of 4-hydroxybenzoic acid as root growth stimulants and the importance of light to this response, Nature (London), 217:870-871.

Wain, R. L., 1977, Chemical aspects of plant disease resistance, Pontif. Acad. Sci. Scr. Varia, 41:483-508.

Wain, R. L., and Wightman, F., 1957, Studies on plant growth-regulating substances. XI. Auxin antagonism in relation to a theory on mode of action of aryl- and aryloxy-alkanecarboxylic acids, Ann. Appl. Biol., 45:140-157.

Wilcox, E. J., and Wain, R. L., 1976, Studies on plant growth-regulating substances. XLIV. The cytokinin activity of 6-benzyloxypurine, Ann. Appl. Biol., 84:403-407.

Wilkins, H., Burden, R. S., and Wain, R. L., 1974, Growth inhibitors in roots of light- and dark-grown seedlings of Zea mays, Ann. Appl. Biol., 78:337-338.

Wilkins, H., Larqué-Saavedra, A., and Wain, R. L., 1973, "Plant Growth Substances," Tokyo, Hirowaka Publ. Co.

Wilkins, H., and Wain, R. L., 1975, The role of root cap in the response of the primary roots of Zea mays L. seedlings to white light and to gravity, Planta, 123:217-222.

Wilkins, S. M., Wilkins, H., and Wain, R. L., 1976, Chemical treatment of soil alleviate effects of soil compaction on pea seedling growth, Nature (London), 259:392-394.
Wright, S. T. C., 1969, An increase in the "Inhibitor-β" content of detached wheat leaves following a period of wilting, Planta, 86:10-20.
Wright, S. T. C., and Hiron, R. W. P., 1969, (+) - Abscisic acid, the growth inhibitor induced in detached wheat leaves by a period of wilting, Nature (London), 224:719-720.

11

CHEMICAL PLANT GROWTH REGULATION IN WORLD AGRICULTURE

R. W. F. Hardy

E. I. du Pont de Nemours and Company
Wilmington, Delaware

INTRODUCTION

The tremendous increases in world crop production during the past twenty-five years were made possible by a system in which agrichemicals as fertilizers and plant protectant chemicals were most important components, while plant growth regulator chemicals were of little significance. This presentation will offer an optimistic view of the future opportunity for plant growth regulators. By 2000 A.D. I predict that plant growth regulators primarily as yield enhancers, but secondarily as quality improvers and production process facilitators, will become as important as fertilizers or plant protectant chemicals for world crop production. Specific topics included in this presentation are:

(1) Strategies for increasing crop production for food, feed, energy, and materials including the relatively undeveloped technology of plant growth regulators.

(2) The current status of plant growth regulators, reasons for their relatively slow development, and their advantages and disadvantages.

(3) Steps in a fundamentally based approach to increase crop production with a tabulation of the many possible limitations or "what's wrong" with two key biological processes--photosynthetic CO_2 fixation and N_2 fixation.

(4) Specific biochemical, physiological, genetic, and agronomic targets for plant growth regulators will be suggested with

a comprehensive tabulation of existing chemicals useful as experimental probes or as commercial plant growth regulators, and

(5) Scientific highlights of selected promising areas for increased crop production including N_2 fixation, photosynthesis, translocation, assimilate partitioning, protection from stress due to air pollutants, and hormonal activity manipulation.

STRATEGIES FOR WORLD CROP PRODUCTION

I have evolved during the past two years a list of assumptions, relevant facts, and strategies for increasing crop production for food, feed, energy, and materials (Hardy, 1976a, 1977a,b,c, 1978a; Hardy et al., 1977b). Plant growth regulators for the major agronomic crops are included as a needed supplemental technology.

The primary emphasis must be on increased crop productivity or increased bioconversion of solar energy to harvested components (Hardy, 1977b,c; Hardy and Havelka, 1977). Current world production of about 1300 MMT must be increased to about 2600 MMT by 2000 A.D., while that of grain legumes which is currently 130 MMT must be increased to about 500 MMT. These increases will be necessary to meet the food demands of the expanded population with the ever increasing demand for animal vs. plant food driven by increased affluence. A high yielding corn field--6000 kg/ha--only converts about 0.2-0.4% of the incident solar energy to harvestable grain, while a high yielding soybean field--1800 kg/ha--converts only about 0.1-0.2%. Assuming no change in crop production area, solar energy conversion must be doubled by cereal grains and quadrupled by grain legumes. This objective is the primary energy one for agriculture and the opportunity here for plant growth regulators is almost unlimited.

Decreased inputs of nonrenewable resources, such as fossil energy, is a secondary objective for crop production. This is a desirable but not essential goal since food is such a primary need that increased allocation of nonrenewable resources for its production must be made if necessary. A crop production strategy which gives primary emphasis to decreased fossil energy input as often suggested rather than increased food production guarantees that the food demands of many people may not be met. Probably one of the best objectives for decreased fossil energy input for crop production would be the development of a new abiological N_2 fixing system in which there would be zero-direct energy input required for the fixation of N_2 vs. the energy intensive biological and Haber processes. A catalyst to convert air to fixed nitrogen, e.g., NO_3^-, at ambient temperature in an irrigation system without any directly added energy may be such a system. It would conserve energy and at the same time supply the increasing quantities of nitrogen fertilizer needed for increased crop production. In addition, plant growth regulators may be useful in conserving use of limited resources, such as fossil energy or even water.

Increased inputs of improved varieties, fertilizers, plant protectant chemicals, irrigation, and possibly mechanization will be required for increased crop productivity in the future as they have in the past. I suggest that these established technologies will require supplementation with new technologies, such as plant growth regulators and genetic engineering (Day, 1977). The effective development of these new technologies in many cases may require a biochemical-physiological-genetic-agronomic focus, such as photosynthesis, assimilate partitioning, senescence, or nitrogen fixation vs. the current predominant commodity orientation, such as rice, wheat, corn, and soybeans.

Technologies suitable for the cash-limited, less developed countries where the objective is high yield with relatively independent labor intensity will often be different from those of the relatively cash-unlimited, more developed countries where the objective is high yield at minimal labor. These differentials suggest that plant growth regulators as other high technology inputs will be at least initially of greater importance to more developed than less developed countries.

The declining ratio of production of high protein grain legumes excluding soybeans to low protein cereal grains during the past decade must be reversed in order to provide high protein foods for people and high protein feed supplements for the projected increased animal production (Hardy et al., 1977a). This suggests that the contribution per unit area of land by plant growth regulators and other inputs must be greater for grain legumes than cereal grains.

Exploratory human nutrition research which during the last quarter century has been somewhat dormant requires a major expansion especially in the areas of chronic (e.g., cardiovascular) and behavioral as opposed to acute (vitamin deficiencies) diseases, and this expanded activity needs to be integrated with crop production research. Plant growth regulators may be useful to improve the nutritional quality of crops.

If economic technologies are evolved for production of significant new amounts of energy and materials (da Silva et al., 1978) from biomass--the biomass refinery--then the demands on increased crop production will greatly exceed those already indicated for cereal grains and grain legumes. The starches and sugars may be currently economically useful fermentation substrates for the synthesis of specific chemicals (Vlitos, see Chapter 21) while in the longer term the huge amount of lignocellulosics dictate that methods must be developed for their use and possibly growth regulators for their production.

CURRENT STATUS OF PLANT GROWTH REGULATORS

Plant growth regulators have been used in agriculture for over forty years (Appendix 1). Induction of flowering in pineapples by ethylene and acetylene was used in the 1930s and since that time there have been a number of additional growth regulators introduced to regulate a number of processes especially in horticultural crops. It is, however, significant that only one or two growth regulators have been introduced that affect major agronomic crops and the total world agrichemical market for plant growth regulators is projected at about \$100 MM in 1980, an insignificant 1% of the projected total world agrichemical market of \$8,000 MM (Fig. 1) (Anonymous, 1977a). This slow development (Anonymous, 1977a, 1978a) of plant growth regulators may be attributed to a variety of factors including: (1) emphasis on an empirical approach similar to that often used in the plant protectant area rather than a more fundamental approach, (2) emphasis on hormones with inadequate consideration of other growth and development molecules and processes, such as enzymes, feedback effects, gene expression, etc., (3) emphasis on horticultural rather than agronomic crops, (4) inconsistency in crop response to growth regulating chemicals, such as TIBA in soybeans or Dinoseb in corn, (5) limited biochemical and physiological knowledge of key plant processes although this is undergoing dramatic improvement, and (6) the difficulties of demonstrating yield improvements vs. the relative ease of recognizing visual effects, such as plant protection or morphological changes.

A number of factors suggest a greatly improved future for plant growth regulators. For example, the many reports (Appendix 2) published on the identification of research objectives and priorities in agriculture and crop production include chemical plant growth regulators as a means of increasing crop productivity. In the report on "Researchable Areas Which Have Potential for Increasing Crop Production," plant growth regulation was one of the six areas selected. Other more practically oriented publications, such as Farm Chemicals and Soybean Digest, indicate the enthusiasm and high expectations for plant growth regulators among farmers and related agriculturists. There is broad interest among many industries in plant growth regulator research (Appendix 3) (Anonymous, 1978b). A Plant Growth Regulator Working Group was organized in 1973 in the United States and a similar professional organization was recently formed in Europe.

Plant growth regulators have inherent advantages over genetic solutions for the regulation of key processes in plants. Their activity should be broad spectrum so that a common key biochemical

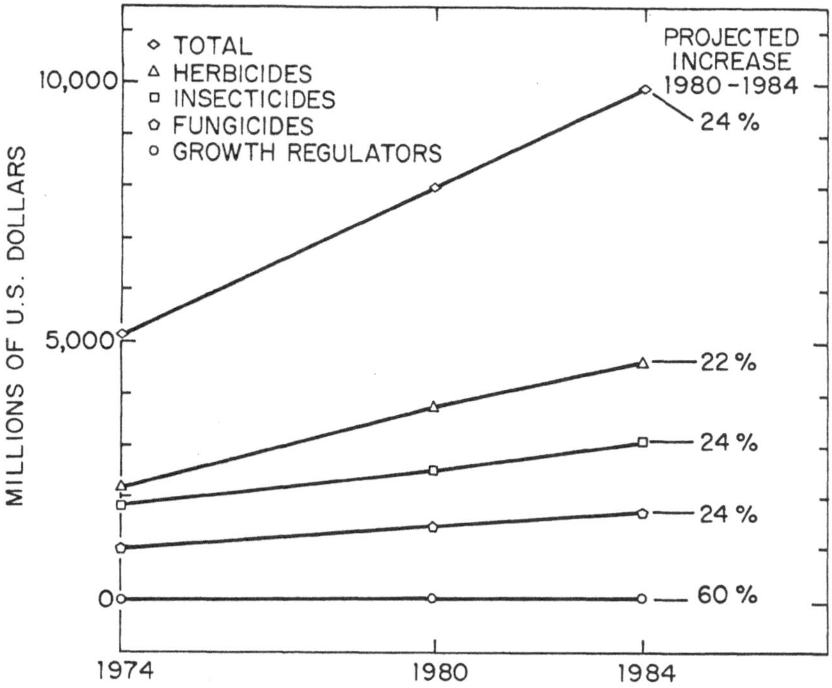

Fig. 1. Current and projected world agrichemical market at the user's level (Anonymous, 1977a) and projected increase 1980-1984. Note low fraction for plant growth regulators but greatest projected increase in this category. Growth regulators include defoliants and dessicants.

process, such as, for example, photorespiration, would be affected by a single chemical in not only different cultivars of the same crop but in different crops and in different geographical locations, enabling a quick impact while genetic manipulation is very tedious and slow. Plant growth regulating chemicals should have a high value in use and be readily acceptable by farmers, who are already familiar with the use and value of plant protectant chemicals and fertilizers. Application of plant growth regulating chemicals would utilize existing equipment. Plant growth regulating chemicals should have a high degree of safety as they are subject to the established procedures for toxicological testing of plant protectant chemicals while new genetically manipulated crops may not be subjected to the same degree of sophisticated toxicological testing (Tucker, 1978). Application of plant growth regulant chemicals at a specific or critical growth time would be possible in order to obtain maximum benefit in regulating a key process whereas genetically modified plants do not allow such timing. Moreover, plant growth regulant chemicals might allow manipulation of the protein or oil content of the crop after planting so as to match more closely the demand for protein or oil. Plant growth regulant chemicals may be effective in extremely low amounts since they are perturbing a specific process rather than completely inhibiting the process.

Plant growth regulant chemicals have some disadvantages relative to genetically manipulated crops. Input of the chemical would be required for each crop whereas a genetically manipulated crop requires only a single initial input of the modified seed. Plant growth regulant chemicals are high technology and would be initially limited to those countries with the infrastructure to enable their implementation. However, both plant growth regulators and genetically engineered crops will require a highly sophisticated environment for their development and successful application.

FUNDAMENTALLY BASED APPROACH FOR INCREASING CROP PRODUCTIVITY

The major advances in crop production have come from empirical rather than fundamentally based approaches. For more sophisticated technologies, such as plant growth regulating chemicals, I suggest that a fundamentally based approach may be more rewarding than an empirically based approach (Hardy, 1977c, 1978a, 1979; Hardy et al., 1977a,b, 1978b). Such an approach may involve six steps. Step 1 involves the identification of possible specific biochemical, physiological, genetic, or agronomic limitations. This information comes from fundamental studies of biological processes. As the information base expands about a biological process, one can suggest limitations or ask "what's wrong with the natural process." The expanding information on, for example, photosynthetic carbon dioxide fixation by ribulose 1,5-bisphosphate carboxylase (RuBPCase) and nitrogen fixation by nitrogenase are making possible the construction of tables of "what's wrongs" (Appendices 4,5) (Hardy, 1977b; Hardy et al., 1978a,b).

For example, at the biochemical level, RuBPCase exhibits substrate promiscuity so that both oxygen and carbon dioxide are competing substrates for the enzyme. Moreover, the affinity of the enzyme for carbon dioxide is inappropriately high for the low ambient partial pressure of carbon dioxide and inappropriately low for the high ambient partial pressure of pO_2. This enzyme makes up as much as 50% of the soluble protein of a leaf and appears to occur in an excessive amount relative to the hundreds of other enzymes required by the plant for growth and development. The enzyme has a low turnover number of about 200 molecules of carbon dioxide fixed per molecule of enzyme per minute. At the genetic level, the occurrence of the genetic information for RuBPCase in two different organelles within the plant cell make manipulation of the enzyme by conventional plant breeding difficult. These are only a few of the limitations that have been revealed by basic studies on the RuBPCase enzyme.

Some of these limitations may represent opportunities for beneficial regulation by plant growth regulators.

Next, it is necessary to assess what is quantitatively important as a "what's wrong" for crop production and what is only a laboratory curiosity so that only those most significant opportunities are pursued as targets for plant growth regulators or other technological inputs. This step, Step 2, is the current major barrier to a fundamentally based approach to increasing crop production. Laboratory scientists have been most effective in providing information that enables tabulations of "what's wrong" but have shown little interest in assessing the quantitative importance of the "what's wrong" under natural crop production conditions. Such assessments must be greatly expanded in the future; moreover, practical solutions are not necessary to make useful assessments. As an example, we have exploited gas phase manipulations--carbon dioxide enrichment or oxygen alteration--to assess the importance in grain legumes of some of the limitations of photosynthetic CO_2 fixation and N_2 fixation (Criswell et al., 1976, 1977; Hardy and Havelka, 1975a,b, 1977; Hardy et al., 1977a,b, 1978b; Havelka and Hardy, 1976; Quebedeaux and Hardy, 1973, 1975, 1976).

In Step 3, specific rapid and simple screens must be developed to select chemical or other solutions to overcome the "what's wrong." In Step 4, these screens must be operated at high capacity to discover possible solutions. A potential solution must have its practicality determined on an economic, safety, and possibly nutritional basis in Step 5. Finally, in Step 6, the effective solution must be implemented into agricultural production systems.

SPECIFIC TARGETS FOR PLANT GROWTH REGULATION

The general targets for plant growth regulation can be subdivided into yield enhancement, quality improvement, and facilitation of production excluding plant protection. The objective of the first is the primary objective for world crop production; that of quality improvement includes nutritional (protein, oil, and sugar) and aesthetic (uniform size and color) characteristics; that of facilitation in many cases relates to a reduction in tedious, time consuming, and expensive labor inputs, such as hand thinning or manual picking of citrus and olives. In Appendix 6, a comprehensive list of specific targets in each of these three categories is provided with a tabulation of chemical agents currently useful as experimental probes or as commercial regulators of these processes.

The range of needs or opportunities for plant growth regulators is relatively unlimited and extends from regulation of seed germination and root growth to regulation of senescence of the mature plant.

In most cases, an effective growth regulant has not yet been found although in, for example, regulation of morphology, a number of active agents have been identified and a few have been commercialized.

This list of plant growth regulating chemicals has been expanded to include some that have not been included heretofore. For example, N-Serve®, which inhibits nitrification, the conversion of ammonia to nitrate in the soil, and thereby indirectly regulates plant growth, is included as a plant growth regulant (Huber et al., 1977). Krenite®, which is uniquely effective as a plant growth regulant for brush control, is included since its effect in regulating growth does not appear until the season following its application and it also avoids the undesirable brownout following application of a herbicide such as 2,4-D. Although the opportunity for plant growth regulation is great (Appendix 6), the significant discoveries for world crop production have yet to be made.

SCIENTIFIC HIGHLIGHTS IN SELECTED AREAS WHERE PLANT GROWTH REGULATION MAY BE OF LARGE POTENTIAL SIGNIFICANCE TO CROP PRODUCTION

Highlights of several areas in which significant scientific advances have occurred in recent years will be described utilizing specific examples from our own laboratory where we have established a significant and diverse group to seek plant growth regulators. Although plant growth regulation research in general has been relatively unsuccessful so far in the discovery of important commercial products for increased crop production, significant plant growth regulators may be most effectively found in my judgment based on an increased fundamental knowledge of the processes that are significant limitations in crop production. Accordingly, various fundamental and practical aspects of nitrogen input, carbon input, translocation, assimilate partitioning, reproductive growth, stress due to air pollutants, senescence, and manipulation of hormone receptor sites will be described.

Nitrogen Input

One of the major factors responsible for increased crop production during the past quarter century is the tenfold increase in the input of fertilizer nitrogen (Hardy and Havelka, 1975b). Additional nitrogen may be provided by expansion of existing or development of new chemical processes or enhancement or extension of the biological nitrogen fixation process (Burns and Hardy, 1975; Hardy, 1975, 1976b, 1977b,c,d, 1978a,b; Hardy et al., 1977a,b; Hardy and Gibson, 1977; Hardy and Silver, 1977; Hardy et al., 1978a).

Explosive scientific advances in biological nitrogen fixation research have revealed that the enzyme nitrogenase is at least as wasteful of energy as is the commercial Haber-Bosch process. Thus, the legume-Rhizobium system (Fig. 2), which is the major biological source of nitrogen for agricultural purposes, consumes 10-20 kg of carbohydrate/kg of nitrogen fixed--a most inefficient fermentation. It is not surprising then that this excessive requirement of energy or carbohydrate by the biological nitrogen fixation system makes the plant and specifically photosynthate production by the plant the major limiting factor for biological nitrogen fixation by all grain legumes so far examined under field conditions (Hardy, 1977c; Hardy and Havelka, 1975a, 1977; Hardy et al., 1977a,b; Havelka and Hardy, 1976; Quebedeaux et al., 1975). Overcoming this photosynthate limitation by CO_2 enrichment of four field grown legumes from an ambient air concentration of about 300 ppm CO_2 to an enriched concentration of 1000-1500 ppm CO_2 during the day from anthesis to senescence produced substantial increases in N_2 fixation (Appendix 7). The increases in most cases are a composite of three factors: (1) a rapid increase in the specific N_2 fixing activity of the nodule, (2) a long-term increase in the mass of nodules, and (3) a delay in the loss of N_2 fixing activity due to nodule senescence. Can plant growth regulators be found that would enable beneficial and practical manipulation of one or more of the above factors so as to increase nitrogen input by biological N_2 fixation in legumes?

The rhizobial-legume symbiosis, as any of the nitrogenase-based N_2 fixing systems, suffers from the promiscuity of nitrogenase in that H_3O^+ is reduced to H_2 as well as N_2 to NH_3 with the consumption of ATP and reductant. Growth regulators that would eliminate this wasteful reduction of H_3O^+ would substantially improve the energy efficiency of biological N_2 fixation.

The discovery of N_2 fixing bacteria associated with the roots of grasses and cereals in the 1960s and early 1970s generated optimism that such systems as the Azospirillum lipoferum and corn might provide substantial quantities of nitrogen for cereal grains. However, the amount of N_2 fixed is only 1-5 kg/ha/yr when measured under in situ conditions--an amount totally inadequate for high yield crop production in which 6000 kg/ha corn may need addition of over 100 kg N/ha. Recently, the Rhizobium bacteria have been shown unexpectedly to associate with the roots of hydroponically grown wheat and rice (Shimshick and Hebert, 1978). Can plant growth regulators make these associations fix adequate nitrogen for high yield by nonlegume cereals and forages?

Some initial steps have been made in the use of recombinant DNA techniques to construct higher plants containing their own N_2 fixing genes. About one-half of the large genetic area for nitrogen fixation containing some now identified 14 genes has been transferred to a plasmid (Cannon et al., 1977). Many steps remain before one can hope to achieve a nitrogen fixing higher plant. In fact, one

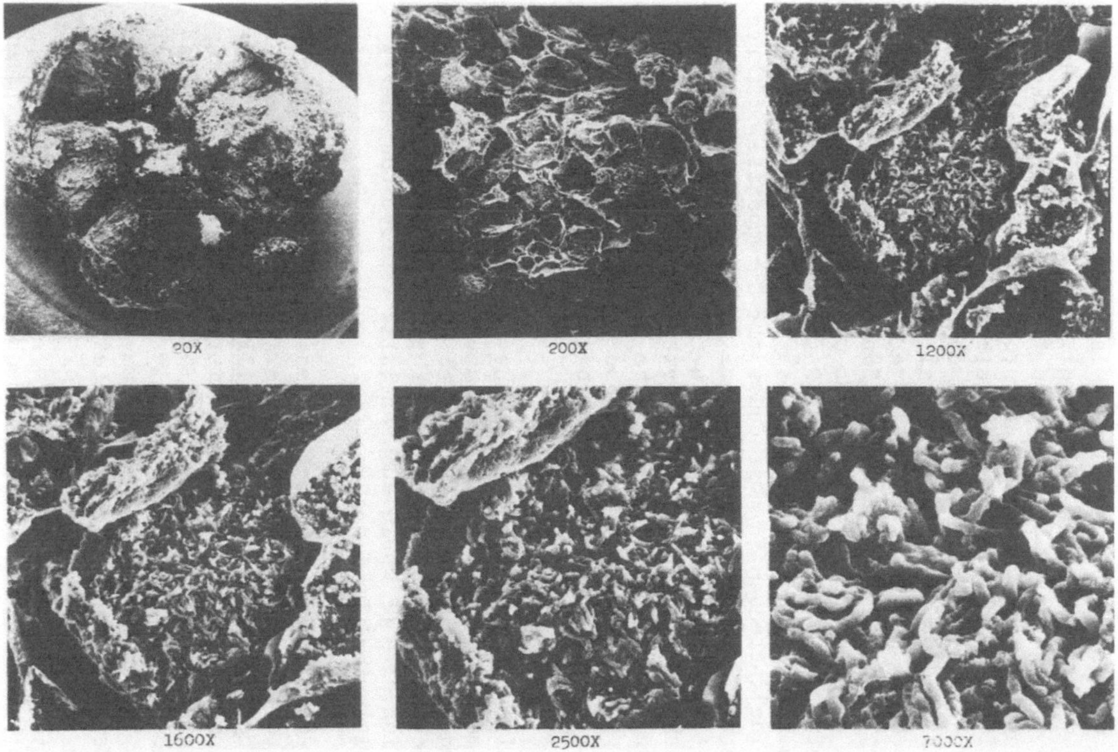

Fig. 2. Scanning electron micrograph of the interior of a freeze cleaved soybean nodule at various magnifications (Hardy, 1977b). Note the densely packed bacteroids containing nitrogenase within the root cells with about 10,000 bacteroids per host legume cell. The huge energy requirement of the bacteroids for growth, N_2 fixation, and a removal of fixed N produces a 10–20 kg drain on plant carbohydrate for each kg of N_2 fixed. Such a wasteful system must have its efficiency improved.

of the major barriers outside the inherent instabilities of the nitrogenase molecule itself is the inability in most cases to generate higher plants from single plant cells. Will plant growth regulators play a critical role in this exciting area of research?

Another naturally occurring nitrogen fixing system is the symbiosis between the water fern Azolla and the blue-green alga Anabaena (Lamborg, 1977). This association has been used empirically to provide nitrogen in paddy-grown rice in the Far East for centuries and is referred to reverently as the "Goddess of Azolla." The independent provision of energy for N_2 fixation by the Azolla-Anabaena association through its own photosynthetic system is an energetic advantage over symbioses in which the crop plant must provide the energy. However, the Anabaena-Azolla system requires additional phosphate and iron and a high innoculation rate. With these requirements, is it economical for high yield crop production? Is there an opportunity here for plant growth regulators?

Alternate nitrogen input systems must be economically competitive with other forms of nitrogen input and must also be sufficiently active to support high yield agriculture. A first attempt at a comparison of the theoretical substitution of fertilizer nitrogen in high yield crop production for a crop such as corn with a yet to be developed symbiosis that biologically fixes nitrogen was economically unfavorable. The assumed economic loss in yield due to the energy required for biological nitrogen fixation did not offset the economic credit for the unused fertilizer nitrogen (Hardy, 1977b). In both, there are costs for distribution and application, but these are assumed to be similar. No cost was assumed for the production of the biological symbiont which, if included, would further worsen the biological case. This comparison further emphasizes the absolute necessity to decrease the energy requirements for biological nitrogen fixation, a problem for which no significant practical solution has so far been reported. The great publication emphasis on reuse of H_2 is probably of only minor significance in the field and may have already been solved by an empirical approach (Evans, 1977). Many of the potential opportunities for new technologies for nitrogen input are summarized in Appendix 8, and plant growth regulators may play a decisive role in their realization.

Carbon Input

The primary reaction in crop production is the utilization of solar energy to convert carbon dioxide to the chemical products of photosynthesis. One of the several undesirable aspects of photosynthesis (Appendix 4) is a process called photorespiration. This process, attributable to the promiscuity of RuBPCase (the carbon dioxide fixing enzyme) toward oxygen as well as carbon dioxide, produces phosphoglycolate, which cannot be directly utilized by the plant. Phosphoglycolate and its products are shuttled among three organelles to enable conversion to a reusable form with the attendant loss of CO_2 back to the atmosphere. Although considerable disagreement exists on the specific steps of the photorespiratory pathway, there is general agreement that the promiscuity of RuBPCase is the primary cause of photorespiration (Chollet, 1977; Ogren, 1977). There has been no demonstrated usefulness to the plant associated with photorespiration and, in fact, the use of various techniques such as carbon dioxide enrichment and O_2 depletion which substantially eliminate photorespiration produced no results that indicate a useful function associated with major photorespiratory activity in plants.

We have utilized carbon dioxide enrichment in field-grown crops and oxygen alteration of laboratory-grown crops to assess the significant waste due to the promiscuity of RuBPCase (Hardy, 1977b,c, 1978a, 1979; Hardy and Havelka, 1975a, 1977; Hardy et al., 1977a,b, 1978b; Havelka and Hardy, 1976; Quebedeaux and Hardy, 1975, 1976). Carbon dioxide enrichment of field-grown legumes from an ambient pCO_2 of about 300 ppm to 1000-1500 ppm from anthesis to senescence during the day has produced dramatic yield increases of about 50-100% in four different grain legumes (Appendix 7). This suggests that an unequaled opportunity for increased crop production exists for a plant growth regulator that would decrease the O_2-promiscuity of RuBPCase and/or increase affinity for CO_2.

Photorespiration is not the only significant already identified limitation of the carbon input system of plants. There are many "what's wrongs" with the photosynthetic system of plants, and some of these represent significant additional opportunities for plant growth regulators. As our biochemical-genetic-physiological-agronomic understanding of the photosynthetic system increases, undoubtedly additional significant opportunities will be found.

Translocation

The translocation of assimilate from sources to sinks is an important but not well-understood area of plant biology. A recent example from our laboratory documents the utility of chemicals as probes to assist in unraveling the complex molecular events in the movement of sucrose from the cell where it is synthesized into the translocation stream (Giaquinta, 1976, 1977a,b, 1978, 1979; Lin and Giaquinta, 1979). The use of PCMBS, which is a nonmembrane-permeating sulfhydryl reagent, revealed that a thiol group on the plasmalemma is involved in the transfer of sucrose from the apoplast or free space to the phloem. In addition, this process of loading sucrose, the major translocatory product of photosynthesis, is driven by vectorial ATPase producing protons which are cotransported with sucrose (Fig. 3). As these molecular events of translocation of

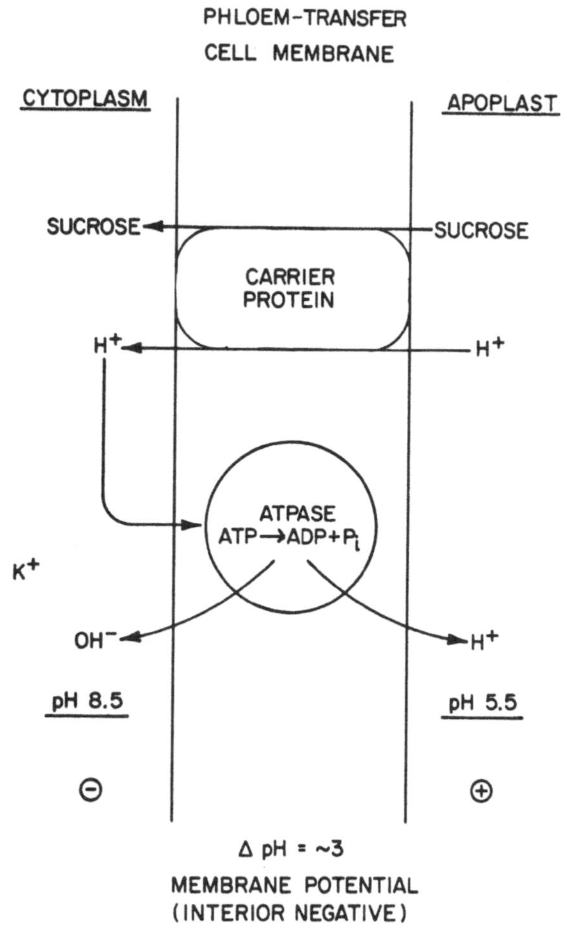

Fig. 3. Model for transport of sucrose from the free space into sieve tubes in which a pH gradient created by a membrane ATPase provides the driving force (Giaquinta, 1977b).

organic solutes as well as uptake of ions are defined, opportunities for plant growth regulators may be found.

Assimilate Partitioning

What factors control the partitioning of assimilate between reproductive and vegetative sinks? In crops where grain is the harvestable product, one would like to optimize the allocation of assimilate to the reproductive sinks while in crops where vegetation is the major objective, such as forage and tuber crops, one would like to maximize the allocation to the vegetative sinks. Experiments a few years ago in our laboratory utilizing altered oxygen concentrations for studies of photorespiration led to the serendipitous discovery that oxygen concentration is a chemical regulator of assimilate partitioning (Fig. 4) (Hardy, 1977c, 1978a; Hardy and Havelka, 1977; Hardy et al., 1977b, 1978b; Quebedeaux and Hardy, 1973, 1975, 1976; Quebedeaux et al., 1975). These experiments demonstrate that concentrations of oxygen less than ambient--21% at sea level--markedly decreased assimilate partitioning into reproductive sinks and that concentrations greater than 21% at least on a short-term basis increase partitioning into assimilate sinks. This oxygen process, which regulates all reproductive growth of higher seed-bearing plants tested such as wheat, sorghum, soybeans, rice, and cotton, is localized within the reproductive structures and may be physical and/or chemical in its mechanism. Its effect is rapid, requiring less than a few hours. Experimental alteration of pO_2 provides a most useful nonsurgical tool to manipulate in a defined manner reproductive sink intensity. Understanding of the mechanism of this critical pO_2 process may reveal opportunities for plant growth regulators to maximize vegetative growth in forages and maximize reproductive growth in grains--a most exciting opportunity.

Stress by Air Pollutants

Ambient concentrations of air pollutants in various agricultural regions may be detrimental to crop production and several crops, such as white beans, potatoes, and other crops, show sensitivity to ozone. Recently in our laboratory a chemical agent EDU or DPX-4891 has been

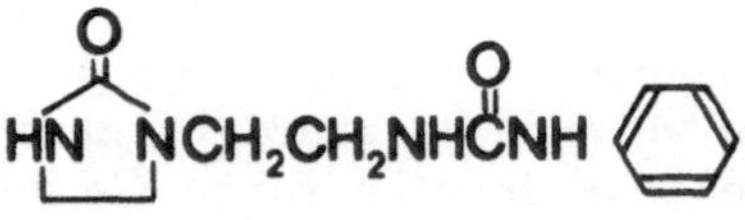

EDU or DPX-4891

found to protect a variety of plants against ozone (Carnahan et al., 1978). The chemical growth regulator provides a most useful probe to assess the quantitative significance of ozone as a yield deterrent under field conditions and may if adequate need exists come to represent a new type of plant growth regulator.

Senescence

On a theoretical basis, the ability to regulate senescence chemically is very desirable. In some crops, such as wheat, where harvesting occurs early relative to the continuing solar energy

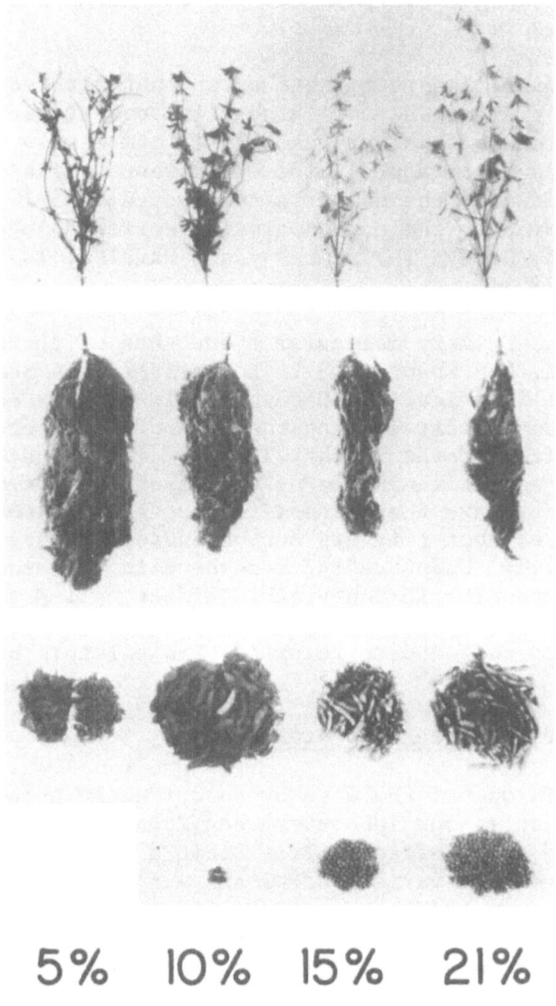

Fig. 4. Oxygen concentration regulates assimilate partitioning into reproductive structures by a recently observed O_2 process localized to reproductive structures (Quebedeaux and Hardy, 1973).

availability, one would like to delay senescence. It can be calculated that an increase of about 3%/day in yield might occur through delayed senescence of the flag leaf in wheat. In soybeans, self-destruction has been suggested as the cause. In double cropping, one may wish to promote senescence in order to better squeeze two crops into a single growing season. Also, one may wish to promote senescence in order to promote field drying of the crop prior to harvesting and thereby decrease the fossil energy cost for post-harvest drying.

Some empirical observations suggest that altered senescence could increase yield. There is a negative correlation between longevity of flag leaf and yields of Triticum aestivum. Part of the increase due to carbon dioxide enrichment of field grown legumes is undoubtedly due to the delay in senescence of 5-10 days that is regularly observed in the carbon dioxide enriched legume but not nonlegume crops (Hardy, 1977a; Hardy and Havelka, 1977; Hardy et al., 1977b, 1978b).

What is the primary molecular event that triggers senescence in plants (Thimann, see Chapter 18)? Recently it has been shown in our laboratory that flag leaf RuBPCase of field-grown wheat undergoes preferential proteolytic loss at the time of senescence prior to that of other soluble proteins in the flag leaf (Wittenbach, 1978, 1979). Why should the essential enzyme of photosynthesis be selectively prematurely lost? Are there specific proteases responsible for this and if there are, what triggers action and/or synthesis of the specific protease? Undoubtedly, somewhere in this complex series of events that results in the visible effect called senescence there is an initiator molecule, and one might anticipate that plant growth regulators could be found to regulate this molecule beneficially.

Manipulation of Hormone Receptor Sites

Ethylene is one of the five or so currently accepted plant hormones. Recently, our laboratory has found that foliar applications of silver salts effectively inhibit a variety of ethylene-mediated effects in a variety of plants (Beyer, 1976a,b,c, 1978). Thus, exposure to ethylene causes defoliation while pre-application of silver inhibits this defoliatory action of ethylene. Similarly, ethylene causes senescence of flowers, such as orchids, while prefoliar application with silver salts renders the plant resistent to ethylene application (Fig. 5). The inhibitory action of ethylene can be antidoted with acetylene which removes the Ag^+ and allows the ethylene response to occur. These and other observations indicate that silver is not inhibiting the biosynthesis of ethylene but rather inhibiting action of endogenous or added ethylene possibly through a reversible perturbation of the yet-to-be-characterized ethylene hormone receptor site. Although a salt such as silver will probably never be a commercial plant growth regulator, it is a most useful probe to assist in detailed understanding of the physiology and possibly even the biochemistry of ethylene hormonal activity. Such approaches may lead to a molecular understanding of hormonal receptor sites and thereby facilitate search for plant growth regulant molecules.

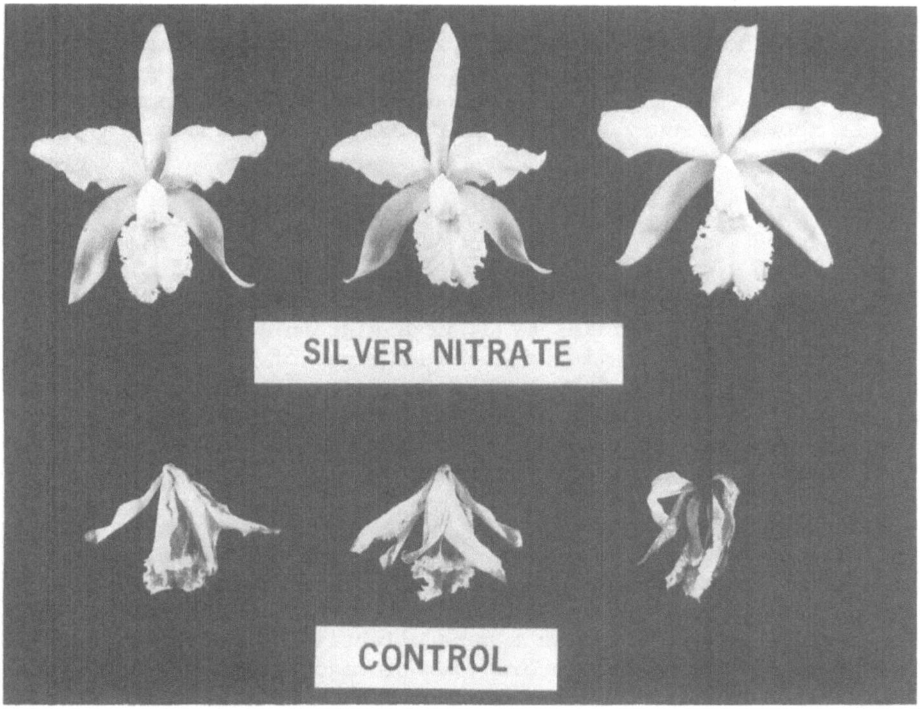

Fig. 5. Foliar treatments with silver nitrate prior to exposure to ethylene inhibits ethylene-mediated senescence (Beyer, 1976a). This is an example of a specific reversible perturbation of a hormone receptor site and demonstrates the powerful potential and selectivity of plant growth regulating chemicals.

Hybridization

Hybrid plants have been effective routes to increased yield in crops such as corn and sorghum as well as providing a built-in proprietariness to encourage commercial breeding. This effect is documented by the commercial activity in corn and sorghum breeding vs. that in soybeans and other cereals where hybrids have not been obtained. Chemical agents have been reported to facilitate hybridization (Appendix 6) but none have been commercialized so far. These agents may be most useful probes for understanding these processes. Chemical agents that would facilitate cross pollination might be most useful in the production of hybrids.

These selected examples of advancing scientific understanding in potentially significant areas of crop production indicate in limited detail the status, opportunity, and power of a more fundamental approach to crop growth regulation than that based exclusively on hormones and an empirical approach which has dominated the past five decades. It seems obvious plant growth regulators that will manipulate some of these key fundamental processes should produce enormous positive impacts on crop production.

SUMMARY

The primary objective in world crop production is to increase productivity of cereal grains by 3%/yr and grain legumes by 5%/yr, and a secondary objective is to decrease input of limited resources into crop production but not at the expense of increased productivity. Plant growth regulators should provide broad spectrum solutions for increasing crop productivity and optmizing use of limited resources such as fossil energy, water, and land.

A fundamentally based approach including asking "what's wrong" at the physiological, biochemical, genetic, and agronomic level coupled with assessment of significance, screen development, discovery of possible solutions, evaluation of their practicality, and implementation is perceived as a more effective route for the discovery of plant growth regulators for our major agronomic crops than an empirical approach.

Although plant growth regulators are an insignificant 1% of world agrichemical sales, it is suggested that they could become as important as other agrichemicals, such as fertilizers and plant protectants.

Several specific targets for plant growth regulation at the yield enhancement, quality improvement, and facilitation of process level are suggested along with a tabulation of existing chemicals useful as experimental probes or commercial regulators.

The exploratory frontier of several types of rate-limiting steps including nitrogen input, carbon input, translocation, assimilate partitioning, air pollutants, senescence, and hormone effects are outlined with, where available, an assessment of the potential offered for major increases in productivity.

A CLOSING PHILOSOPHY

Maximized economic harvest vs. maximized survival is the objective of crop research in the years ahead as it has been in the past. Plants have evolved many "inefficient" systems (CO_2 fixing system, biological N_2 fixation, etc.) where the objective of the pre-agricultural era was an abundance of redundancies or multiple fail safe systems to enable maximum survival in the multi-organism natural (hostile) environment, while the objective of plant growth regulation and plant breeding is to manipulate these "inefficient" systems so as to maximize economic harvest in an increasingly synthetic (fertilizers, irrigation, cultural practices) and protected (plant protectant chemicals) environment with conservation of limited resources of water, land, and fossil energies.

REFERENCES

Anonymous, 1975, Entering the age of plant growth regulators, Farm Chem., 138:15-26.

Anonymous, 1977a, A look at world pesticide markets, Farm Chem., 140: 38-43.

Anonymous, 1977b, "Plant Growth Regulator Handbook," Plant Growth Regulator Working Group, E. F. Sullivan, Great Western Sugar Co., Longmont, Colo.

Anonymous, 1977c, "Proceedings of 4th Annual Meeting Plant Growth Regulator Working Group," Plant Growth Regulator Working Group, E. F. Sullivan, Great Western Sugar Co., Longmont, Colo.

Anonymous, 1978a, How regulation is impacting on pesticide research, Farm Chem., 141:26-34.

Anonymous, 1978b, PGRWG sustaining members, Plant Growth Regulator Bulletin, 6:17-22.

Beyer, E. M., Jr., 1976a, A potent inhibitor of ethylene action in plants, Plant Physiol., 58:268-271.

Beyer, E. M., Jr., 1976b, Ethylene antidote, HortScience, 11:174.

Beyer, E. M., Jr., 1976c, Silver ions: A potent antiethylene agent in cucumber and tomato, HortScience, 11:195-196.

Beyer, E. M., Jr., 1978, A method for overcoming the antiethylene effects of Ag^+, Plant Physiol., 62:(in press).

Burns, R. C., and Hardy, R. W. F., 1975, "Nitrogen Fixation in Bacteria and Higher Plants," Springer-Verlag, New York.

Cannon, F. C., Riedel, G. E., and Ausubel, F., 1977, Recombinant plasmid that carries part of the nitrogen fixation (nif) gene cluster of *Klebsiella pneumoniae*, Proc. Natl. Acad. Sci. U.S., 74:2963-2967.

Carnahan, J. E., Jenner, E. L., and Wat, E. K. W., 1978, Prevention of ozone injury to plants by a new protectant chemical, Phytopathology, 68:1225-1229.

Chollet, R., 1977, The biochemistry of photorespiration, Trends Biochem. Sci., 2:155-159.

Criswell, J. G., Havelka, U. D., Quebedeaux, B., and Hardy, R. W. F., 1976, Adaptation of nitrogen fixation by intact soybean nodules to altered rhizosphere pO_2, Plant Physiol., 58:622-625.

Criswell, J. G., Havelka, U. D., Quebedeaux, B., and Hardy, R. W. F., 1977, Effect of rhizosphere pO_2 on nitrogen fixation by excised and intact nodulated soybean roots, Crop Sci., 17:39-44.

Day, P. R., 1977, Plant genetics: Increasing crop yield, Science, 197:1334-1339.

Evans, H. J., 1977, Loss of energy during the fixation of atmospheric nitrogen by nodulated legumes, in: "Report of the Public Meeting on Genetic Engineering for Nitrogen Fixation," A. Hollaender, ed., U.S. Government Printing Office, Washington, D.C.

Giaquinta, R. T., 1976, Evidence for phloem loading from apoplast. Chemical modification of membrane sulfhydryl groups, Plant Physiol., 57:872-875.

Giaquinta, R. T., 1977a, Possible role of pH gradient and membrane ATPase in the loading of sucrose into the sieve tubes, Nature, 267:369-370.

Giaquinta, R. T., 1977b, Phloem loading of sucrose. pH dependence and selectivity, Plant Physiol., 59:750-755.

Giaquinta, R. T., 1978, Source and sink leaf metabolism in relation to phloem translocation, Plant Physiol., 61:380-385.

Giaquinta, R. T., 1979, Phloem loading of sucrose. Involvement of membrane ATPase and proton transport, Plant Physiol., in press.

Hardy, R. W. F., 1975, Fertilizer research with emphasis on nitrogen fixation and century III technology, in: "Proceedings and Minutes of the 24th Annual Meeting of the Agricultural Research Institute," Agricultural Research Institute, Washington, D.C.

Hardy, R. W. F., 1976a, Nitrogen and carbon input and distribution for increased crop production, in: "New York Academy of Sciences Symposium on Food and Nutrition in Health and Disease," December 1976, Philadelphia.

Hardy, R. W. F., 1976b, Potential impact of current abiological and biological research on the problem of providing fixed nitrogen, in: "Proceedings of the 1st International Symposium on Nitrogen Fixation," W. E. Newton and C. J. Nyman, eds., Washington State Univ. Press, Pullman.

Hardy, R. W. F., 1977a, Increasing crop productivity, in: "European Seminar on Biological Solar Energy Conversion Systems," May 1977, Grenoble-Autrans, France.

Hardy, R. W. F., 1977b, Increasing crop productivity: Agronomic and economic considerations on the role of biological nitrogen fixation, in: "Report of the Public Meeting on Genetic Engineering for Nitrogen Fixation," A. Hollaender, ed., U.S. Government Printing Office, Washington, D.C.

Hardy, R. W. F., 1977c, Rate-limiting steps in biological photoproductivity, in: "Genetic Engineering for Nitrogen Fixation," A. Hollaender et al., eds., Plenum Press, New York.

Hardy, R. W. F., 1977d, Nitrogen fixation, in: "McGraw-Hill Yearbook of Science and Technology," McGraw-Hill Book Co., New York.

Hardy, R. W. F., 1978a, New technologies to increase world crop productivity, in: "Energy, Food, Population and World Interdependence," American Chemical Society, Washington, D.C.

Hardy, R. W. F., 1978b, Food, famine, and nitrogen fixation, "1979 Yearbook of Science and the Future," Encyclopedia Brittanica, Inc., Chicago.

Hardy, R. W. F., 1979, Chemical horizons in crop production, in: "Food from the Chemical Viewpoint," American Chemical Society, Washington, D.C.

Hardy, R. W. F., and Gibson, A. H., eds., 1977, "A Treatise on Dinitrogen Fixation. Section IV. Agronomy and Ecology," John Wiley & Sons, New York.

Hardy, R. W. F., and Havelka, U. D., 1975a, Photosynthate as a major factor limiting nitrogen fixation by field-grown legumes with emphasis on soybeans, in: "Symbiotic Nitrogen Fixation in Plants," P. S. Nutman, ed., Cambridge Univ. Press, London.

Hardy, R. W. F., and Havelka, U. D., 1975b, Nitrogen fixation research: A key to world food?, Science, 188:633-643.

Hardy, R. W. F., and Havelka, U. D., 1977, Possible routes to increase the conversion of solar energy to food and feed by grain legumes and cereal grains (crop production): CO_2 and N_2 fixation, foliar fertilization, and assimilate partitioning, in: "Biological Solar Energy Conversion," A. Mitsui et al., eds., Academic Press, New York.

Hardy, R. W. F., and Silver, W. S., eds., 1977, "A Treatise on Dinitrogen Fixation, Section III, Biology," John Wiley & Sons, New York.

Hardy, R. W. F., Criswell, J. G., and Havelka, U. D., 1977a, "Investigations of possible limitations of nitrogen fixation by legumes: 1) methodology, 2) identification, and 3) assessment of significance," W. E. Newton, J. R. Postgate, and C. Rodriguez-Barruero, eds., Academic Press, London.

Hardy, R. W. F., Havelka, U. D., and Quebedeaux, B., 1977b, Increasing crop productivity; the problem, strategies, approach, and selected rate limitations related to photosynthesis, in: "Proceedings of the 4th International Congress on Photosynthesis, Photosynthesis '77," D. O. Hall, J. Coombs, and T. W. Goodwin, eds., The Biochemical Society, London.

Hardy, R. W. F., Bottomley, F., and Burns, R. C., 1978a, "A Treatise on Dinitrogen Fixation, Sections I and II, Inorganic and Physical Chemistry, Biochemistry," John Wiley & Sons, New York.

Hardy, R. W. F., Havelka, U. D., and Quebedeaux, B., 1978b, The opportunity for and significance of alteration of ribulose 1,5-bisphosphate carboxylase activities in crop production, in: "Photosynthetic Carbon Assimilation," H. W. Siegelman, ed., Plenum Publishing Co., New York.

Havelka, U. D., and Hardy, R. W. F., 1976, Legume N_2 fixation as a problem in carbon nutrition, in: "Proceedings of the 1st International Symposium on Nitrogen Fixation," W. E. Newton and C. J. Nyman, eds., Washington State Univ. Press, Pullman.

Huber, D. M., Warren, H. L., Nelson, D. W., and Tsai, C. Y., 1977, Nitrification inhibitors--New tools for food production, BioScience, 27:523-529.
Lamborg, M. R., 1977, The role of blue-green algae enhancing crop production, in: "Report of the Public Meeting on Genetic Engineering for Nitrogen Fixation," A. Hollaender, ed., U.S. Government Printing Office, Washington, D.C.
Leopold, A. C., and Kriedemann, P. E., 1975, "Plant Growth and Development," McGraw-Hill Book Co., New York.
Lin, W., and Giaquinta, R. T., 1979, Evidence for dual sites of fusicoccin-mediated plasmalemma H^+ efflux, Plant Physiol., in press.
Nickell, L. G., 1978, Plant growth regulators, Chem. Eng. News, 56:18-34.
Ogren, W., 1977, Increasing carbon fixation by crop plants, in: "Proceedings of the 4th International Congress on Photosynthesis, Photosynthesis '77," D. O. Hall, J. Coombs, and T. W. Goodwin, eds., The Biochemical Society, London.
Quebedeaux, B., and Hardy, R. W. F., 1973, Oxygen as a new factor controlling reproductive growth, Nature, 243:477-479.
Quebedeaux, B., and Hardy, R. W. F., 1975, Reproductive growth and dry matter production by Glycine max (L.) Merr. in response to oxygen concentration, Plant Physiol., 55:102-107.
Quebedeaux, B., and Hardy, R. W. F., 1976, Oxygen concentration: Regulation of crop growth and productivity, in: "CO_2 Metabolism and Crop Productivity," R. H. Burris and C. C. Black, eds., University Park Press, Baltimore.
Quebedeaux, B., Havelka, U. D., Livak, K. L., and Hardy, R. W. F., 1975, Effect of altered pO_2 in the aerial part on symbiotic N_2 fixation, Plant Physiol., 56:761-764.
Shimshick, E. J., and Hebert, R. R., 1978, Adsorption of Rhizobia to cereal roots, Biochem. Biophys. Res. Commun., in press.
da Silva, J. G., Serra, G. E., Moreira, J. R., Concalves, J. C., and Goldemberg, J., 1978, Energy balance for ethyl alcohol production from crops, Science, 201:903-906.
Tucker, W., 1978, Of mites and men, Harper's, August:43-58.
Wittenbach, V. A., 1978, Changes in proteolytic activity and the level of RuBPCase in the flag leaf of wheat during grain development and senescence, Plant Physiol., 61S:136.
Wittenbach, V. A., 1979, Breakdown of ribulose bisphosphate carboxylase and change in proteolytic activity during dark-induced senescence of wheat seedlings, Plant Physiol., in press.

Appendix 1. Plant Growth Regulators[1]

Time	Growth Regulator	Use
1932	C_2H_4, Ethylene C_2H_4, Acetylene	Pineapple flowering
1940	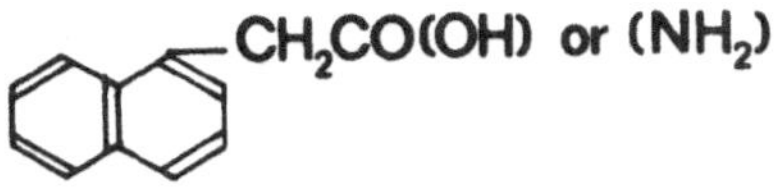	Fruit set and drop
	Naphthalene Acetic Acid or Amide	
	Fruitone-N® Tre-Hold® Transplantone® Amid-Thin W® Niagara Stik®	
	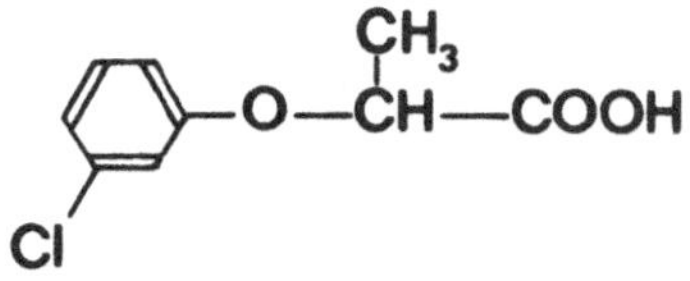	
	2-(3-Chlorophenoxy)Propionic Acid	
	Fruitone® CPA®	
	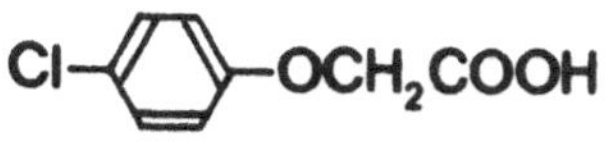	
	4-Chlorophenoxyacetic Acid	
1950	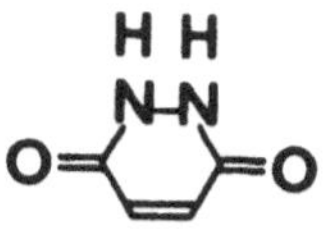	Sucker control in tobacco Sprouting inhibition of potatoes and onions Turf growth inhibitor
	Maleic Hydrazide	
	MH-30® Sprout Stop® Sucker Stuff® De-Cut®	

Appendix 1 (cont'd.)

Time	Growth Regulator	Use
1955	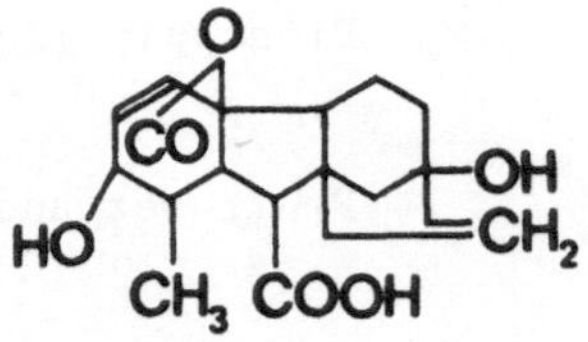 Pro-Gibb® Gib-Sol® Gib-Tabs® Gibrel® Activol® Barelex®	Thompson seedless grape Berry size, etc.
1960	$(CH_3)_3\overset{+}{N}CH_2CH_2Cl \quad Cl^-$ Chlormequat Chloride Cycocel®	Wheat dwarfing
1965	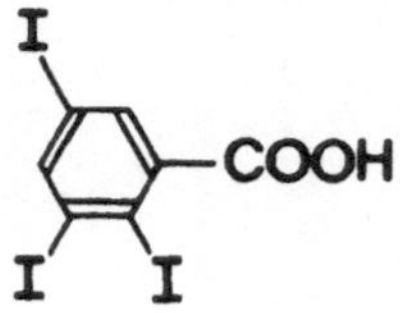 2,3,5-Triiodobenzoic Acid TIBA - Regim 8®	Soybean dwarfing (discontinued)
	$(CH_3)_2NNH\overset{O}{\overset{\|}{C}}CH_2CH_2COOH$ Daminozide Alar® Kylar® B-Nine	Size and color of various fruits and peanuts
	$CH_3(CH_2)_{6-8}COOH$ Off-Shoot®	Tobacco sucker control

Appendix 1 (cont'd.)

Time	Growth Regulator	Use
1970	$Cl-CH_2CH_2PO_3H_2$ Ethephon Ethrel® Cepha®	Ripening of various fruits, color enhancer Latex flow of rubber enhancer
1975	$CH_3CH_2O\underset{O^-}{\overset{O}{\overset{\|}{P}}}\overset{O}{\overset{\|}{C}}NH_2\ NH_4^+$ Ammonium Ethyl Carbamoyl Phosphonate Krenite®	Brush control
	$HO\overset{O}{\overset{\|}{C}}CH_2N(CH_2\underset{O-H}{\overset{O}{\overset{\|}{P}}}-OH)_2$ Glyphosine Polaris®	Sugarcane ripener
	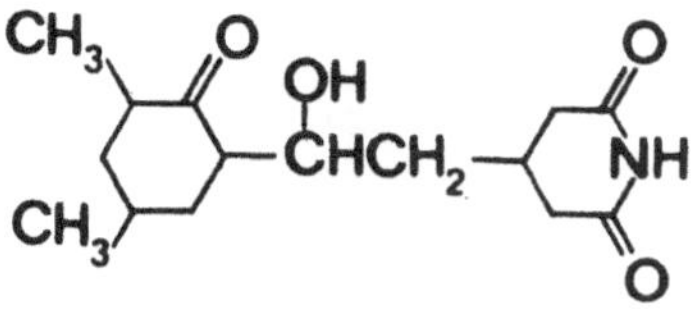 Cycloheximide Acti-Aid®	Citrus harvest aid
	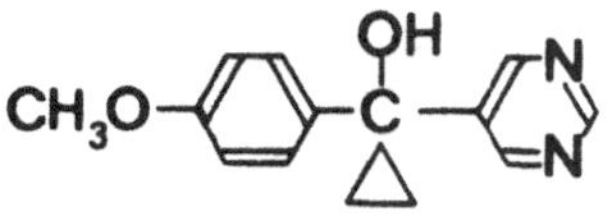 Ancymidol A-Rest®	Ornamental dwarfing

Appendix 1 (cont'd.)

Time	Growth Regulator	Use
	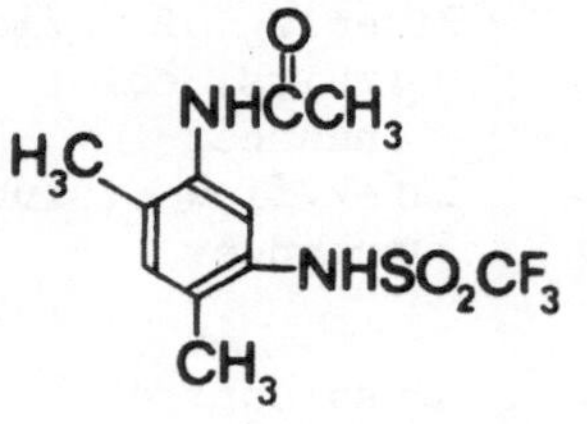 Mefluidide Embark®	Turf growth inhibitor
	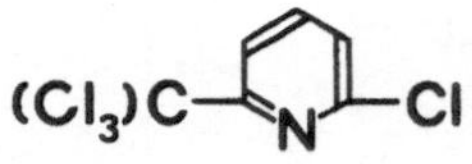 2-Chloro-6-Trichlomethylpyridine N-Serve®	Nitrification inhibitor
	$(CH_3OC_2H_4O)_3SiCH_2CH_2Cl$ Etacelasil Alsal®	Olive harvest aid
	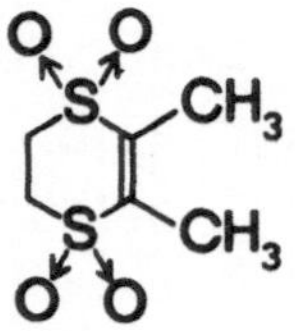 2,3-Dihydro-5,6-Dimethyl-1,4-Dithiin-1,1,4,4-Tetraoxide Harvade®	Cotton defoliant Potato dessicant
	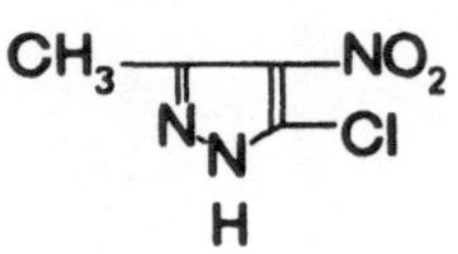 5-Chloro-3-Methyl-4-Nitro-H-Pyrazole Release®	Citrus harvest aid

Appendix 1 (cont'd.)

Time	Growth Regulator	Use
	HON=CH-CH=NOH Glyoxal Dioxime or Ethanediol Dioxime Pik-Off®	Citrus harvest aid
1980	? ? ? ? ?	

[1]Anonymous, 1975, 1977b,c; Hardy, 1979; Leopold and Kriedemann, 1975; Nickell, 1978.

Appendix 2. Publications in Which Plant Growth Regulators Are Discussed

1. Weaver, R. J., 1972, "Plant Growth Substances in Agriculture," W. H. Freeman and Co., San Francisco.
2. Leopold, A. C., and Kriedemann, P. E., 1975, "Chemical Modification of Plants in Plant Growth and Development," 2nd ed., McGraw-Hill Book Co., New York.
3. Brown, A. W. A., Byerly, T. C., Gibbs, M., and San Pietro, A., eds., 1975, "Crop Productivity--Research Imperatives," Michigan Agricultural Experiment Station, East Lansing, and C. F. Kettering Foundation, Yellow Springs, Ohio.
4. Anonymous, 1975, Entering the age of plant growth regulators, Farm Chem., March:15-26.
5. Scrimshaw, N. S., Wang, D. I. C., and Milner, M., 1975, "Protein Resources and Technology--Status and Research Needs--Summary and Research Recommendations," U.S. Government Printing Office, Washington, D.C.
6. Plant growth regulators, in: "Potential Increases in Food Supply Through Research in Agriculture--Researchable Areas Which Have Potential for Increasing Crop Production," J. L. Ozbun et al., New York State College of Agriculture and Life Sciences, Cornell Univ., Ithaca, N.Y., 1976.
7. Crop productivity, in: "Supporting Papers: World Food and Nutrition Study," Vol. 1, National Academy of Sciences, Washington, D.C., 1977.
8. Plant Growth Regulator Working Group, 1977, "Plant Growth Regulator Handbook," E. F. Sullivan, Great Western Sugar Co., Longmont, Colo.
9. Plant Growth Regulator Working Group, 1977, "Proceedings 4th Annual Meeting Plant Growth Regulator Working Group," E. F. Sullivan, Great Western Sugar Co., Longmont, Colo.
10. Jobman, D., 1977, Soybean growth regulation--It'll still be awhile, Soybean Digest, May:14-15.
11. Nickell, L., 1978, Plant growth regulators, Chem. Eng. News, 56:18-34.
12. Hardy, R. F. W., 1979, Chemical horizons in crop production, in: "Food from the Chemical Viewpoint," American Chemical Society, Washington, D.C.

Appendix 3. Industrial Support for Plant Growth Regulator Research[1]

Amchem Products, Inc.	HRL Sciences, Inc.
American Crystal Sugar Co.	ICI Americas, Inc.
American Cyanamid Corp.	Kalo Laboratories, Inc.
American Hoechst Corp.	3M Co.
BASF Wyandotte Corp.	Mobil Chemical Co.
Celpril Industries, Inc.	Monsanto Co.
Chemagro, Mobay Chemical Corp.	NOR-AM Agricultural Products, Inc.
Chevron Chemical Co.	Rhodia, Inc.
Ciba-Geigy Corp.	Rohm and Haas Co.
Diamond Shamrock Corp.	Sandoz, Inc.
Dow Chemical Co.	Shell Development Co.
E. I. du Pont de Nemours & Co.	Spraying Systems Co.
Eli Lilly and Co.	Stauffer Chemical Co.
Fisons Corp.	Trans Agra Corp.
FMC Corp.	Union Carbide Corp.
GAF Corp.	Uniroyal, Inc.
Great Western Sugar Co.	Velsicol Chemical Corp.
W. R. Grace & Co.	

[1]Based on PGRWG sustaining members (Anonymous, 1978b).

Appendix 4. What's Wrong with RuBPCase and Ancillary Components of the Photosynthetic CO_2 Fixing System for Crop Production[1]

Biochemistry

- Large Molecular Weight (560,000)
- Multicomponent (? Altered Ratios)
- Increased Complexity from Bacteria to Higher Plants
- Multiple Active Sites with No Reported Effect of One Site on Another
- Activation Requirements--pH, Mg^{+2}, CO_2, Light
- Allosteric Behavior
- Activator Role of Small Subunit?
- Synthesis of Small Subunit in Cytoplasm and Large Subunit in Chloroplast and Subsequent Transfers
- Cleavage of Subunit Precursor
- Substrate Promiscuity (O_2, CO_2, ?)
- High K_m for CO_2 (~ 10 μM) vs. ambient pCO_2 and Increases with Temperature
- Low K_m for O_2 (~ 200 μM) vs. ambient pO_2 and Decreases with Temperature
- Disagreement on Importance of Oxygenase as Source of Glycolate
- Kinetic Differences of RuBPCase in vitro vs. in vivo
- Inability to Directly Use Phosphoglycolate
- No Reported Chemicals that Alter Carboxylase:Oxygenase Ratio
- Form of Substrate--CO_2 vs. HCO_3^-
- Differential Solubility of O_2 and CO_2 with Temperature
- Limitations Other than pCO_2--RuBP, ATP, Reductant

---

[1]Hardy et al., 1978a,b.

Appendix 4 (cont'd.)

- Low Turnover Number (~ 200)
- Excessive Amount (up to 50% of Soluble Protein)
- Functional vs. Nonfunctional (Stored) Form?
- Regulation?--P_i, Starch, Sugar Phosphates
- Stability
- Chloroplast Localization

Genetics

- Nuclear and Chloroplast Genes
- Repressors and/or Inducers for Nuclear and Chloroplast Genes?
- Number of Genes and Gene Dose?
- Limited Identified Diversity--*Panicum*, Rye (tetraploid vs. diploid)
- Failure of Conventional Breeding--*Atriplex*
--Tobacco
--Soybeans
--Wheat
- Failure of Conventional Breeding--*Atriplex*, Tobacco, Soybeans, Wheat
- Failure of Induced Mutation--Soybeans
- Unconventional Genetics--?

Physiology

- Low Relative Rate of Photosynthesis in C_3's
- High Compensation Point
- Post-Illumination Burst of CO_2
- Common Port for CO_2 and H_2O (X 100's H_2O molecules lost/ CO_2 molecule fixed)
- Closure of Stomates by Elevated pCO_2

Appendix 4 (cont'd.)

- Intercellular CO_2 Resistance
- Absence of CO_2 Transport System in C_3's
- Need for a CO_2-Pumping System with Attendant Energy Needs in C_4's
- Need for Specialized Organelles-Peroxisomes
- Slow Adaptation to Increased Light Intensity
- Competition with Other ATP- and Reductant-Requiring Enzymes
- Effect of Light Quality?
- Inactive in Dark
- Inappropriate Quantitative Relationship to Other Enzymes?
- Proteolytic Destruction and Senescence
- Alteration with Age?
- Photorespiration α 1/Leaf Expansion
- Sucrose as Main Export Product
- Effects of Sink (pO_2, Sink Removal, Pod Growth)--Molecular Nature of Signal (Hormone?)--Altered Leaf Angle and Stomate Opening
- Greater Rate of Translocation in C_4 vs. C_3
- Low Photosynthetic Rate in Cultured Cells
- Assay Limitations

Agronomy

- Low Ambient pCO_2
- High Diffusivity of CO_2 Even in Crop Canopy
- Low Relative Growth Rate of C_3's

- Inadequate Photosynthesis for Reproductive Growth and N_2 Fixation in High Protein Legumes (Self-Destruction Hypothesis)

- Photosynthesis not Correlated with Yield but with Leaf Thickness

- Harvest Index Usually Greater for C_3 than C_4

- Variable Leaf Area Index

Appendix 5. What's Wrong with Nitrogenase and Ancillary Components of the Biological N_2 Fixing System for Crop Production[1]

Biochemistry

- Large Molecular Weight (300,000)
- Multicomponent
- Optimum Component Ratio
- Single(?) Active Site
- Allosteric Characteristics
- O_2 Lability of Each Component
- O_2 Inhibition of Reaction
- Special O_2 Handling Molecules and Systems--LHb
- Temperature Instability
- Biphasic Arrhenius Plot with High Apparent Activation Energy at $\leq$ 18-20°
- Mo, Fe, and S Content
- Systems for Uptake and Storage of Mo and Fe
- Activating Factor in Some Cases
- Low Turnover (50-100)
- Electrons Required for Reduction
- Special Electron Donors--Ferredoxin or Flavodoxin
- High Redox Potential (NADPH/NADP $\geq$ 100)
- High Direct ATP Requirement
- ADP Inhibition
- High ATP:ADP Ratio $\geq$ 10
- High ATP-Generating Capacity

---

[1]Hardy, 1977b.

Appendix 5 (cont'd.)

- Substrate Promiscuity--H^+ Reduction
- Re-utilization of H_2
- NO_3^- Inhibition
- Special NH_3 Incorporation System
- Export vs. Incorporation of NH_3 by Microsymbiont
- Ancillary Molecules for Development of Symbioses--Trifoliin

Genetics

- Repression by fixed N-NH_4^+
- Large Number of Genes for nif and Associated Activities (~ 14)
- Large Size of Above Genes
- Prokaryotic Occurrence (Limitation?)
- Plasmid Location in Rhizobium

Physiology and Agronomy

- Low pO_2 Required in Most Cases
- Microsymbiont N_2 Fixation not Representative of Symbiotic Activity by Rhizobium
- Inefficient Coupling to Plant with Free-Living Organism or Associations not Involving the Plant
- High and Inefficient Use of Carbohydrate (10-20 kg CH_2O/kg N) Fixed in Various Legumes
- Photosynthetic Inefficiency of Host Crops
- Inferior Competitive Ability of Microsymbiont vs. Reproductive Sinks for Plant Carbohydrate
- Evolution of H_2--Lack of H_2 Re-utilization System.
- Insignificant for Most Cereals (1-10 kg N/ha·yr) with Possible Exception of Azolla-Anabaena for Rice

Appendix 5 (cont'd.)

- Inadequate Amount for High Yield Grain Legumes (75-100 kg N/ha vs. 300-600)

- Inhibition by Fixed N as Occurs in High Fertility Soils

- Special Structure--Nodules

- Need for a Multiplicity of Organisms and/or Strains Dependent on Crop, Cultivar, Soil, Climate, etc., vs. Fertilizer N Where One Form Is Applicable to All Cases

- Problem of Manufacture, Storage, Handling, and Application of Labile Organisms

- Competition Between Applied and Endogenous Bacteria

- Persistence of Endogenous Bacteria

- Susceptibility to Pathogens and Chemicals

Policy

- Inadequate Proprietariness to Encourage Adequate Investment in Exploration, Development, and Implementation of Biological Solutions

Appendix 6. Specific Targets for Plant Growth Regulation and Chemicals Used as Experimental Probes or Commercial Regulators[1]

<u>Yield Enhancement</u>	
Seed Germination, Tuber Sprouting, Emergence, Breaking of Dormancy	Benzyladenine, Kinetin, Light Quality, Pro-Gib®, Gib-Sol®, Gibnel®, Activol®, Banelox®
Root Growth and Shape	Rootone®, Hormodin®, Transplantone®
Vegetative Growth and Retardation	Embark®, B-Nine®
Morphology (Height, Shape, Leaf, Size, LAI)	Cycocel®, Regim 8®, Stemtrol, Atrinal, BAS08300E, DPX-1840, Sustar, Alar®, A-Rest®, Morphactin, MH-30
Nitrogen Input (Fertilizer; Soil--Mineralization, Nitrification, Denitrification, Volatilization, Leaching; Plant--NO_3^- Uptake and Reduction, N_2 Fixation)	Ammonia, Urea, Nitrate, N-Serve®
Ion Uptake Other than N	
Carbon Input (CO_2 Fixation, Photorespiration, Sugar and Starch Biosynthesis, Respiration)	CO_2 Fertilization
Flowering	Ethrel®, BOH (Bromeliads) Floraltone® (Apples) Light Quality
Translocation and Assimilate Partitioning (Loading, Movement, Unloading)	
Reproductive Growth	pO_2
Tuber Formation	

[1]Anonymous, 1975, 1977b,c; Hardy, 1979; Leopold and Kriedemann, 1975; Nickell, 1978.

Appendix 6 (cont'd.)

Stress Coping (Water, Temperature, Air Pollutants)	ABA, DPX-4891
Senescence	
Latex Flow	2,4-D, Ethrel®, Cepha®
<u>Quality Improvement</u> (Nutrition, Esthetics, etc.)	
Starch	
Sugar--Beets	
--Cane	Polaris®, Mon-8000, Embark®, Cycocel®, Ripenthol®
Protein--Quantity	N-Fertilizer
--Quality	
Oil--Quantity	
--Quality	
Uniformity	Promalin®, Alar®
Color	Alar®, Ethrel®, Cepha®
Parthenocarpy in Cucurbits	Morphactin®, DPX-1840
Inhibition of Sprouting	MH-30®, Sprout Stop®
Tobacco Sucker Control	MH-20, Sucker Stuff®, Off Shoot®, De-Cut®
Defoliation of Cotton	DEF, Folex®, Harvade®, ABA
Dessication of Potatoes	Paraquat®, Harvade®
Tillering of Mature Tobacco	Ethrel®
Flower Preservation	Everbloom, Flora Life, Ag^+
<u>Facilitation</u> (Reduction of Labor Input)	
Harvest Aids--Citrus	Acti-Aid®, Release®, Pik Off®, CGA-13586
Thinning	NAA-800, Amid-Thin®, Fruitone®, 4-CPA, Sevin®

Appendix 6 (cont'd.)

Prevention of Premature Fruit Drop	Fruitone® T, Tre-Hold®, Niagara Stik®
Synchronous Ripening	Ethrel®, Cepha®
Brush Control	2,4,5-T, Krenite®
Hybridization	Ethrel®, DPX-3778, Mendok®

Appendix 7. Increased N_2 Fixation and Yield of Legumes with Aerial Enrichment of CO_2 from Anthesis to Senescence[1]

	N_2 Fixation kg N_2/ha[2]	Grain Yield kg/ha[2]
Soybeans	76/427	3003/5946
Peas	88/128	3446/5262
Beans	8/12	2930/4666
Peanuts[3]	58/102	3472/4205

[1]Hardy, 1977c; Hardy and Havelka, 1977; Hardy et al., 1977a,b, 1978a,b.

[2]Value for ambient air/Value for CO_2-enriched.

[3]Erect growth habit in chambers prevents normal pegging and senescence was frost initiated.

Appendix 8. Past and Current and Possible Future Alternate Technologies[1]

Generation	Technology	Period of Initial Impact
1	Legumes as Green Manures	Biblical Times
2	Recycling of Nitrogen-Containing Wastes	Biblical Times
3	Mined Nitrates as Nitrogen Fertilizers	19th Century
4	Inoculation of Legumes with Rhizobia	19th Century, 4th Quarter
5	Synthetic Nitrogen Fertilizer by Haber-Bosch Process	20th Century, 1st Quarter
6	Nitrogen-Responsive Crops--Corn, Rice, Wheat	20th Century, 2nd & 3rd Quarters
7	Multiple-Cropping and Inter-Cropping of Legume and Nonlegume Crops	?
8	Rhizobial Inoculation Technology	?
9	High Efficiency of Fixed Nitrogen Use by Crops, e.g., Soil Nitrogen Transformation Effectors	?
10	Nitrogen Fertilizer Responsive Legumes or Systems, e.g., Foliar Fertilization	?
11	Enhanced Nitrogen Fixation by Crops by Microsymbiont Derepressed for Fixed Nitrogen	?
12	Enhanced Nitrogen Fixation by Crops with Improved Photosynthate Available to Microsymbiont, e.g., Inhibitors of Photorespiration	?

Appendix 8 (cont'd.)

Generation	Technology	Period of Initial Impact
13	Non-Rhizobial N_2 Fixing Associated Symbioses for Nonlegume Crops, e.g., *Spirillum*-Corn	??
14	Mycorrhizal Associations Containing Endosymbiotic Diazotrophs	??
15	N_2 Fixing Infective but Non-Pathogenic Pathogens, e.g., *Agrobacterium*, *Erwinia*	??
16	Naturally Occurring but Undiscovered N_2 Fixing Systems, e.g., *Rhizobium*-*Trema*	??
17	Synthetic Nitrogen Fertilizer by Zero-Direct Energy Input Process	??
18	Extension of Rhizobial N_2 Fixing Association to Nonlegume Crops	???
19	Transfer of Genetic Information for N_2 Fixing System to Crop Plants	????
20	Synthetic Gene that Codes from Small, Stable (oxygen and temperature), High Turnover, Absolute Substrate Specificity (no H_3O^+ reduction), Zero-Direct Energy Requiring (no ATP) N_2 Fixing Enzyme with Appropriate Repression by Fixed N	??????

[1]Hardy, 1975, 1976b, 1977b,c,d, 1978a,b; Hardy et al., 1977b.

12

REGULATION OF FLOWER INDUCTION AND FRUIT DEVELOPMENT

Ger J. H. Bennink

Department of Plant Physiology
University of Amsterdam
The Netherlands

INTRODUCTION

Man's interest in flowering seems to go far back in history. In the oldest works of art we find flowers and plants decorating temples, palaces, and houses. During the Middle Ages handwritten books were decorated with beautiful black and white and even colored drawings in which flowers often perform an ornamental function. Later on beautiful paintings show us how interested man was in the works of nature. Often plants and flowers were used as symbols. Nowadays they still play an important role, not only in our garden, but also to express our feelings toward our friends and toward people around us. At all major events in our lives (e.g., birth, birthday, success in study and work, jubilee, and finally the funeral) flowers are used to express joy or appreciation. Another reason for interest in flowering is the pleasure we get in awaiting a good harvest while looking at an orchard or a field flowering abundantly.

Man's interest in studying flowers originally had anatomical and morphological aspects. Later on, about seventy years ago, man started to find out how the plant produces flowers. Since then numerous papers, books, reviews, short studies, and case histories on the subject of flower induction and the phenomenon of photoperiodism have come out. In preparing this chapter I made use of many excellent reviews which contained a lot of specialized information on this subject. Of these I can mention only a minor part: Biale (1978), Evans (1969), Hillman (1962), Jennings (1977), Lang (1961), Murneek and Whyte (1948), Salisbury (1963), Salisbury and Ross (1978), Vince-Prue (1975), and Zeevaart (1976).

THE DISCOVERY OF PHOTOPERIODISM

The phenomenon of photoperiodism was detected, demonstrated, and described for the first time by W. W. Garner and H. A. Allard in 1920 in the United States. The crucial experiments were done with tobacco (*Nicotiana tabacum* cv Maryland Mammoth) and soybean (*Glycine max* cv Peking). In tobacco they observed that the cultivar Maryland Mammoth remained vegetative during the growing season and that flowering took place in winter and early spring. In soybean they observed that all plants flowered in the month of September in spite of different sowing times spread over the period from the beginning of May to the beginning to August.

From these observations followed by experiments in which the plants were kept at different day-lengths they proved that the relative length of day and night was the only factor that determined flowering or not flowering.

After these experiments with tobacco and soybean, Garner and Allard studied a wide variety of field, garden, and ornamental plants as to their response to photoperiods of various length. Not only did they study flowering in the experiments, but they also gathered a lot of information about the influence of day-length on vegetative growth, on the formation of bulbs and tubers, on pigment formation, on abscission, and on other physiological aspects of plant growth.

Based on the observations the plants were classified into short-day plants (SDP), long-day plants (LDP), and day-neutral plants (DNP). It soon appeared that a fourth group had to be added--a group of plants that only comes to flowering during intermediate day-length, remaining vegetative when days are either too short or too long. These plants only flower at a day-length of intermediate duration (e.g., 12-14 hours) and don't flower at day-lengths of less than 12 hours and more than 14 hours. To this group belong *Phaseolus polystachyus* and *Saccharum spontaneum* (sugarcane).

Later on it came out that there were also plants that did not flower at intermediate day-length but produced normal flowers at day-lengths shorter than 12 hours and also at day-lengths longer than 14 hours. This group was called ambiphotoperiodic plants (e.g., *Chenopodium rubrum* [goosefoot] and *Setaria verticillata* [bristle grass]). At the same time it appeared that there were dual day-length plants: long-short-day plants (LSDP), such as *Kalanchoe laxiflora*, and short-long-day plants (SLDP), such as *Trifolium repens*. LSDP require for flowering a number of long days followed by a number of short days such as occur at the end of summer and the beginning of fall. SLDP require a number of short days followed by a number of long days such as occur in spring.

At the present time the following classification is used:

short-day plants	SDP
long-day plants	LDP
day-neutral plants	DNP
intermediate plants	
ambiphotoperiodic plants	
long-short-day plants	LSDP
short-long-day plants	SLDP.

In reviews and handbooks lists of plants have been mentioned belonging to the different groups. In these lists, too, we can find the critical day-length, that is the duration of the day-length in the 24-hour period during which the different types will flower. However, we must keep in mind that the critical day-length often depends on environmental conditions, namely, temperature, light intensity, age of the plant, nutrient level, and on the need for vernalization. Vernalization is the need for a cold treatment during development. Such a treatment is necessary for a great number of plants: cereals, biennials, fruit trees. Moreover, species exist that only need a single inductive cycle for flowering, such as *Xanthium*, while other species, such as *Chrysanthemum morifolium*, need a number of inductive cycles for flowering.

Thus, we must conclude that in the plant kingdom a wide variety of flowering types exist in their response to light and other factors.

THE PERCEPTION OF DAY-LENGTH

Moshkov and Chaylakhyan, in the thirties, and later on other investigators clearly demonstrated that the leaves of the plant are the organs for perception of day-length. It was found that the individual leaves were not always sensitive to the light stimulus. It appeared to be necessary for the leaf to have reached a certain ripeness. In most species the fully expanded young leaf is most sensitive; however, there are species in which half-expanded leaves, very young leaves, and even cotyledons are very sensitive to the light stimulus. Also, a seedling needs a minimum number of leaves for flowering response. This number of essential leaves varies greatly--from a seedling with only two cotyledons (Japanese morning glory) to a whole tree full of leaves.

Thus the plant needs for flowering a certain ripeness of leaves and meristems. The time at which they become ripe also varies greatly.

THE NIGHT INTERRUPTION

In 1938 Bonner and Hamner did experiments with SDP and LDP in which they hoped to demonstrate the importance of the dark period both for LDP and SDP. From their experiments it appeared that a light break in the middle of the night inhibits flowering in SDP and promotes flowering in LDP. This night-interruption phenomenon, as it was called, required only a few minutes low intensity white light to be effective. Of the whole spectrum, red light was more effective than light of other wavelengths. During the fifties it came out that the red light effect during the dark period could be reversed by far-red illumination. The conclusion is that the dark period plays a very important role in flowering both in SDP and in LDP. In this night-interruption phenomenon the low energy reaction (LER) of phytochrome is involved.

TIME MEASUREMENT

During the last decade experiments have produced results which support the idea that photoperiodic time measurement is coupled to an endogenous rhythmic oscillation. It could be demonstrated that phytochrome in the Pfr form either promoted or inhibited flowering. This promotion or inhibition depended on an endogenous circadian timer. It is thought that phytochrome phases the rhythm. However, how phytochrome is coupled to this biological clock remains unknown even now. Other investigators have the idea that possibly other mechanisms are involved in time measurement (e.g., the concept of dark reversion of phytochrome). We must conclude that though a lot of work has been done on the biological clock, no definite answer has been given to its riddle.

PHOTOPERIODISM AND A FLOWERING HORMONE

During the thirties it was demonstrated that the leaf detects the photoperiod and, as we know, the meristem produces the flower. From Chaylakhyan's experiments with SDP in which the leaf was enclosed in a black paper envelope and the rest of the plant kept under LD conditions, and also from experiments in which Chaylakhyan grafted induced plants to noninduced plants under LD conditions, he concluded from the resulting flowering response that the stimulus was a hormone transported in the sapstream from the leaf to the meristem and even from one plant to the other in the case of grafted plants. Chaylakhyan proposed the name florigen for this hypothetical hormone.

Grafting experiments have been done by several investigators (e.g., Melchers, Lang, Zeevaart, and many others). The results lead to the conclusion that florigen is probably produced in all flowering plants under favorable conditions and is transported in the sapstream. It might be possible that instead of one single flowering hormone we must think of more than one positive acting florigen. Other investigations led to interest in not only flowering hormones but at the same time in flowering inhibiting substances. Experiments in which extracts of induced and noninduced plants were examined for effects on flowering have been done. However, until now, success was limited and as yet no one has identified florigen or any of the inhibiting substances. In Zeevaart's opinion (1976), the lack of a convenient and reliable bioassay for the floral stimulus is the major handicap.

PLANT HORMONES AND GROWTH REGULATORS

Instead of accepting the hypothetical flowering hormone, Cholodny introduced in 1939 the idea that plant growth substances (auxins) might be responsible for initiating the generative state of the plant. This idea was the start of experiments in which plants under noninductive conditions were treated with plant hormones and growth regulators, not only for initiating flowering but also for inhibiting the flowering process. Cholodny's theory is founded on the knowledge that plant hormones influence nearly all aspects of plant growth and development. The results from this kind of investigation, still in full progress in several laboratories, are often very positive on that point, but it appears to be impossible to find general rules for the effects of the plant hormones since there are so many exceptions to the rules.

The conclusion from these experiments must be that none of the known plant hormones can claim to be a florigen in spite of their pronounced effects on growth and development and flowering per se. However, in agriculture and in horticulture a lot of practical information about the use of growth regulators became available for promoting flowering, for fruit development, for seed production, and for all kinds of vegetative physiological reactions in the plant.

FLOWER DEVELOPMENT AND FRUIT GROWTH

In the flowering process there exists more than initiation. After induction the top meristem starts growing and differentiating, resulting after some time in a flower with stem, calyx, corolla, androecium, and gynoecium. Considering flower initiation and flower development in connection with day-length the flowering plants can be divided into four groups, as shown in Table 1. From this table we must again say that there is a wide diversity in flower development among plants. We must add to this that the number of essential daily cycles also shows a very great diversity; for example,

Table 1

Group	Needed for Initiation	Needed for Development	Species
1	photoperiod(s)	day-neutral	Kalanchoe, Fuchsia
2	day-neutral	photoperiod(s)	Phaseolus vulgaris
3	photoperiod(s)	photoperiod(s)	
a	photoperiod(s) SD	photoperiod(s) SD	Xanthium, Glycine
b	photoperiod(s) LD	photoperiod(s) LD	Lolium
4	photoperiod(s)	photoperiod(s)	
a	photoperiod(s) SD	photoperiod(s) LD	Fragaria
b	photoperiod(s) LD	photoperiod(s) SD	Callistephus chin.

Chrysanthemum morifolium cv Luyona needs at least 24 SD cycles (Bennink, 1974). If it recieves less than 24 SD cycles this plant only produces "crown buds," or stems provided only with bracts. The same effect was found in a great number of other plants, where abortion of flowers was often observed or flowers were found with sterile anthers or sterile ovules.

In order to acquire information about factors controlling the fertility of flower organs, several attempts have been made to cultivate excised flower buds on a special culture medium. In these experiments it was demonstrated that in excised buds the development of anthers and ovules is controlled by plant hormones: auxins, gibberellins, and cytokinins. The normal development of these organs was influenced by an alteration in concentration in one of these three groups of hormones. This means that we must keep in mind that the effect of the daily light-dark regime on fertility might be mediated by a change in vivo in one or more of the endogenous plant hormones. Not only fertility but also sex expression in flowers, that is the production of either male or female flowers, appears to be under influence of day-length. Further research showed that this phenomenon probably is regulated by plant hormones. Most effective seem to be auxins and ethylene, which favor femaleness in a variety of plants. One such plant is Cucumis sativus, in which it is of great economic importance to produce female flowers and no male flowers since in this vegetable the taste of parthenocarpic fruits is much better than the natural product. In *Cucumis sativus* it appeared that the interaction between auxins, ethylene, gibberellins, and abscisic acid played an important role in sex expression. From experiments on fertility and on sex expression we must conclude that probably the daily light regime is responsible for changing the relative endogenous concentrations of known plant hormones. These relative endogenous concentrations are very difficult to estimate, especially inside the relevant cells. Consequently we are not very well informed about the relative concentrations in different species, but we may assume that a certain diversity exists in these concentrations.

VEGETATIVE GROWTH

Not only is reproductive growth controlled by the relative length of light and dark, but also many aspects of vegetative growth not linked with flowering are under photoperiodic control--formation of bulbs, tubers and roots, leaf growth, leaf movements. The perception of the stimulus for these photoperiodic phenomena appeared to take place in the leaf. In these cases no stimulus, no specific hormone, could be isolated and identified.

Summarizing the preceding information about photoperiodism we can say:

(1) In flowering response a very wide diversity of plant types can be found.

(2) Also in ripeness for flowering a wide diversity of plant types was observed.

(3) In the night-interruption phenomenon the low energy reaction of phytochrome is involved.

(4) Time measurement in photoperiodism is linked with circadian rhythmicity and with phytochrome.

(5) Flowering may be controlled by a flowering hormone that has until now not been isolated nor identified.

(6) Plant hormones and growth regulators affect the flowering process, but no general rules can be given.

(7) Plant hormones affect fertility and sex expression in developing flowers.

(8) In flower development a diversity of reaction types can be found in relation to the light-dark regime.

(9) In photoperiodic phenomena concerning vegetative growth the leaf of the plant is the place for perception, but no specific hormone(s) could be identified.

In considering the literature on photoperiodism I had the feeling of walking in a street that led only to a dead end, but then one gets the same feeling reading recent reviews and recent handbooks such as those by Zeevaart, 1976; Biale, 1978; Salisbury and Ross,

1978. When we compare the state of our knowledge about photoperiodism, and especially about the induction of flowering, at this moment with the situation ten or twenty years ago, we must say that no promising steps forward have been made and that we have reached a standstill. When we compare the present situation with that in 1948 when Murneek and Whyte's symposium on "Vernalization and Photoperiodism" was published, we must conclude that some progress has been made, especially in the field of phytochrome. However, the big questions are still the same:

What is the flowering hormone?
What happens in the cells of the apex?
How is time measured?
How is the information about day- and night-length "translated?"
How is flower development regulated?

Answers to these and many other questions concerning photoperiodism cannot be given. Apparently the problem of photoperiodism is too complex, and it seems as if research in this field has decreased. Therefore it is urgently necessary that someone make a breakthrough; alternatively, we must retrace our steps and look for a new way of approaching the problem.

REGULATION OF FLOWERING

During the late thirties, auxins and, later on, other plant hormones and growth regulators became available. This was the start of research in agriculture and horticulture into the effects of growth substances on crop production. In 1940 it was found that a treatment with NAA inhibited the pre-harvest apple drop. In the same period workers discovered that pineapple plants sprayed with NAA were stimulated to flower earlier and, what was very important, they flowered synchronously, so that the fruit harvest could be predicted and made more efficient. Similar results were obtained with ornamental bromeliads by application of NAA, 2,4-D, ethylene, or ethrel. By this treatment the plants could be induced to flower much earlier and simultaneously, so that the marketing time could be planned.

In rosette plants with a LD requirement for flowering, gibberellins, especially GA_3, are used to promote flowering. The use of gibberellins has been studied very intensively. In connection with the GA-effect the use of the growth retardants Amo-1618, CCC, and B9 was developed. These substances are used to lower the endogenous GA-content in the plant, resulting in growth retardation of the shoots and at the same time stimulation of flowering (e.g., in fruit trees and in *Chrysanthemum*). Gibberellins and also auxins stimulate fertilization, fruit set, and fruit growth. In various plants such as tomatoes, strawberries, blueberries, cherries, figs, and grapes it seems that treatment with auxins, gibberellins, cytokinins, ethrel, growth retardants, and growth regulators, or a combination of two or more substances, could promote parthenocarpic fruit set. By these treatments, which are very specific for the different species, spectacular increases in yield and quality have been obtained.

The application of these substances at the correct concentration and at a specific time during development is thought to regulate the transport system in a way such that more photosynthetic products are mobilized and brought to the developing fruits. Other uses of growth regulators are the promotion of fruit thinning and flower thinning in apple and pear and the stimulation of abscission of, for example, cherries in connection with mechanical harvesting.

During the last decade the use of ethrel, a substance that produces ethylene in the plant, has become popular. It is used alone or in combination with Fruitone-T, a synthetic auxin. In this combination a spray applied to apples causes a fine color of the apples, a uniform ripening, and inhibition of the pre-harvest drop.

In general we can say that the use of a large number of natural and synthetic growth regulators has very much increased the harvest of products in agriculture and horticulture. The professional skill of the farmers appears to be very important in the use of these substances; there is a need for explicit instructions about their use and also about the problems that can arise when they are used incorrectly.

Research into the application of growth regulating substances has been done on an empirical basis, and we have only a limited understanding of how the effects are brought about. It would seem that endogenous development is controlled by a dynamic equilibrium between several plant growth substances, but how this is translated into the morphological response is completely unknown. However, the worldwide need for higher food production together with the energy crisis and the difficulties involved in supplying fresh water to large areas of the world means new approaches and new methods in growing cereals, fruit, and vegetables are necessary. Research is needed not only on an empirical basis into the uses of fertilizers, antitranspirants, substances controlling photosynthesis, and growth regulators, but it is also very important to study the physiological reactions taking place in the whole plant, namely, photosynthesis, respiration, transport, transpiration, vegetative and generative growth, and development. This basic knowledge is necessary before we can understand how activating and inhibiting substances interfere with the plant processes.

WHOLE-PLANT PHYSIOLOGY

When an annual plant has flowered, been pollinated, and has produced ripe seeds, it stops growing and dies. However, if the flowers are cut off immediately after having withered, then the plant continues producing flowers. When a biennal such as Digitalis purpurea (foxglove), starts flowering and the flowerstalk is cut off just above the leaves, the plant immediately initiates new side stalks with flowers. However, if the flower stalk is removed after the seeds begin to ripen, then the plant does not form new flowers, though the conditions are still suitable for flowering.

In Erodium (stork's-bill) when the plant has flowered and pollination has occurred the small flower stalks in the umbel bend down and the fruits grow out until they have the shape of the head of a stork with the bill in an upright position in the umbel. At this stage the middle part of the fruit stem becomes very thin and dries out. Later the fruit, still in an upright position, dries out as well and then suddenly the fruits are thrown away.

From these examples and numerous others we get the feeling that the different parts of the plant receive a signal or signals telling them how the situation is in other parts of the plant. The plant as a whole seems to be informed about what happens in its parts. Unfortunately, we have very little information on how plant development is integrated and coordinated.

Perhaps some insight into the problem can be obtained by looking at the culture of apple trees. Long ago it was already common knowledge that for cultivating apples it was necessary to graft a small part of the shoot of a cultivar onto a receptor. Until 1925 only seedlings were used as receptors. The quality of these seedlings was often very poor and the results were variable. In the twenties and thirties a lot of research into the quality of the receptor trees was performed and a good stock of receptors was obtained. These receptor stems are cultivated by vegetative reproduction. At this moment in the Netherlands M9 is often used as a receptor. M9 has the quality of being a very slow grower combined with the ability to induce high fertility in the grafted shoots. This means that a two- or three-year-old tree already produces a lot of flowers and fruits.

At the same time a special technique of pruning has been developed, which results in a tree that is about two meters high and one meter in diameter. When trees are planted at the correct distance from each other, given nutrients at the right moment, and the branches bent in a particular manner then the crop production per unit area is appreciably enhanced, compared with the conventional horticultural technique.

People working in this field know exactly how to bend down the branches at the right time to get good flower buds which are more resistant to bad conditions in early spring. At the right time new shoots are cut away, for it is known that pruning at the wrong time induces the tree to grow extra unwanted shoots. In these trees it is also known that growth regulators should be used only if absolutely necessary and then only at the right moment (e.g., for suppressing growth of the shoot, for inhibiting the drop of the apples, for getting optimal color, and for influencing the process of ripening). From looking at the work being done in the orchards we get the idea that the fruit tree is acting as a whole and that all activities in the plant are integrated. Another important aspect of growing apple trees is the grafting of single buds or shoots onto receptors. When the graft starts growing one can always see where the graft was made, for the stem in this place shows a pronounced thickening that remains during the whole life of the tree. The same has been found in grafting experiments with vegetables (e.g., Cucumis sativus) and also with some ornamentals. This shows that an interaction takes place between the two individuals when they are brought together. In a number of combinations, after the initial growth of the graft, the upper part dies, sometimes after a growth period of three of four years. This too appears to be an interaction between the graft and receptor. This interaction is perhaps comparable with the warding-off mechanism seen when incompatible tissue is transplanted onto another animal. However, no evidence for such an immunogenic-like reaction has been found. On the other hand it is known in some plants, such as Phaseolus vulgaris and Pisum sativum, that phytoalexins play a role in disease resistance. Phytoalexins are usually not present in healthy tissues or they are present in very low concentrations. They are usually synthesized after infection only at the area of infection (e.g., phaseollin in the bean plant and pisatin in peas). Furthermore, there is also increasing evidence for a recognition mechanism being present in the stigma which allows intraspecific pollination but not interspecific pollination. However, there is no reason to equate these reactions with the immunological system of higher animals.

The observations in foxglove, in stork's-bill, in grafting and growing fruit trees, the existence of mechanism of recognition, and the existance of phytoalexins may direct our attention to the whole-plant physiology. This is the way in which in the whole plant all aspects of the physiological reactions are integrated and coordinated, that is, the integration between photosynthesis, respiration, photorespiration, mineral nutrition, water uptake, transport, hormone production, vegetative and generative development, and senescence.

We know a lot about these reactions from a biochemical point of view. But we must ask ourselves: "How do these phenomena work together in the whole plant?" "What system is involved in the integration?" We know that the rates of action during the day and night are not always the same. Even large differences have been found, as has been mentioned by Dr. Lenz (see Chapter 9), in photosynthesis in fruiting and nonfruiting trees.

Whatever this system may be and however it works, I do believe that such a system for integration exists. I believe that the plant as a whole "knows" what happens in the different parts and that the plant is able to change the pattern of physiological reactions according to the environmental conditions.

Several times the word "signal" has been mentioned here. What is meant by "a signal from shoot to root" and "a signal from one part to another part in the plant?" Signals are mentioned even within cells, and in this case I must think of what was said by Dr. Laetsch (see Chapter 26) about the chloroplast and the envelope of the chloroplast: Several substances active within the chloroplast in the process of photosynthesis are produced in the cytoplasm and are transported through the envelope exactly to the right place. What is that signal that directs these substances to the right place? I think we have no idea about this, but it is most important to know about these signals, about integration and coordination, and about the role of plant hormones in this. If we understand what happens it might be easier to interfere, that is, to direct the plant into a special process such as into the production and transport of more assimilates, into flowering, or to prevention of senescence.

I cannot give you a plan of attack in this field. I bring this forward as a subject for discussion. It appears to me that it is very important to know how photoperiodism fits in the whole of reactions taking place in the plant. Therefore, study of whole-plant physiology may open new doors.

REFERENCES

Bennink, G. J. H., 1974, Flower development in Chrysanthemum under long-day conditions by injections with the cytokinin benzyladenin, in: "Plant Growth Substances 1973," 8th International Conference on Plant Growth Substances, Hirokawa Publ. Co., Inc., Tokyo.

Biale, J. B., 1978, On the interface of horticulture and plant physiology, Ann. Rev. Plant Physiol. 1978, 28:1-23.

Evans, L. T., 1969, "The Induction of Flowering; Some Case Histories," Macmillan of Australia, South Melbourne.

Hillman, W. S., 1962, "The Physiology of Flowering," Holt, Rinehart and Winston, New York.

Jennings, D. H., 1977, "Integration of Activity in the Higher Plant," Cambridge Univ. Press, Cambridge.

Lang, A., 1961, Physiology of flower initiation, in: "Encyclopedia of Plant Physiology," Vol. 15, W. Ruhland, ed., Springer Verlag, Berlin.

Murneek, A. E., and Whyte, R. O., 1948, "Vernalization and Photoperiodism," Chronica Botanica Co., Waltham, Mass.

Salisbury, F. B., 1963, "The Flowering Process," Pergamon Press, Oxford.

Salisbury, F. B., and Ross, C. W., 1978, "Plant Physiology," 2nd ed., Wadsworth, Belmont, Calif.

Vince-Prue, D., 1975, "Photoperiodism in Plants," McGraw-Hill, London and New York.

Zeevaart, J. A. D., 1976, Physiology of flower formation, Ann. Rev. Plant Physiol. 1976, 27:321-348.

13

THE ROLE AND EFFECTIVENESS OF STIMULATIVE-INHIBITIVE REGULATORS ON EARLY AND LATE BLOOMING OF FRUIT TREES

N. Kaska

University of Cukurova
Adana, Turkey

INTRODUCTION

To be able to control the opening of buds has been one of the most important interests of fruit tree physiologists for centuries. They have been looking for a magic substance, chemical, etc. to help reach this goal. The search for this substance or chemical has been carried out in nearly every fruit growing part of the world by pomologists, who have performed many experiments and added much valuable information to our knowledge of this subject. The pomologists in the temperate zone, where spring frosts (especially the late ones) often kill the flowers, were interested in finding a way to delay flowering. On the other hand, the physiologists in the subtropical zone, where the winters are warm and therefore the chilling requirements of many deciduous trees are not satisfied, were looking for efficient rest breaking agents. At first glance, the objectives of these two types of scientists look quite opposite, but in fact they are the same: to be able to control bud openings. The best way to approach developing this magic substance or chemical was, of course, to study the plants: how was the plant controlling blooming? Therefore, the efforts of physiologists were concentrated on determining the control mechanism of blooming in plants. Eventually they came to the conclusion that the magic substance is in the type of phytohormone or plant growth regulator.

This article discusses the need, the research efforts, and the work still to be done to master control of bud opening in fruit trees. We will examine four parts of the problem: (1) delaying of flower bud openings, (2) mechanism of bloom delay, (3) breaking of rest and early flowering, and (4) mechanism of bud-break.

DELAYING OF FLOWER BUD OPENINGS

Late spring frosts are the most dangerous phenomenon for fruit growers. Some places have severe late frosts annually; in others late frosts are not so frequent. However, when they occur they kill nearly all the flowers and as a result no yield is obtained. Of course, the most useful preventive measures have to be taken before establishing the orchard or vineyard; that is, to carefully select frost free sites and late blooming species and varieties. However, even in locations assumed to be safe or with relatively safe varieties, the trees are subjected to frost damages from year to year.

In some districts where the occurrence of frost is inevitable, the growers are trying to heat the orchards, or installing wind machines or overhead sprinklers to protect the flowers or the fruitlets. Of course these measures are rather expensive and therefore the economics of using them must be considered. Lately, overhead sprinkling or misting has been used to delay bloom. Although a delay of 8 to 17 days in apple and 15 days in peach has been obtained, maturity has been delayed and substantial tree losses sustained (Lipe et al., 1977; Buchanan et al., 1977; Stang et al., 1978).

Auxins and Maleic Hydrazide

In fruit trees (especially in stone fruits), the materials used most extensively to delay bloom are plant growth regulators. Among the first used substances were Na or K salts of the auxins of indol, naphtalen, and phenoxy acetic acid groups (Table 1). The history of bloom delay by growth regulators goes back to 1939. As can be seen from the table, the auxins were used either in the spring before blooming or in the summer and autumn months of the previous year. In these experiments stone fruits were generally used. Since the results were sometimes conflicting or not satisfactory, physiologists looked for a plant growth inhibitor such as maleic hydrazide (MH). This substance was applied to apples, pears, strawberries, raspberries (White and Kennard, 1950; Kennard et al., 1951), peaches and apricots (Okasha and Crane, 1963) (Table 1). Maleic hydrazide was found to be effective in delaying the opening of flower buds (with some damage to the leaves and twigs) in strawberry and raspberry and ineffective in the other fruit trees tested.

Gibberellic Acid

Around 1960 two compounds attracted the attention of researchers in the area: gibberellic acid (GA) and succinic acid, 2,2-dimethyl hydrazide (alar). Work on these substances is still going on.

Table 1. Effects of Auxins and Maleic Hydrazide in Delaying the Opening of Buds in Fruit Trees

Fruit Species	Applied Material	Concentration (ppm)	Time of Application	Bloom Delay (Days)	Author
Peach, Pear	IAA, IBA		Prebloom	No delay	Mitchell and Cullinan, 1942
Apple, Pear	KNA	100;330;1000	Sept.	Some delay	Hitchcock and Zimmerman, 1943
		200;400;800	July, Aug., Sept.	14 (Fruit bud) 19 (Leaf bud)	"
Plum, Cherry, Peach	KNA, NANA		Aug., Sept., Oct.	2	Marth et al. (White and Kennard, 1950)
Cherry	NAA, 2,4-D		Sept.	7	Tukey and Hammer (Tukey, 1954)
Apple, Grape, Strawberry, Black Raspberry	MH	1000;1500;2000 3000	Spring	24 to 38 (in Raspberry)	White and Kennard, 1950
Black and Red Raspberry	MH	50 to 2000	Spring	7 to 18 (in Black Raspberry)	Kennard et al., 1951
Apricot, Peach	MH	1000 to 2000	May	No delay in the following year	Okasha and Crane, 1963

Gibberellic acid is still the growth regulator used most extensively to delay bloom. The first GA trials with the idea of prolonging dormancy and thus delaying bloom were done in pome fruits (Brian et al., 1959) and grapes (Weaver, 1959) (Table 2). In the following years, more studies were carried out in stone fruits. Among the stone fruits special attention was paid to peaches. Many workers applied GA in autumn and obtained some satisfactory results in not only delaying the blossoming but at the same time in thinning the flower buds and increasing their winter hardiness. They generally used concentrations up to 200 ppm. The longest delaying effect was obtained in Redhaven peach (14 days) with the application of 200 ppm GA foliar sprays in August.

Alar

Alar, the other compound commonly used for this purpose, also gave satisfactory results in stone and pome fruits (Table 3). In nearly all these trials alar was applied during the previous summer and fall or in the spring before flowering. The investigators generally claimed that they obtained good results and were able to delay blossoming 1 to 13 days.

Ethephon

First results on the bloom delaying effect of ethephon were reported by Bukovac et al. (1969). They found that the flower buds of the ethephon treated branches of Montmorency sour cherries opened after 2 to 5 days, depending on the concentration of the chemical (Table 4). The same type of effect was obtained by Proebsting and Mills (1973) with three sweet cherry varieties. In Ankara conditions Özbek et al. (1974) carried out experiments to delay blooming in six important Turkish apricot varieties. In addition to the other growth regulators, they also used ethephon in summer, fall, and spring. The delaying effect was obtained by the fall applications. When ethephon was applied in March, a few early bud openings were observed in nearly all the varieties. Although the bloom delaying effect of ethephon looks positive, its side effects make it not very desirable to use. Among these side effects in apricots are rather severe gummosis, bud drops, dieback, and size decrease in flowers (Özbek et al., 1974; Gülşen, 1975; Kaşka, 1977).

Abscisic Acid

In recent years quite a lot of investigations have been carried out to clarify the dormancy mechanism in the buds, seeds, bulbs, etc. of various plant species. Among the results of these studies was the discovery that abscisic acid appears to be a dormancy regulating

Table 2. The Results of Gibberellic Acid Applications to Delay Bloom in Fruit Trees

Fruit Species	Variety	Applied Material	Concentration (ppm)	Time of Application	Bloom Delay (Days)	Author
Cherry	--	GA	50	Aug.,Nov.	No effect or 1-3 weeks	Brian et al.,1959
Peach	Fay Elberta	GA	50 to 500	Before the flower induction time	Insufficient effect	Bradley and Crane,1960
Apricot Almond Plum	Royal Jordanola President	GA GA GA	-- -- --	" " "	50 ppm completely stopped the development of flower buds	"
Cherry	Bing	GA	--	"	Very few flowers could develop	"
Pear	Bartlett	GA	10 to 500	Sept.,March,Apr.	No effect	Griggs and Iwakiri,1961
Peach	Elberta	KGA	80;240	Sept.	3 to 7 days	Proebsting and Mills,1964
Peach	Redhaven, Golden Jubilee	KGA	50;80	July,Aug.	1	Edgerton,1966
Almond	Peerless, Nonpareil, Mission	GA	100;200	Aug.,Sept.	2 to 7	Hicks and Crane,1968
Peach	Loadel, Fortuna, Palora, Peak, Halford	GA	50;100;200	End of July	2 to 11	Brown et al.,1968
Peach	Real George	--	200	Autumn	Full bloom delayed	Marlangeon,1969
Peach	Redskin	KGA	150	Sept.	5	Stembridge and LaRue,1969
Peach	Helberta Giant	GA	50;100;150 150	July Aug.,Sept.	3 to 7 7 to 10	Konarli,1970
Peach	Gage Elberta Redhaven Loring	GA GA GA	200 200 200	July Aug. Sept.	-- 14 --	Corgan and Widmoyer,1971
Peach	Hale	GA	150 to 250	July,Aug.	--	Konarli,1972
Peach	Hale, Fowler	GA	50;100;200	Sept.	1 to 2	Özçagiran,1972
Almond	Texas, 105-1, 17-1, 17, 5	GA	100;200;300	--	1 to 7	"
Peach	Redskin	KGA	75	After leaf fall	Some delay	Painter and Stembridge,1972
Peach	3 varieties	GA	50;500	June Aug.	Efficient No effect	Clanet and Borsani,1973
Apricot	6 Turkish varieties	GA	50;100;200	Autumn	2 to 4	Özbek et al.,1974
Apricot	4 varieties	GA	200	Sept.	2	Gülşen,1975

Table 3. Results of Alar Applications in Delaying the Bloom of Fruit Trees

Fruit Species	Variety	Applied Material	Concentration (ppm)	Time of Application	Bloom Delay (Days)	Author
Peach	Cardinal	Alar	2000;4000;6000	Oct.	2	Guerriero et al.,1971
Peach	Hale	Alar	500;1500;3000	Feb.	?	Konarli and Yavuz,1968
Peach	Redhaven, Golden Jubilee	Alar	2000	July	1	Edgerton,1966
Pear	Bartlett	Alar	1000 to 4000	Sept.-Oct.	13	Griggs et al.,1965
Pear	Barlett	Alar	1000;2000;3000		?	Griggs and Iwakiri,1968
Pear	Bartlett, Anjou	Alar	500;1000;2000; 3000	Summer	No effect	Griggs and Iwakiri,1968
Apple	McIntosh R. I. Greening	Alar	1000;5000;10,000 500;2000	Pinkbud Stage Preharvest	0 to 3 1 to 3	Edgerton and Hoffmann,1965
Apple	Cleopatra	Alar	2000	Nov.	No effect	Martin et al.,1968
Apple	Golden Delicious	Alar	3000;10,000	Sept.,Oct.	Reduced percentage of blooming	Stembridge and Ferrée,1969
				Jan.,March	Negligible effect	
Apricot	6 Turkish varieties	Alar	1000;2000;4000 8000	Summer,Fall Spring	1 to 6	Özbek et al.,1974
Apricot	Précoce de Boulbon, 3 Turkish varieties	Alar	1000 to 8000	Summer,Fall Spring	2 3-6	Gülşen,1975
Stone Fruits		Alar			Some delay	Guerriero and Scalabrelli,1977

Table 4. Effect of Ethephon and Abscisic Acid on Delaying the Blooming

Fruit Species	Variety	Applied Material	Concentration (ppm)	Time of Application	Bloom Delay (Days)	Author
Sourcherry, Plum	Montmorency	Ethephon	2000;4000	Preharvest	3 to 5	Bukovac et al.,1969
Sweet cherry	Bing, Chinook, Rainier	Ethephon	250 to 500	Sept.	3 to 5	Proebsting and Mills,1973
Apricot	6 Turkish varieties	Ethephon	2000;4000	End of Aug.	2 to 6	Özbek et al.,1974 Kaşka,1977
Apricot	Précoce de Boulbon, 3 Turkish varieties	Ethephon	2000;4000	Sept.,Oct.	2 to 6	Gulşen,1975
Stone fruits		Ethephon		Fall sprays	Delayed bloom	Dennis,1977
<u>Cornus stolonifera</u>		Ethephon	250;500;1000;2000	Sept.,Oct.	3 to 7	Fuchigami,1977
Apricot	6 Turkish varieties	ABA	10;25;50;100 25;50;100	Spring injection Soaking the branches in ABA solution	Delaying or stopping the opening of both leaf and fruit buds	Özbek et al.,1974 Kaşka,1977
Apple		ABA	100 to 1000		Some delay	Powell,1977

substance. This substance is common in all woody and herbaceous plants and their different organs. So it was thought for a time that physiologists had found the "magic substance" to control the opening of buds. But, unfortunately, during the last few years some findings "casted doubt on the involvement of ABA in the control of winter bud dormancy" (Mielke and Dennis, 1978). However, the effect of ABA in delaying the opening of buds keeps alive some hope for the future. In our experiments with apricots (Table 4) we have shown that ABA is able either to delay or to stop the opening of both flower and leaf buds (Özbek et al., 1974; Kaşka, 1977). The problem facing us is the weak penetration and rather slow movement of ABA basipetally and acropetally. In these applications no toxic effect was observed.

MECHANISM OF BLOOM DELAY

We have seen that the opening of buds can be delayed by the application of some growth regulating agents. Although some of these delays are rather short, it should be remembered that sometimes a bloom delay of even one day may be enough to save the whole crop.

Now the question arises: how do these agents act? Do they stop or slow down the growth and development of buds after their application? If so, how? In order to find some answers to these questions, two types of experiments were carried out in our laboratories: (1) study of the growth and development of the floral organs, and (2) study of the changes in the promoter and the inhibitor contents of buds from the time of application of the substance until the following spring. Gülşen (1975) has found that after the application of alar and GA the growth and development of the floral parts are slower than those of a control during the above mentioned time. She also observed late defoliation in the treated trees. Study of the changes of endogenous growth regulator levels by the oat coleoptile test in the September alar-treated buds revealed that in five varieties out of six, at the end of January when the chilling requirements had been satisfied, the amount of ABA-like substances was consistently higher than in the controls.

The bloom-delay effect of GA was explained by Bradley and Crane (1960) and Corgan and Widmoyer (1971) as the delaying of the flower induction and differentiation time. On the other hand, the results of Stembridge and LaRue (1969) and Painter and Stembridge (1972) are in accordance with the results of Gülşen (1975). They suggest that late defoliation due to GA application causes the buds to enter the winter rest late and consequently satisfaction of the chilling requirements takes place later than in the untreated buds. This results in late opening of buds. However, in places where the winters are long, such as Central Anatolia, this assumption may be refuted. During such a long winter period even the varieties with the longest chilling requirement cannot be faced with the lack of chilling. It seems, therefore, that some other mechanism is involved.

The effects of ethephon on the bloom-delay mechanism seem to be the result of damage to the branches and the buds. For example, especially at high doses (i.e., 4000 ppm), ethephon was killing some of the buds, defoliating the branches, and causing gummosis in apricots. This weakening of the trees may cause late opening of buds.

BREAKING OF REST AND EARLY FLOWERING

In areas like the Mediterranean coastline, South Africa, California, Florida, etc., the winters are warmer and shorter than in the other temperate zone countries. In those places the satisfaction of the chilling requirements of buds of fruit or ornamental trees creates some unavoidable problems such as irregular bud break, formation of smaller leaves, uneven opening of flower buds, bud shedding, late maturity, etc. Due to these undesirable problems yield is lowered and economic problems are created. The best way to avoid these problems is to grow trees with low chilling requirements. But unfortunately not all such trees give good quality fruits. Therefore, some technique or method must be found to shorten or break dormancy. A lot of rest breaking agents are known (Tables 5 and 6). For delaying blossoming, GA was supposed to be one of the most effective growth regulators. Then, along came kinetin, which seemed as effective as GA. The combination of a growth regulator with one of the rest breaking agents is reported to be even more beneficial than one or the other used alone. Indoleacetic acid (IAA) was found to be inefficient in breaking the rest of buds. Dinitro-ortho-cresol (DNOC) as a winter spray with mineral oil emulsion is used in many warm countries. Thiourea is accepted by the horticulturists as a good rest breaking agent for peach. However, since it may damage flower buds in especially weak trees the growers must be very careful. It should not be sprayed earlier than 4 to 5 weeks prior to the expected start of the blossoming and the rate of application should not exceed 10 kg/ha. Erez et al. (1971) demonstrated that DNOC-mineral oil+thiourea, DNOC-mineral oil+GA, and KNO_3+ thiourea are the most efficient combinations of these rest breaking agents. The investigators suggest that the combinations of pairs of the three compounds, DNOC-mineral oil, thiourea, and KNO_3, can give best results in commercial use. Erez et al. (1971) also noted that when combined treatments include an oil spray, the aqueous solutions must be applied before the oil spray.

The efficiency of all these dormancy breaking growth regulators and agents is increased when applied to buds that have been chilled for a while. If the chemicals are sprayed too early they may not be

Table 5. The Effects of Growth Regulators Alone or in Combination with Other Regulators or Agents on Breaking the Dormancy of Fruit Tree Buds

Fruit Species	Variety	Applied Material	Concentration (ppm)	Time of Application	Bud Opening (%)	Author
Peach	Elberta	IAA*	100;500	Jan. 4	None	Lavee,1973
Peach	Elberta	Kinetin*	100;500	Jan. 4	3.6 and 2.6	Lavee,1973
Peach	Elberta	GA*	100;500	Jan. 4	3.7 and 9.1	Lavee,1973
Peach	Elberta	(GA+IAA)*	(100+100), (100+500)	Jan. 4	5.8 and 1.3	Lavee,1973
Peach	Elberta	(GA+Kinetin)*	(100+100), (100+500)	Jan. 4	7.1 and 7.0	Lavee,1973
Peach	Redhaven	IAA**	200	Feb. 23	63.3(T.), 23.8(L.)	Erez et al.,1971
Peach	Redhaven	GA**	200	Feb. 23	75.6(T.), 45.4(L.)	Erez et al.,1971
Peach	Redhaven	Kinetin**	200	Feb. 23	77.0(T.), 27.0(L.)	Erez et al.,1971
Peach	Elberta	(GA+TU)**	(100+10,000)	Jan. 1	17.3	Erez et al.,1971
Peach	July Elberta	GA**	200	Feb. 24	50.0	Erez et al.,1971
Peach	July Elberta	Kinetin**	200	Feb. 24	64.0	Erez et al.,1971
Peach	July Elberts	(TU+GA)**	(5000+200)	Feb. 24	69.0	Erez et al.,1971
Peach	July Elberta	(W.W.+GA)**	(40,000+200)	Feb. 24	64.0	Erez et al.,1971
Peach	Robin	GA**	200	Feb. 25	41.0	Erez et al.,1971
Peach	Robin	(GA+DNOC)**	(200+20,000)	Feb. 25	71.0	Erez et al.,1971
Peach	Robin	(GA+TU)**	(200+10,000)	Feb. 25	67.0	Erez et al.,1971
Apple	Golden Delicious	Ethephon*	1000	Jan. 4	31.0	Paiva and Robitaille,1978
Apple	Golden Delicious	CGA 15281*	1000	Jan. 4	34.0	Paiva and Robitaille,1978

*in vitro; **in vivo; T - terminal bud; L - lateral bud; W.W.- (winter wash) parlatox; TU - thiourea; DNOC - dinitro-ortho-cresol

Table 6. Dormancy Breaking Effects of DNOC, Thiourea, and Winter Wash (Parlatox) in Fruit Trees

Fruit Species	Variety	Applied Material*	Concentration (ppm)	Time of Application	Bud Opening (%)	Author
Peach	July Elberta	W.W.	40,000	Feb. 24	42.0	Erez et al.,1971
Peach	July Elberta	TU	2000	Feb. 24	72.0	Erez et al.,1971
Peach	July Elberta	TU	20,000	Feb. 24	62.0	Erez et al.,1971
Peach	Robin	DNOC	2000	Feb. 25	42.0	Erez et al.,1971
Peach	Robin	TU	10,000	Feb. 25	40.0	Erez et al.,1971
Peach	Robin	TU	20,000	Feb. 25	57.0	Erez et al.,1971
Peach	Robin	(DNOC+TU)	(2000+10,000)	Feb. 25	70.0	Erez et al.,1971
Peach	Robin	W.W.	50,000	Feb. 20	66.0	Erez et al.,1971
Peach	Robin	(TU+W.W.)	(20,000+50,000)	Feb. 20	84.0	Erez et al.,1971
Peach	Robin	(TU+DNOC)	(20,000+2000)	Feb. 20	69.0	Erez et al.,1971
Japanese plum	Santa Rosa	W.W.	50,000	Jan. 25	2.4	Erez et al.,1971
Japanese plum	Santa Rosa	TU	10,000	Jan. 25	2.6	Erez et al.,1971
Japanese plum	Santa Rosa	(TU+W.W.)	(10,000+50,000)	Jan. 25	3.3	Erez et al.,1971
Apricot	Canino	W.W.	50,000	Feb. 4	3.6	Erez et al.,1971
Apricot	Canino	TU	20,000	Feb. 4	3.9	Erez et al.,1971
Apricot	Canino	(TU+W.W.)	(20,000+50,000)	Feb. 4	3.9	Erez et al.,1971
Apple	Golden Delicious	W.W.	50,000	Feb. 22,March 29	2.1	Erez et al.,1971
Apple	Golden Delicious	TU	20,000	Feb. 22,March 29	2.8	Erez et al.,1971
Apple	Golden Delicious	(TU+W.W.)	(20,000+50,000)	Feb. 22,March 29	3.4	Erez et al.,1971
Grapevine	Perlette	TU	20,000	Jan. 11	12.2	Erez et al.,1971

*W.W. (winter wash) parlatox; TU - thiourea; DNOC - Dinitro-ortho-cresol

effective. On the other hand if they are applied too late they may cause some damage and may even delay bud opening (Hill and Campbell, 1949).

MECHANISM OF ARTIFICIAL BUD BREAK

As described previously, some agents such as mineral oil, DNOC, or thiourea can break the rest in the buds of fruit trees. The mineral oils cover the buds entirely and thus most likely interfere with the oxygen supply to the cells, thereby starting an anaerobiosis in the buds. The bud-break effect of dinitro compounds has also been attributed to the respiration mechanism of buds.

The modes of action of other rest breaking agents are also not yet clearly explained. However, there are some clues that they may activate or stimulate the growth promoters. For instance, according to Wareing and Williers (Leopold and Kriedemann, 1975), in the germination of seeds thiourea may cause an increase in gibberellinlike substances in the seed. It apparently does not cause a decrease in the inhibitory substances present.

CONCLUSION

Even after all of these studies have been carried out and the results evaluated, it is still rather difficult for us to say that bloom delay by growth regulators can be controlled precisely by men. Therefore the magic substance(s) is (are) still waiting to be discovered. However, there is no doubt that plant physiologists have come a long way in unraveling the secrets of plant behavior. Now, for instance, we know that the efficiency of the "bloom delayers" is increased when they are applied around bud differentiation time. It seems that if the buds get the above-mentioned effect at the right time, bloom is delayed without much influence of ambient temperature. But it should be noted that by applying a bloom delaying substance nearly a year before, we are already accepting the occurrence of the frost next spring. In this case we want to let the tree bloom late anyway. I suppose that, right now, breeding should be more helpful to the growers. That is, by crossing and selection late blooming and frost hardy varieties can be obtained. From especially the selection point of view, Turkey is a very rich source. For instance Dokuzoguz and Gülcan at Ege University have been working for many years on such a selection program with almonds.

In case of bud break, it is apparent that the pomologists are in a better position. Efficient bud-breaking agents and growth regulators are being sold commercially. The problem we face is to find the best application time, suitable concentrations, and useful combinations of different bud-breaking agents and growth regulators.

Breeding efforts for short chilling varieties have also been more efficient than the delaying efforts. Several examples of the results of breeding versus delaying can be shown from California, Florida, Israel, South Africa, etc. I would like to mention here that such a selection project for short chilling apricot was started last year in our department and we have found 18 promising trees so far.

REFERENCES

Bradley, M. V., and Crane, J. C., 1960, Gibberellin induced inhibition of bud development in some species of Prunus, Science, 131:825-826.

Brian, P. W., Petty, J. H. P., and Richmond, P. T., 1959, Extended dormancy of deciduous woody plants treated in autumn with gibberellic acid, Nature, 184:69.

Brown, J. R., Crane, J. C., and Beutel, J. A., 1968, Gibberellic acid reduces cling peach flower buds, Calif. Agr., 22:7-8.

Buchanan, D. W., Bartholic, J. F., and Biggs, R. H., 1977, Manipulation of bloom and ripening dates of three Florida grown peach and nectarine cultivars through sprinkling and shade, J. Amer. Soc. Hort. Sci., 102:466-470.

Bukovac, M. J., Zuccani, F., Larsen, R. P., and Kesner, C. D., 1969, Chemical promotion of fruit abscission in cherries and plums with special reference to 2-chloro-ethylphosphonic acid, J. Amer. Soc. Hort. Sci., 94:226-230.

Clanet, H., and Borsani, O., 1973, The action of gibberellic acid on shoot growth and flower bud formation in peach trees, practical consequences, Hort. Abst., 43:1826.

Corgan, J. M., and Widmoyer, F. B., 1971, The effect of gibberellic acid on flower differentiation, date of bloom, and flower hardiness of peach, J. Amer. Soc. Hort. Sci., 96:54-57.

Dennis, F. G., 1977, Dormancy and hardiness of fruit trees, Hort-Science, 12:444.

Edgerton, L. J., 1966, Effect of gibberellin and growth retardants on bud development and cold hardiness of peach, Proc. Amer. Soc. Hort. Sci., 88:197-203.

Edgerton, L. J., and Hoffmann, M. B., 1965, Some physiological responses of apples to N-dimethyl amino succinamic acid and other growth regulators, Proc. Amer. Soc. Hort. Sci., 86:28-36.

Erez, A., Lavee, S., and Samish, R. M., 1971, Improved methods for breaking rest in the peach and other deciduous fruit species, Amer. Soc. Hort. Sci., 96:519-522.

Fuchigami, L. H., 1977, Ethephon-induced defoliation and delay of spring growth in Cornus stolonifera Michx., J. Amer. Soc. Hort. Sci., 102:452-454.

Griggs, W. H., and Iwakiri, B. T., 1961, Effect of gibberellin and 2,4,5,-Trichlorophenoxypropionic acid sprays on Bartlett pear trees, Proc. Amer. Soc. Hort. Sci., 77:73-89.

Griggs, W. H., and Iwakiri, B. T., 1968, Effect of succinic acid 2,2-dimethyl hydrazide (alar) sprays used to control growth in "Bartlett" pear trees planted in hedgerows, Proc. Amer. Soc. Hort. Sci., 92:155-166.

Griggs, W. H., Iwakiri, B. T., and Bethell, R. S., 1965, B-nine fall sprays delay bloom and increase fruit set on Bartlett pears, Calif. Agr., 19:8-11.

Guerriero, R., Loreti, F., and Vitagliano, C., 1971, The effects of growth regulators on peach flowering date, Hort. Abst., 41:8405.

Guerriero, R., and Scalabrelli, G., 1977, Several trials for delaying bloom in stone fruit trees by SADH and other growth regulators, in: "I.S.H.S. Symposium on Growth Regulators in Fruit Production," Poznan, Poland.

Gülşen, Y., 1975, The effect of alar, gibberellic acid and ethrel on the apricot flower bud development (Ph.D. thesis in Turkish), A.Ü.Z.F., Ankara, Turkey.

Hicks, J. R., and Crane, J. C., 1968, The effect of gibberellin on almond flower bud growth, time of bloom and yield, Proc. Amer. Soc. Hort. Sci., 92:1-6.

Hill, G. G., and Campbell, G. K. G., 1949, Prolonged dormancy of deciduous fruit trees in warm climates, Emp. Jour. Exp. Agr. V., 17:259-264.

Kaşka, N., 1977, Delaying of flowering in apricots by ethrel and abscisic acid, in: "I.S.H.S. Symposium on Growth Regulators in Fruit Production," Poznan, Poland.

Kennard, W. C., Tukey, L. B., and White, D. G., 1951, Further studies with maleic hydrazide to delay blossoming of fruits, Proc. Amer. Soc. Hort. Sci., 58:26-32.

Konarli, O., 1970, Effect of gibberellic acid in stopping blooming, J. Yalova Hort. Rest. Inst., 3:49-54 (in Turkish).

Konarli, O., 1972, Effect of gibberellic acid on the delaying of flowering and thinning of Hale peach, J. Yalova Hort. Res. Inst., 5:22-27 (in Turkish).

Konarli, O., and Yavuz, S., 1968, Effect of N-dimethyl amino succinamic acid on bloom delaying in peaches, J. Yalova Hort. Res. Inst., 1:83-85 (in Turkish).

Lavee, S., 1973, Dormancy and bud break in warm climates; Considerations of growth regulator involvement, Acta Horticulturae, 34: 225-233.

Leopold, A. C., and Kriedemann, P. E., 1975, "Plant Growth and Development," McGraw-Hill, New York.

Lipe, W. N., Wilke, O., and Newton, O., 1977, Freeze protection of peaches by evaporative cooling in the post-rest, pre-bloom period, J. Amer. Soc. Hort. Sci., 102:370-372.

Marlengeon, R. C., 1969, Efectos del acido giberelico y de otras drogs sobre la permanencia del follje Verde otonal y la induccion de resistencie a Heleda en flores de duraznero, Phyton, B. Aires, 26:113-122.

Martin, D. T., Levis, L., and Cerny, J., 1968, The effect of alar on fruit cell division and other characteristics in apples, Proc. Amer. Soc. Hort. Sci., 92:67-70.

Mielke, E. A., and Dennis, F. G., Jr., 1978, Hormonal control of flower bud dormancy in sour cherry (*Prunus cerasus* L.). III. Effects of leaves, defoliation and temperature on levels of abscisic acid in flower primordia, J. Amer. Soc. Hort. Sci., 103:446-449.

Mitchell, J. W., and Cullinan, F. P., 1942, Effects of growth regulating chemicals on the opening of vegetative and floral buds of peach and pear, Plant Phys., 17:16-26.

Okasha, K. A., and Crane, J. O., 1963, Vegetative and fruit responses of the apricot and peach to maleic hydrazide, Proc. Amer. Soc. Hort. Sci., 83:234-239.

Özbek, S., Kaşka, N., Erdogan, M., Kaynak, L., and Kaleli, Ş., 1974, Investigations on bloom delaying of apricot by some growth regulators, TÜBİTAK publications No. 240 TOAGS., No. 34, Ankara, Turkey.

Özçagiran, R., 1972, Investigations on thinning and bloom delaying in fruit trees by some chemicals (Assoc. Prof. Thesis), Univ. of Ege, Faculty of Agriculture, Izmir, Turkey.

Painter, J. W., and Stembridge, G. E., 1972, Peach flowering responses as related to time of gibberellin application, HortScience, 7:389-390.

Paiva, E., and Robitaille, H. A., 1978, Breaking bud rest on detached apple shoots: Interaction of gibberellic acid with some rest-breaking chemicals, HortScience, 13:57-58.

Proebsting, E. L., Jr., and Mills, H. H., 1964, Gibberellin-induced hardiness responses in Elberta peach flower buds, Proc. Amer. Soc. Hort. Sci., 85:134-140.

Proebsting, E. L., Jr., and Mills, H. H., 1973, Bloom delay and frost survival in ethephon-treated sweet cherry, HortScience, 8:46-47.

Stang, E. J., Ferree, D. C., Hall, F. R., and Spotts, R. A., 1978, Overtree misting for bloom delay in "Golden Delicious" apple, J. Amer. Soc. Hort. Sci., 103:82-87.

Stembridge, G. E., and Ferree, M. E., 1969, Immediate and residual effects of succinic acid, 2,2-dimethyl hydrazide (alar) on young "Delicious" apple trees, J. Amer. Soc. Hort. Sci., 94: 602-604.

Stembridge, G. E., and LaRue, J. H., 1969, The effect of potassium gibberellate on flower bud development in the Redskin peach, J. Amer. Soc. Hort. Sci., 94:492-495.

Tukey, H. B., 1954, "Plant Regulators in Agriculture," John Wiley and Sons, New York.

Weaver, R. J., 1959, Prolonging dormancy in *Vitis vinifera* with gibberellin, Nature, 183:1198-1199.

White, I. G., and Kennard, W. C., 1950, A preliminary report on the use of maleic hydrazide to delay blossoming of fruits, Proc. Amer. Soc. Hort. Sci., 55:147-151.

Zimmerman, P. W., and Hitchcock, A. E., 1942, Contribs. Boyce Thompson Inst., 12:321.

14

STRUCTURE-ACTIVITY RELATIONSHIPS OF SOME NEW GROWTH RETARDANTS

E. N. Karanov

M. Popov Institute of Plant Physiology
Bulgarian Academy of Science
Sofia, Bulgaria

The first growth retarding substance was discovered approximately thirty years ago by Mitchell et al. (1949). Since then much work has been done on the effects of growth retarding chemicals on the growth and developmental processes of plants. Methods for applying retardants have also been developed and studies have been made on the mode of action of these growth regulators.

The field of retardants is so broad and touches so many aspects of plant growth and development processes that a short article can deal with only some of them. The following pages are concerned particularly with structure-activity relationships of some new growth retarding substances.[1]

QUATERNARY TETRAALKYLAMMONIUM SALTS

Paul and Göring (1974) have studied the growth retarding activity of compounds with the following structure:

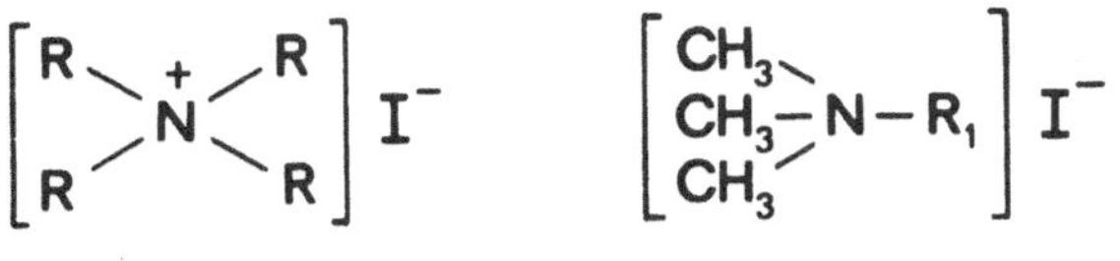

[1]Abbreviations: CCC--N-(2-chloroethyl)-ammonium chloride; Alar--mono-N, N, dimethylhydrazide of succinic acid; AMO-1618--N-(4-hydroxy-5-isopropyl-2-methylphenyl)-trimethylammonium chloride, 1-piperidine carboxylate; BOH--β-hydroxyethylhydrazine; MH--cyclic hydrazide of maleic acid.

where R = n-alkyl radical containing C_1 to C_5 atoms, and R_1 = n-alkyl radical containing C_1 to C_{10} atoms. They established on wheat seedlings that in the case of tetraalkylammonium halides, the activity falls sharply with increasing to C_3 the number of C-atoms in the alkyl radicals. The activity of N-alkyltrimethylammonium halides increases linearly with increasing the number of C-atoms in the alkyl chain from C_1 to C_{5-6} atoms. Further increasing the number of C-atoms in the alkyl radical results in parabolic reduction of activity.

QUATERNARY ARYLTRIALKYLAMMONIUM SALTS

The growth activity of these retardants was discovered during 1964 (Cathey and Stuard, 1961; Downing et al., 1964), but detailed structure-activity relations were studied in R. L. Wain's laboratory (Knight et al., 1969; Wain, 1972). The structure of the compounds studied is as follows:

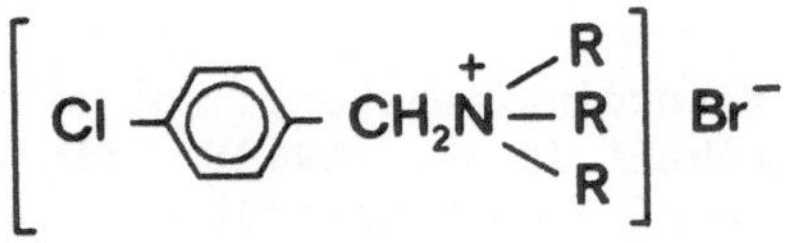

where R = n-alkyl containing C_1 to C_7 atoms. It was established in wheat, pea, and bean tests that activity appears when C_3 atoms are present in the alkyl radical and reaches its maximum at C_4. Further increasing the length of the alkyl chain, depending on the test object, leads to weak activity or phytotoxicity. The introduction of a Cl-atom into the phenyl ring increases the activity, with substitution in the 4- or 3-position being most effective. Incorporation of a second Cl-atom into the ring leads to a greater rise of activity, but only when one Cl-atom is in the 3- or 4-position. Replacement of the phenyl ring by 1- or 2-naphthyl did not remarkably alter the activity. When an oxygen bridge was introduced between the methylene group and the ring, activity was markedly reduced. N-(4-chlorobenzyl)-tri-n-butylammonium bromide (B-4) and the corresponding 1-naphthyl analog were considered to be compounds of practical importance.

QUATERNARY AMMONIUM (+)-LIMONENE DERIVATIVES

Newhall (1969; 1971) and Newhall and Pieringer (1966; 1967; 1972) studied the retarding activity of (+)-limonene derivatives with the following structure:

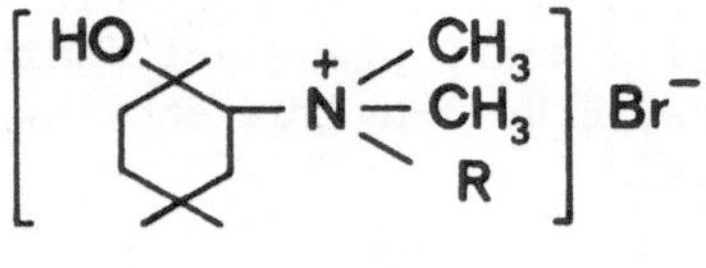

where R = n-alkyl chain containing C_1 to C_{10}, C_{12}, and C_{18} atoms. Using a bean test, enhancement of retardant activity was observed with increasing length of the alkyl radical from C_2 to C_7 atoms, but further increasing the number of C-atoms led to weak activity, and with C_{12} atoms the activity disappeared. The heptyl derivative was the most active. Using an alfalfa seedlings test, activity increased from C_2 to C_9 atoms and decreased after introduction of C_{10} atoms.

In comparing the activity of the compounds containing single and double bonds between the 8- and 9-position, it was established that saturation of the bond increases activity (Newhall, 1969).

High growth retarding activity is also shown by some quaternary benzyl derivatives of (+)-limonene (Newhall, 1971; Newhall and Pieringer, 1966, 1967; Pieringer and Newhall, 1968) with structure:

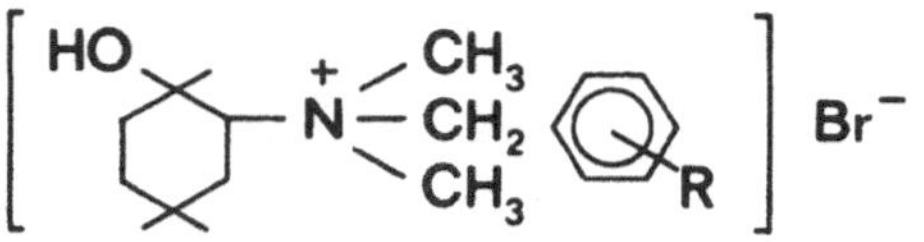

where R = -H, -Cl, $-CH_3$.

Introduction of a Cl-atom into the benzyl ring enhances activity, with substitution into the 2- or 4-position being most effective. High activity was shown also by 4-methylbenzyl-, 2, 4-dichlorobenzyl, and 3, 4-dichlorobenzyl derivatives (Newhall and Pieringer, 1966; Pieringer and Newhall, 1970). Optical activity has no influence on the retarding effect (in comparing (+)- and (-)-limonene derivatives) in the bean test. Three pure geometrical isomers of $\Delta^{8(9)}$-p-menthene derivatives (derived from (+)-limonene) showed that they possess different retarding activity, but when applied in mixtures, the effects were additive (Newhall and Pieringer, 1972).

QUATERNARY AMMONIUM 2-HYDROXYCYCLOHEXYL DERIVATIVES

Studying the action of 2-hydroxycyclohexylammonium derivatives Newhall (1974) found high activity of the following structures:

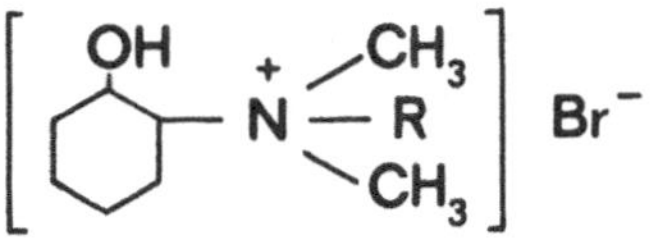

where R = n-alkyl radical containing C_7 to C_{16} atoms. Depending on the test object and the length of the alkyl chain the following structure-activity correlations were established: In tests with cucumber rootlets and alfalfa seedlings C_{11} and C_{12} derivatives possess highest activity. Using a test based on the retardation of the second internodium of bean seedlings, the highest activity occurred in the C_7 to C_{11} derivatives, with the most active substances being octyl and nonyl derivatives. Using grapefruit seedlings, the best compounds were two-decyl and dodecyl derivatives. The mentioned compounds generally exceed the activity of Alar. The results are in broad agreement with those found for (+)-limonene derivatives, except that for a high activity the cyclohexanol derivatives must have a longer alkyl chain (with C_3 to C_4 atoms).

QUATERNARY AMMONIUM DERIVATIVES OF α- AND β-IONONE, ISOPHORONE, AND OTHER TERPENOIDES

The retarding activity of these compounds was reported by Haruta et al. (1972, 1974a,b,c). It was shown that N, N, N-trimethyl-3-(2', 6', 6'-trimethyl-2'-cyclohexene-1'-yl)-2-propenylammonium iodide (a derivative of α-ionone, structure A), N, N, N-trimethyl-1-methyl-3-(2', 6', 6'-trimethyl-1'-cyclohexene-1'-yl)-propylammonium iodide (a derivative of β-ionone, structure B), and N, N, N-trimethyl-2-(3', 5', 5'-trimethylcyclohexenyl)-ethylammonium iodide (a derivative of isophorone, structure C) exceed the activity of AMO-1618 (Haruta et al., 1972, 1974b).

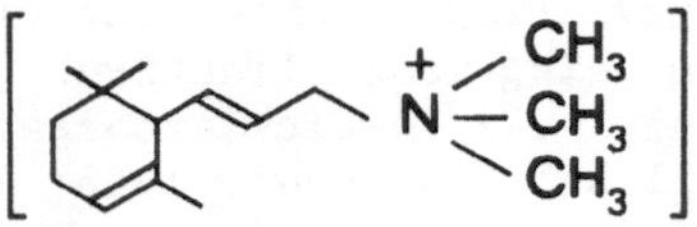

Structure A

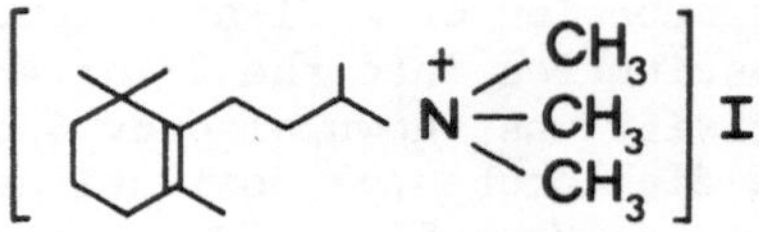

Structure B

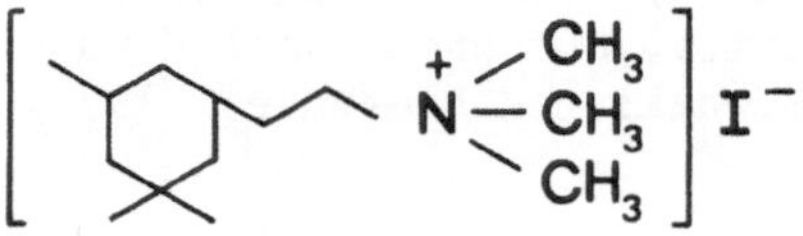

Structure C

By testing numerous derivatives of these compounds on rice seedlings and cucumber hypocotyls it was found that the presence or absence of a double bond in the ring system or in the alkyl chain between the ring and a quaternized N-atom does not influence the activity. On the other hand, compounds in which the trimethylammonium group is directly bonded with the cycle are inactive. Compounds with a longer alkyl chain (stearyl, heptyl, and lauryl radicals) possess, as a rule, high activity.

In another set of experiments (Haruta et al., 1974a) the effect of replacing a methyl group attached to the quaternized N-atom by n-alkyl-, halogen-n-alkyl-, hydroxy-n-alkyl-, allyl-, propargyl, 4-chlorobenzyl, 2, 4-dichlorobenzyl, and 3, 4-dichlorobenzyl was investigated. Besides the tests mentioned, a tomato hypocotyl test was employed. Most of the compounds tested were highly active. Substitution of the $-CH_3$ group with a higher alkyl radical in all the three basic structures as a rule decreases activity. With rice seedlings highest activity was obtained with the propargyl radical ($-CH_2C{\equiv}CH$) in structure A and by the $-CH_3$ group in structure B. In the cucumber hypocotyl test highest activity was exhibited by compounds with $-CH_2CH_3$ and $-CH_2CH_2Br$ radicals in structure A and with $-CH_3$ and $-CH_2C{\equiv}CH$ radicals in structure B. The last compound was most active also in the tomato hypocotyl test. Substitution of two methyl groups, attached to the quaternary N-atom with pyrrolidinium, piperidinium, and morpholinium rings in the basic structure A, revealed that pyrrolidinium derivatives were slightly more active than the initial structure. N, N, N-trimethyl-1-methyl-3-(2', 6', 6'-trimethyl-2'-cyclohexene-1-yl)-2-propenylammonium iodide (a derivative of α-ionone, structure A) was proposed for practical use.

The derivatives of trimethylaminoacetohydrazide chloride (Girard's reagent) are interesting from a structural point of view.

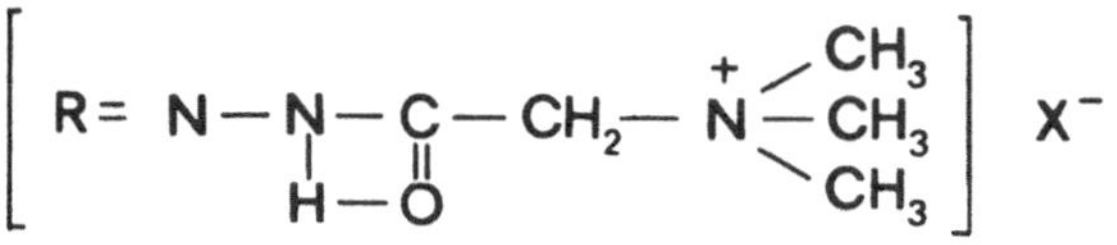

where X = Cl- or I, and R = $(CH_3)_2CH{=}$, $CH_3(CH_2)_4CH{=}$,

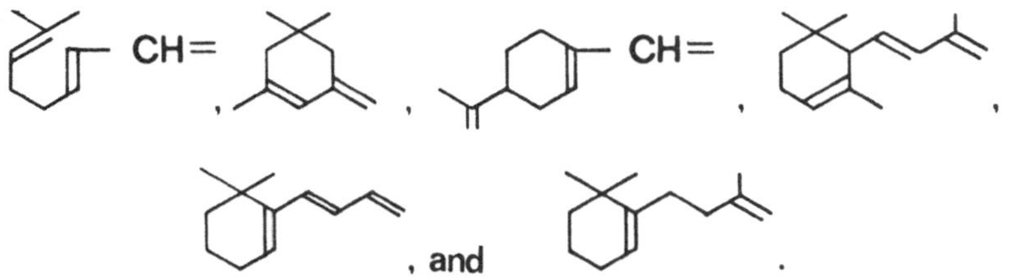

And these compounds contain the trimethylammonium radical, which occurs in CCC and AMO-1618, and the system C-C-N-N, which occurs in Alar, BOH, CO-11, and MH (Haruta et al., 1974b).

It was found that all these compounds containing the terpenoid moeity exceed the activity of Alar in the rice seedlings test. Highest activity was obtained by α- and β-ionone derivatives.

TRIMETHYLHYDRAZONIUM SALTS

Nagao and Tamura (1971) have studied the retardant activity of compounds with the following structure:

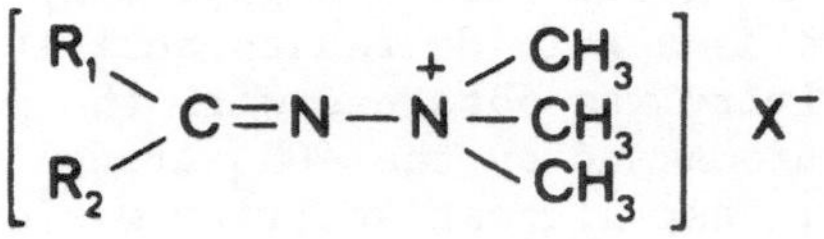

where, when X = -I and R_2 = -H, R_1 = $-CH_3(CH_2)_{10}$ (A)

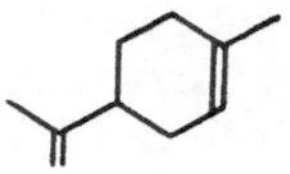 (C), 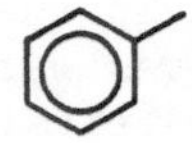 (D), and 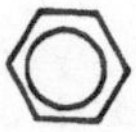 -CH=CH- (E).

When X = -I and R_2 = $-CH_3$, R_1 = 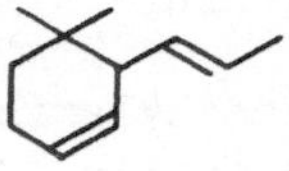 (F) and 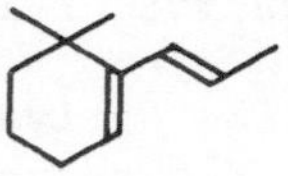 (G),

and when X = -Cl and R_2 = -H, R_1 = 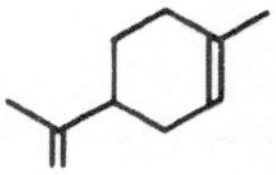 (H).

It was shown in the rice seedling test that the activity of compounds A, C, F, G, and H slightly exceeds that of Alar. In the wheat seedling test, highest activity was exhibited by A, C, and G; in the cucumber hypocotyl test, strongest action was observed for A, C, F, and G. It is noteworthy that in the wheat seedlings test F was inactive while in the cucumber hypocotyl test the same compound showed highest activity.

QUATERNARY PYRROLIDINIUM, PIPERIDINIUM, MORPHOLINIUM, PRINIDINIUM, AND QUINOLINIUM SALTS

Göring and Paul (1974) have established retardant activity in N-methyl-N-alkylpyrrolidinium iodides:

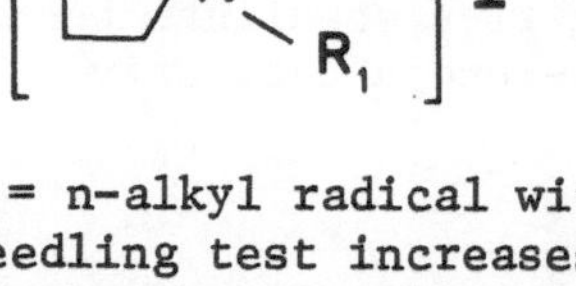 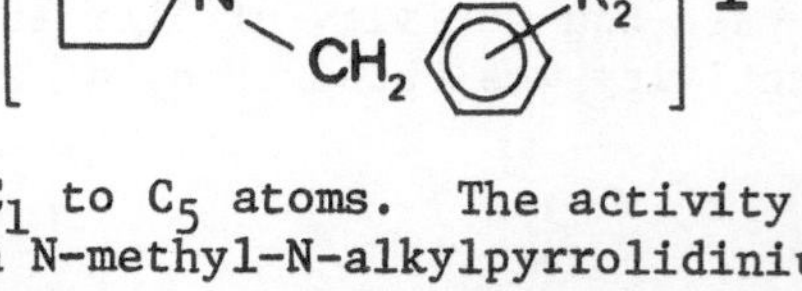

where R = n-alkyl radical with C_1 to C_5 atoms. The activity in the wheat seedling test increases in N-methyl-N-alkylpyrrolidinium iodide with lengthening the alkyl radical to C_3 or C_4 atoms, and then falls with further increasing the number of C-atoms. With N_1,

N_2-dialkylpyrrolidinium iodide the activity falls sharply when R = C_4. N, N-dimethylpyrrolidinium iodide has approximately the same activity as CCC, as Buchenauer et al. (1973) have also established.

Wain's laboratory (Chamberlain et al., 1976) has investigated the retardant action of some N-methyl-N-chloroalkyl and N-methyl-N-chlorobenzyl-pyrrolidinium halides of the basic structure:

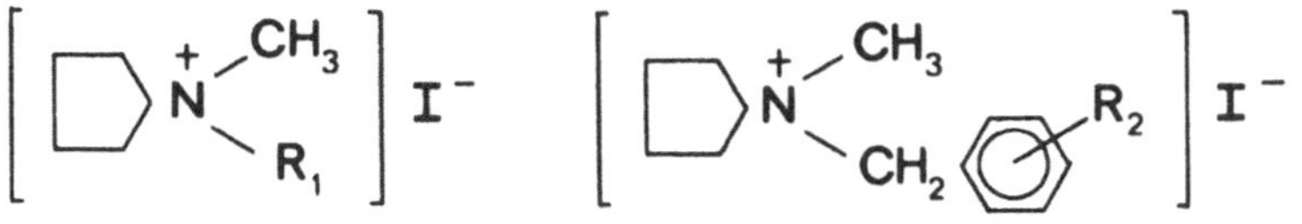

where R_1 = $-CH_2Cl$, $-CH_2CH_2Cl$, $-CH_2CH_2CH_2Cl$, $-CH_2CH(CH_3)CH_2Cl$, and R_2 = 2-, 3-, and 4-Cl-, 2, 3-, 2, 4-, 2, 5-, 2, 6-, and 3, 4-Cl_2.

It was shown with wheat seedlings that among chloroalkyl substituted derivatives highest activity was exhibited by N-methyl-N-chloromethyl-pyrrolidinium bromide. Lengthening of the alkyl radical led to reduction of the activity, when the chloromethyl derivative was found to be by the 2-, 4-, 2, 3-, and 2, 4-derivatives. The same relationships were established for the retardant activity of N-methyl-N-chlorobenzylpiperidinium and N-chlorobenzylpryridinium halides.

On the other hand, Wain and his coworkers found N-methyl-N-3-chlorobenzylpyrrolidinium and N-methyl-N-3-chlorobenzylpiperidinium halides to be completely inactive on the wheat seedlings, although they possess high activity by the bean seedlings test.

Hüppi et al. (1976) have found retardant properties to be exhibited by N-alkyl-N-(3, 7-dimethyloctyl)-piperidinium iodide.

Karanov and Vassilev (1974) have investigated the action of some quaternary N-alkylpyridinium, N-alkylquinolinium, and N-benzylpyridinium halides of the following structure:

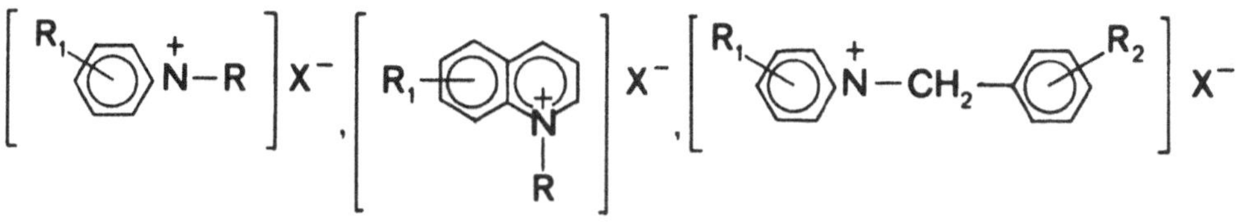

where R = methyl-, ethyl-, n-propyl-, allyl-, n-butyl-, n-hexyl-; R_1 = hydrogen- or methyl-; R_2 = chlorine; and X = halide.

They found that for high activity of N-alkylpyridinium and N-alkyl-quinolinium halides, in a tall pea test, the alkyl group must contain C_1 to C_3 atoms in the alkyl moiety. The introduction of a

$-CH_3$ group in the pyridilium and quinolinium rings enhances the activity of the compounds, and its position in the ring is not important. Methyl substitution in the molecule of N-benzylpyridinium halides, however, has little effect on activity. Introduction of a Cl-atom into the benzyl radical increases action, most effectively by substitution in the 4-position. Some of the derivatives tested were more active than CCC.

The derivatives of N-alkylpyridilium, N-alkylquinolinium, and N-benzylpyridilium halides were highly active in retarding chlorophyll degradation in isolated discs of mature radish leaves in the dark. For high activity the alkyl radical of N-alkylpyridilium and N-alkylquinolinium halides must not be higher than methyl. Higher homologues induce phytotoxic symptoms. Introduction of a Cl-atom in the ortho position of the benzyl ring of N-benzylpyridilium halides increases activity.

In other investigations Karanov (1978) and Barth et al. (in press) examined the growth retarding activity of some derivatives of piperidineacetanilide having the basic structure:

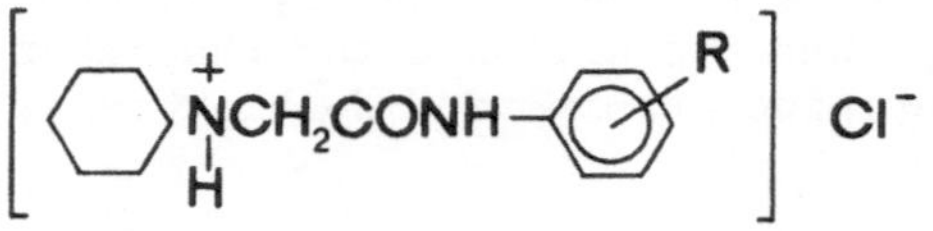

where R = -H; 2-, 3-, and $4-CH_3-$; 2-, 3-, and $4-OCH_3-$; 2-, 3-, and $4-OC_2H_5$; 2-, 3-, and $4-CF_3-$; 2-, 3-, and 4-F-; 2-, 3-, and 4-Cl; and 4-Br; 3-I; 2-, 3-, and $4-NO_2-$.

These derivatives contain in their structure in addition to the quaternized N-atom typical for the retardant activity, the -C = O and -N-H- groups which occur in herbicides performing their action through inhibition of the Hill reaction (Moreland, 1969).

It was shown in the pea test that these substances possess high retardant activity; some of them exceed the activity of CCC when used at only one-tenth the concentration. Introduction of substituents into the anilide ring of hydrochlorides of piperidineacetanilides as a rule increased the activity. $-CH_3$, Cl-, and Br- substitution led to the highest activity, $-NO_2$, $-OCH_3$, and $-OC_2H_5-$ groups having little effect.

The derivatives of piperidineacetanilide were found to delay the chlorophyll degradation in detached radish leaves. For high activity, substitution into the 3- or 4-position in the anilide ring is necessary. Among the hydrochlorides of piperidineacetanilides highest activity was exhibited by -Cl and -Br- substituted compounds, and the lowest activity by compounds substituted with $-CH_3$.

SULPHONIUM SALTS

The retardant activity of these compounds has been reported for the first time by Knight et al. (1969). The substances have the following structure:

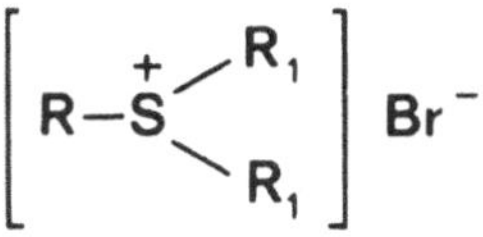

where R = benzyl-, chlorobenzyl-, naphthylmethyl-, and allyl-; R_1 = $-CH_3$ or n-C_4H_9-; when R_1 = $-CH_3$, R = $C_6H_5CH_2$-, 2-, 3-, and 4-$ClC_6H_4CH_2$-; 2, 3-, 2, 4-, 2, 5-, and 2, 6-$Cl_2C_6H_3CH$-, $C_{10}H_7CH_2$-, and $CH_2CH = CH_2$-; when R_1 = n-C_4H_9-, R = $C_6H_5CH_2$-, 3- and 4-$ClC_6H_4CH_2$-, and $C_{10}H_7CH_2$-.

All benzylsulphonium and chlorobenzylsulphonium bromides showed higher activity in wheat seedling tests as compared with those using pea and bean seedlings. In most cases, however, retardant activity is accompanied by some inhibition of the root system and phytotoxicity and only S-allyl-S, S-dimethylsulphonium bromide showed comparable activity to CCC and AMAB with no phytotoxic effects.

Bokarev et al. (1971) have established that S-(2-bromethyl)-dimethylsulphonium bromide exceeds the activity of CCC by 3 to 4 times when applied to the tall peas varieties. A high activity was also obtained for some acetylcholine halides, betainchloride, dimethylprotiotein chloride, dimethyltetin chloride, and others. These substances generally exceed the activity of CCC.

DERIVATIVES OF ALIPHATIC DICARBOXYLIC ACIDS

To these derivatives belong Alar and CO-II, whose structural properties have been discussed by Cathey (1964).

Karanov et al. (1974a,b, 1975a,b, 1976) and Karanov and Christova (1975) have recently reported the retardant activity of mono- and dialkyl itaconic acid esters.

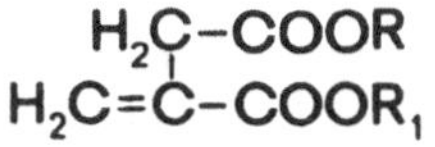

where R and R_1 = -H and/or $-CH_3$, $-C_2H_5$, n-C_3H_7-, iso-C_3H_7-, n-C_4H_9-, iso-C_4H_9-, sec-C_4H_9-, and $CH_2C_6H_5$. It was shown by the tall peas test that most of the substances used exceed the activity of Alar. Itaconic acid esters exhibit a high activity provided the R and R_1 groups contain C_1 to C_4 atoms. Itaconic acid esters delay the aging processes in detached leaves, higher activity being exhibited by diesters with C_1 to C_2 atoms in the alkoxy moiety.

OTHER NEW RETARDANTS

The growth retarding activity of some other types of compounds has been reported in recent years. According to Beyer (1972), 3, 3a-di-hydroxy-2-(4-methoxyphenyl)-8H pyrazolo-(5,1a) isoindol-8-on(DPX 1840), which is an active inhibitor of auxin transport, has a retarding activity. According to Snel and Gramlich (1973), Furuta et al. (1972), and other investigators α-cyclopropyl-α-(4-methoxyphenyl)-5-pirimidinemethanol (Ancymidol) suppresses the growth of some ornamental plants.

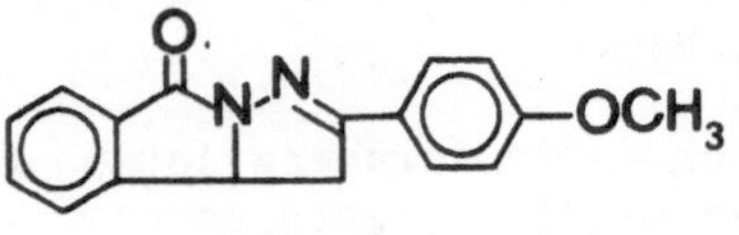

DPX 184O

Aigami et al. (1977) have reported the retardant activity of some hydroxy-4-homoisotwistanes and of some polycyclohexanols structurally related to them (1978).

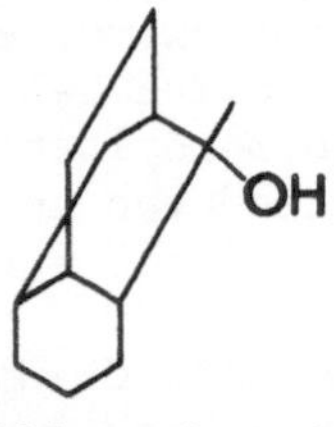

hydroxy-Y-homoisotwistanes

According to Wain (1972), 3, 5-dichlorophenoxyacetic acid shows retardant activity in tomato plants. The same effect is exhibited by 3-(3, 5-dichlorophenoxy)-butyric and 2-(3, 5-dichlorophenoxy)-ethylamine, which, according to Taylor and Wain (1978), convert in tomato plants to 3, 5-dichlorophenoxyacetic acid.

Retardant effects are shown by some anticytokinins such as 4-substituted 7-(β,D-ribofuranosil)-pirolo-(2, 3-d)-pirimidines (Iwamura et al., 1976).

In general, the research on structure-activity relationships published in recent years and the summarized data from Cathey's review (1964) make it possible to outline some basic structural requirements for growth retarding activity:

1. Quaternary ammonium moeity;
2. Quaternary phosphonium moiety;
3. Dialkylsulphonium moiety;
4. -C-C-N-N- system.

Modifications of the quaternary ammonium group such as replacing the trialkylammonium group with alkylpyrrolidinium, alkylpiperidinium, alkylmorpholinium, piridinium, and quinolinium moieties, and substitution of an alkyl group of the alkyl radicals attached to the quaternized N-atom by an amino group or chlorobenzyl radical, can retain or increase the growth retarding activity. The remainder of the quaternary ammonium type molecule may vary (alkyl, halogen alkyl, substituted benzyl, terpenoid moiety, etc.), but such substitution may lead to enhancement of activity and phytotoxicity or to reduction of the retardant action.

Itaconic acid derivatives, homotwistane derivatives, and ancymidol are of interest in that they are retardants with completely different structural types; further research on these compounds to determine their mode of action would appear to be warranted.

REFERENCES

Aigami, K., Ynamoto, Y., Fujikura, Y., Ohsugi, M., and Takaishi, N., 1978, Phytochem., 17:804.
Aigami, K., Ynamoto, Y., Takaishi, N., and Fujikura, Y., 1977, Phytochem., 16:41.
Barth, A., Karanov, E., et al., In press.
Beyer, E. M., 1972, Pl. Physiol., 50:322.
Bokarev, K. S., Karanov, E., and Ivanova, R. P., 1971, USSR pat. N 369887.
Buchenauer, H., and Erwin, D. C., 1973, Z. Pflanzenkrankh. und Pflanzenschutz, 80:575.
Cathey, H. M., 1964, Ann. Rev. Pl. Physiol., 15:271.
Cathey, H. M., and Stuard, N. W., 1961, Bot. Gaz., 123:51.
Chamberlain, V. K., Chamberlain, K., and Wain, R. L., 1976, Ann. Appl. Biol., 82:589.
Downing, C. R., Felton, S. L., and Melton, T. M., 1964, Abs. Am. Soc. Hort. Sci., 25:471.
Furuta, Tok, Jones, W. Clay, Mock, T., Humphrey, W., Mair, R., and Breece, J., 1972, Calif. Agr., 26:10.
Göring, H., and Paul, E., 1974, in: "Proceedings of the International Symposium on the Biochemistry and Chemistry of Plant Growth Regulators" (Cottbus, German Republic, September 24-26, 1974), Klaus Schreiber, H. R. Schütte, and G. Sembdner, eds., Institut für Biochemie der Pflanzen, Akademie der Wissenschaften der DDR, Berlin.
Haruta, H., Yagi, H., Iwata, T., and Tamura, S., 1972, Agr. Biol. Chem., 36:881.

Haruta, H., Yagi, H., Iwata, T., and Tamura, S., 1974a, Agr. Biol. Chem., 38:417.
Haruta, H., Yagi, H., Iwata, T., and Tamura, S., 1974b, Agr. Biol. Chem., 38:141.
Haruta, H., Yagi, H., Iwata, T., and Tamura, S., 1974c, Agr. Biol. Chem., 38:877.
Hüppi, G. A., Bocion, P. F., and da Silva, W. H., 1976, Experientia, 32:37.
Iwamura, H., Kumazavwa, Z., Eguchi, J., Mogami, M., and Okuda, S., 1976, Agr. Biol. Chem., 40:1653.
Karanov, E., 1978, Dr. Sc. Thesis, Bulg. Acad. Sci., Sofia.
Karanov, E., and Christova, L., 1975, C. R. Acad. Bulg. Sci., 28: 1097.
Karanov, E., and Vassilev, G., 1974, in: "Proceedings of the International Symposium on the Biochemistry and Chemistry of Plant Growth Regulators" (Cottbus, German Republic, September 24-26, 1974), Klaus Schreiber, H. R. Schütte, and G. Sembdner, eds., Institut für Biochemie der Pflanzen, Akademie der Wissenschaften der DDR, Berlin.
Karanov, E., Vassilev, G., and Christova, L., 1975a, C. R. Acad. Sci. Agr. Bulg., 8:1085.
Karanov, E., Vassilev, G., Christova, L., and Pogoncheva, E., 1974a, in: "Proceedings of the International Symposium on the Biochemistry and Chemistry of Plant Growth Regulators" (Cottbus, German Republic, September 24-26, 1974), Klaus Schreiber, H. R. Schütte, and G. Sembdner, eds., Institut für Biochemie der Pflanzen, Akademie der Wissenschaften der DDR, Berlin.
Karanov, E., Vassilev, G., Christova, L., Pogoncheva, E., and Planchkova, S., 1974b, Bulg. pat. N 26120.
Karanov, E., Vassilev, G., Christova, L., Pogoncheva, E., and Fam Thi Shang, 1976, in: "Design and Mechanism of Action of Antimetabolits," Sofia.
Karanov, E., Vassilev, G., and Pogoncheva, E., 1975b, C. R. Acad. Bulg. Sci., 28:1097.
Knight, B. E. A., Taylor, H. F., and Wain, R. L., 1969, Ann. Appl. Biol., 63:211.
Mitchell, J. W., Wirwill, J. W., and Weil, L., 1949, Science, 110: 252.
Moreland, D., 1969, in: "Progress in Photosynthesis Research," 111: 1693.
Nagao, M., and Tamura, S., 1971, Agr. Biol. Chem., 35:1635.
Newhall, W. F., 1969, Nature, 223:965.
Newhall, W. F., 1971, J. Agr. Food Chem., 19:294.
Newhall, W. F., 1974, J. Agr. Food Chem., 22:465.
Newhall, W. F., and Pieringer, A. P., 1966, J. Agr. Food Chem., 14:23.
Newhall, W. F., and Pieringer, A. P., 1967, J. Agr. Food Chem., 15:488.
Newhall, W. F., and Pieringer, A. P., 1972, HortScience, 7:254.

Paul, E., and Göring, H., 1974, in: "Proceedings of the International Symposium on the Biochemistry and Chemistry of Plant Growth Regulators" (Cottbus, German Republic, September 24-26, 1974), Klaus Schreiber, H. R. Schütte, and G. Sembdner, eds., Institut für Biochemie der Pflanzen, Akademie der Wissenschaften der DDR, Berlin.

Pieringer, A. P., and Newhall, W. R., 1968, J. Agr. Food Chem., 16:523.

Pieringer, A. P., and Newhall, W. R., 1970, J. Amer. Soc. Hort. Sci., 95:53.

Snel, M., and Gramlich, J., 1973, Meded. Fac. Landbouwwetensch. Rijkuniv. Gent., 38:1033.

Taylor, H. F., and Wain, R. L., 1978, Ann. Appl. Biol., 89:271.

Wain, R. L., 1972, in: "Plant Growth Substances, 1970," D. J. Carr, ed., Springer-Verlag, Berlin.

15

PLANT GROWTH RETARDANTS: PRESENT AND FUTURE USE IN FOOD PRODUCTION

A. Skytt Andersen

Royal Veterinary and Agricultural University
Copenhagen, Denmark

INTRODUCTION

This article on the subject of growth retardants (GRs) will try to answer the following questions:

(1) What is a growth retardant?
(2) How do growth retardants affect plants?
(3) What do we use growth retardants for?
(4) Is it sensible to use growth retardants?
(5) Is it possible to envisage other uses of growth retardants?
(6) Is it possible to envisage new growth retardants?

First we must define the term growth retardant. The following definition will do although it may have to be strained a bit at times:

A GR is a chemical which causes reduction in height or volume of plants without a reduction in yield.

An ideal GR should thus be one which gives rise to a small, compact but otherwise fully developed plant. The reduction of growth should occur in organs (stems, petioles, peduncles) which are of little or no consequence for the part of the plant we intend to harvest.

Why would anyone in his right mind wish to restrict the growth of plants when all other agricultural practice seems to be directed toward the increase of plant growth? The philosophy behind growth retardation is as follows:

(1) No need to grow tall unused stems.
(2) Better weather resistance.
(3) Reduction of water use.
(4) Less damage due to mechanical soil treatment.
(5) Easier harvest.
(6) Better canopy shape for energy collection.

(1) In many crops, exemplified by cereals, the stem (straw) is a nuisance which is burned or removed at great expense to the farmer, therefore the less straw the better.

(2) Tall thin plants, again the cereals are the example, do not withstand adverse weather conditions such as rain, wind, and hail. Shorter plants will stand up better and the destruction of harvestable grain will be reduced. This is the main reason for using GRs in the cereal fields, i.e., restriction of lodging.

(3) In addition to the effects on lodging, some researchers have noticed a reduced water requirement of GR-treated plants. Of course this is a very interesting aspect which would, if it holds true, be of far greater significance on a worldwide scale than lodging control.

(4) If plants with runners or hypogaeus fruit stalks such as the peanut (Arachis) could be restricted in the space used for these organs, closer planting and better land use would be the result. Furthermore, these more compact plants would resist traffic by soil treatment machinery (or hand hoes) better.

(5) The easier harvest of small plants is self evident, not only for the lodging plants but also for other types of plants--machines can be smaller, more energy efficient.

TYPES OF CHEMICALS PRESENTLY IN USE OR IN THE EXPERIMENTAL STAGE

The following is a description of a number of growth retardants presently in use. It is not an exhaustive list, but rather one which stresses group characteristics where such are evident.

The concept of GR was apparently not conceived theoretically before the manufacture and use of these compounds began. The chemicals more or less happened to appear in various industrial screening programs primarily designed to detect and test new herbicides. The basic plant physiological research lags behind the screeners and the practical people by long periods of time and in a number of cases we have not yet begun to unravel the mechanisms underlying the observable effects. We are far from the pharmaceutical industry goal of tailoring molecules for particular usefulness in particular problem areas on the basis of solid evidence in plant biochemistry. A list of compounds capable of reducing plant height includes molecular structures ranging from the rather simple ethephon to the intricate ring systems of dikegulac or ancymidol (Fig. 1).

The most widespread useful GRs presently are CCC, cycocel, chlorcholinchloride, chlormequat, or whatever you prefer to call it, as far as cereal crops and certain ornamentals are concerned, and alar, alias B-9, N,N-dimethyl succinic acid, SADH, or daminozide, for other crops including peanuts, fruit trees, and other ornamentals (Fig. 1).

Chlormequat is by far the most widely used chemical growth retardant today. Since it appeared about twenty years ago as a curiosity--an antigibberellin, which the plant physiologists/horticulturists played with--and the purpose of this article is to look forward another twenty years, I have gone back to the early papers on CCC from 1960 to see what people thought then.

These first papers in Plant Physiology mentioned nothing about the possible use of growth retardants although I am sure Tolbert and Wittwer must have had some thoughts regarding them. When they assumed the guise of agriculturalists or horticulturists, they then had many more ideas (Tolbert, 1960; Wittwer, 1968).

Since it thus seems not to be appropriate for a plant physiologist to prophesy, you may regard me as an agri-horticulturist for the purposes of this article.

GROUPS OF COMPOUNDS WITH GR ACTIVITY

It is rather difficult to group the GRs homogenously due to the haphazard manner in which they have been discovered. The following paragraphs give a limited description of the groups of chemicals which are presently known to exhibit GR activity taken in the order of importance today (Table 1).

Quaternary Ammonium or Phosphonium Compounds

Chlormequat, AMO-1618, and other not commercially available compounds of this group all contain 5-valent nitrogen (Fig. 1) (see Corcoran, 1975, for details) and Phosphon D contains a similarly positioned phosphorous. The more complex compounds of this group have not achieved widespread use due to their limited range of sensitive plant species and their high persistence in soils (Sullivan, 1977). In contrast to these carbamates the simplest of the quaternary ammonium compounds (CCC, chlormequat) has been widely used both on an experimental and a commercial scale.

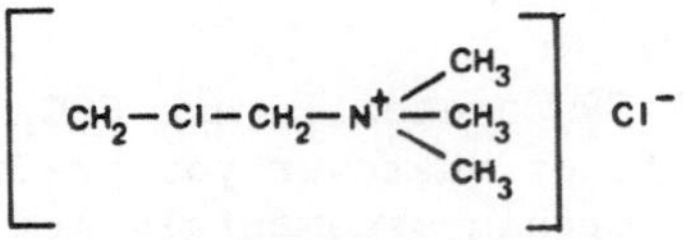

CHLORMEQUAT

CCC, CYCOCEL

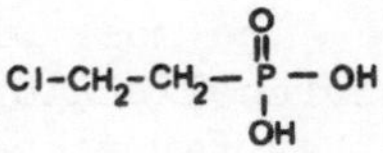

ETHEPHON

CEPHA ETHREL

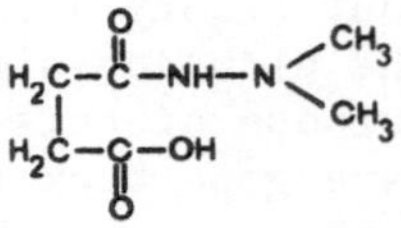

DAMINOZIDE

BENINE, ALAR, SADH

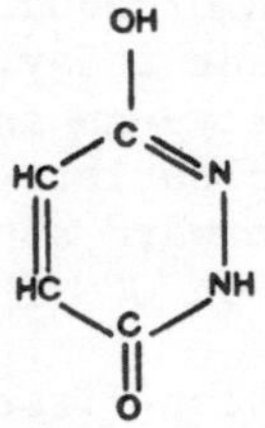

MALEIC HYDRAZIDE

MH - 30 SLO-GRO

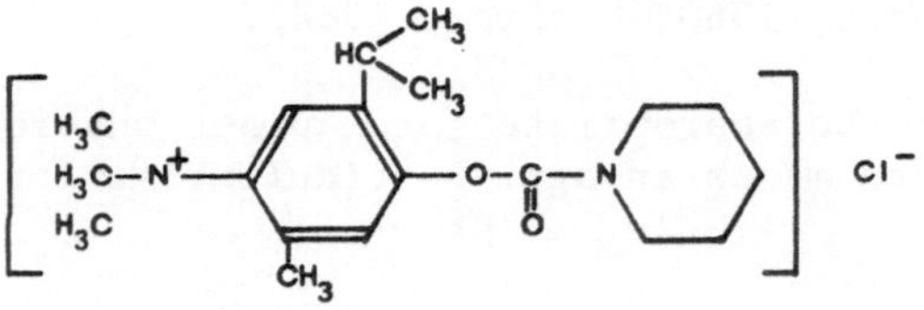

AMO 1618 CARBAMATE

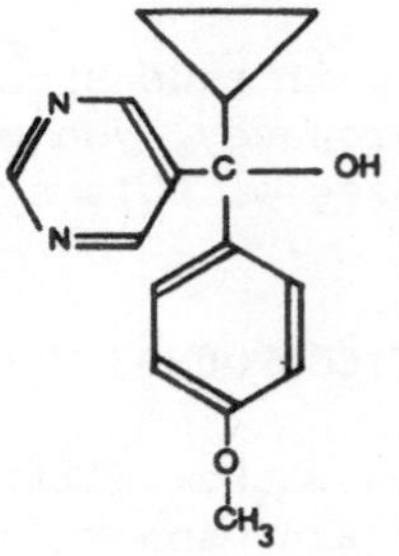

ANCYMIDOL

REDUCYMOL

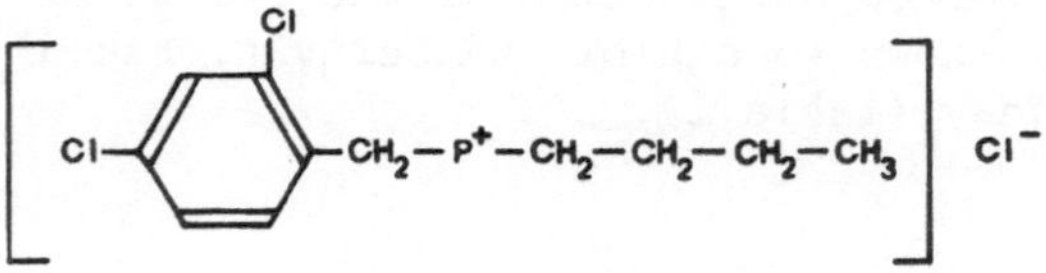

PHOSPHONIUM

PHOSPHON D

Fig. 1.

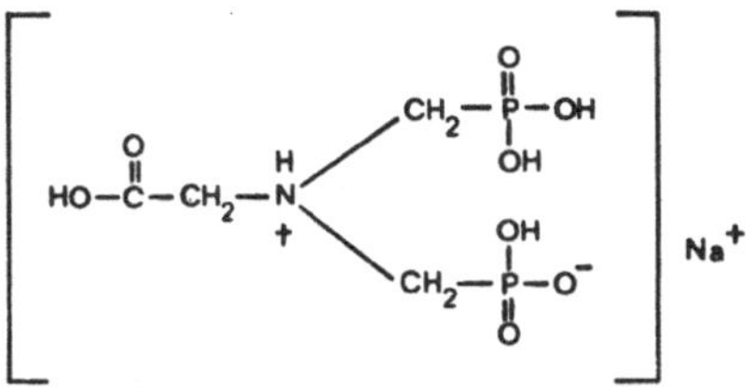

GLYPHOSINE

POLARIS

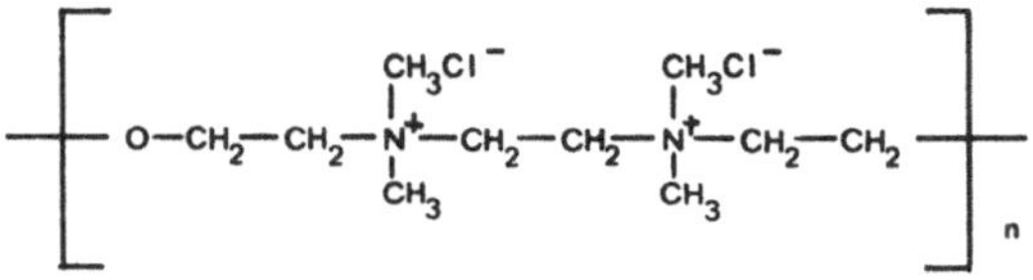

POLYIMINOETHYLENE

BUALTA

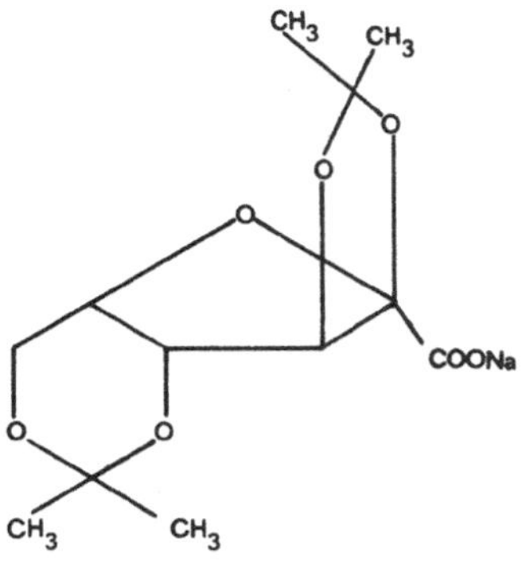

DIKEGULAC

ATRINAL

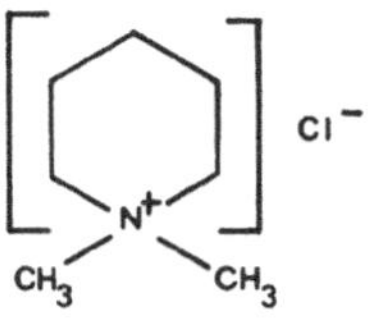

MEPIQUAT

TERPAL

Fig. 1. (cont'd.)

Table 1. Types of Growth Retardants

Original Code Names	Approved or SUGGESTED Common Names	Examples of Trade Names	Reference	Principal Uses 1978 EXPERIMENTAL
EL 3855	Chlormequat*	Cycocel CCC	Tolbert, 1960 Jung and Schott, 1974	Lodging control, wheat
AMO 1618	Carbamate*	--	Douglas and Paleg, 1978	none
	Phosphonium*	Phosphon D	see lit. Moore, 1967	Ornamentals
B-995	Daminozide*	Alar B-Nine Kylar	Jung, 1973	Fruit trees Tomatoes Peanuts
AMCHEM 66-329	Ethephon*	Ethrel Cepha Terpal	Andersen, 1970 Jindal et al., 1975 BASF, 1977	Latex flow Fruit abscission LODGING CONTROL, BARLEY
MH 30	Maleic hydrazide*	Slo-gro Antergon	Noodèn, 1969	Grasses Potatoes Onions Tobacco
EL 531	Ancymidol*	Reducymol A-Rest	Coolbaugh and Hamilton, 1976	Ornamentals
RO 7-6145	Dikegulac*	Atrinal	Sachs et al., 1975	Woody ornamentals

CP 41 845	Glyphosine*	Polaris	Anonymous, 1976/1977	Sugarcane
	"POLYIMINOETHYLENE"*	Boalta	Sullivan, 1977	Sugarcane
BAS 08300 W	Mepiquat*	Terpal	BASF, 1977	LODGING CONTROL, BARLEY
	Piproctanylium-Br**	Stemtrol	Sullivan, 1977	Ornamentals
		Alden	BASF, 1977	Ornamentals, Cotton
IT 3299	Flurenol** Morphactin	EMD-IT	Schneider, 1970	Grass-seed stalk inhibition
CPA 448	CPA**	Fruitone	Sullivan, 1977	Pineapple crown growth
	TIBA**	Floraltone	Sullivan, 1977	Trees
P 293	OXATIIN**		Sullivan, 1977	TREES? POTATOES
MBR 12325	Mefluidide**	Embark	Wu and Santelmann, 1977	PEANUT, GRASSES
PP 528	TETRAZOLACETATE**		Grausland, 1975	PEANUT
RH 531	Pyridone** CCDP		Yib et al., 1971	CEREALS, TOMATOES
DMC 28 979	PROPIONITRIL**	Orthonil	Wu and Santelmann, 1977	PEANUTS
BAS 0640 W	Hydrazoniums**		Jung, 1967	CEREALS, COTTON

Table 1. (cont'd.)

Original Code Names	Approved or SUGGESTED Common Names	Examples of Trade Names	Reference	Principal Uses 1978 EXPERIMENTAL
BAS 0660 W	Morpholiniums**		Jung, 1973	CEREALS
Q 58 a.o.	LIMONENES**		Corcoran, 1975	BEANS
SKF 7732 A_3 a.o.	TRISPHOSPHATES***		Corcoran, 1975	
	TWISTANOL***		Aigami et al., 1978	CUCUMBER
TD 6817	?		Wu and Santelmann, 1977	PEANUTS
ABG 3030	NITROPYRAZOL***			
CP 70139	Glyphosate	MON 8000	Anonymous, 1976/1977	Sugarcane ripener
	Abscisic acid			

*Chemical structure depicted in Fig. 1.

**Chemical structure depicted in Fig. 2.

***Chemical structure depicted in Fig. 3.

Chemically chlormequat is a choline derivative with Cl substitution; also, the Br substituted compound is active and a substitution is essential for activity. It is now well established that the quaternary ammonium compounds interfere with gibberellin biosynthesis (Frost and West, 1977) or utilization (Coolbaugh and Hamilton, 1976) as well as other biochemical processes (Douglas and Paleg, 1978).

Chlormequat is highly water soluble and it is persistent in soils, but not from one season to the next. The rate of disappearance is influenced by soil types and temperature (Linser et al., 1963). It has a toxicity to animals with a range of LD_{50} oral between 0.5-1.0 g kg^{-1} (Sullivan, 1977). This toxicity has been reduced in some newer formulations and in conjunction with lower application rates there are promises of near-freedom from toxicological restrictions in the future.

Daminozide

The compound succinic acid dimethylhydrazide (Fig. 1), commonly known as benine, B-9, or alar is a very different compound from CCC with no strong nucleophilic substituents or reactive groups. It is an ionizable, highly water-soluble free acid, but the metal or amide salts are also active GRs. Other compounds with related chemical structure have been tested for GR activity, but none has reached the market yet.

Daminozide is as nontoxic as one could hope; it is in the range of sodium chloride with an LD_{50} oral of 8-10 g kg^{-1}. It is nearly non-persistent in soils since it is rapidly consumed by microorganisms and leaves no noxious residues (Sullivan, 1977). In plants it is more stable and distributed systematically throughout the plant regardless of point of entry. The uptake of daminozide is much easier through the roots than through the leaves because of ionic characteristics of the compound in solution (Schönherr and Bukovac, 1978). There is some controversy regarding the mode of action of daminozide. Auxin, gibberellin, and ethylene synthesis and translocation have been found to react to daminozide application (Moore, 1967; Jung, 1967).

Ethephon

Ethephon (Fig. 1) and a few related substances have generally been regarded as growth regulators that induce senescense and fruit drop, and enhance latex flow from rubber trees (Abeles, 1973). These effects are due to its ability to cause internal ethylene formation in plant tissues. This picture is, however, changing rapidly. Depending on time of application, ethephon can provoke very different results. As shown in earlier publications one of the main effects of ethephon on young pea plants is a reduction in final height of these plants and a thickening of the basal stems (Andersen, 1970). This effect is going to be utilized in one of the newer developments in the GR field: A mixed formulation. We are now entering a stage of development which occurred some 10 or 15 years ago in the herbicide area. It is a type of GR of which the future will bring many specially designed mixtures which need to be applied at very exact developmental stages to get the desired response (BASF, 1977).

The chemical characteristics of ethephon are amply described and well known; toxicity (LD_{50} 4 g kg^{-1}) is rather low, but inhalation dangers may exist at very low air concentrations (Sullivan, 1977).

Maleic Hydrazide

Maleic hydrazide (MH) (Fig. 1) is one of the oldest GRs. Although its main use is as a herbicide, it does have potential as a GR. There is clear evidence that MH acts in the plant by inhibition of cell division, especially in roots (Noodèn, 1969). It is freely movable in the plant but accumulates in meristems. MH is comparatively nontoxic (LD_{50} oral 1400 mg kg^{-1}, Sullivan, 1977) and is rapidly metabolized in soils. There are, however, other environmental problems with compounds which interfere with mitosis and DNA synthesis which may account for the limited use of this compound. According to one source MH is only active toward monocotyledons (Schneider, 1970), but other sources describe its main target plants as potatoes, tobacco, and citrus (Sullivan, 1977)

Ancymidol

Ancymidol (Anonymous, 1972) is presently only used in ornamentals due to the high price of the compound, which is only partially offset by the low active concentrations, in the μg l^{-1} range. It is only slightly soluble in water (650 mg l^{-1}) and the toxicological characteristics of the compound are good (LD_{50} o ~ 5 g kg^{-1}, Sullivan, 1977). In plants ancymidol is distributed evenly throughout the plant following root or shoot uptake. It retards the growth of stem cells of a number of plant species without changes in leaf number, size, or shape. In soil ancymidol is leached fast, but still it is more effective when applied as a soil drench than when sprayed on the leaves (Adriansen, 1975). The effect is produced through inhibition of gibberellic acid (GA) synthesis at a late stage, after kaurene (Coolbaugh and Hamilton, 1976) (Fig. 1).

Dikegulac

Dikegulac (Fig. 1) is a newly developed growth retardant primarily used in woody plants (Sachs et al., 1975). Chemically it is an isopropylgulonate derivative of very complex character, highly water soluble and nontoxic (LD_{50} o 18 g kg^{-1}). The persistence in soils depends on soil type, moisture, and temperature. In the plant dikegulac moves freely with no accumulation in specific areas (Sullivan, 1977). Reduction in plastid rRNA has been found in one species after dikegulac treatment, but the investigators doubt that it is a primary effect (Gressel and Cohen, 1977).

Glyphosine

Closely related to a selective herbicide, glyphosate, glyphosine (Fig. 1) is presently being investigated for one specific purpose only--sugarcane "ripening" (Anonymous, 1976/1977). It is a highly water soluble, partly systemic GR which is persistent (1 to 2 months) in soil and plants, but not taken up into plants from soil. Toxicological properties of glyphosine have been examined in detail: LD_{50} o is 4 g kg^{-1} and no mutagenic or teratogenic effects have been observed. There is presently no indication of mode of action of glyphosine.

Mepiquat

Mepiquat (Fig. 1), the chloride of N,N-dimethylpiperidinium, is one of the future GRs which is presently being tested extensively in field trials. These trials are primarily aimed at lodging control in barley, which is practically insensitive to the more commonly used GRs. Effect is achieved through the previously mentioned mixture with ethephon in a formulation called Terpal (BASF, 1977). Alone mepiquat has very little effect on spring barley at least under Danish conditions (Larsen, 1977). Mepiquat is also of interest to cotton growers as a means of shaping the plants for better light penetration through the canopy (Schneider, 1970).

Morphactins

This class of compounds has several members with growth regulator activity. Officially they are called flurenols (Fig. 2) and some of them have been introduced commercially, but their use is presently limited. Their toxicity (LD_{50} o) is in the range of 6-10 mg kg^{-1}, but they are rapidly degraded in soil and water (Sullivan, 1977). Morphactins are active and nontoxic to plants over a wide concentration range (Schneider, 1970). They affect plants through alterations of hormonal balance, although the particular hormone which is affected is not known. There has been reported increased ethylene synthesis (Khan et al., 1977), which may inhibit auxin transport through interference with auxin receptor sites (Gaither, 1975).

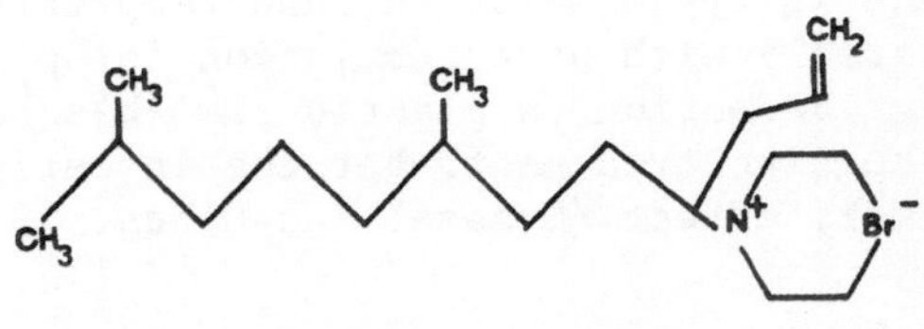

PIPROCTANYLIUM

STEMTROL

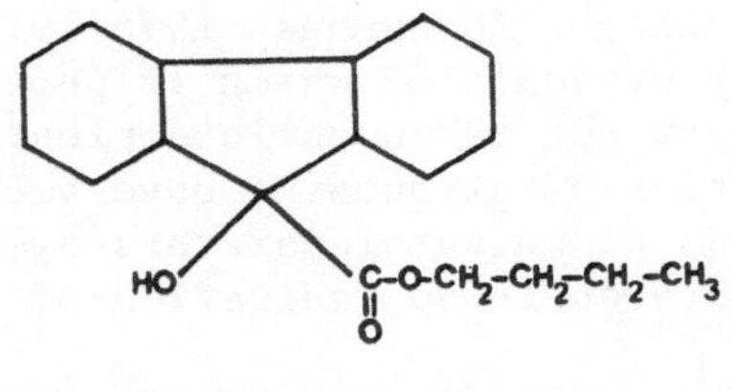

FLURENOL MORPHACTIN

EMD - IT

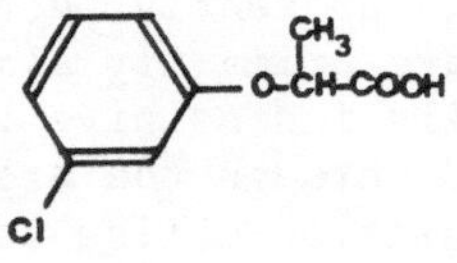

CPA

FRUITONE

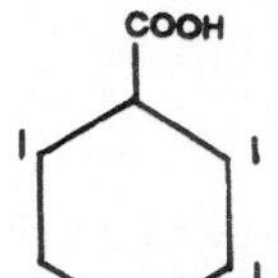

TIBA

FLORALTONE

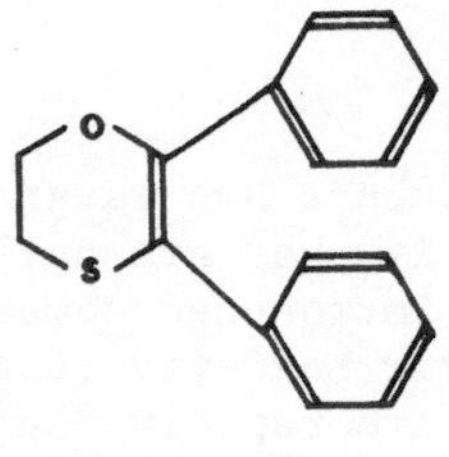

OXATIIN

Fig. 2.

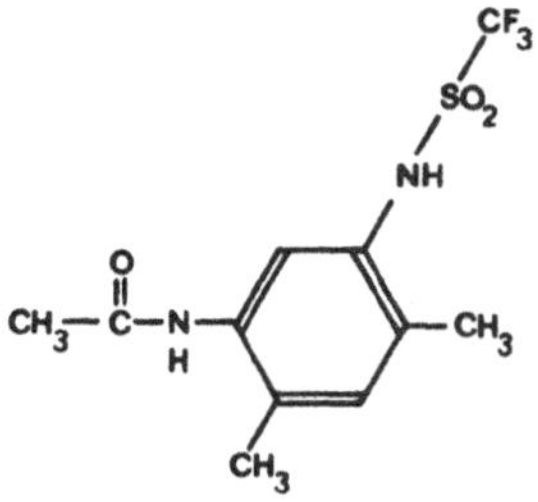

"MEFLUIDIDE"

EMBARK

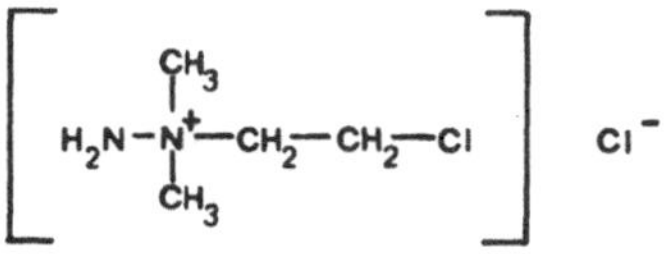

CMH
HYDRAZONIUM

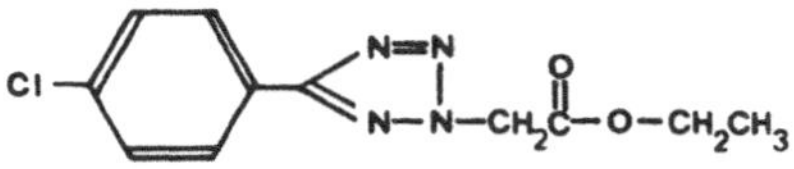

TETRAZOLACETATE

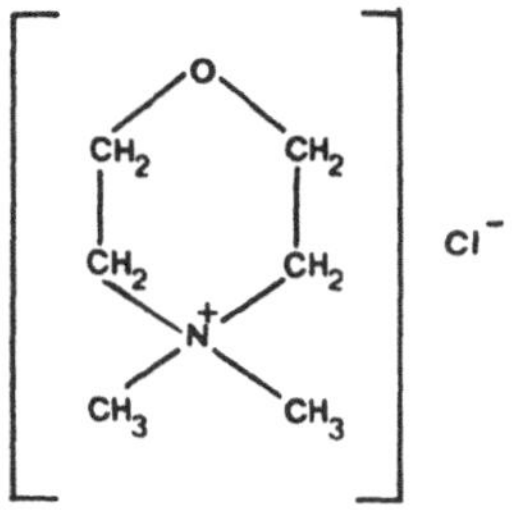

MORPHOLINIUM
DMC

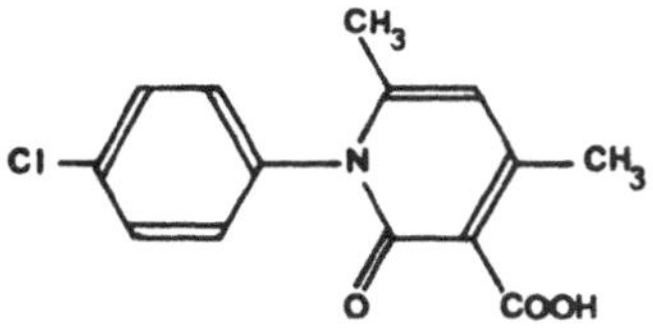

PYRIDONE

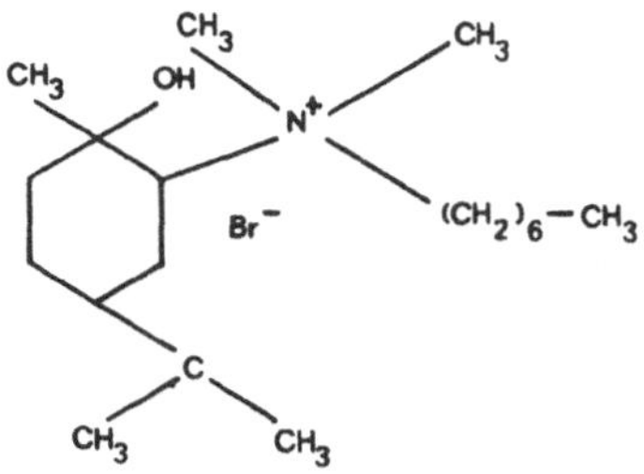

LIMONENE

Q 58

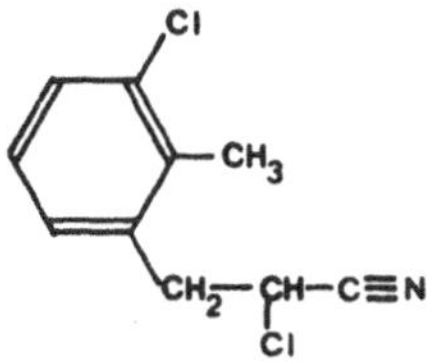

DMC 28979

ORTHONIL

Fig. 2. (cont'd.)

CPA

2-(3-chlorophenoxy) propanoic acid (Fig. 2) is also a weak herbicide, and its only use for growth retardation is in pineapples where the crown growth is reduced giving rise to large fruits (Sullivan, 1977). CPA does not move within the plant once it has entered through the leaves.

TIBA

Triiodobenzoid acid (Fig. 2) is well known in plant physiology as an auxin transport inhibitor. It has found limited use as a growth regulator if not exactly retardant; especially as an aid to regulate the growth of young fruit trees (Sullivan, 1977). TIBA also affects fruit tree flowering, and has been tested on other crops such as peanuts (Wu and Santelmann, 1977).

Oxatiin

Whereas all the preceding compounds had at least one commercial application, oxatiin (Fig. 2) and the following compounds or groups of compounds are strictly experimental, and the range of their possible use is presently unknown. Even the name given here is not approved. Oxatiin is almost insoluble in water and not very toxic (LD_{50} o = 3 g kg^{-1}). It has been tested for disbudding and general reduction of apical dominance in fruit trees (Cathey, 1974).

Mefluidide

Mefluidide (Fig. 2) is a substituted sulfonyl aminophenylacetamide which has been tested on peanuts (*Arachis hypogaea*) for control of peduncle growth (Wu and Santelmann, 1977). It proved to have the additional effect of causing the leaflets to fold. There was no indication of yield reduction while the plant height and canopy width were reduced almost to the same extent as with daminozide, which had the unwanted effect of reducing yield.

"Tetrazolacetate"

This is another new compound whose common name has not even been suggested yet (Fig. 2). It has been tested on peanuts with mixed results (Wu and Santelmann, 1977).

Pyridones

Pyridones (Fig. 2) have been tested extensively on cereal crops, tomatoes, and trees (Yib et al., 1971; Larsen, 1977) for lodging control and growth retardation. The compound is rather nontoxic (LD_{50} o 1.5 g kg^{-1}), water soluble, and stable in soils. Results, however, are not encouraging and the present status of the experimental compound is that it is on the verge of withdrawal.

Propionitril

When propionitril was used experimentally on peanuts (Wu and Santelmann, 1977) it had a limited GR effect and yields were unaffected. No other details about the compound are presently available.

Hydrazoniums

Closely related to chlormequat, these compounds (Fig. 2) have been extensively investigated by Jung and coworkers (Jung, 1967, 1973), who reported effects similar in magnitude to chlormequat regarding the height of wheat and barley plants. None of the publications mention anything about yield or lodging control. The effect of the hydrazonium compounds is presumably a blocking of GA synthesis.

Morpholiniums

More complex molecules than the hydrazoniums, but also ammonium-ion containing compounds, the morpholiniums (Fig. 2) have been undergoing trials in cereals other than wheat--in maize, cotton, and a number of horticultural plants (Jung and Schott, 1974). In independent experiments at three Danish experiment stations during two years and with several spring barley varieties some reduction in height was found but very little if any increase in yield (Yib et al., 1971).

Limonenes

Limonenes (Fig. 2) are also quaternary ammonium compounds, but in contrast to most other growth retardants these are found naturally in citrus peel among other places. To give maximum GR activity the alkyl chain must have 6 to 8 carbons (Corcoran, 1975).

"Trisphosphates"

These experimental compounds (Fig. 3) with code numbers preceded by SK and F were introduced 10 to 15 years ago as regulators of flowering in short-day plants (Corcoran, 1975). Some of these regulators also have retardant effects, but none has yet reached the market. It has been postulated that it is through inhibition of sterol biosynthesis that the trisphosphates exert their effect (Corcoran, 1975).

"Twistanols"

Very recently a Japanese group reported on the testing of a new group of compounds structurally related to homoisotwistanol, di- and tricyclic alkanols (Fig. 3). Some of the structures completely inhibited the growth of cucumber hypocotyls in concentrations around 10^{-4} M (Aigami et al., 1978).

TD 6817

This is an experimental compound of which nothing is known chemically, but it has been tested on peanut plants with slight GR effect and some increase in yield (Corcoran, 1975).

Abscisic Acid

The natural growth retardant abscisic acid (ABA) has of course been extensively investigated as a possible useful compound, but its stability in solution and in plants is too low to warrant any use of this hormone. It follows a common pattern, whereby none of the other endogenous hormones are used in their naturally occurring state in any capacity.

It is possible that substitutions in the molecule could render it more stable and give it better uptake into intact plants. One such analog has been tested as a growth retardant (Blaydes and Saus, 1978). It is not a synthetic, but a fungal product which inhibits auxin-induced growth in coleoptile segments.

AGRICULTURAL APPLICATIONS

Lodging Control

Presently the greatest quantities of growth retardants used for the retardation of growth during specific stages of wheat growth are those used for lodging control. This is the case especially in

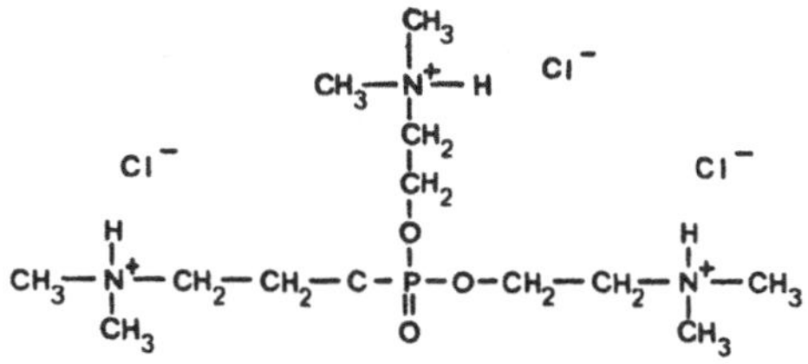

"TRISPHOSPHATE" SKF 7994 A3

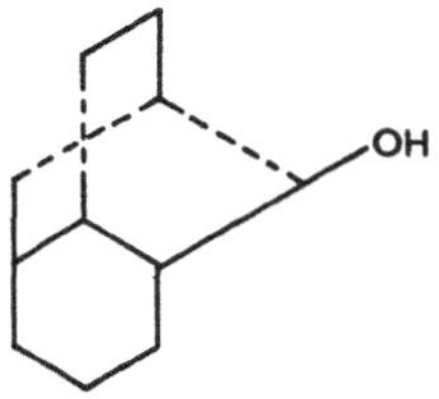

"TWISTANOL"

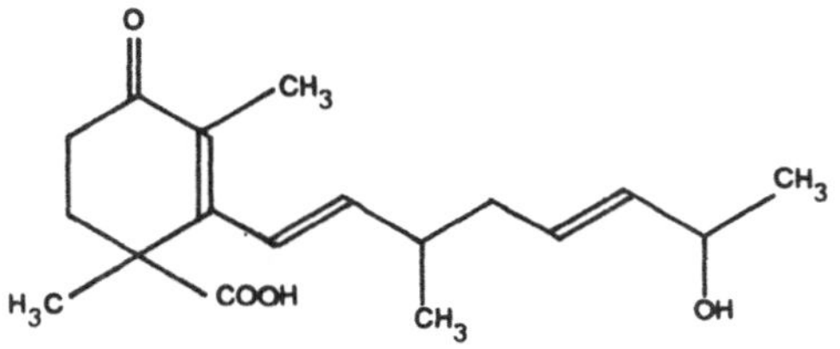

TRISPORIC ACID

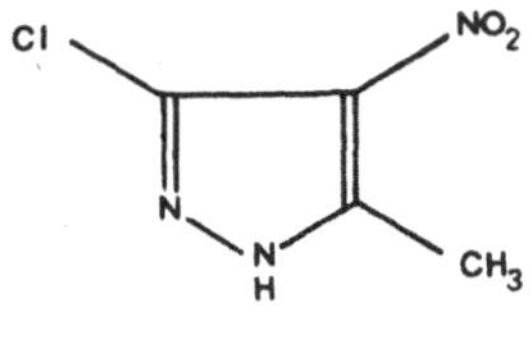

NITROPYRAZOL ABG 3030

Fig. 3.

northern Europe where the climate often is less favorable for cereals. The use of growth retardants is no simple matter. It does not always pay, due to the unpredictability of weather and the fact that the positive effects on yield are often dependent on heavy N fertilization, irrigation, or disease control measures. Although wheat is one of the most important cereals, a longstanding drawback of GRs is that wheat is the only cereal that has responded to treatments. In the future it will probably be possible through the use of specific mixtures of GRs to control the lodging of the other cereals. This is of particular interest in areas that are marginal for growing these crops.

Several studies have been made of the plant characteristics which may favor or disfavor lodging. One of the most thorough investigations is that of Oda et al. (1966). Total plant height is not all that is important for lodging; therefore, it is perhaps misleading to try to correlate any reduction in plant height with better yield through lodging control. Through measurements of a number of characters in 200 cultivars of wheat and barley (Oda et al., 1966), it was possible to correlate lodging resistance with the following parameters:

(1) <u>Bending momentum at breaking (M)</u>
(2) <u>Bending-rigidity (EI)</u>
} culm stiffness (dw. l^{-1} g. cm^{-1}),

of which 1 is calculated from the breaking stress and the external and internal diameters of the culm at node 1, and 2 from Young's Modulus (E) and the secondary momentum of inertia (I). Thus if the dry weight of the culm is high and culms are thick at the base bending rigidity will increase. Lodging resistance is calculated as

$$L_R = \frac{WM}{l^2 w}$$

where w is dry weight of culm (per tiller), W fresh weight, and l length of culm. The morphological and anatomical effects of GR are to reduce l and to increase M through changes in stem anatomy. It is possible to measure these parameters in experiments where lodging is absent due to good weather or in greenhouse experiments. A slightly different method and apparatus have been used by Linser (1968). Lodging can occur in two different stages of cereal development. "Root lodging," the most widespread, is a bending of the culms just above the soil surface. Stem lodging occurs as a bending of internodes 7 to 8 after heading (Pinthus, 1973). Early treatments of cereal plants help relieve the root lodging while late treatments may decrease the stem lodging, though the latter may not be a profitable undertaking (Table 2).

Table 2. Effects of Lodging

Lodging Affects:	
Total grain yield	Decreased 17-40%
Straw yield	Decreased 21-25%
Carbohydrate accumulation	Decreased 10-17%
Kernel number/head	Decreased
Kernel weight	Decreased 8-15%
N Content in grain	Increased 3-20%
Milling quality	Decreased
Malting quality	Decreased
Baking quality	No effect
Grain drying experiment	Increased 20-30%

One of the main problems in lodging control is timing of the application. Many experiments have given the general results that stage 6 to 7 (Feekes scale) is best for control of root lodging and about 9 is best for control of head lodging (BASF, 1977). Another problem is that so far only wheat has responded to growth retardants with any significant increase in yield. This is, according to some chemical companies, going to change in the future. New regulators are being developed that will be effective in all cereals including barley which has been very difficult to retard. One of the promising compounds or formulations is a mixture of mepiquat and ethephon (trade name in some areas Terpal). This compound is presently undergoing field trials in the barley growing areas of northern Europe.

Wünsche (1977) and Larsen (1977) have examined the parent compounds morpholinium and ethephon separately for the growth retardant effects on cereals under Scandinavian conditions. They found very little effect of morpholinium on any of the cereals. Several cultivars of the four small cereals grown were tested, but only in oats was there an effect of ethephon on plant height (Wünsche, 1977) without concomitant reduction in yield.

Trees

There are basically two areas in which GRs can be of use in tree growing. One is for reducing the size of fruit trees to facilitate easier harvest, and the second, which is more hypothetical, is to control lodging or windfall in tree farms.

Fruit trees of many species often have growth characteristics which are unsatisfactory for easy harvest of fruits--or they require extensive pruning to obtain a tree of the desired shape and size. This has in the past been amended by grafting the cultivars with the desired fruits onto root stocks with the desired growth habit. Grafting is an expensive and often difficult process which can be eliminated through propagation by cuttings. The resulting trees may not have the best growth habit. This can, however, for several species be achieved through regular use of growth retardants (Grauslund, 1975). Daminozide has proven to be best for reduction of apple tree size while other species respond better to chlormequat.

An added advantage of GR treatments of apple trees is an increase in number of flowers; however, the fruit size is generally reduced.

Cold Hardening

A number of plant species have been prospective candidates for use in areas where they cannot survive due to low temperatures. Many treatments have been tried to increase cold hardiness, among them the growth retardants. The theoretical background for this is the observation that increased frost or chilling resistance in individual plants or cultivars often can be correlated to

--stunted growth habit (wheat, Blaydes and Saus, 1978)
--smaller leaves (wheat, Roberts, 1971)
--leaf angle (wheat, Roberts, 1971)
--reduction of GA-like substances (*Acer*, Irwing and Lamphear, 1968)
--higher sugar content (citrus, Young, 1971)
--cessation of cambial activity (citrus, Young, 1971)
--decrease in water content in tissues (citrus, Young, 1971)
--dormancy (strawberry, Freeman and Carne, 1970)
--permeability of membranes (Kacperska-Palacz et al., 1969; Young, 1971)
--sulfhydryl groups (cabbage, Kacperska-Palacz et al., 1969)
--increased ascorbic acid contents (tomato, Michniewics et al., 1965).

Which results have been obtained after GR treatments? In laboratory experiments it has been possible to increase frost or cold tolerance in wheat with chlormequat (e.g., Roberts, 1971). Two distinct types of experiments are involved here: Treatments of prehardened plants or treatments of unhardened plants. In the former GRs can increase the hardiness while the latter are far less responsive, even though the changes in some of the above mentioned characters are similar in the two types of plants.

Problems in this area are many. It is often stated that plants survive cold better after treatments, but die later, when growth should have taken place; much more research is evidently needed before cold hardening with chlormequat can be generally used in the winter wheat fields. The observations on winter wheat suggest, according to Roberts (1971): "Important changes in hormones other than gibberellins may be involved in cold hardening." It is, however, possible that there may be some indirect effects on winter survival under field conditions. I here refer to the known results on early plant modifications: less damage due to snow or ice cover in winter cereal crops treated with known or coming GRs. Smaller, sturdier plants with thicker basal stems will be better covered by snow and more resistant to ice breakage.

Many other crop plants have been used in experiments on frost or cold hardening. Some examples are: cabbage (Kacperska-Palacz et al., 1969), strawberry (Freeman and Carne, 1970), oats (Rawlinson, 1971), tomato (Michniewics et al., 1965), bean (Michniewics et al., 1965), and rape (Kacperska-Palacz et al., 1969). The main thrust of the experimentation was done during the latter half of the sixties. There is presently not much activity on that front, but nearly all experiments have been done with chlormequat or daminozide. It is necessary for the newer GRs to be examined over a broad range of species as well before it is clear whether the procedure will be of any future significance for agriculture.

In citrus trees, or rather young cuttings or seedlings, only the application of maleic hydrazide (MH) had any effect on cold hardiness of prehardened plants. ABA, chlormequat, daminozide, and ethephon had no effect on survival (Young, 1971). It is not clear whether this use of MH could be helpful since there was no record of the later growth of the treated trees.

Drought Resistance

From a long list of traits assembled by Pinthus (1973) for the purpose of modifications to restrict water use in a crop plant we can select a few that are amenable to manipulation by the application of growth retardants today and some that may be coming tomorrow:

--High photosynthetic rate
--Increased albedo (hairs)
--Stomatal physiology
--Water use efficiency
--Canopy shape
--Reduced vegetative phase
--Modified root structure

Already in 1966 Plaut and Halevy (1966) observed an increased drought resistance of wheat plants after treatment with chlormequat. Later investigations in Australia (Singh et al., 1973) have shown the complexity of the problem: It was not possible to detect any influence of chlormequat on leaf water potential or water uptake. There was, however, a pronounced effect on proline accumulation, but only during stress and since the plants were smaller the actual amount of proline per pea plant was similar in treated and nontreated plants. This of course may have implications for water relations of the leaf cells, enabling the GR treated plants to recover from stress with less damage to the functions of the leaf cells.

In pea plants, Lee et al. (1974) have tried to increase drought resistance of two cultivars (one drought resistant) with daminozide, and have examined the effects on a number of physiological processes. For wheat Singh et al. (1973) found no change due to the GR in water uptake or leaf water content of the pea plants under stress conditions. The drought susceptible cultivar ("Alaska") showed relative increase in growth during stress after daminozide treatment perhaps due to increased RudP carboxylase activity. It is probable that some of the effect in pea plants also is due to proline accumulation, since we have found that pea plants react to ABA treatments with proline accumulation just as cereal plants do (Rajagopal and Andersen, 1978).

Several other crops are under active investigation regarding the amelioration of water stress effects through growth retardants. These crops include cotton, bean, tomato, and pineapple (see Lee et al., 1974; Singh et al., 1973).

Salt Stress

Since salinity problems often result in symptoms and effects similar to those resulting from drought, salt stress resistance logically may be reduced by GR treatments. Only a few investigations have centered on this important aspect, one of which is by Imbamba (1973), who worked with cowpeas (Vigna unguiculata). Dry matter production was reduced by saline conditions and by chlormequat treatments, but salt stressed plants, growing in 0.15 M NaCl, were somewhat relieved by chlormequat treatments. There was, however, by no means a reversal of the salt stress by chlormequat.

Sugarcane Ripening

In many sugarcane growing areas of the world there are poor conditions for the ripening process to take place. Ripening is a cessation of growth usually brought about by some sort of shock environmental conditions, such as drought, lack of available nutrients, or low temperature. With ripening, vegetative growth ceases and internodes become short. The ripe sugarcane contains more, and more easily recoverable, sucrose.

The development of a sugarcane ripener has been of great interest especially for use in areas where the environmental conditions for ripening are poor. One such sugarcane ripener is glyphosine, which when sprayed on actively growing canes induces a growth retardation similar to the ripening process (Anonymous, 1976/1977). Other compounds have been examined for the same use, but are reported to have limited effect (Anonymous, 1976/1977; Sullivan, 1977). The change in sugar percentage is especially notable in the upper parts of the plants. It is clear that glyphosine is the "first generation" compound and the producing company (Monsanto) is actively working on newer and even more effective compounds such as CP 70139, MON 8000, and other formulations of glyphosate, which have a broader variety range and a higher rate of sugar increase. These compounds, which probably will be of increased importance in the coming years, are all less toxic both to plants and other organisms than glyphosine (Sullivan, 1977).

Tomatoes

Besides obtaining a shorter, sturdier plant which stands up better and is easier to harvest mechanically at least, there are the advantages from chlormequat and ancymidol treatments that the number of flowers in the first cluster is increased and the percentage of aborted flowers at anthesis is reduced (Abdul et al., 1978). Treatment time is important; the plants must be in a stage where they have less than six leaves of 2 cm length. Perhaps there is also a possibility of changing phyllotaxy with growth retardants. It has been shown that tomato (and pepper) plants normally have a distribution of 50% right-"handed" and 50% left-"handed" plants and that in some cultivars the right-handed ones yield up to 25% more fruits than the left-handed ones (Bible, 1976). It has also been shown, albeit in a totally unrelated species, *Echinodorus*, a water plant, that phyllotaxy is subject to change with treatments with chlormequat or daminozide (Charlton, 1974). Perhaps someone should try this on some crop plants, especially tomato.

There seems to be a great potential for the use of growth retardants in agriculture if what we want is to increase food and fiber production (Table 3), but a note of warning from the perspective of academe is in order: We must be very cautious of those of our fellow scientists who are subtly or not so subtly on the payrolls of those giant companies which live and live well from the production of chemicals. These firms have an enormous interest in the potential market for growth retardants which exists in the world of agriculture. Therefore, some of them do not hesitate to use all means of persuasion toward consultants, extension agents, agriculture teachers, and other "influential people." We must not let the chemical industry induce us to lower the "acceptance treshhold," by which I mean that there must be an extensive testing and analysis period before the release

Table 3. Present and Future Uses of Growth Retardants

Lodging control--wheat, cotton, tomatoes, barley
Fruit tree shaping
Sugarcane maturation
Peanut peduncle growth
Strawberry runner control
Reduction of apical dominance
Induce dormancy
Increase frost, drought, salt resistance

of the chemicals for general use. I regret to say that some companies appear too eager and some countries too lax in their regulations or requirements in this respect. It would be tragic indeed if we, in our eagerness to put our findings to a greater use, promulgate an ecological disaster similar to the DDT adventure.

REFERENCES

Abdul, K. S., Canham, A. E., and Harris, G. P., 1978, Effects of CCC on the formation and abortion of flowers in the first inflorescence of tomato, Ann. Bot., 42:617-625.

Abeles, F. B., 1973, "Ethylene in Plant Biology," Academic Press, New York.

Adriansen, E., 1975, Wuschhemmung von Tofpflanzen in Fliessrinnen, Gartenwelt, 76:275-276.

Aigami, K., Inamoto, Y., Fujikura, Y., Ohsugi, M., and Takaishi, N., 1978, Plant growth retardant activity of polycycloalkanols structurally related to 4 homoisotwistanols, Phytochem., 17: 804-805.

Andersen, A. S., 1970, Plant growth modification by 2-chlorethyl phosphonic acid (ethrel). I. Apical dominance in "Alaska" pea plants regulated by ethrel and benzyladenine, Yearbook Roy. Vet. & Agri. Univ., 70:30-40.

Anonymous, 1972, Technical Report on A-REST, Ancymidol, a Plant Growth Regulator, Elanco Products, Indianapolis, Ind.

Anonymous, 1976/1977, Sugar cane ripener, Seminar Proceedings, 1976-1977, Monsanto Agricultural Products Company, St. Louis, Mo.

BASF, 1977, Terpal (BAS 098 OOW) Technical Information, October, 1977, BASF, Limburgerhof, Germany.

Bible, B. B., 1976, Non-equivalence of left handed and right phyllotaxy in tomato and pepper, HortScience, 11:601-602.

Blaydes, O. F., and Saus, F. L., 1978, Inhibition of coleoptile elongation by trisporic acids, Plant & Cell Physiol., 19:519-521.

Cathey, H. M., 1974, Influence of a substituted oxatiin, a localized growth inhibitor on stem elongation, branching and flowering of plants, Abs. in HortScience, 9:300.
Charlton, W. A., 1974, Studies in Alismataceae. V. Experimental modification of phyllotaxis in pseudostolons of Echinodorus tenellus by means of growth inhibitors, Can. J. Bot., 52:1131-1142.
Coolbaugh, R. C., and Hamilton, R., 1976, Inhibition of ent-kaurene oxidation and growth by α-cyclopropyl-α(p-methoxyphenyl)-5-pyrimidine methyl alcohol, Plant Physiol., 57:245-248.
Corcoran, Mary R., 1975, Gibberellin antagonists and antigibberellins, in: "Gibberellins and Plant Growth," H. N. Krishnamoorthy, ed., John Wiley & Sons, New York.
Douglas, T. J., and Paleg, L. G., 1978, AMO 1618 and sterol biosynthesis in tissues and subcellular fractions of tobacco seedlings, Phytochem., 17:705-712.
Freeman, J. A., and Carne, I. C., 1970, Use of succinic acid 2,2-dimethylhydrazide (alar) to reduce winter injury in strawberries, Can. J. Plant Sci., 50:189-190.
Frost, R. G., and West, C. A., 1977, Properties of kaurene synthesis from Marah macrocarpus, Plant Physiol., 59:22-29.
Gaither, D. H., 1975, Auxin and the response of pea roots to auxin transport inhibitors: Morphactin, Plant Physiol., 55:1082-1086.
Grausland, J., 1975, Vaekstregulatorer til frugtraeer II. Growth regulators on fruit trees II. SADH/young trees (Dan. with Eng. Summary), Tidsskr. f. Planteavl., 79:37-50.
Gressel, J., and Cohen, N., 1977, Effects of dikegulac, a new growth regulator, on RNA synthesis in Spirodela, Plant & Cell Physiol., 18:255-259.
Imbamba, S. K., 1973, Response of cowpeas to salinity and (2-chloroethyl)-trimethyl ammonium chloride (CCC), Physiol. Plant., 28:346-349.
Irwing, R. M., and Lamphear, F. O., 1968, Regulation of cold hardiness in Acer negundo, Plant Physiol., 43:9-13.
Jindal, K. K., Andersen, A. S., and Dalbro, S., 1975, Ethylene production in alar treated apple branches, Physiol. Plant., 34:26-29.
Jung, J., 1967, Hydrazoniumsalze als Wachstumsregulatoren, Landwirt. Forsch., 20:221-228.
Jung, J., 1973, Zur Wirkung synthetischer Wachstumsregulatoren aus der Oniumgruppe, Z. Acker-u. Pflanzenbau, 137:258-269.
Jung, J., and Schott, P. E., 1974, Möchlickkeiten der Anwendung von Wachstumsregulatoren in de Pflanzenbau, Z. Acker-u. Pflanzenbau, 140:312-324.
Kacperska-Palacz, A., Blaziak, M., and Wciślińska, B., 1969, The effect of growth retardants CCC and B-9 on certain factors related to cold acclimation of plants, Bot. Gaz., 130:213-221.
Khan, A. R., Andersen, A. S., and Hansen, J., 1977, Morphactin and adventitious root formation in pea cuttings, Physiol. Plant., 39:97-100.

Larsen, K. E., 1977, Vaekstregulering i byg (growth retardation in barley), Tidsskr. f. Planteavl., 81:122.

Lee, K. C., Campbell, R. W., and Paulsen, G. M., 1974, Effects of drought stress and succinic acid 2,2-dimethylhydrazide treatment on water relations and photosynthesis in pea seedlings, Crop Sci., 14:279-282.

Linser, H., 1968, Influence of CCC on lodging and behaviour of cereal plants, Euphytica (suppl.), 1:215-238.

Linser, H., Kuhn, H., and Bohring, J., 1963, Zur Frage der Nachwirkung von Chlorcholinchlorid, Bodenkultur, 14:111-117.

Michniewics, M., Kentzer, T., Kriesel, K., and Purzycka, B., 1965, The effect of CCC on frost resistance of tomato and bean plants, Acta Soc. Bot. Pol., 34:181-190.

Moore, T. C., 1967, Kinetics of growth retardant and hormone interactions in affecting cucumber hypocotyl elongation, Plant Physiol., 42:677-684.

Noodèn, L. D., 1969, The mode of action of maleic hydrazide: Inhibition of growth, Physiol. Plant., 22:260-270.

Oda, K., Suzuki, M., and Odagawa, T., 1966, Varietal analysis of physical characters in wheat and barley plants relating to lodging and lodging index, Bull. Nat. Inst. Ag. Sci. (Tokyo), D 15:55-91.

Pinthus, M. J., 1973, Lodging in wheat, barley and oats: The phenomenon, its causes, and preventive measures, Adv. in Agron., 25:210-263.

Plaut, Z., and Halevy, A. H., 1966, Regeneration after wilting, growth and yield of wheat plants, as affected by two growth retarding compounds, Physiol. Plant., 19:1064-1072.

Rajagopal, V., and Andersen, A. S., 1978, Does abscisic acid influence proline accumulation in stressed leaves?, Planta, in press.

Rawlinson, C. J., 1971, Effect of an organo-mercurial fungicide, chlormequat and decenylsuccinic acid on frost hardiness and seedling diseases of oats, Ann. Appl. Biol., 67:223-234.

Roberts, D. W. A., 1971, The effect of CCC and gibberellins A_3 and A_7 on the cold hardiness of Kharkov 22 MC. Winter Wheat, Can. J. Bot., 49:705-711.

Sachs, R. M., Hield, H., and deBie, J., 1975, Dikegulac: A promising new foliar applied growth regulator for woody species, HortScience, 10:367.

Schneider, G., 1970, Morphactins: Physiology and performance, Ann. Rev. Plant Physiol., 21:499-536.

Schönherr, J., and Bukovac, M. J., 1978, Foliar penetration of succinic acid dimethyl hydrazide: Mechanism and rate limiting step, Physiol. Plant., 42:243-251.

Singh, T. N., Aspinall, D., and Paleg, L. G., 1973, Stress metabolism IV. The influence of (2-chloroethyl)trimethylammonium chloride and GA on the growth and proline accumulation of wheat plants during water stress, Aus. J. Biol. Sci., 26:77-86.

Sullivan, E. F., 1977, "Plant Growth Regulator Handbook," Plant Growth Regulator Working Group, Great Western Sugar, Co., Longmont, Colo.

Tolbert, N. E., 1960, (2-chloroethyl)trimethylammonium chloride and related compounds as plant growth substances. II. Effect on growth of wheat, Plant Physiol., 35:380-385.

Wittwer, S. H., 1968, Chemical regulators in horticulture, HortScience, 3:163-166.

Wu, C. H., and Santelmann, P. W., 1977, Influence of six plant growth regulators on Spanish peanuts, Agron. J., 69:521-522.

Wünsche, U., 1977, Influence of growth retarding substances on cereals. III. Field experiments with CCC, DMC and CEPA on wheat, rye, barley and oats, Z. Acker-u. Pflanzenbau, 145: 238-253.

Yib, R. Y., McNulty, P. J., Seidel, M. C., and Viste, K. L., 1971, Plant growth regulating properties of 3-carboxy-2-pyridones, HortScience, 6:460-461.

Young, R., 1971, Effect of growth regulators on citrus seedling cold hardiness, J. Am. Soc. Hort. Sci., 96:708-710.

16

POSSIBILITIES FOR OPTIMALIZATION OF PLANT NUTRITION BY NEW AGROCHEMICAL SUBSTANCES--ESPECIALLY IN CEREALS

J. Jung

BASF Agricultural Research Centre
Limburgerhof, Federal Republic of Germany

INTRODUCTION

When discussing measures for further increasing crop production by optimalizing plant nutrition, it is natural to start by asking to what extent the productivity of crop plants can be increased under specific conditions. It is well known that the yield level of one and the same plant can vary considerably under the various cultivation conditions found in world agriculture. The factors responsible for these variations in productivity may be such that they cannot be influenced by realistic production techniques. Frequently, however, in the traditional cultivation areas of a crop, growth factors are involved that can be substantially influenced and optimalized by appropriate measures.

How great the variation in the biological photoproductivity of one and the same plant is can be seen merely from a comparison of the average yield of a certain cultivation area or country with the individual maximum yields of the particular area. This can be vividly demonstrated particularly in the case of the cereal species that dominate in the production of food and fodder and which account for usage of approximately 50% of the world's agricultural area (apart from permanent pasture). According to Hageman (1977), for example, the record yield for wheat in the United States is 209 bu/a = 141 dt/ha. The average yield for the same variety of wheat in the same area, in the State of Washington, was 100 bu/a = 67.5 dt/ha. Compared with the average yield of wheat in the United States, the maximum yield mentioned was seven times as high.

Top yields of over 100 dt/ha are nowadays being recorded more and more frequently in wheat, particularly in the maritime climate of northwest Europe; they represent approximately twice the normal average yields in this region. Whether these yields already constitute the complete utilization of the genetic yield potential of the plant is doubtful rather than certain. Via an analysis of the yield-forming organs originally produced by the wheat plant, Aufhammer (1976) arrives at a theoretical grain yield potential of 225 dt/ha.

Thus today's wheat varieties are apparently adjusting themselves anatomically and morphologically to a synthesis capacity which can only be partially realized physiologically during further development. Therefore, reduction of the yield-forming organs sets in corresponding to the particular conditions of development (Fig. 1). It is quite possible to diminish the extent and effect of this reduction in yield-determining components (ear-bearing stalks per unit of area, number of grains per ear, and grain weight) on the grain yield, agrochemical agents proving not least effective in this respect.

This article consists of a discussion of some of the extensive endeavors and activities in the agrochemical industry to improve plant nutrition as a condition for the formation of higher yields. This does not, however, only involve development work, which has already led to results of practical value to the farmer. It seems, especially for those who will read this, quite justifiable also to deal with the directions of operations and optimalization trials which have been accepted by farmers, though only to a limited extent for certain reasons, such as economic ones.

Possibilities or starting points for the further optimalization of the nutrition of plants as a condition for increased production are still to be seen:

(1) in the further development of <u>direct</u> measures for nutrient supply (especially increased utilization and improved adaptation to the plant's needs within a given time),

(2) in <u>flanking</u> agrochemical measures with a favorable influence on the action of the nutrients (especially growth regulators).

FURTHER DEVELOPMENT OF DIRECT MEASURES FOR IMPROVING THE PLANT'S NUTRIENT SUPPLY

The dominating measure for increasing crop production in this century has been the improved nutrition of crop plants through the supply of mineral fertilizers. The importance of fertilizers for crop production can be easily seen from the increase in their consumption. In western Europe, for example, the classical field for fertilizer development and application, the consumption of fertilizers

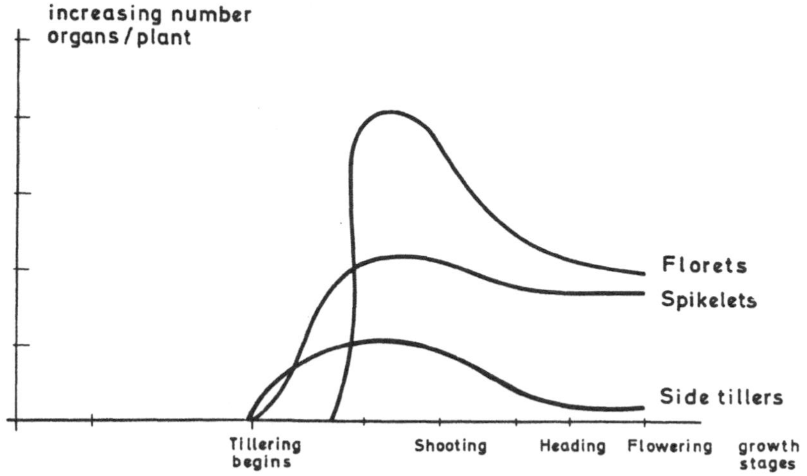

Fig. 1. The development of the number of yield-forming organs in the winter wheat plant (Aufhammer, 1976).

has increased more than tenfold since 1910. Crop production has approximately doubled during this period.

Fertilizers account for only about 10% of farming costs in western Europe but their effect on productivity is certainly 50%. For the United States Bond (1977) states that in the period 1940-1955 about 60% of the increases in crop production are attributable to the use of fertilizers. Even during the period of the rapid adaptation of other farm technologies from 1955-1964, the contribution of the application of fertilizers to the increase in yields is estimated to have been 36%.

From 1940-1974 the value of the increase in yields achieved with fertilizers is given as $293 billion (U.S.) at a cost of $42 billion (benefit:cost ratio = $7 crop value for each dollar spent for fertilizer). How this dominant factor has developed for the increase in crop production in the United States in comparison to other farm inputs can be seen from Fig. 2.

Since fertilization is considered to be so important for increasing crop production, a comparison of fertilization intensity and yield performance in various parts of the world, taking approximate account of the infrastructure, is very instructive. An example given in Table 1, in which wheat and rice are taken as the indicator crops, shows that in many parts of the world the decisive increases in yield are to be expected for some time to come from the conventional possibilities of optimalizing plant nutrition.

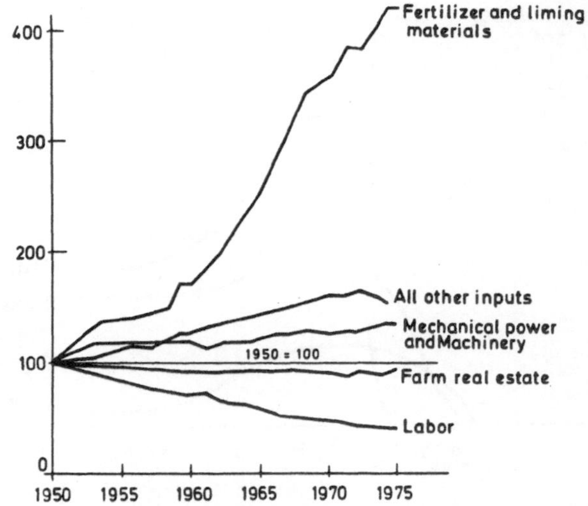

Fig. 2. Use of selected farm inputs (Bond, 1977).

However, both at low and high fertilization levels, there is a current optimalization problem for many plant nutrients, namely the improvement of their efficiency by increasing their utilization or their uptake by the plant. Thus, according to Wittwer (1977), utilization values of about 50% are assumed for the nitrogen supplied by mineral fertilizers and of 25-35% for phosphorus and potassium under the application conditions in the United States. This optimalization problem is extremely complex, since the causes of the limited utilization of the various plant nutrients naturally differ considerably.

Questions of Optimalizing Nitrogen Nutrition

The increase in the use of nitrogen in world agriculture, which has risen from 4 million tons in 1950 to 10 million tons in 1960 to as much as 45 million tons in 1977, underlines the significance of this nutrient which is so important to crop production. Successful attempts have constantly been made to optimalize the effect of nitrogen, particularly by developing appropriate fertilizers and efficient methods of application. There has always existed interest in explaining and quantifying the losses which, until recently, in the case of this nutrient, had been considered to be mainly due to displacement into deeper soil layers--outside the zones accessible to the plant roots. Particularly in lysimeters (one of which has been in operation for fifty years at our Experimental Station) results have been obtained which illustrate the greater importance of vegetative cover or rotation for the level of losses from N leaching (Jürgens-Gschwind and Jung, 1977). For temperate climatic

Table 1. Fertilization Intensity and Yield Relations 1974-1975[1,2]

Region	Fertilizer Application in kg/ha				Yield Performance Ratio to World Average (= 100)	
	N	P_2O_5	K_2O	Total	Wheat	Rice
Developed Countries	41.28	28.67	24.65	94.60	140	239
N. America	33.22	18.23	16.94	68.39	128	209
W. Europe[3]	44.86	31.24	28.75	104.85	199	227
Oceania	4.25	20.79	4.83	29.87	86	209
Others	47.56	51.42	42.58	141.56	89	253
Developing Countries	10.60	5.10	3.05	18.75	83	81
Africa	2.19	1.61	1.12	4.92	50	54
Latin America	13.76	10.87	6.87	31.50	92	77
Near East	14.52	6.36	0.58	21.46	84	163
Far East	13.76	4.20	3.17	21.13	85	81
Others	10.07	2.40	3.14	15.61	53	93
Centrally Planned Economies (CPE)	35.25	18.04	18.54	71.83	84	131
CPE Asia	31.07	11.49	4.67	47.22	87	130
CPE Europe + USSR	37.26	21.21	25.25	83.72	82	156
World	25.79	15.12	13.23	54.14	100	100

[1]Non-European countries: Only arable farming and permanent crops data.

[2]Fertilizer consumption, agricultural area, and yields according to 1975 FAO Yearbook.

[3]With reference to the total agricultural area.

conditions these can be given as, on an average, 5% of the nitrogen supplied.

However, the losses of gaseous N caused by denitrification (as the result of the formation of N_2, N_2O, and NO in the biological reduction of NO_3 and NO_2) appear to be considerably higher, especially under certain conditions; only recently has this become increasingly apparent. These losses are estimated, by Huber et al. (1977) for example, to average 20% (see Fig. 3).

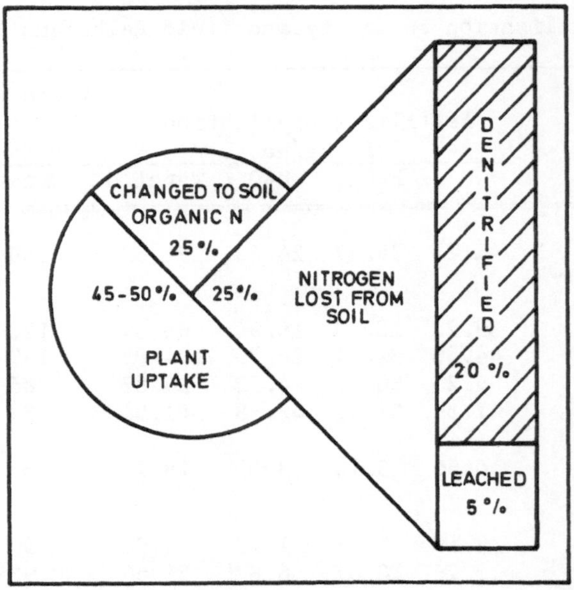

Fig. 3. Theoretical fate of nitrogen applied to soil (Huber et al., 1977).

Probably some 120 million tons of soil nitrogen and applied fertilizer nitrogen escape worldwide per year in the gaseous form as a result of the microbial process of denitrification and are thus lost to crop production (Wittwer, 1977); this is approximately three times as much as the world consumption of synthetically fixed fertilizer nitrogen.

Reduction of denitrification losses. One of the concepts for solving this problem consists in curbing nitrification by the use of substances with a specific influence on the *Nitrosomonas* species, so-called nitrification inhibitors (see Fig. 4).

In the meantime a number of compounds with an inhibitory action on nitrification have been described (Bundy and Bremner, 1974), only a few of which are listed in Table 2. The compound Nitrapyrin (Goring, 1962) has been subjected to the most intensive study so far.

As can be easily demonstrated in laboratory tests, this compound completely inhibits nitrification, the duration of action being strongly influenced by the rate of application (Fig. 5).

After this concentration-dependent period of action, nitrification restarts relatively quickly on a full scale. Moreover, it can be shown by means of soil respiration (i.e., the production of CO_2)

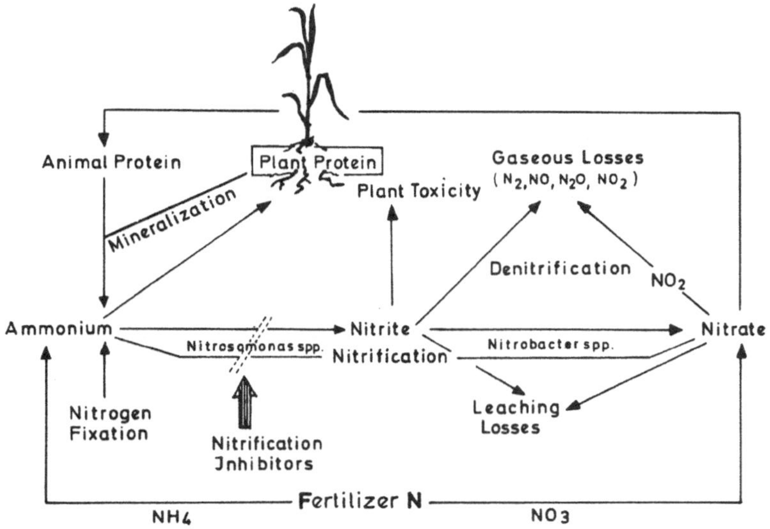

Fig. 4. Point of attack by nitrification inhibitors in nitrogen cycle.

Table 2. Compounds with an Inhibitory Effect on Nitrification

<u>Nitrapyrin</u>	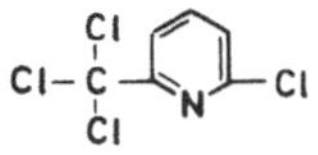	2-chloro-6-trichloromethyl-pyridine
<u>AM</u>	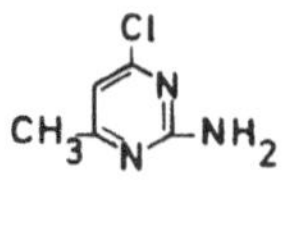	2-amino-4-chloro-6-methyl-pyrimidine
<u>ST</u>	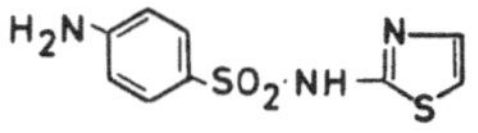	2-sulfanilamidothiazole
<u>DCS</u>	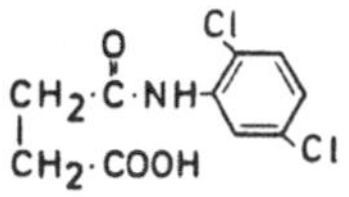	N-2,5-dichlorophenylsuccinamic acid

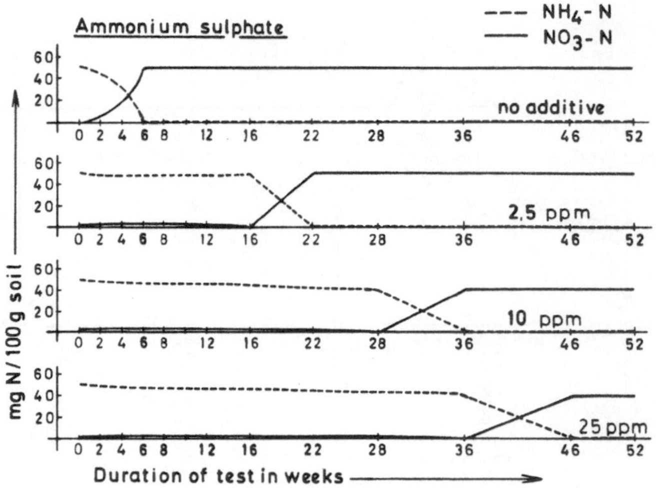

Fig. 5. Effect of increasing rates of Nitrapyrin on nitrification. Loamy soil (Alt-Wiesloch).

that the general microbial activity in the soil is not adversely affected while the nitrification is being inhibited (Fig. 6). The favorable effect of the nitrification inhibitor on the action and utilization of the ammonium form of nitrogen naturally depends to a considerable extent on how greatly a particular soil is susceptible to denitrification on account of permanent or temporary factors. To illustrate this, an example of a pot experiment with ryegrass (Lolium perenne) is given in Fig. 7.

Stabilization of the nitrogen in the ammonium form also means that a reduction of the N leached into deeper soil layers can be expected on soils having a sufficiently large cation exchange capacity. However, how greatly this effect depends on the type of soil will be shown by the results of an experiment with soil columns given in Fig. 8.

If the cation exchange capacity of a soil is sufficiently high, it is possible to apply nitrogen in the fall if a nitrification inhibitor is used, and this is already being recommended in the United States for anhydrous ammonia. In particular, it could have advantages from the point of view of labor and storage.

The nutrient uptake and metabolism of the plant are affected by whether the nitrogen is offered as an anion (NO_3^-) or as a cation (NH_4^+). Thus, a one-sided supply of NH_4 encourages antagonism among the cationic nutrients whereas a supply of nitrate diminishes it. The particular form of N offered can also exert a strong influence on the synthesis rate of organic acids in the plant.

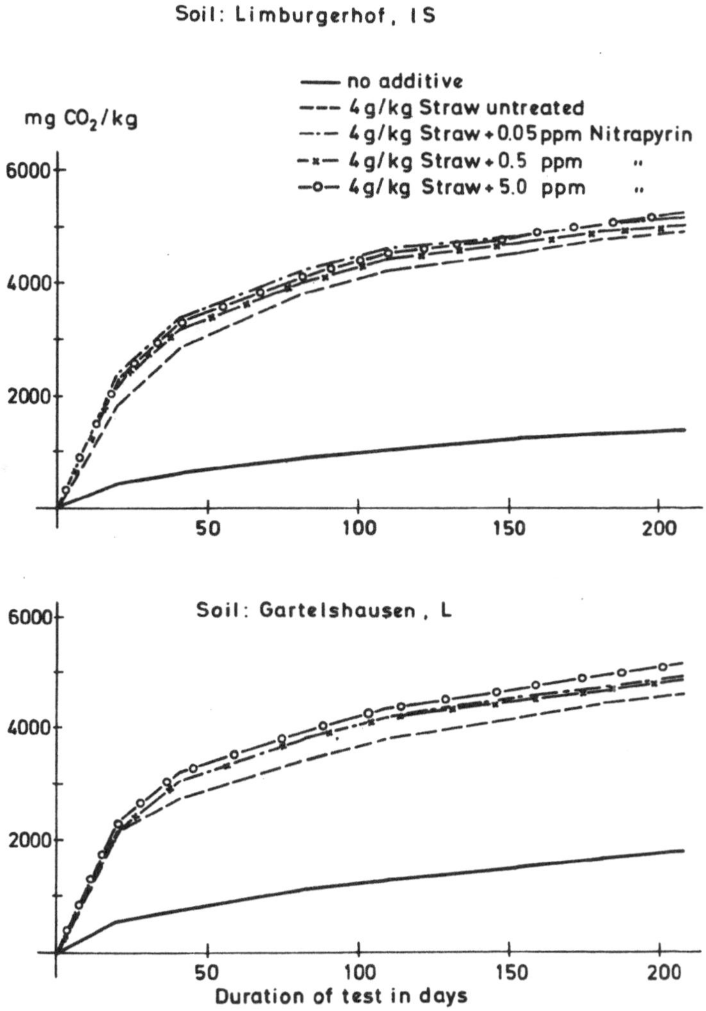

Fig. 6. Influence of Nitrapyrin on soil respiration.

These interrelationships and questions will have to be investigated more intensively in the future in combination with the application of nitrification inhibitors particularly under normal farming conditions. For the time being, emphasis should be placed on the possibility of reducing the accumulation of nitrate in certain crops by inhibiting nitrification in the soil. There is no doubt that the interesting concept of the use of nitrification inhibitors for optimalizing nitrogen nutrition, particularly by reducing losses not only from denitrification but also from leaching, can be assumed, and that this concept will be expanded further in the coming years.

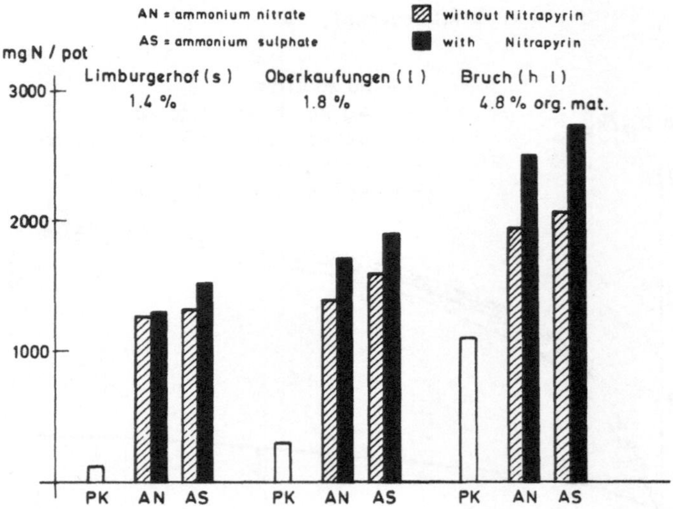

Fig. 7. Nitrogen uptake from ammonium nitrate and ammonium sulphate under the influence of Nitrapyrin (pot trial with ryegrass).

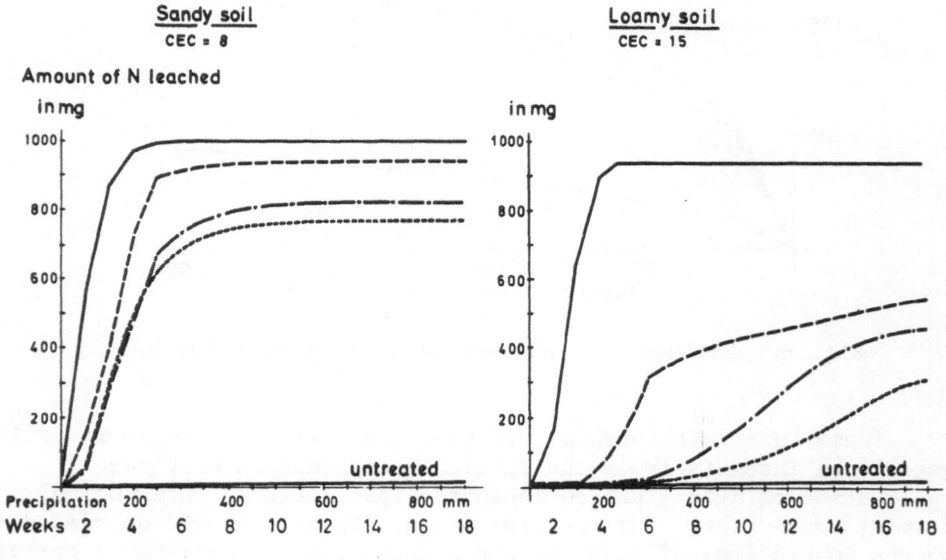

Fig. 8. Influence of Nitrapyrin on the N leaching from soil columns (70 cm).

"Controlled" supply of nitrogen to the plant. Besides minimizing losses, there is another possibility for optimalizing nitrogen nutrition by adapting the supply as far as possible to the needs of the plant during growth. A concept which has been adopted by agricultural chemistry for some time consists in the development of fertilizers with limited solubility, i.e., slow-release nitrogen fertilizers. Fertilizers of this type have been produced in particular on the basis of urea-aldehyde reaction products. The best known are: polymethylene ureas (Ureaform), crotonylidene diurea (CDU), and isobutylidene diurea (IBDU). Until now, these fertilizers (if one disregards Japan, where they are also used in rice) have been introduced virtually only in horticulture and landscaping or, in isolated cases, in special crops. The reason for this limited use is their relatively high price in comparison to normal nitrogen fertilizers.

In addition to the organic nitrogen compounds with limited solubility, a further concept of controlled nutrient supply has been developed which consists in coating the granules of readily soluble fertilizers with film-forming materials which influence the diffusion. This involves building up a kind of "metering coating" of certain polymer substances as well as plasticized elementary sulphur. By means of the coating principle it is possible to influence the release not only of nitrogen but also other nutrients; this technology, therefore, can also be applied to compound fertilizers.

The point in time at which the nutrients are made available or released to the soil solution can be varied within wide limits, as can be seen from the levels of yield given for Lolium in Fig. 9.

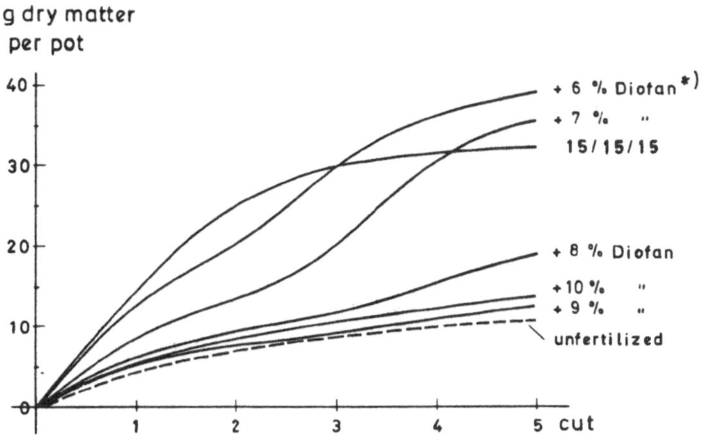

Fig. 9. Effect of plastic-coated NPK fertilizer on yield.

At present, technological development and agronomical evaluation are being concentrated on sulphur-coated urea (SCU), the basic work of the Tennessee Valley Authority (Rindt et al., 1968; Blouin et al., 1971) providing the lead in this field. Urea, which, at higher rates of application, is tolerated by plants only to a limited degree on account of its hydrolysis in the soil and which also causes losses of gaseous N when it is applied to the surface, can have its mode of action substantially modified as can be seen from Fig. 10, a and b.

In principle, the concept of coating fertilizers with film-forming materials offers increasing possibilities of optimalizing nutrient supply. However, in view of the present cost of their manufacture, it remains to be seen to what extent use of these substances will develop.

Endeavors to adapt the supply of nitrogen to the needs of the plant, which is so important particularly in intensive cereal farming, have been made in recent years by the timing of the N-fertilization, i.e., by splitting up the total amount of N into several (generally three) separate applications. In view of the higher costs of slow-release fertilizers, this method will remain the standard solution for normal agricultural crops in the future. It is also greatly promoted by recent developments in application techniques and equipment.

Phosphate and Micronutrients

Regrettably, we cannot presently go deeper into the question of the plant's generally relatively low utilization of phosphate. At the moment there are hardly any realistic aspects of how this problem can be solved by agrochemical means. Results with organic phosphates, which initially reveal substantially quicker diffusion in the soil, as for example glycerophosphate, have only slight relevance for broader application in practice.

This is all the more likely to apply to the covalent phosphorus-nitrogen compounds, for which it was originally assumed there would be improved P utilization by the plant and different mobility in plant and soil on account of their chemical form differing from that of previous fertilizer phosphates. This class of compounds, which includes in particular phosphoroxitriamide and phosphorus nitrilamide with extremely high contents of P and N (for example 72% P_2O_5 + 42% N), has not so far fulfilled these expectations in our tests.

Increasing attention is also being paid to the supply of micronutrients in intensive cereal cropping. At least temporary deficiency situations appear to occur frequently, particularly in the course of later growth when there is a spontaneously high requirement. Consequently the application of micronutrients via foliar fertilizers,

a) Urea

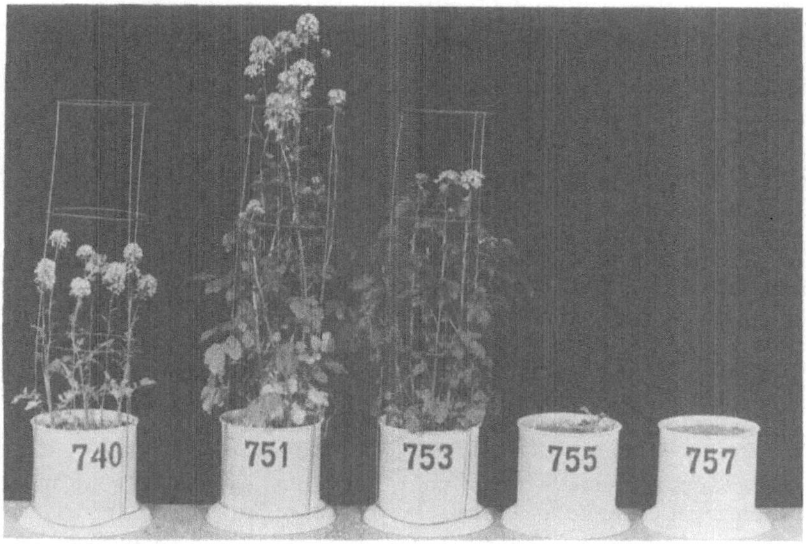

0 0.75 1.5 3.0 4.5
(g N per pot)

b) SCU

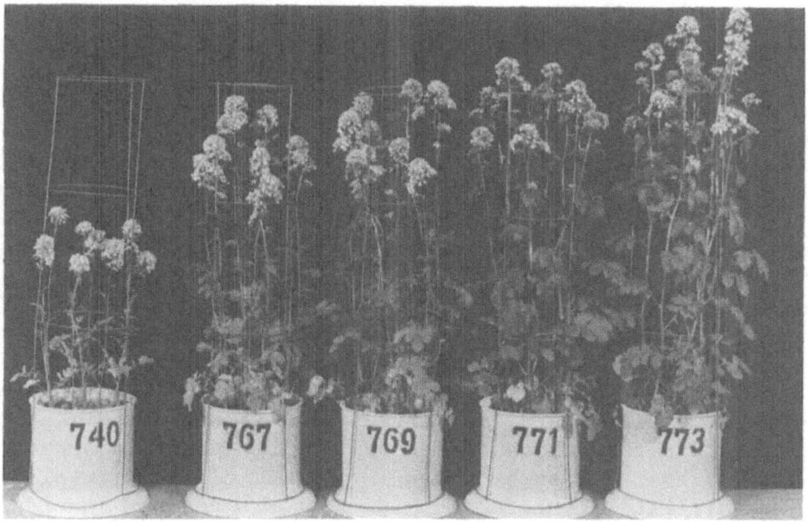

0 0.75 1.5 3.0 4.5
(g N per pot)

Fig. 10. Effect of increasing urea rates in normal and coated (SCU) form (*Sinapis alba*).

which occasionally contain the cationic nutrients in the form of chelates, is being introduced more often.

FLANKING AGROCHEMICAL MEASURES WITH A POSITIVE INFLUENCE ON THE EFFECT OF THE NUTRIENTS

Measures for Improving the Resistance of Cereals to Lodging and the Functioning of Assimilating Organs

It is characteristic of some plant nutrients that their effect on yield formation follows an optimum curve. The course of this curve cannot be influenced fundamentally but rather in degrees. The yield curve obtained from increasing rates of N in cereals depends on the standing ability of the particular species or variety of cereal and on how long the assimilating organs of the plant remain functional.

The effectiveness of any nutrient, but especially of nitrogen, diminishes when the cereal lodges or grain formation is impaired by leaf or ear diseases. These limiting factors in intensive cereal farming result from the complex interrelationships of plant, soil, macroclimate, and microclimate as well as rotation, with the particular nutrient supply, however, also exerting at least an indirect influence. Lodging is one of the principal problems in intensive cereal cultivation that has an unfavorable effect particularly when it occurs in the early reproductive stage of development, as shown for example by the results of Weibel and Pendleton (1961) given in Fig. 11. Apart from the losses in yield, which not infrequently lie between 20-40%, the quality of the grain is adversely affected and harvesting is considerably impeded. Therefore, it is essential in intensive wheat cultivation to keep the crop standing until harvest. By the introduction of the growth regulator chlorocholinechloride (CCC = Chlormequat) as a stalk strengthener, therefore, it has proved possible to make an important contribution to optimalizing nitrogen fertilization especially in intensive cereal cultivation in Europe (Linser et al., 1961; Jung and Sturm, 1964; Bruinsma et al., 1965).

The losses in yield that can result from the impaired functioning of the assimilating organs caused by leaf and ear diseases are no less serious than those caused by lodging. This is supported, for example, by the results shown in Fig. 12 of field trials in which wheat was artificially infected with *Septoria nodorum* in order to quantify the extent of the reduction in yield resulting from attack by this widespread ear disease, also in relation to the supply of nitrogen (Bockmann and Partsch, 1975).

State of development in wheat. The application of the growth regulator CCC in combination with increased nitrogen dressings has

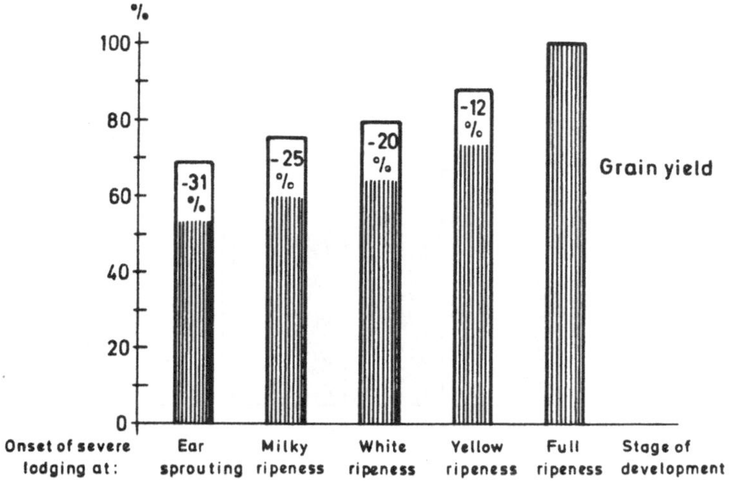

Fig. 11. Effect of artificially induced lodging on grain yield in winter wheat (Weibel and Pendleton, 1961).

become a standard technique in many wheat growing areas of Europe. In the Federal Republic of Germany about 60% of the area under wheat is nowadays treated with this growth regulator. As an "antigibberellin," CCC increases the standing ability of wheat, on the one hand by reducing the length of the stalk--especially of the lower internodes--and, on the other by increasing the diameter of the stalk and strengthening its wall.

Practically all the wheat varieties which have so far been tested react to this growth regulator, although to different degrees. Generally the short-straw varieties react more vigorously than the long-straw ones. In order to achieve an optimum effect, the rate of application must be adjusted to the variety, and in addition the growth stage and the local cultivation conditions must be taken into consideration. When CCC is used properly it definitely offers possibilities for optimalizing the nitrogen yield curve in wheat cultivation, as shown by the example in Fig. 13 of trials by Dilz (1966) carried out during the introductory phase of this growth regulator in the Netherlands.

Apart from being used in the temperate climate of Europe, CCC has either already found considerable acceptance in practice in other areas or produced positive results in trials. It is not always the improvement in standing ability or the prevention of lodging that is conspicuous, but frequently other effects of this compound as well. Thus, widespread use of CCC in the USSR as a seed treatment can be attributed to the fact that this increases the winter resistance of wheat seedlings. The improved overwintering of wheat treated with

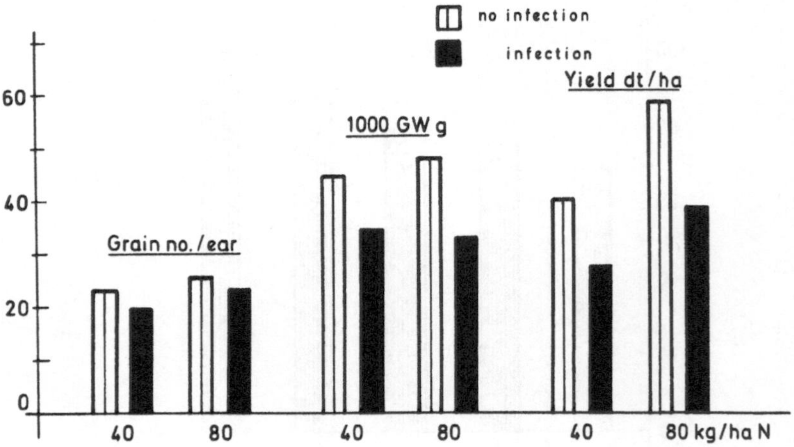

Fig. 12. Effect of Septoria infection on the various yield components of winter wheat ("Werla" variety) at 40 and 80 kg/ha N (Bockmann and Partsch, 1975).

CCC was shown by us (Jung, 1965) earlier in a model trial. Treatment of both the seed and the soil with CCC produced a clear growth advantage for the treated plants up to the end of tillering in the spring.

Zadoncev et al. (1977) emphasize particularly the lowering of the tillering node after seed treatment with CCC as the reason for improved wintering under field conditions (see Fig. 14). The seed treatment carried out in the USSR in 1974 over an area of 2 million hectares of winter and spring wheat underlines the practical significance of the effect of this treatment under the conditions of application here.

This reference to the inclusion of CCC in wheat cultivation operations under the continental climatic conditions of eastern Europe may be taken as a starting point for some remarks about its use under completely different climatic and cultivation conditions, namely in the Mediterranean climate. A number of the results obtained so far (Pinthus and Rudich, 1967; El-Fouly and Fawzi, 1970; Atanasiu and Westphal, 1971; Hassan et al., 1975) disclose the possibility of raising yields with CCC even under these climatic and cultivation conditions. Emphasis should be laid here on the substantially consistant observation that the increased yields are frequently attributable to the greater number of ear-bearing stalks per plant or unit of area, to the larger number of grains per ear, and evidently to retardation of senescence.

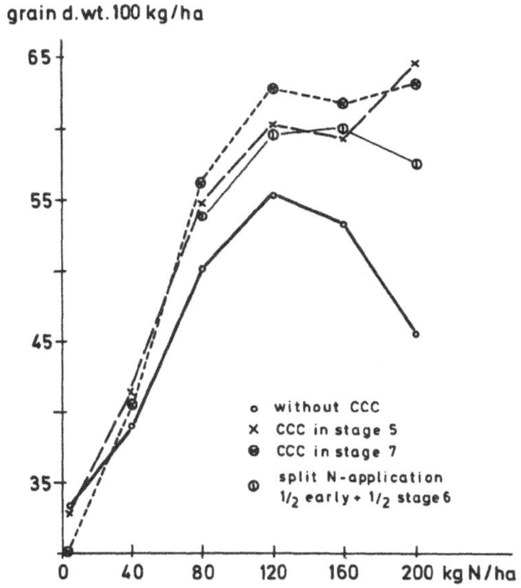

Fig. 13. Yield curves (without CCC depression of yield with 160 and 200 kg N/ha; with CCC still increasing yields with these nitrogen dressings) from field trials with winter wheat according to Dilz, 1966.

Vig et al. (1975) report increases in grain yield of 10-20% as the result of the application of CCC in wheat under the cultivation conditions in the Indian state of Punjab, whereas Lowe and Carter (1971) disclose that, under Australian conditions, CCC produced an increase in ear-bearing stalks and the number of grains per ear equal to that already mentioned for the Mediterranean. Relatively little is reported about the results obtained with CCC in the great wheat growing countries of the United States and Canada, although Appleby et al. (1966) mentioned some time ago the significant increases in yield achieved with three long-strawed wheat varieties in contrast to a short-strawed one.

In addition to the so-called "physiological" form of lodging, increasing attention has recently had to be paid to the parasitic variant which is mainly caused by the Cercosporella herpotrichoides fungus and which is primarily attributable to the close sequence of certain cereal species in the rotation. Even before lodging damage occurs, there can be an adverse influence on the transport of nutrients and water in the cereal plant as the result of tissue damage at the base of the stalk. Additional treatment with systemic fungicides has therefore also been introduced on a considerable scale as a further flanking measure to improve the action of

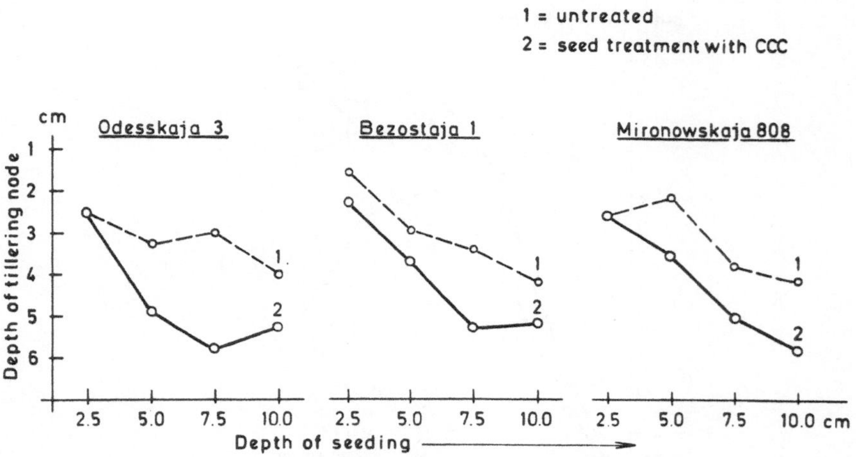

Fig. 14. Depth of the tillering node of wheat in relation to seed treatment with CCC and the depth of seeding (Zadoncev et al., 1977).

nutrients, especially N. At present, mainly fungicides of the benzimidazole and thiophanate types are being used for this purpose.

This measure can counteract the effect of one-sided cereal crop rotations on the spread of "foot" diseases, and the level of yield achieved with appropriate nitrogen dressings and CCC treatment can be consolidated and raised further. An example to illustrate this is given in Table 3 (Sturm, 1976).

In addition to the measures for improving the standing ability and the additional advantages which this involves for the transport of nutrients and water in the cereal plant, the longest possible functioning of the assimilating organs (leaves, stalks, and ears) and their protection from disease are decisive, in the final analysis, for the grain yield.

Of the "critical" development phases of the cereal plant the grain filling period deserves special attention. The assimilates required for the grain filling are produced during a relatively short period from organs of which only a few are capable of assimilation. This important time is the period of development of the top (flag) leaf, the upper parts of the stalk, and the glumes, with only 5-10% of the total assimilates deposited in the grain originating (according to Evans, 1975) from the pre-flowering period. Any disturbance in the photosynthetic activity of the plant organs just mentioned (insolation, supply of water and nutrients, lodging, or parasitic attack) is therefore bound to have an adverse effect on the grain formation and the yield.

Table 3. Influence of Increasing N Dressings, Combined with a CCC + Fungicide Treatment for Stabilizing the Stalk, on the Yield of Wheat in dt/ha (Mean of Three Trials)

Dressings kg/ha	Untreated	CCC	CCC + Systemic Fungicide in g.s. 5/6
90+40	73.7	79.3	83.0
90+60	74.9	80.4	84.0
90+40+60	77.3	81.8	87.9

A very important contribution to cereal cultivation in practice is to be seen in the fact that it has been possible to quantify somewhat more accurately the production of matter in the generative phase of certain cereal species in relation to anatomical-physiological factors and time. In particular the experiments by Stoy (1973) have provided the surprising information that half the assimilates deposited in the grain are synthesized by the plant within merely two weeks, about 30-40 days after heading (see Table 4).

In Fig. 15 the time schedule of the deposition of the assimilates in the grain is set in relation to the plant's nitrogen uptake, which also reaches a peak during this phase.

It goes without saying that both processes should proceed as optimally as possible for the formation of the grain yield. However, this is only possible when the assimilation organs are fully functional.

Particular attention must be paid to powdery mildew (*Erysiphe graminis*) and glume blotch (*Septoria nodorum*) as pathogenic disturbance factors in the assimilation performance in intensively fertilized, dense cereal stands. Particularly the latter infection can cause heavy losses in yield by reducing the thousand grain weight.

It cannot come as a surprise that the application of fungicides in intensive cereal cultivation is finding rapid acceptance and in some countries is already being practiced on 50% of the area under cereals. The fungus pathogens covered by the generic term "leaf and ear diseases" are combatted by fungicides from various classes of chemical compounds, of which only benzimidazoles, chlorinated imides of thiocarboxylic acid, morpholines, thiophanates, thiocarbamates, and triazols should be mentioned here.

Table 4. Relative Proportion of ^{14}C Assimilates Produced at Various Times After Heading and Discovered in the Grains on Ripening (Expressed as % of the Accumulated ^{14}C Content of the Grains at Ripening); Spring Wheat (Stoy, 1973)

	Days After Heading			
	1-14	15-28	29-42	43-56
Average of 10 varieties	5.6	24.9	52.7	16.9

The use of the plant growth regulator CCC and appropriate fungicides, together with the application of herbicides for eliminating broadleaved and grass weeds as an already integrated measure, has constituted the introduction in intensive wheat cultivation of important agrochemical aids for increasing yields on the basis of a high supply of nutrients. Agriculture can avail itself of these possibilities in relation to the intensity of farming and the economic situation--or it can dispense with them.

In any case a concept is offered here that can serve as a model for a considerable proportion of the area under wheat cultivation in the world; however, it is a model developed with particular reference to the temperate and maritime climates and the varieties of wheat normally grown there today. Its adaptation to other climatic conditions will--where there is a realistic basis--require modifications.

Precisely where a very high level of yield has been achieved by appropriate fertilization, the flanking or added agrochemical measures can lead to considerable combined effects, as can be seen from the example in Fig. 16.

State of development in other cereal species. The flanking measures for increasing the effects of fertilization on assimilation are not quite as far advanced in the other cereal species as they are in wheat. Whereas suitable fungicides are also available for these other cereal species, there are no appropriate plant growth regulators or they are still under development. For this reason, lodging in barley, rye, oats, and rice over wide areas is also a problem restricting nitrogen fertilization and thus yield levels.

It is known that CCC does not generally increase the resistance of barley and rice to lodging. In the case of rye and oats the action is considerably weaker than in wheat but it frequently leads at least to a gradual reduction in the damage from lodging in these species of cereal. There is, then, an obvious need to look for

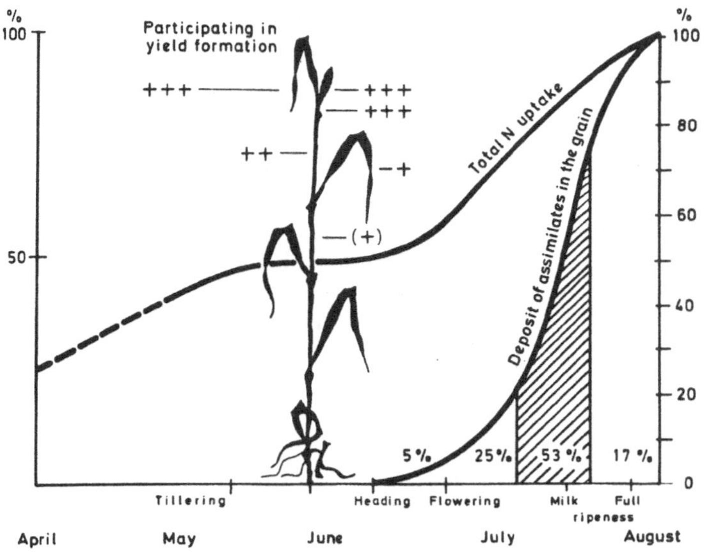

Fig. 15. Deposit of assimilates in the grain and N uptake of the wheat plant.

further compounds that might have a more pronounced action on the cereal species which exhibit a weaker reaction to CCC.

In this connection, it should first of all be remembered that Tolbert (1960a,b) in his investigations into the action of quaternary ammonium compounds came to the conclusion that the growth regulating properties of this class of compounds are primarily attributable to the trimethyl ammonium cation and that furthermore the intensity of action also depends on the length of the carbon chain (optimal length = C_2).

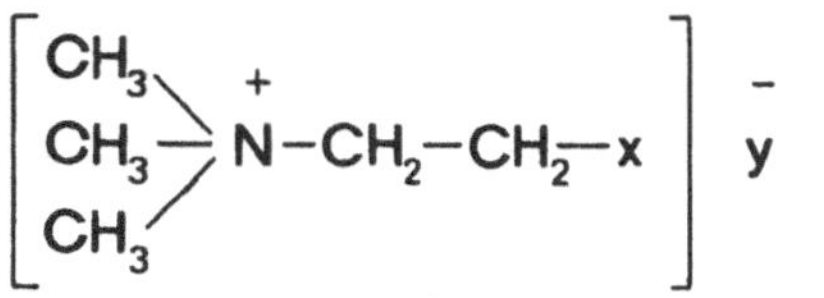

In the screening of several hundred mono-, di-, and trimethyl ammonium compounds at our Research Station it has been possible to substantially confirm Tolbert's conclusion. To supplement the known growth regulating compounds of the ammonium group, other classes of highly active substances have been found which also belong to the group of "onium compounds," i.e., have a positively charged central atom. For example, substances with an action similar to CCC had already been found earlier in the group of hydrazonium and

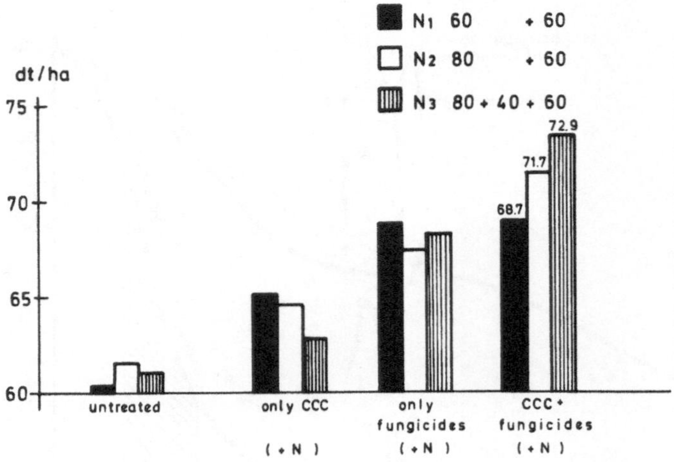

Fig. 16. Increased yields from the use of CCC and fungicides with 3 different rates of N dressing (winter wheat 1977-- 5 trials).

morpholinium compounds at BASF's Research Laboratories (König, 1968; Jung, 1967, 1970), in particular:

N-dimethyl-N-β-chloroethyl-hydrazonium chloride = CMH

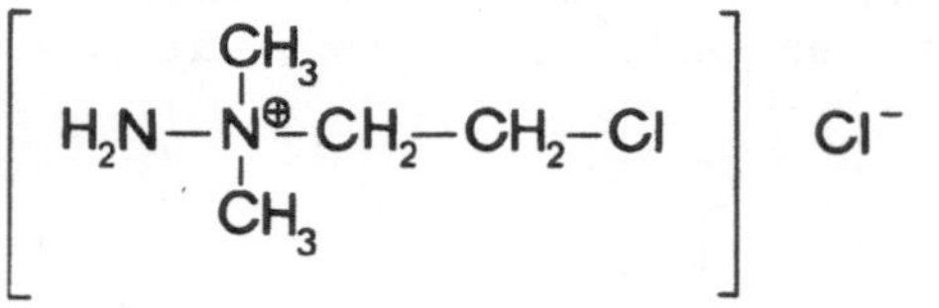

(BAS 06400 W)

N-dimethyl-morpholiniumchloride = DMC

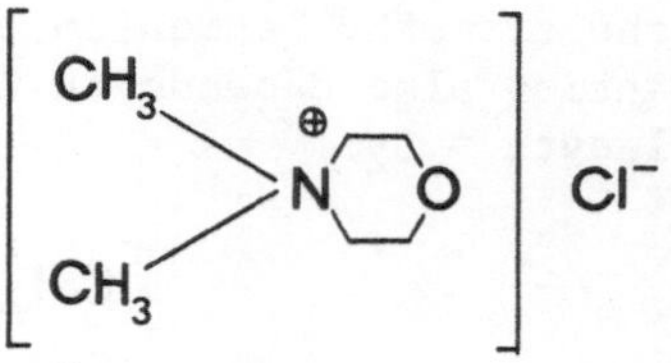

(BAS 06600 W)

Recently a new group of growth regulating substances has been found in the class of pyridazinium and piperidinium salts (Zeeh et al., 1974; Jung and Dressel, 1977). From the large number of substances screened in the first test, compounds have emerged with a high growth regulating activity as well as some with none at all as a result of slight modifications to the molecule (Table 5). Observations up to now have shown 1,1-dimethylpyridazinium bromide (DPYB) and 1,1-dimethylpiperidinium chloride (DPC) to have the most pronounced activity.

Table 5. Relative Activity of Pyridazinium and Piperidinium Derivatives in the Wheat Seedling Assay

Compound	Relative value	Compound	Relative value
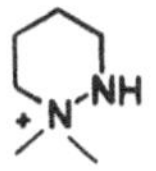	100	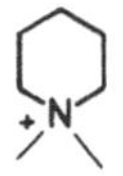	100
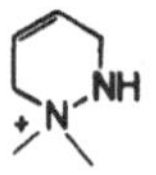	100	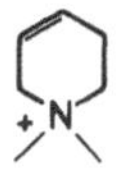	100
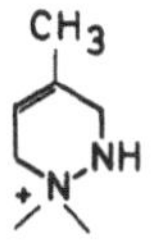	85	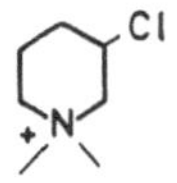	95
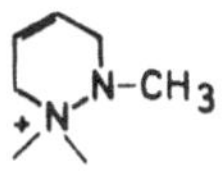	70	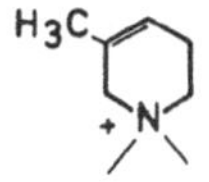	70
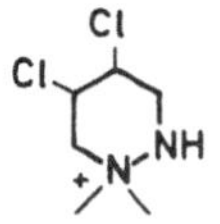	40	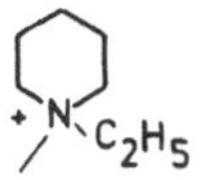	65
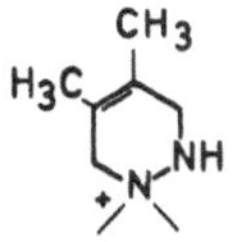	0	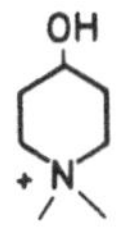	0

1,1-dimethylpyridazinium bromide = DPYB

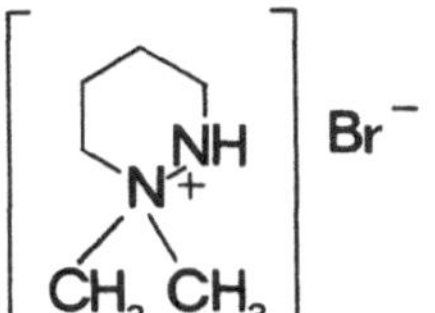

(BAS 08500 W)

1,1-dimethylpiperidinium chloride = DPC

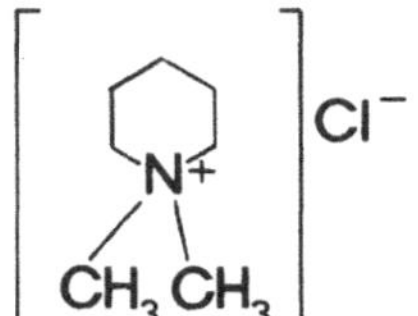

(BAS 08300 W)

It is not possible to go into details here of the spectrum of action of these substances from the onium group. However, it should be mentioned that, in view of the graduations in action, an expansion can be expected. For example, DPC is in an advanced state of testing as the basic substance of a stalk stabilizer for barley and rye. In field trials during the vegetation period last year and this year when there was a pronounced lodging tendency, the corresponding trial product (BAS 09800 W) brought about a considerable increase in the standing ability, particularly of winter barley.

It is also worth mentioning in this connection that DPC has particularly pronounced growth regulating properties in cotton (Jung et al., 1975). These can be utilized to restrain too vigorous vegetative growth when there are particularly favorable nutrition or growth conditions. The advantages of this "plant architecture" are directed in particular to simplifying the mechanical harvesting of cotton. However, the advantages do not merely affect the technical side of harvesting; they also affect the yield. There are already certain indications that this method of influencing growth will bring about an optimalization similar to that produced by the application of CCC in wheat.

Potential growth regulators for cereals are also to be seen in some substances from the group of the so-called ethylene generators, of which 2-chloroethyl phosphonic acid = Ethephon should be mentioned in particular (Kühn et al., 1977). Recently this compound has already been used in some areas as a stalk stabilizer for rye (Hoffmann et al., 1975).

Further Desirable Optimization by Means of Growth Regulating Substances

Influencing root growth. The influence on plant growth of growth regulators is not restricted to the shoot, but also, at least to a limited extent, to the root system. Naturally the uptake of both water and nutrients can be favorably influenced by stimulated root growth.

In world cereal cultivation water is no doubt the primary limiting factor in the formation of yield. There has therefore been no lack of ideas as to how the supply of water to the cereal plant can be improved, particularly in the critical reproductive phase, without water being furnished directly. The primary idea here is the application of specific active substances which either have a direct influence on the plant's water balance or promote the plant's ability to absorb water via a better developed root system.

Even though no "root regulator" is available at present, the probability of finding such a substance should be assessed relatively favorably. Some growth regulators are known to have a noticeable effect on root development or at least on the root/shoot ratio. Thus, gibberellins tend to have an adverse effect on root growth, the "antigibberellins" a favorable one. Higher grain yields resulting from the use of CCC in non-lodging wheat stands can surely be attributed in part to the better utilization of water in dry years.

Certain substances are also known to provide starting points for a direct influence on the plant's water balance. The opposing effects of abscisic acid (ABA) on stomatal opening have provoked investigations into the possibility of using this substance as an antitranspirant (Milborrow, 1969). However, ABA exhibits relatively labile behavior in the plant, as can be seen from the example from our trials given in Fig. 17. As in the case of the auxins, however, it will probably not be impossible to find substances which have a longer duration of action with a similar effect.

Influence of growth regulating substances on yield-determining processes in the reproductive period. In addition to certain nutrients, especially N, Mg, Fe, Mn, and Cu, the growth regulators of the onium group, in particular, exert an influence on the assimilation apparatus which consists in increasing the content of chlorophyll and other leaf pigments. The obvious question whether this also has a favorable influence on the rate of assimilation cannot be answered adequately yet. Isolated results do not support such a connection (Jung, 1973). If, however, an increased pigment content is linked to a prolonged functioning of the assimilation apparatus--which is frequently to be observed after treatment with onium compounds--an overall higher assimilation performance is to be expected virtually via delayed senescence.

Increasing attention has been paid recently not only to the intensity of assimilation but also to assimilate partitioning and the source-sink relations which become effective in this connection (Yoshida, 1972; Evans, 1975; Hageman, 1977; Hardy, 1977).

An important question for the formation of the grain yield in cereals is how the plant controls the direction and intensity of the streams of assimilates in the period of grain fill. There is not much information available on this so far but what there is is illuminating.

As a result of their investigations into barley caryopses, Michael and Seiler-Kelbitsch (1972) provided a possible explanation for this phenomenon in that they were able to show correlations between grain size and cytokinin content of the growing grain. This result underlines the importance of growth regulating substances for the formation of yield and it can be assumed that an exogenous influence by means of appropriate active ingredients is fundamentally possible (Herzog and Geisler, 1977). This could open up a very important field of activity for increasing cereal yields.

At present, opinions are divided on the relative significance of assimilation intensity and assimilate partitioning (transport and distribution) for the grain yield. However, it is agreed that the duration of photosynthesis during grain fill is a dominant factor in the level of yield. From this, Hageman (1977) draws the following

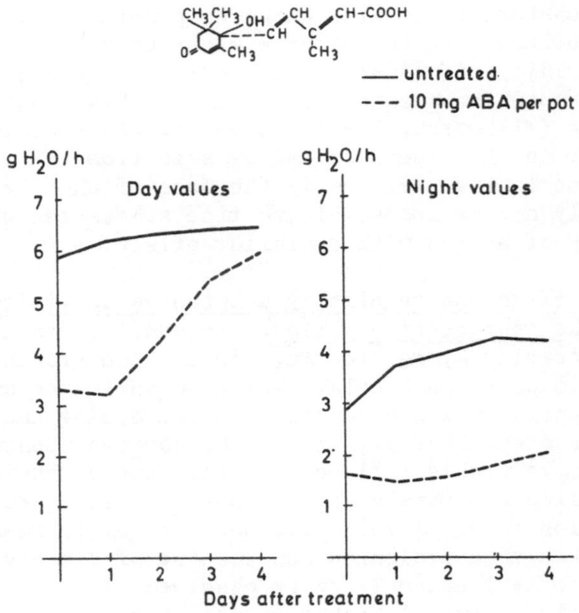

Fig. 17. Influence of abscisic acid (ABA) on the transpiration rate of sunflowers.

conclusion: "Because of the large number of factors (sink number and capacity, feedback inhibition, hormonal levels, changes in environment, leaf structure, area, and enzymatic composition) that have been associated with photosynthetic rates, perhaps it is not surprising that the photosynthetic rates and yields are not closely related. A growth regulator that would extend the duration of grain fill appears to be the most promising research lead, as this involves only the control of the onset of the reproductive events, the identification and control of the 'senescence signal" and the precise determination of maturity."

These objectives can be regarded as perfectly realistic, especially as some of the known growth regulators have already shown that they can exert a significant influence on the course of development in the reproductive phase (ethylene generators and onium compounds). How far metabolism, which is directly linked to photosynthesis, can be deliberately influenced by growth regulators is a question that should not be discussed in detail here. It should merely be recalled that photorespiration in particular has recently frequently been discussed as a limiting factor in the rate of assimilation. It is uncertain whether this metabolism phenomenon will be subject to influence by growth regulators. The inhibition of the glycolate synthesis by glyoxylate, an intermediate of the glycolate oxidation (Oliver and Zelitch, 1977), might possibly be a first step in this direction.

FINAL REMARKS

Of the possibilities shown here for optimalizing plant nutrition by means of agrochemical measures, some have been of a more topical nature, others of a more futurological nature. Some of the themes touched on here do not therefore belong before a forum of those actually engaged in agriculture but should appear on a checklist with which plant research workers will no doubt have to concern themselves well beyond the approaching turn of the millennium.

There are, however, justified hopes that the future-oriented beginnings will also contribute to an increased utilization of the genetic yield potential of crop plants as mentioned at the start; after all, today's agrochemical techniques in intensive cereal cultivation were nothing more than beginnings a few years or decades ago.

REFERENCES

Appleby, A. P., Kronstadt, W. E., and Rohde, C. R., 1966, Influence of 2-chloroethyltrimethylammonium chloride (CCC) on wheat (Triticum aestivum) when applied as a seed treatment, Agron. J., 58:435-437.

Atanasiu, N., and Westphal, A., 1971, Die Wirkung von CCC (Chlorcholinchlorid) auf Wachstum und Ertragsbildung von türkischen Weizensorten, Z. Acker- u. Pflanzenbau, 132:267-280.

Aufhammer, W., 1976, Für die Ertragsbildung kritische Wachstumsstadien bei der Getreidepflanze, DLG-Mitt., 14:780-783.

Blouin, G. M., Rindt, D. W., and Moore, O. E., 1971, Sulfur coated fertilizer for controlled release: Pilot plant production, Agr. Food Chem., 19:801-808.

Bockmann, H., and Partsch, G., 1975, Zusammenhänge zwischen Stickstoffdüngung und Pflanzenkrankheiten im intensiven Getreidebau, Mitt. Landbau BASF, 2/75.

Bond, B. Z., 1977, Fertilizer for the nation, in: "Proceedings TVA Fertilizer Conference 1977," pp. 88-93.

Bruinsma, J., de Vos, N. M., and Dilz, K., 1965, Effects of (2-chloroethyl) trimethylammonium chloride (CCC) on growth and development of cereal plants, "Zeventiende Internationaal Symposium over Fytofarmacie en Fytiatrie," pp. 1990-2006.

Bundy, L. G., and Bremner, J. M., 1974, Inhibition of nitrification in soils, Proc. Soil Sci. Am., 37:396-398.

Dilz, K., 1966, Stikstofbemesting van granen, Stikstof, 51:174-187.

El-Fouly, M. M., and Fawzi, A. F. A., 1970, Durch Chlorocholinchlorid induziertes Ansteigen des Körnerertrages von Weizen, Pest. Sci., 1:129-131.

Evans, L. T., 1975, The physiological basis of crop yield, in: "Crop Physiology," L. T. Evans, ed., Cambridge Univ. Press, Cambridge.

Goring, C. A., 1962, Control of nitrification by 2-chloro-6-(trichloromethyl)-pyridine, Soil Sci., 93:211-218.

Hageman, R. H., 1977, Factors effecting yield of cereal grains via physiological processes, in: "Proceedings of 4th Annual Meeting Plant Growth Regulator Working Group," Plant Growth Regulator Working Group, E. F. Sullivan, Great Western Sugar Co., Longmont, Colo.

Hardy, R. W. F., 1977, Rate-limiting steps in biological photoproductivity, Basic Life Sci., 9:369-399.

Hassan, H. M., El-Fouly, M. M., Bassiony, S. Z., and Attia, K. A., 1975, Response of wheat to combined treatment of chlormequat and 2,4-D on plant properties and CCC-residue contents, Z. Acker- u. Pflanzenbau, 141:55-70.

Herzog, H., and Geisler, G., 1977, Einfluß von Cytokininapplikation auf die Assimilateinlagerung und die endogene Cytokininaktivität der Karyopsen bei zwei Sommerweizensorten, Z. Acker- u. Pflanzenbau, 144:230-242.

Hoffmann, G., Schulzke, D., Heyter, F., Kramer, W., and Kühnel, F., 1975, Camposan, ein neuer Halmstabilisator in Winterroggen, Nachrichtenbl. Pflanzenschutz DDR, 28:249-252.

Huber, D. M., Warren, H. L., Nelson, D. W., and Tsai, C. Y., 1977, Nitrification inhibitors--New tools for food production, Bioscience, 27:523-529.

Jung, J., 1965, Über den Einfluß von CCC auf die Überwinterung von Weizen und dessen Halmlänge, Z. Acker- u. Pflanzenbau, 122: 9-14.

Jung, J., 1967, Hydrazoniumsalze als Wachstumsregulatoren, Landwirt. Forsch., 20:221-228.

Jung, J., 1970, Über die wachstumsregulierende Wirkung von N-Dimethylmorpholiniumchlorid - DMC, Z. Acker- u. Pflanzenbau, 131:325.

Jung, J., 1973, On the biological action of new synthetic growth regulators of the onium group, in: "Proceedings 8th International Conference on Plant Growth Substances," Tokyo.

Jung, J., and Dressel, J., 1977, Pyridazinium- und Piperidiniumsalze als Wachstumsregulatoren, Z. Pflanzenern. Bodenkde., 140:375-386.

Jung, J., and Sturm, H., 1964, Wachstumsregulierende Wirkung von Chlorcholinchlorid (CCC), Landwirt. Forsch., 17:1-9.

Jung, J., Würzer, B., and von Amsberg, H., 1975, Biological activity of new onium compounds in cotton and other crops, Abstr. Papers, Am. Chem. Soc., 170 Meet., Abstract of paper 69, Pesticide Div.

Jürgens-Gschwind, S., and Jung, J., 1977, Lysimeteruntersuchungen in der Großanlage Limburgerhof, Mitt. Landbau BASF, 1/77.

König, K. H., 1968, N,N-Dimethylhydrazoniumsalze als neue Wachstumsregulatoren, Naturwiss., 55:217.

Kühn, H., Schuster, W., and Linser, H., 1977, Halmverkürzung bei Winterroggen durch kombinierte Anwendung von CCC und Ethephon, Z. Acker- u. Pflanzenbau, 145:22-30.

Linser, H., Mayer, H. H., and Bodo, G., 1961, Über die Wirkung von Chlorcholinchlorid auf Sommerweizen, Die Bodenkultur, 12:279-280.

Lowe, L. B., and Carter, O. S., 1971, Grain yield and quality of wheat as affected by Chlormequat (2-chloroethyltrimethyl ammonium chloride), Am. Appl. Biol., 68:203-211.

Michael, G., and Seiler-Kelbitsch, H., 1972, Cytokinin content and kernel size of barley grains as affected by environmental and genetic factors, Crop Sci., 12:162-165.

Milborrow, B. V., 1969, The occurrence and functions of abscisic acid in plants, Sci. Prog. (Oxford), 57:533-545.

Oliver, D. J., and Zelitch, J., 1977, Increasing photosynthesis by inhibiting photorespiration with glyoxylate, Science, 196: 1450-1451.

Pinthus, M. S., and Rudich, J., 1967, Increase in grain yield of CCC-treated wheat (Triticum aestivum) in the absence of lodging, Agrochimica XI, 6:565-570.

Rindt, D. W., Blouin, G. M., and Getsinger, J. G., 1968, Sulfur coating on nitrogen fertilizer to reduce dissolution rate, J. Agr. Food Chem., 16:773-778.

Stoy, N., 1973, Assimilatbildung und -verteilung als Komponenten der Ertragsbildung beim Getreide, Angew. Botanik, 47:17-26.

Sturm, H., 1976, Trends in der Pflanzenernahrung, bezogen auf Stickstoff, Mitt. Landbau BASF:159-185.

Tolbert, E., 1960a, (2-Chloroethyl)-trimethylammonium chloride and related compounds as plant growth substances. I. Chemical structure and bioassay, J. Biol. Chem., 235:475-479.

Tolbert, E., 1960b, (2-Chloroethyl)-trimethylammonium chloride and related compounds as plant growth substances. II. Effect on growth of wheat, Plant Physiol., 35:380-385.

Vig, A. C., Sekhon, G. S., Gupta, V. K., and Dass, B., 1975, Chemical composition of wheat (Triticum aestivum) C-306 as affected by Cycocel (2-chloroethyl-trimethyl ammonium chloride) and nitrogen application, Technology, 12:30-34.

Weibel, R. O., and Pendleton, J. W., 1961, Effect of artificial lodging on winter wheat grain, Agron. J., 56:187-188.

Wittwer, S. H., 1977, Agricultural science and world food production, in: "Proceedings of 4th Annual Meeting Plant Growth Regulator Working Group," Plant Growth Regulator Working Group, E. F. Sullivan, Great Western Sugar Co., Longmont, Colo.

Yoshida, S., 1972, Physiological aspects of grain yield, Am. Rev. Plant Physiol., 23:437-464.

Zadoncev, A. I., Pikus, G. R., and Grincenko, A. L., 1977, "Chlorcholinchlorid in der Pflanzenproduktion," VEB Deutscher Landwirtschaftsverlag, Berlin.

Zeeh, B., König, K. H., and Jung, J., 1974, Development of new plant growth regulators with biological activity related to CCC, Kemia (Helsinki), 9:621-623.

17

GROWTH REGULATORS AND ASSIMILATE PARTITION

P. F. Wareing

Department of Botany and Microbiology
University College of Wales
Penglais, Aberystwyth, Dyfed, UK

INTRODUCTION

As has already been pointed out (Wareing, see Chapter 8), crop yield depends not only upon the total dry matter production (biomass) by the crop, but also upon the proportion of the total dry matter which constitutes the harvested part of the crop, the so-called "harvest-index." It is generally accepted that the increased yield of crop plants over that of their wild ancestors is primarily due to the improved distribution of dry matter to the harvested part of the plant, rather than to increased production of total dry matter. Hence a better understanding of the processes controlling the partition of assimilates within the plant is of paramount importance for the further improvement of crop yields.

The partition of assimilates within the plant appears to be determined by the demand of the various "sinks" arising either from the utilization of assimilates in growth or their accumulation in the form of insoluble reserves, such as starch, lipids, and proteins. However, there is normally competition between the various sinks within the plant, as shown by the fact that pruning, disbudding, or fruit-thinning lead to increased growth of the remaining sinks. There is much evidence that various types of sink differ in their competitive ability and that, for example, developing flowers and fruits have high competitive ability, and have priority of demand on neighboring leaves and even on more distant sources of assimilates.

Little is known as to what determines the competitive ability of a sink, but evidently each sink has a certain "mobilizing ability" whereby it can "pull" or "attract" assimilates against the competing abilities of other sinks. However, there is considerable evidence that endogenous growth regulators may play an important role in determining the mobilizing ability of a sink.

It is now well established that endogenous growth substances are required for all aspects of normal growth, so that these growth substances must be essential for sink activity wherever this involves the utilization of assimilates in growth. Moreover, it would seem significant that sites of active growth, such as young, growing leaves and fruits, contain high levels of endogenous growth substances, such as auxins, gibberellins, and cytokinins. Hence adequate levels of endogenous growth substances are required for all aspects of normal growth and their importance in sink activity would not be in question even if they played no other role. However, there is now considerable evidence that growth substances such as auxins and cytokinins may be important in determining the "pulling power" or mobilizing ability of sinks, independently of any indirect effects they may have by affecting the demand for assimilates in growth.

GROWTH REGULATORS AND MOBILIZING ABILITY

There is now a well-established body of evidence that application of exogenous growth substances to nongrowing tissues can lead to increased movement of assimilates to the point of application and their accumulation there. Thus, application of cytokinin to detached tobacco leaves resulted in the movement of amino acids toward the site of application and this effect did not appear to be dependent upon increased metabolic demand (e.g., in protein synthesis) as a result of application of the growth substance (Mothes et al., 1959). Again, application of indoleacetic acid (IAA) to decapitated mature (nongrowing) internodes of dwarf bean or pea stimulates the movement of ^{14}C-sucrose from a site several cm remote from the point of hormone application (Booth et al., 1962; Davies and Wareing, 1965; Patrick and Wareing, 1973). The normal duration of these latter experiments was 12 hr and over this period there was no detectable increase in internode length or of dry weight of the terminal 1 cm of the internode to which the growth substance was applied. Hence there was no detectable stimulation of growth over the period of the experiment. Moreover, there was no increase in the respiration rate, or of the rate of incorporation of ^{14}C-leucine into protein in the internode tissue at the point of hormone application (Patrick and Wareing, 1972, 1976).

Several other lines of evidence also seem to indicate that increased mobilization of ^{14}C-sucrose in response to applied IAA is not the result of increased metabolic demand in response to hormone application. Thus, the rate of metabolism of ^{14}C-sucrose in decapitated internodes was found to be unaffected by treatment with IAA (Patrick and Wareing, 1976). Moreover, the levels of sucrose appeared to be higher in stems treated with IAA than in untreated stems. Again, when 1-cm stem segments from decapitated internodes pretreated with or without IAA were then immersed in ^{14}C-sucrose solution, the uptake of ^{14}C-sucrose was not increased but reduced by pretreatment with IAA (Patrick and Wareing, 1976).

Thus, in various types of experiment no evidence could be obtained that application of IAA to decapitated internodes results in a detectable increase in the general rate of metabolism or in the demand for sucrose in the stem tissues immediately below the point of hormone application. Hence it would seem that the transport of ^{14}C-sucrose during the 12 hr following hormone application is not due to increased metabolic demand in the ground tissues at the site of application. It would appear, therefore, that the growth substance is affecting some other step in the process of phloem transport.

This conclusion is supported by the results of an experiment in which ^{14}C-sucrose was supplied at various distances from the site of IAA application; it was found that when ^{14}C-sucrose was supplied at the site of IAA application its uptake was unaffected by the presence of IAA; but when the distance between the sites of hormone and sucrose application was increased to 2 cm or more, then IAA greatly increased the movement of ^{14}C-sucrose (Johnston and Wareing, unpublished). Thus, IAA only increases the movement and accumulation of ^{14}C-sucrose at the site of application when phloem transport is involved.

The question arises as to whether IAA acts at its immediate point of application or along the path of ^{14}C-sucrose transport, i.e., whether it acts only locally at the sink or on the phloem throughout the path of transport. It is not possible to distinguish between these two alternatives when IAA is applied to the distal (upper) end of a decapitated internode, since there is then basipetal movement of IAA from the point of application. However, application of IAA to the basal end of a stem section also stimulates the basipetal movement of ^{14}C-sucrose toward this point, although there is very little acropetal movement of IAA away from its point of application. In this type of experiment therefore, the IAA can only be acting locally at the site of application. On the other hand, there is also evidence that when IAA is applied to the upper end of a decapitated internode, the IAA transported away from the site of application can also affect phloem transport (Patrick and Wareing, 1978).

THE POSSIBLE MECHANISM OF AUXIN-DIRECTED TRANSPORT

If the local effect of IAA at the site of application is not due to increased metabolic demand and is only exerted when long-distance transport of ^{14}C-sucrose is involved, it would appear that the IAA must be stimulating the transfer of ^{14}C-sucrose from the sieve tubes into the surrounding ground tissue. This latter process appears to occur via the apoplast (Glasziou and Gayler, 1972), so that it involves transfer across two membrane systems, viz., (1) transfer across the plasmalemma of the sieve tube into the apoplast ("unloading") and (2) uptake from the apoplast into the symplast of the sink tissue, the rate of which will be measured by its sink activity. Therefore, IAA and cytokinin may stimulate the unloading process from the sieve tubes into the apoplast and/or active uptake by the ground tissue from the apoplast. It is probable that both unloading from the phloem and uptake by the sink tissues are active processes.

Hitherto it has been difficult to envisage how growth substances might promote the active transport of sucrose across membranes. However, it has recently been proposed that loading into the phloem involves the proton co-transport of sugars. Following the earlier demonstration that the uptake of sugars by microorganisms involves proton co-transport (Tanner et al., 1977), it has been suggested (Giaquinta, 1977a,b) that the loading of sugars into phloem involves the establishment of a pH gradient between the apoplast (pH 5-6) and the sieve tube (pH 8-8.5) across the plasmalemma of the sieve tube. It is postulated that the proton gradient across the plasmalemma provides the driving force for sucrose uptake, and is maintained by an ATP-driven proton-extrusion system. A charged complex (sucrose-H^+ carrier) is held to be driven across the membrane by the electrical potential difference generated by the proton extrusion mechanism.

A very similar model for phloem loading has also been suggested by Malek and Baker (1977), who showed that the loading of ^{14}C sugars into the phloem of <u>Ricinus communis</u> is stimulated by low pH and by K^+. A model was proposed for a proton co-transport of sugars from the apoplast driven by a linked proton efflux/K^+ influx pump which is ATP energized. Moreover, these authors have subsequently shown (Malek and Baker, 1978) that fusicoccin, and to a lesser extent IAA, stimulate phloem loading of ^{14}C-sucrose in the petiole of <u>Ricinus</u>. This result is consistent with other evidence that fusicoccin and IAA apparently stimulate proton secretion in <u>Avena</u> coleoptiles and other growing tissues. There is indeed considerable evidence that the promotion of cell extension growth by IAA may involve the stimulation of an electrogenic proton pump coupled with passive K^+ uptake (Cleland and Rayle, 1978). The nature of this pump remains to be elucidated, but there are good reasons for thinking that it may involve an ATP-ase. Thus, current views regarding the mode of action of fusicoccin and IAA derived from studies of their action in promoting cell extension correspond closely with the hypothesis that phloem loading involves proton co-transport of ^{14}C-sucrose and with the observation that such loading is stimulated by fusicoccin and IAA.

Now, these ideas seem to provide a clue as to the possible mechanism of IAA-promoted transport which, as suggested above, seems to involve stimulation by IAA of the transfer of ^{14}C-sucrose from the sieve tubes into the surrounding ground tissue. It seems very likely that "unloading" involving transfer of sucrose across the sieve tube membrane is an active process, and a mechanism very similar to that proposed for phloem loading can be suggested by postulating that this process involves proton "anti-port" transport of sucrose, i.e., that a sucrose-H^+ carrier is involved in which the direction of transport of sucrose is opposite to that of the protons, so that as protons move inward sucrose is transported out of the sieve tube into the apoplast, from which it is taken up by the surrounding cells of the ground tissue, possibly by proton co-transport. If unloading is an active process requiring the establishment of a pH gradient by an ATP-ase, it seems very likely, on the grounds stated above, that this process would be stimulated by IAA. If this conclusion is valid, it follows that IAA is probably involved in the normal process of phloem loading and unloading, and that the phenomenon of hormone-directed transport is not just an artifact.

EFFECTS OF CYTOKININS AND GIBBERELLINS

Most of the studies on the effects of growth substances on long distance transport of assimilates have been carried out with auxins, especially IAA. The earlier studies on the mobilizing ability of cytokinins generally involved transport over relatively short distances in leaf tissue (Mothes et al., 1959). However, there have been a few studies on the effects of other types of growth substance involving transport of assimilates over several cm of stem tissue. Thus, Hew et al. (1967) demonstrated the effects of gibberellic acid on long distance transport of assimilates in soybeans. Earlier studies on the effects of kinetin and gibberellic acid applied in lanolin to decapitated pea seedlings suggested that they have relatively little effect compared with that of IAA (Davies and Wareing, 1965), but later studies indicated that they can act synergistically with IAA in *Phaseolus* (Seth and Wareing, 1967), and subsequent work has shown that they can have quite a marked effect on transport of ^{14}C-sucrose when applied in aqueous solution (Johnston and Wareing, unpublished; Mulligan and Patrick, 1978).

Thus, the effects of growth substances on the mobilization of assimilates do not appear to be confined to auxins, and further detailed studies will be required to determine how similar effects are brought about by very different types of growth substance. Recent work suggests that gibberellic acid acts only at the point of application (Mulligan and Patrick, 1978), whereas when IAA is applied to the upper end of a decapitated internode it has remote effects, as well as those at the point of application (Patrick and Wareing, 1978).

HORMONE-DIRECTED TRANSPORT AND THE PARTITION OF ASSIMILATES

The importance of endogenous growth substances as factors affecting "sink activity" cannot be doubted, irrespective of their mode of action; insofar as cytokinins and auxins appear to be essential for cell division and cell expansion in callus cultures, and gibberellins are apparently essential for many aspects of normal growth in the intact plant, the presence of adequate levels of these growth substances is a necessary condition for sink activity involving growth.

There is no doubt that growth rate is sometimes limited by the levels of one or more types of growth substance, as shown by the responses to applied growth substances; indeed, the concept of "hormonal control" depends upon the assumption that the levels of a given growth substance are limiting and hence regulate the growth rate (Wareing, 1977). Thus, there is good evidence that geotropic and phototropic curvatures are hormonally controlled, which implies that the levels of endogenous growth substances in the growing regions of stems and roots are probably limiting. Again, the growth responses of genetic dwarf varieties (e.g., of pea or maize) and of seedless grapes to applied gibberellins indicates that the levels of endogenous gibberellins are limiting in such cases. However, the number of instances in which growth and crop yield can be increased by applied growth substances is relatively few, suggesting that the growth of many organs, such as fruits or storage organs (tubers, rootstocks), is not normally limited by endogenous hormone levels. This conclusion is consistent with the fact that growing tissues, such as developing embryos, normally contain high levels of endogenous growth substances.

On the other hand, the growth of specific organs is very commonly limited by competition with other sinks for assimilates and mineral nutrients, as shown by the effects of pruning, fruit thinning, and other agricultural and horticultural practices. Hence, there would seem to be potential scope for increasing the harvest index and hence yield by increasing the competitive ability of the usable parts of the crop. The factors determining the competitive ability of growth centers are not fully understood, and our approach to this problem will depend upon what hypothesis we adopt regarding the mechanism of phloem transport, and specifically as to the mechanism of transfer of assimilates from the sieve tubes to the sink tissues.

According to the "pressure flow theory," phloem transport depends on the removal of sucrose and other metabolites from the sieve tubes at the sinks, and it is commonly assumed that such removal is determined by the demand for assimilates for growth and metabolism. As we have seen, the transfer of sucrose from the sieve tubes into the sink cells appears to involve transport across at least two membranes and if such transfer is controlled by the "metabolic demand" of the sink, then presumably the factor regulating the rate of this process is the concentration gradient of sucrose between the sieve tube and the sink tissues. So far as the author is aware, there is no evidence bearing directly on this hypothesis, and it would probably be very difficult to obtain any.

However, our studies on hormone-directed transport described above suggest that, under the experimental conditions adopted, sucrose movement is not determined directly by the metabolic demand, since more than 50% of the accumulated ^{14}C activity is still in the form of ^{14}C sucrose. Thus, it is possible, from the experimental evidence already presented, that transfer from the sieve tubes into the sink tissues is an active, energy-dependent process which is under hormone control. If this hypothesis is valid, then the competitive ability of a sink will depend more directly upon its hormonal status than upon the rate of utilization of assimilates, and the effects of growth substances are only indirect. In view of the importance of sink activity and competitive ability in determining yield it is clearly of vital importance that we should fully understand their physiological basis, not only in relation to the use of growth regulators but also in designing rational breeding programs.

To obtain partition of a greater proportion of assimilates to the usable part of the plant two broad alternative strategies are possible: (1) to increase the competitive ability of the usable part or (2) to decrease the competitive abilities of other parts. It may be possible, in time, to develop techniques for applying growth stimulants specifically to the usable parts of the plant and thereby to increase their competitive ability and yield, but the immediate possibilities seem to be rather limited, and to be restricted mainly to parthenocarpic fruits. The alternative strategy is to inhibit competing sinks, as is already practiced with apples and pears by inhibiting vegetative growth with retardant and hence increasing flower initiation (Batjer et al., 1964). When we have a better understanding of the role of growth substances in assimilate partition, this in itself may suggest new types of growth retardants to be tested and new "screening" methods.

It is commonly considered that the use of growth regulators and breeding are alternative ways of achieving the same end, as in the case of the use of growth retardants or semi-dwarf varieties for reducing stem height in wheat. However, we should also consider the possible combined use of both approaches. Thus, the application of growth substances to "normal" fruits (i.e., with seeds) may not increase growth because endogenous growth substances are already present at nonlimiting levels, and the limiting factor may be the rate of DNA or protein synthesis or some other aspect of growth not directly under hormonal control. It is possible that genetic variation exists with respect to the rates of the limiting processes and that screening methods involving the application of growth regulators might reveal genotypes which would increase yield in response to applied growth substances. Certainly, there is no doubt that there is considerable intraspecific variation with respect to responses to applied growth regulators, as is well known for stem growth and for parthenocarpy with respect to gibberellins and auxin, respectively. Thus, it may be possible to breed varieties which will give, for example, larger fruits in response to applied growth substances, where there is little response in existing varieties.

REFERENCES

Batjer, L. P., Williams, M. W., and Martin, G. C., 1964, Effects of N-dimethyl amino succinamic acid (β-nine) on vegetative and fruit characteristics of apples, pears and sweet cherries, Proc. Amer. Soc. Hort. Sci., 85:11-16.

Booth, A., Moorby, J., Davies, C. R., Jones, H., and Wareing, P. F., 1962, Effects of indolyl-3-acetic acid on the movement of nutrients within plants, Nature (London), 194:204-205.

Cleland, R. E., and Rayle, D. L., 1978, Auxin, H^+-excretion and cell elongation, Bot. Mag. (Special issue), 1:125-140.

Davies, C. R., and Wareing, P. F., 1965, Auxin-induced transport of radiophosphorus in stems, Planta (Berlin), 65:139-156.

Giaquinta, R., 1977a, Possible role of pH gradient and membrane ATPase in the loading of sucrose into the sieve tubes, Nature (London), 267:369-370.

Giaquinta, R., 1977b, Phloem loading of sucrose. pH dependence and selectivity, Pl. Physiol., 59:750-755.

Glasziou, K. T., and Gayler, K., 1972, Storage of sugars in stalks of sugar cane, Bot. Rev., 38:471-490.

Hew, C. S., Nilson, C. D., and Krotkov, G., 1967, Hormonal control of translocation of photosynthetically assimilated ^{14}C in young soybean plants, Amer. J. Bot., 54:252-256.

Malek, F., and Baker, D. A., 1977, Proton co-transport of sugars in phloem loading, Planta (Berlin), 135:297-299.

Malek, F., and Baker, D. A., 1978, The effect of fusicoccin on proton co-transport of sugars in the phloem loading of Ricinus communis L., Plant Sci. Letters, 11:233-239.

Mothes, K., Engelbrecht, L., and Kulaeva, O., 1959, Über die Wirkung des Kinetins und Stickstoffverteilung und Eiweisssynthese in isiolerten Blättern, Flora (Jena), 147:445-464.

Mulligan, D. R., and Patrick, J. W., 1978, Gibberellic acid-promoted transport of assimilates in stems of Phaseolus vulgaris L., Planta (in press).

Patrick, J. W., and Wareing, P. F., 1972, "Plant Growth Substances 1970," Springer-Verlag, Berlin.

Patrick, J. W., and Wareing, P. F., 1973, Auxin-promoted transport of metabolites in stems of Phaseolus vulgaris L., J. Exp. Bot., 24:1158-1171.

Patrick, J. W., and Wareing, P. F., 1976, Auxin-promoted transport of metabolites in stems of Phaseolus vulgaris L. Effects at the site of hormone application, J. Exp. Bot., 27:969-982.

Patrick, J. W., and Wareing, P. F., 1978, Auxin-promoted transport of metabolites in stems of Phaseolus vulgaris L. Effects remote from the site of hormone application, J. Exp. Bot., 29:359-366.

Seth, A. K., and Wareing, P. F., 1967, Hormone directed transport of metabolites and its possible role in plant senescence, J. Exp. Bot., 18:67-77.

Tanner, W., Komor, E., Fenzl, F., and Decker, M., 1977, Sugar-proton cotransport systems, in: "Regulation of Cell Membrane Activities in Plants," E. Marrè and O. Ciferri, eds., North-Holland Publishing Co., Amsterdam.

Wareing, P. F., 1977, Growth substances and integration in the whole plant, Symp. Soc. Exp. Biol., 31:337-365.

18

STOMATAL APERTURE AND THE SENESCENCE OF LEAVES

Kenneth V. Thimann, Nasir Malik, and Sergio Satler

The Thimann Laboratories
University of California
Santa Cruz

The senescence of isolated leaves of the seedling of Victory oats has been under study in our laboratory for some eight years. When the leaves are detached and placed in the dark, proteolysis begins in about 6 hours and after 20-24 hours the breakdown of chlorophyll begins. By 72 hours (at 24°C) almost 60% of both the chlorophyll and the protein have disappeared (Tetley and Thimann, 1974). In white light the process is generally similar but much slower; after 72 hours in 200 foot-candles of fluorescent lights such leaves have lost only about 20% of their protein and 10% of their chlorophyll (Thimann et al., 1977). At first this delaying effect of light was ascribed to the photosynthetic production of reducing sugar, and it was found that infusing the leaves with glucose or sucrose did delay senescence, as had been reported by earlier workers (Marré et al., 1966). However, three facts mitigated against this explanation. First, the action of light reached saturation at 150 f-c, or 1500 lux, while photosynthesis is barely saturated at 10 times this intensity. Second, the concentration of glucose needed to delay senescence comparably to the effect of light was several times higher than that actually present in the leaf. Third, and most critical, DCMU[1] at 10^{-5} M totally inhibited the photosynthetic production of sugars, yet had no influence at all on the delaying effect of light. This observation not only proved that sugar formation was not the cause of the light effects but it raised acutely the problem of how light is acting.

The action of kinetin in delaying or preventing senescence in the dark had been tentatively ascribed to its tightening the coupling

[1]3-(3,4-dichlorophenyl)-1,1-dimethyl urea.

between respiration and phosphorylation, a theory with which many other observations fitted well. In parallel, then, it was suggested (Thimann et al., 1977) that the action of light could be due to cyclic photophosphorylation, which had been shown to be insensitive to DCMU, and to be saturated at much lower light intensities than photosynthesis proper (Good, 1977). We have now examined the light effect further and have encountered a surprising result.

First, additional evidence has been obtained to support the concept that phosphorylation plays a role in controlling senescence. Both methylamine and NH_3 are known to inhibit photophosphorylation (Good, 1977). The maintenance of chlorophyll after 4 days in light was about 95% of the initial value, and in the same light in the presence of 100 mM methylamine was only 45%, i.e., little more than in the dark. Ammonia had similar effects at slightly higher concentrations (Fig. 1).

Next, direct determinations of the ATP content of the leaves have been made by the luciferin-luciferase method (Strehler and McElroy, 1957; Patterson et al., 1970). Strict precautions were taken to prevent the action of ATPase by freezing the leaves in liquid nitrogen, transferring the powder to boiling water, and holding the extract frozen until measurement. The results in Table 1 show that in the dark the ATP level falls to about one-third of the initial value, while in the light it is maintained and even somewhat increased. What is more, after five days with kinetin in the dark the ATP level is twice that of the dark controls. This concentration of kinetin maintains about 75% of the chlorophyll content. Thus the

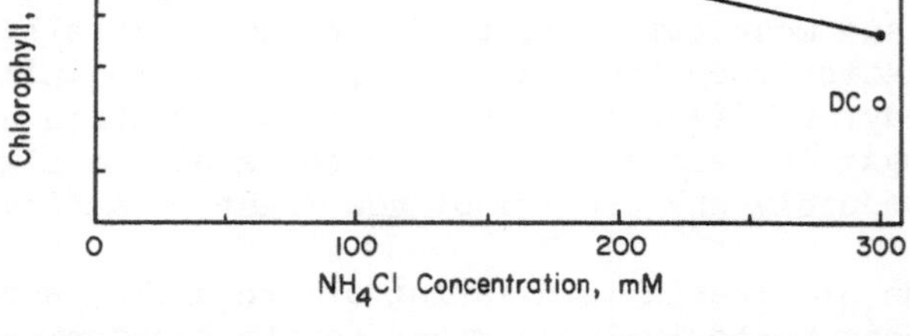

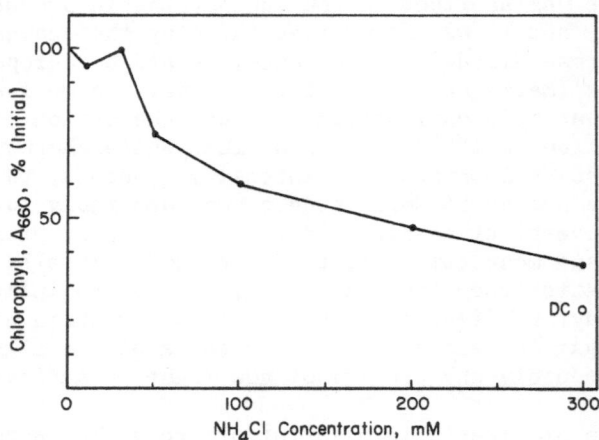

Fig. 1. Chlorophyll contents of detached oat leaves after 4 days in light on ammonium chloride solutions. DC, chlorophyll content in dark controls.

Table 1. ATP and Chlorophyll Levels in Oat Leaf Segments After 5 Days' Incubation[1]

	Initial Value	Light	Dark	Dark with Kinetin (3 ppm)
Picomoles of ATP per mg fresh weight	170	187	76	120
ATP as percent of initial	100	110	44.7	70.6
Chlorophyll A_{660}	0.861	0.776	0.080	0.641
Chlorophyll as percent of initial	100	90.2	9.3	74.4

[1]Mean of six complete experiments.

role of phosphorylation in both kinetin action and in the effect of light is supported; ATP declines in the dark, along with senescence, and it is maintained by light or by kinetin, both of which prevent senescence.

Now, however, Kasamo (1976) has reported that leaves from which the epidermis has been peeled do not senesce normally, and Kuraishi (1976) has shown that if discs from mature leaves of several dicotyledonous plants which have stomata only on one side are floated with the stomatal surface downwards, i.e., in contact with the solution, kinetin does not inhibit their senescence. This and other observations (Kuraishi and Ishikawa, 1977) led to the suggestion that cytokinins may exert their effect on senescence by opening the stomata. But substances that open and close the stomata have been known for some time and until now there has been no suggestion that they modify senescence. Some of these reagents were therefore tested on detached oat leaves in dark and light.

Phenylmercuric salts were shown to cause stomatal closing by Zelitch and Waggoner (1962). Fig. 2 shows the progress of diffusion resistance, determined by porometer, on the leaves floating on phenylmercuric nitrate in dark and in light. Controls in light evidently open their stomata wide at first and then slowly and partially close them. In the dark they remain closed for 3 days and then partially reopen. Phenylmercuric nitrate causes tight closure both in light and in dark, followed by partial reopening on the third day. The lower figure shows the changes in chlorophyll content of these leaves. In the light chlorophyll is maintained for 3 days, then decreases; in the dark it decreases steadily after

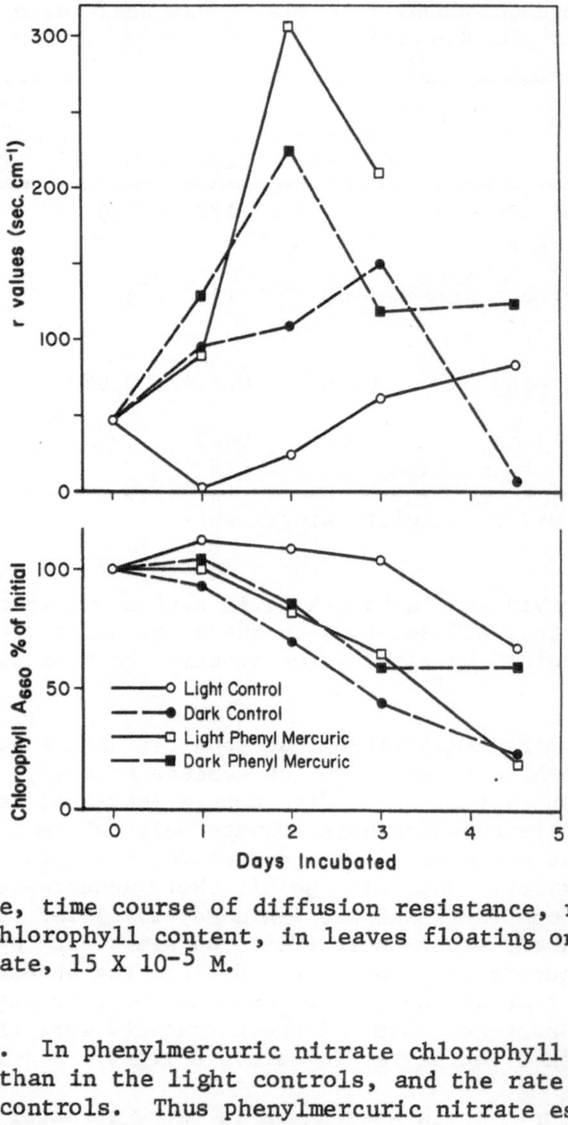

Fig. 2. Above, time course of diffusion resistance, r, and below, of chlorophyll content, in leaves floating on phenylmercuric nitrate, 15 X 10^{-5} M.

the first day. In phenylmercuric nitrate chlorophyll decreases much more rapidly than in the light controls, and the rate is close to that in dark controls. Thus phenylmercuric nitrate essentially prevents the light effect on senescence.

Abscisic acid (ABA) is also known to cause rapid stomatal closure. In our floating leaf segments the porometer rate on ABA became very slow for the first 2 days but then increased somewhat; on the average the aperture for the 4 days was nearly that of the dark controls. Table 2 shows that correspondingly the chlorophyll loss was nearly that in the dark, and proteolysis was much greater than in light, being about one-half as fast as in the dark. Sugar content in light was not influenced, which further supports the

Table 2. Analysis of 3 cm Leaf Segments of 7-Day-Old *Avena* Seedlings After 4 Days in Light (Data as Percent of the Light Control)

Treatment of Leaves	Chlorophyll	Free Amino Nitrogen	Reducing Sugar
On water in light	100.0	100	100.0
On ABA in light[1]	26.7	183	117.0
On water in dark	18.0	253	50.7
On ABA in dark[1]	28.9	139	34.9

[1]Abscisic acid 30 mg per liter.

Table 3. The Effect of Kinetin (3 mg per Liter) on Diffusion Resistance and Loss of Chlorophyll in White Light

	On Water	On Kinetin
	Diffusion Resistance, r	
Day 0	3.0	2.7
Day 1	3.2	2.0
Day 2	14.7	2.2
Day 3	20.0	2.4
Day 4	34.0	3.1
Day 5	73.0	18.0
	Chlorophyll Content, Percent of Initial	
Day 5	46.4	115.0

earlier conclusion that sugar content does not correlate with senescence.

It was seen in Fig. 2 that the stomata tend to close slowly after 2 days in light. The action of kinetin on senescence is additive to that of light (Thimann et al., 1977). Is it additive in its effect on stomatal aperture? Table 3 shows that kinetin at 3 ppm maintains full opening in light for 4 days; r values of about 2 are maximal. The chlorophyll content is correspondingly fully maintained and even increased over the initial value. Fig. 3

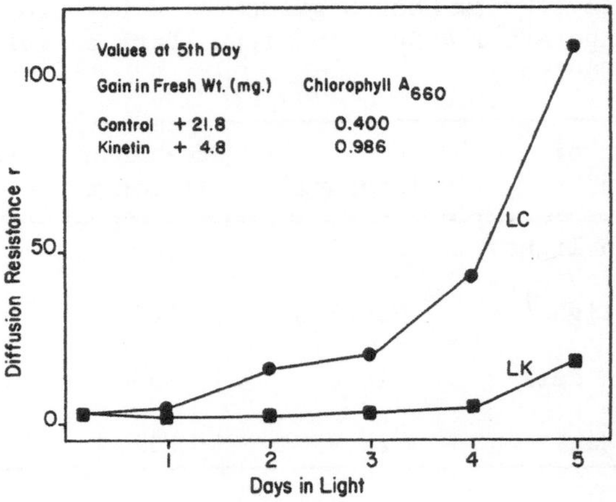

Fig. 3. Time course of diffusion resistance, r, in leaves floating on kinetin, 3 ppm (LK), and controls (LC), both in white light throughout.

presents these values and also shows (data on fig.) that the wide-open stomata decrease the normal gain in wieght due to water uptake.

Determination of mean stomatal opening by diffusion porometer calls for comment because porometer readings have sometimes been considered inferior to direct observation, but the long narrow stomata of the Gramineae make such direct observation very difficult in oat leaves. In addition, the opening, in some leaves at least, is not rectilinear, so that quantitation of the opening would be virtually impossible from direct measurements (cf. Shiraishi et al., 1978).

The above experiments on leaves in the light have been supplemented by experiments with stomatal opening in the dark. Turner and Graniti (1969) found fusicoccin to cause opening in the dark. Fig. 4 confirms this and shows that fusicoccin (kindly given by Prof. E. Marré of Milan University) maintains maximal opening for 2 days in darkness. Strikingly, at 100 ppm it correspondingly maintains the chlorophyll at nearly the level of controls in light. The dashed lines show also that the level of free amino acids, i.e., the proteolysis typical of senescence in the dark, is greatly decreased.

Kinetin, which classically maintains chlorophyll and prevents proteolysis in the dark, has also been reported by several workers to open stomata, and again we have repeatedly confirmed this on our own material.

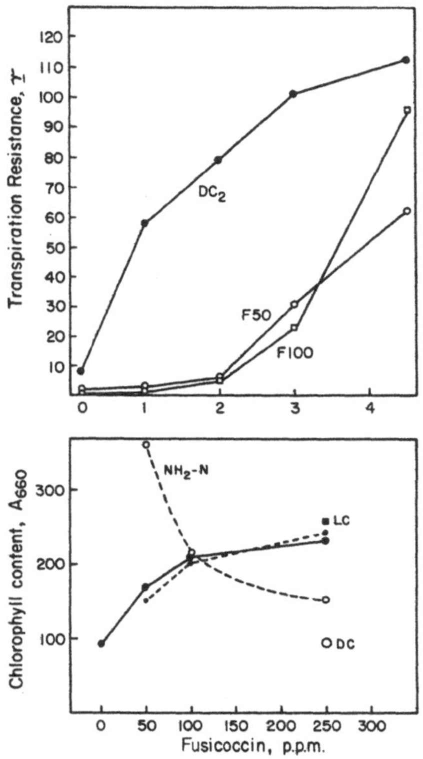

Fig. 4. Above, time course of diffusion resistance, r, of leaves kept for 4 days in the dark with and without fusicoccin at 50 and 100 ppm. Below, chlorophyll content (closed circles) and free amino acid content (open circles) after the fourth day in the dark, as function of fusicoccin concentration. LC and DC, chlorophyll contents in light and dark controls, respectively.

Senescence and stomatal aperture are thus closely parallel, in light and in dark, with four different reagents of unrelated chemical nature, two causing opening and two causing closing. Which is cause and which is effect remains to be seen. And, if the action of photophosphorylation is borne out too, as seems clear, then the three processes, senescence, transpiration, and photophosphorylation, will appear as interconnected parts of the same syndrome.

ACKNOWLEDGMENT

This research was supported in part by a grant (PCM 768-3126) from the National Science Foundation, USA.

REFERENCES

Good, N. E., 1977, Uncoupling of electron transport from phosphorylation in chlorplasts, in: "Encyclopedia of Plant Physiology," new series, Vol. V, Photosynthesis, A. Trebst and V. Avron, eds., Springer-Verlag, Berlin and New York.

Kasamo, K., 1976, The role of the epidermis in kinetin-induced retardation of chlorophyll degradation in tobacco leaf discs during senescence, Plant and Cell Physiol., 17:1297-1307.

Kuraishi, S., 1976, Ineffectiveness of cytokinin-induced chlorophyll retention in hypostomatous leaf discs, Plant and Cell Physiol., 17:875-885.

Kuraishi, S., and Ishikawa, F., 1977, Relationship between transpiration and amino acid accumulation in Brassica leaf discs treated with cytokinins and fusicoccin, Plant and Cell Physiol., 18:1273-1279.

Marré, E., Schwendiman, M., and Lado, P., 1966, Ricerche sull'invecchiamento in foglie recise. I. Effetto protettivo degli zuccheri e della luce sui sistemi fotosintetico e respiratorio de foglie recise di Solanum tuberosum, Rend. classe sci. fis. mat. e nat. (Acad. dei Lincei), ser. #8, 40: 1089-1094.

Patterson, J. W., Brezonik, P. L., and Putnam, H. D., 1970, Measurement and significance of ATP in activated sludge, Env. Sci. and Tech., 4:569-575.

Shiraishi, M., Hashimoto, Y., and Kuraishi, S., 1978, Cyclic variations of stomatal aperture observed under the scanning electron microscope, Plant and Cell Physiol., 19:637-645.

Strehler, B. L., and McElroy, W. D., 1957, Assay of ATP, in: "Methods in Enzymology," Vol. 3, S. P. Colowick and N. O. Kaplan, eds., Academic Press, New York.

Tetley, R. M., and Thimann, K. V., 1974, The metabolism of oat leaves during senescence. I. Respiration, carbohydrate metabolism and the action of cytokinins, Plant Physiol., 54:294-303.

Thimann, K. V., Tetley, R. M., and Krivak, B. M., 1977, The metabolism of oat leaves during senescence. V. Senescence in light, Plant Physiol., 59:448-454.

Turner, N. C., and Graniti, A., 1969, Fusicoccin, a fungal toxin that opens stomata, Nature, 223:1070-1071.

Zelitch, I., and Waggoner, P. E., 1962, Effect of chemical control of stomata on transpiration and photosynthesis, Proc. Nat. Acad. Sci., USA, 48:1101-1108, 1297-1299.

19

MODERN CHROMATOGRAPHIC METHODS FOR THE IDENTIFICATION AND QUANTIFICATION OF PLANT GROWTH REGULATORS AND THEIR APPLICATION TO STUDIES OF THE CHANGES IN HORMONAL SUBSTANCES IN WINTER WHEAT DURING ACCLIMATION TO COLD STRESS CONDITIONS

Frank Wightman

Carleton University
Ottawa, Ontario, Canada

ABSTRACT

The early development and recent use of gas-liquid chromatography (GLC) and high performance liquid chromatography (HPLC) for the qualitative and quantitative analysis of growth regulators in plant extracts is reviewed in this paper. It will be shown how recent improvements in both GLC and HPLC procedures which give excellent separation of the different growth regulators in ether, ethyl acetate, and butanol extracts, when combined wherever possible with the use of gas chromatography-mass spectrometry for conclusive identification of each growth regulator, now provide plant physiologists with modern techniques for carrying out rapid qualitative and quantitative analyses of the growth regulators found in extracts from plants taken at different stages in their growth and development, or at different stages in their response to changing environmental conditions. In a final section of the paper, the application of analytical GLC techniques to studies of the changes in growth regulating substances in two varieties of winter wheat during acclimation of the tissues to cold temperature conditions will be described.

INTRODUCTION

The qualitative and quantitative determination of endogenous plant growth regulators has for many years been a time-consuming, multi-step process. It has usually involved lengthy extraction and solvent purification procedures, followed by paper or thin-layer chromatography to separate the growth regulators, which are then tentatively identified by chromogenic reagents, or quantitatively determined by bioassay techniques. Such lengthy procedures, however, frequently result in appreciable losses during solvent fractionation and chromatography which have not always been taken into account in the final quantitative estimates. Furthermore, many of the chromogenic procedures and bioassay tests employed are only generally specific for the class of growth regulator under investigation and do not differentiate between individual compounds within any one group of naturally occurring substances. For these reasons, then, it has been virtually impossible to conduct a well-replicated study involving the analysis of several growth regulators in extracts of plants taken at various stages of development. Consequently, many studies have been made in which only one type of growth regulator, such as 3-indolylacetic acid (IAA), abscisic acid (ABA), or zeatin, has been measured during certain phases of plant development, and this has led to attempts to explain growth regulation or other physiological processes in terms of changing levels of the one growth substance which has been analyzed. Current views suggest, however, that the regulation of plant development is not controlled by any single substance, but rather by sequential changes in the activity of several regulatory substances, which is probably related to their changing concentrations. If this is the case, then rapid and sensitive methods of analysis are clearly required to investigate reliably the changing amounts of the different growth regulators in a plant at various stages of growth and development.

Development of new forms of liquid chromatography, namely gas-liquid chromatography (GLC) and high performance liquid chromatography (HPLC), now provide rapid and highly sensitive methods for analyzing the many growth regulators present in plants. This article will review the early use of these modern chromatographic techniques in quantitative studies examining the role of individual growth regulators in certain phases of plant development, and will show how recent improvements in both GLC and HPLC procedures now provide plant physiologists, for the first time, with the opportunity of carrying out rapid qualitative and quantitative analyses of the many growth regulators present in extracts from plants taken at different stages of development. It should be emphasized, however, that the identification of growth regulators based solely on co-chromatography with authentic compounds during GLC or HPLC separations can only be regarded as provisional. Although both these methods are excellent separatory procedures and have detector systems that are highly sensitive to most growth regulating substances, more rigorous chemical characterization is still required to provide conclusive proof of the presence of each regulator substance in a plant extract, and this can best be achieved by combined gas chromatography-mass spectrometry (GC-MS) (Gaskin and MacMillan, 1978). Unfortunately, the capital cost of a GC-MS system is beyond the financial resources of most plant physiologists, but whenever access to such a facility is possible, the provisional identification of different growth regulators in a plant extract by GLC or HPLC analyses based on co-chromatography with authentic compounds should be confirmed at some stage in the work by GC-MS.

At the same time, it should be recognized that while conclusive identification of the growth regulators in a plant extract is a desirable aim, much of our present day understanding of the physiological and biochemical action of plant growth regulators has come over the last 25 years from the examination of plant extracts using only paper or thin-layer chromatography in combination with chromogenic and bioassay techniques. While these older separatory methods now appear to some plant physiologists/biochemists to leave much to be desired in terms of reliable identification of the growth regulators under study, nevertheless, where careful chromatographic and bioassay examination has been made of the changes in amounts of one or more growth regulators during growth and development, and especially when ^{14}C-labeled precursors have been employed in biochemical studies, much valuable information has been obtained on the metabolism and probable physiological roles of the various growth regulators. Indeed, with very few exceptions, the recent reexamination of some of the known hormone-regulated growth processes employing GC-MS analysis of plant extracts has not shown the earlier chromatographic data and conclusions on the nature of the growth regulator involved to be wrong.

There is therefore good reason to conclude that while rigorous chemical identification of each growth regulator present in a growing plant, or plant organ, is a desirable biochemical aim, careful time-course studies of the changing levels of the main growth regulators in a developing leaf or fruit, for example, is also equally desirable if we are to obtain a better understanding of the possible sequential control these substances may exert on the physiological processes associated with growth and development. If such investigations must be performed without the help of a GC-MS facility, then providing the GLC or HPLC analytical methods employed are very selective for each growth regulator, as can be achieved for example when temperature programming procedures are used with GLC, combined with different forms of derivatization of the plant extract and the use of different detector systems, then studies of this kind while only providing provisional identification of the different growth regulators can still yield much useful information on the hormonal regulation of plant growth and development.

GAS-LIQUID CHROMATOGRAPHY OF THE GROWTH REGULATOR IN PLANT EXTRACTS

Early work exploring the possible use of gas-liquid chromatography for the purification of plant extracts prior to identification and quantification of the indole constituents by spectrophotofluorimetry was reported in the same year by Stowe and Schilke (1964) and Powell (1964). The work of Stowe and Schilke clearly demonstrated the potential of these two physico-chemical techniques for the separation and identification of sub-microgram amounts of authentic samples of a range of indole compounds known to occur in plants, and Powell's investigations showed how the two procedures could be used to analyze the indole auxins present in acidic and neutral methylene chloride extracts of homogenized maize seeds and cabbage heads. Powell's gas chromatographic results showed the presence of 3-indolylacetic acid (IAA) in maize seeds and of 3-indolylacetonitrile (IAN) in cabbage tissue, which confirmed the findings of earlier workers who used classical chemical techniques for isolating these two indole auxins from much larger amounts of tissue (Berger and Avery, 1944; Jones et al., 1952). Although investigations of the best column substrates for optimum gas chromatography of indolic methyl esters were later reported by Stowe and coworkers (Grunwald et al., 1967; Grunwald et al., 1968), it was several more years before further gas chromatographic studies were made to demonstrate the occurence of IAA in growing root and shoot tissues, and in many of the more recent studies, identification of IAA was conclusively demonstrated by combined GC-MS.

In view of its relatively high melting point, IAA must first be converted to a more volatile derivative before GLC analysis. The choice of derivative depends on the nature of the detector system employed in the gas chromatograph. The IAA derivative used by Stowe and Powell in their early work and still widely used today is the methyl ester of IAA (Me-IAA) obtained by reacting IAA (or extract containing IAA) with an ethereal solution of diazomethane, when methylation occurs at the carboxyl group (Schlenk and Gellerman, 1960). This ester is readily detected in the GC-column effluent by a flame ionization detector (FID), which is the most widely used detector system because it has sensitivity limits approaching 1 ng for almost all organic compounds. This ester was used in the identification of IAA in maize seeds (Powell, 1964), in tobacco shoots (Bayer, 1969), and in flower buds, flowers, and fruits of daffodil (Edelbluth and Kaldewey, 1976), where identification was based on co-chromatography with authentic Me-IAA and spectrophotofluorimetry. Me-IAA was also employed for identifying IAA in maize roots (Elliott and Greenwood, 1974) and in shoots of Douglass fir (DeYoe and Zaerr, 1976) using GC-MS procedures.

A more sensitive GC-detector is the electron-capture detector (ECD), but since it only responds to substances that readily capture electrons, when used for IAA detection it is necessary to convert any IAA present in a sample, after methylation, to a halogenated derivative. Fluorinated derivatives of Me-IAA have proved suitable for ECD analysis and the procedure has been shown to have a lower limit of sensitivity of approximately 100 pg. Fluorination occurs at the imino group of IAA, and Seeley and Powell (1974) utilized both heptafluorobutyryl (HFB) and trifluoroacetyl (TFA) derivatives of Me-IAA for demonstrating the presence of IAA in apple seeds. Rivier and Pilet (1974) used the HFB derivative of Me-IAA to identify IAA by mass fragmentography in the cap and apical tissues of maize roots, whereas Hopping and Bukovac (1975) produced the TFA ester of Me-IAA for their GC-MS identification of IAA in *Prunus* fruits.

Trimethylsilyl (TMS) esters of IAA have been used successfully in the GLC detection of IAA by FID. This ester is formed by the reaction of IAA with a silylating agent, usually *bis*-trimethylsilylacetamide (BSA) or *bis*-(trimethylsilyl) fluoroacetamide (BSTFA), and silylation occurs at both the carboxyl and imino groups (Fig. 1). The *bis*-TMS ester has been used extensively in both GLC and GC-MS analyses of IAA, particularly so in work reported over the last five years. It was first employed by Bridges et al. (1973) in their identification and localization of IAA in the primary root of maize seedlings and by Bandurski and Schulze (1974, 1977) in their GC-MS identification of IAA in the seed and shoot tissues of a range of cereal, legume, and other plants. Similarly, *bis*-TMS-IAA was the derivative used to demonstrate IAA in the phloem sap of castor bean plants (Hall and Medlow, 1974), in cotton ovules (Shindy and Smith, 1975), in the shoots and lateral buds of kidney bean seedlings (White et al., 1975; Hillman et al., 1977), and in lettuce seeds (Robertson et al., 1976). In all the above studies on IAA, the choice of derivative used was most probably related to the type of detector system employed, and to convenience of preparation. Although production of the *bis*-TMS derivative using BSTFA is the simplest method of esterification and results in a stable product, formation of the methyl ester using diazomethane often gives more consistent results when many samples are being analyzed for IAA. The main problem encountered in preparing TMS derivatives is the occasional incomplete drying of the extract prior to silylation; a slight trace of water will lead to solidification of the reaction mixture and gradual destruction of the derivative. A possible disadvantage of using methylation as the derivatization procedure is that Me-IAA has been shown to be present in citrus fruit extracts (Takahashi et al., 1975), and hence estimations of IAA in total methanol or acetone plant extracts, based on methylated IAA, might not allow for a contribution from the naturally occurring ester. However, if estimates of free IAA are determined from acidic ether or ethyl acetate fractions of the original plant extract, then any natural Me-IAA present could easily be removed from the original extract by first partitioning with ether at neutral pH. At the same time, it should be pointed out that except for the work of Takahashi et al. (1975), no other investigations including many carried out in my laboratory have reported any evidence for the presence of Me-IAA as a naturally occurring constituent of plant extracts.

With regard to the isolation and provisional identification of other auxin substances in plants by GLC, Bayer (1969) was the first to report the presence of 3-indolylpropionic acid (IPA) in tobacco

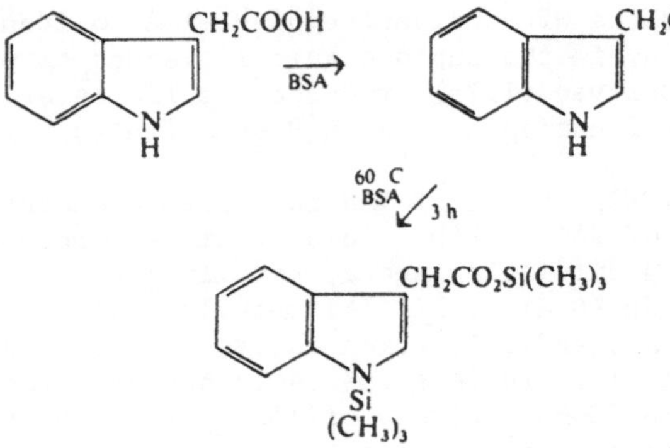

Fig. 1. Derivatization of IAA using the silylating reagent, BSA, to produce the bis-TMSi ester (from McDougall and Hillman, 1978b)

shoot extracts and this finding has been confirmed in my laboratory in a detailed GLC-study, employing both methylated and silylated derivatives, of the auxin substances present in developing tobacco leaves (Wightman, 1977). This investigation simultaneously revealed the presence of 3-indolylacrylic acid (IAcA) and phenylacetic acid (PAA) in tobacco leaves and also demonstrated the presence of PAA in appreciable amounts in ether extracts from a range of shoot tissues, which fully confirmed earlier results from biosynthetic studies in my laboratory demonstrating the conversion of L-phenylalanine-3-^{14}C to phenylacetic acid-^{14}C in shoots from the same range of plants (Wightman, 1973; Wightman and Rauthan, 1974). Although the auxin, 4-chlorindolylacetic acid, and its methyl ester were first identified in immature pea seeds by TLC procedures followed by infrared, NMR, and mass spectrometry (Marumo et al., 1968a,b, 1971), the natural occurrence of the methyl ester of this highly active auxin in developing pea seeds harvested from plants grown in water culture containing radioactive chloride has recently been conclusively demonstrated by Engvild et al. (1978) using combined GC-MS.

In many of the gas chromatographic studies so far described, the prime emphasis of the investigation was the purification and rigorous demonstration of the occurrence of IAA in the seeds or vegetative tissue under examination. Although quantitative data were also usually reported, based on ion monitoring when GC-MS was used or the isotope dilution technique of Bandurski and Schulze (1974), little or no attempt was made in most of these studies to investigate changes in the level of IAA or other auxin substances during the subsequent growth and development of the plant organ under study. Two recent exceptions are the GLC and GC-MS investigations by Hillman et al. (1977) on the changing level of IAA in developing lateral buds of kidney bean shoots in relation to the mechanism of apical dominance, and the examination by analytical GLC of the changing levels of several auxin substances in tobacco leaves during their growth and development (Wightman, 1977) as shown in Fig. 2.

Although IAA was the first natural growth regulator to be investigated by gas chromatography, much of the early use of this sensitive analytical procedure in growth regulator research centered around the work of MacMillan and coworkers on the separation and identification of the gibberellins in plant extracts (Cavell et al., 1967; MacMillan, 1968; Crozier et al., 1971). These early GLC studies of plant gibberellins were primarily concerned with the careful purification and chemical identification of the gibberellin under investigation and consistent with this chemical approach,

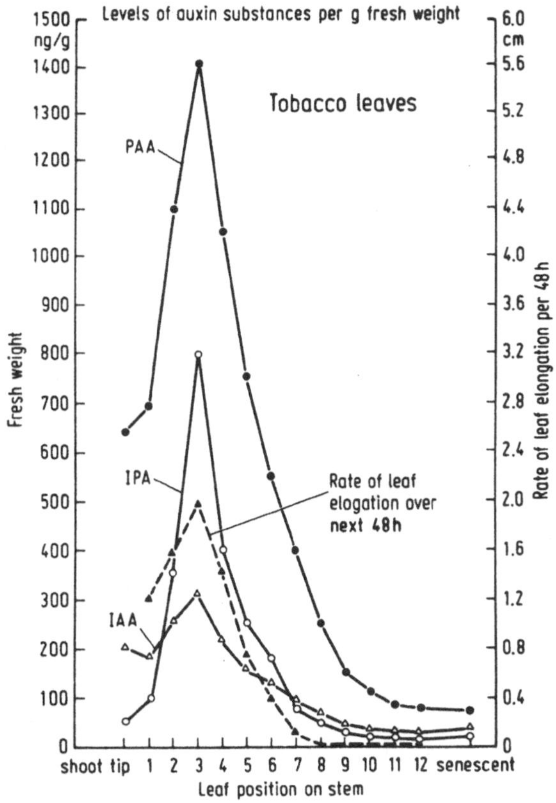

Fig. 2. Changes in endogenous levels of 3-indolylacetic acid (IAA), 3-indolylpropionic acid (IPA), and phenylacetic acid (PAA) in tobacco leaves at different stages of development; as determined by analytical GLC examination of acidic ether extracts using temperature programming procedures and co-chromatography with authentic standards (from Wightman, 1977).

MacMillan and coworkers pioneered the development of combined gas chromatography-mass spectrometry (GC-MS) for the rigorous characterization of gibberellins and other growth regulators in plant extracts (MacMillan, 1968, 1972; Gaskin and MacMillan, 1968; Bowen et al., 1973; Gaskin et al., 1973; Frydman et al., 1974). GC-MS provides the conclusive chemical identification that is lacking when GLC alone is used for analyzing a plant extract since by mass spectrometry, it is possible to identify a compound by virtue of its molecular weight and characteristic fragmentation pattern. When this procedure is combined with gas chromatography, the effluent from the GC column is led into the source of the mass spectrometry and any compound present in the effluent is then ionized and the ions rapidly analyzed to provide the mass spectrum for the compound. In some instruments, a portion of the ions is intercepted before analysis to provide a total ion current (TIC) profile, which is a measure of the amount of compound in the source at any given time and corresponds to the more conventional methods of GLC detection such as flame ionization. In other instruments, the TIC data is collected and processed directly by a computer to give the mass spectrum in the form of a line diagram where intensities of the ions are expressed as percentages either of the most intense peak (base peak) or of the total ion current. To obtain an identifiable mass spectrum the minimum amount of compound in the column effluent can vary between 50 ng and 50 pg, depending upon the sensitivity of the mass spectrometry to the type of compound under analysis.

A typical mass spectrum obtained by the GC-MS procedure is that given by the bis-trimethylsilyl ester of IAA, shown in Fig. 3. The fragmentation pattern consists of the molecular ion (M^+) occurring at m/e 319, the base ion at m/e 202, and other ions occurring at m/e 304, 130, and 73. Characterization of this compound in a silylated plant extract by GC-MS can be made either by obtaining a full scan showing the detailed fragmentation pattern of the compound (and this will probably include some interfering ions), or by multiple ion monitoring where only 3 or 4 prominent ions of the compound are monitored, along with the GC retention time of the compound.

The application of GC-mass fragmentography to the quantitative analysis of the different growth regulators in a plant extract is still in its infancy although it has been used successfully to determine the levels of four gibberellins in maturing pea seeds (Frydman et al., 1974), of IAA in lateral buds and shoot tissues of *Phaseolus vulgaris* (Hillman et al., 1977; McDougall and Hillman, 1978a), of both IAA and ABA in the root cap and apical tissues of maize roots (Rivier and Pilet, 1974; Rivier et al., 1977), and of GA_4 and GA_9 (gibberellins) in wheat chloroplasts (Browning and Saunders, 1977). Such quantitative determinations have usually been achieved by comparing the peak height of the base ion (single peak monitoring) with a calibration curve constructed by plotting the amount of the authentic substance injected as a function of the peak

Table 1. Average Values for the IAA and ABA Content of Different Regions of the Maize Root as Determined by Mass Fragmentography (from Rivier and Pilet, 1974; Rivier et al., 1977)

Root Sections from the Tip (mm)	Number of Sections in Each Extract	Number of Replicate Extracts	Fresh Weight (mg/section)	Dry Weight (mg/section)	IAA (μg)		ABA (μg)	
					Kg^{-1} Fresh Weight	g^{-1} Dry Weight	Kg^{-1} Fresh Weight	g^{-1} Dry Weight
I: <0.05 (root cap)	1,000	2	0.263	0.035	356.6	2.67	36.1	0.27
II: 0.05–1.0 (meristem)	1,000	2	0.370	0.058	179.9	1.16	66.5	0.43
III: 1.0–4.0 (region of cell elongation)	500	4	4.122	0.561	76.5	0.56	33.3	0.25
IV: 4.0–10.0 (region of cell elongation)	250–400	5	8.858	0.695	114.8	1.46	24.9	0.32

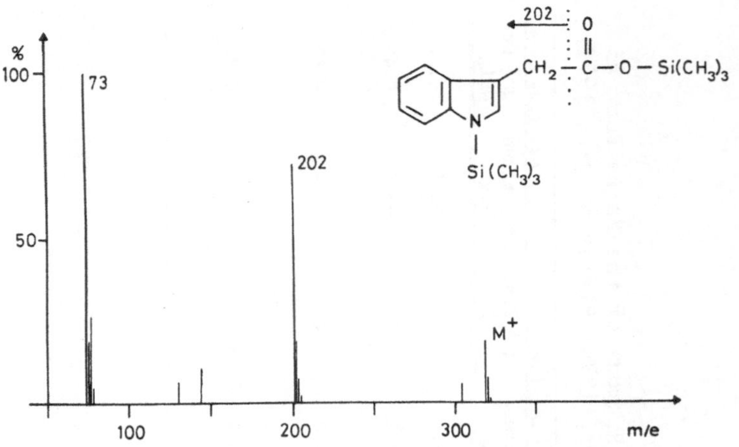

Fig. 3. Mass spectrum of the bis-trimethylsilyl ester of IAA.

height of the base ion, which normally results in a linear calibration curve. Quantitative estimations based on multiple peak height monitoring can be carried out in the same manner using calibration curves constructed for each of the ion peaks used in the analysis. The few quantitative studies so far carried out using GC-mass fragmentography have certainly produced interesting results, such as the evidence for the involvement of GA_9, GA_{17}, GA_{20}, and GA_{29} in the embryogenesis of pea seeds as reported by Frydman et al. (1974) (Fig. 4), the differing levels of IAA and ABA in the root cap and apical tissues of maize roots (Table 1) as shown by Rivier and coworkers (1974, 1977), and the surprising rise in IAA levels in lateral buds of Phaseolus seedlings after removal of the shoot apex (Table 2) revealed by the investigations of Hillman et al. (1977). This latter interesting finding contrasts strikingly with previous views on the nature of the hormonal mechanism underlying the inhibition of lateral bud development by the apical bud.

The natural occurrence of the growth inhibitor substance abscisic acid (ABA) has also received extensive study by GLC procedures and some of the most convincing early demonstrations on the use of this excellent separatory technique for growth regulator analysis came from investigations on the levels of ABA in dormant shoot and fruit extracts. Thus, Saunders and coworkers were the first to demonstrate the detection of ABA in xylem sap from willow shoots by GLC (Lenton et al., 1968) and this report was soon followed by the GLC-identification of ABA in cotton fruits by Davis et al. (1968) and by the conclusive identification of the inhibitor in crude plant extracts using combined GC-MS (Gaskin and MacMillan, 1968). Although ECDs have been most frequently used in the identification of ABA in shoot, leaf, and bud extracts because of

Table 2. Endogenous IAA Levels of *Phaseolus* Lateral Buds in Axils of Primary Leaves. Decapitation was Performed 24 Hours Prior to Harvesting. Total Dry Weights of Tissue Harvested per Treatment Are Given in Brackets (from Hillman et al., 1977)

Experiment Number	Age of Plants (days)	Number per Treatment	GC-MS Method*	μg IAA g^{-1} Dry Weight		pg IAA Bud^{-1}	
				Intact	Decapitated	Intact	Decapitated
1	18	2,500	SIM	0.08 (0.18)	0.13 (0.15)	2.9	3.9
2	18	5,000	SIM	0.06 (1.8)	0.14 (2.1)	10.8	29.4
3	20	1,500	SIM	0.02 (0.5)	0.03 (0.6)	3.3	6.0
4	20	1,500	SIM	0.02 (0.75)	0.03 (1.3)	5.0	13.0
5	25	1,500	SIM	0.04 (0.6)	0.13 (0.6)	8.0	26.0
6	25	2,000	MPM	0.06 (0.55)	0.08 (0.75)	8.2	15.0

*SIM = base ion monitoring; MPM = molecular ion monitoring.

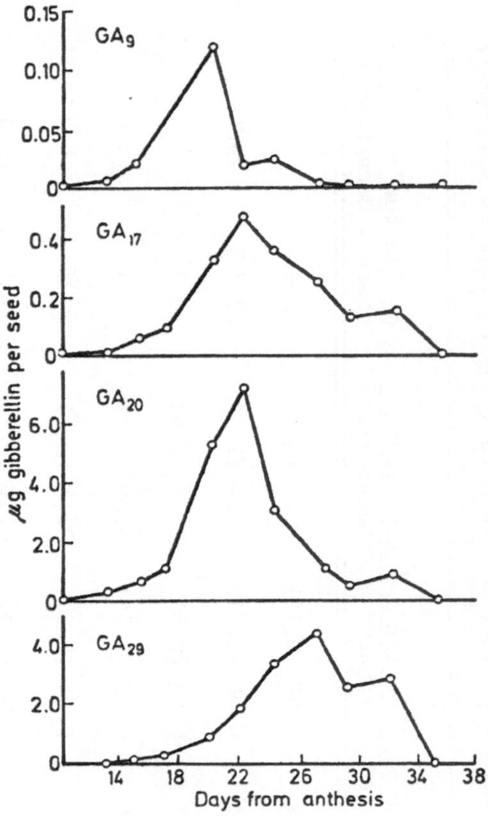

Fig. 4. Changes in endogenous levels of GA_9, GA_{17}, GA_{20}, and GA_{29} during embryogenesis of pea seeds (var. Progress No. 9); as determined by GC-MS and GC-SICM examination of selected fractions from TLC-purified acidic ethyl acetate extracts. Note differing scales on ordinates (from Frydman et al., 1974).

their high sensitivity to Me-ABA (e.g., Seeley and Powell, 1970; Mizrahi et al., 1971; Zabadal, 1974; Loveys and Kriedemann, 1974; Loveys et al., 1974; Harrison and Saunders, 1975; Beardsell and Cohen, 1975; Harrison and Walton, 1975; Loveys, 1977; Quarrie, 1978), other GLC investigations of ABA have successfully employed FIDs (e.g., Davis et al., 1968; Lenton et al., 1968, 1971, 1972). We have found the dual heated FIDs in our Pye Series 104 Gas Chromatograph to be highly sensitive to ng amounts of Me-ABA, just as they are to similar trace quantities of the methyl- or TMS-esters of other known endogenous growth regulators (Wightman, 1977; Phipps and Wightman, 1977).

The methyl ester of ABA (Me-ABA) is the derivative most frequently used in GLC and GC-MS studies since methylation of ABA-containing extracts using diazomethane has consistently given reliable results, whereas silylation of similar extracts has sometimes failed to esterify the ABA or produced a variable amount of products (Saunders, 1978). Moreover, the methyl ester of the naturally occurring cis,trans-isomer of ABA (cis-Me-ABA) can be readily converted to its trans,trans-geometrical isomer (2,trans-Me-ABA) by simply subjecting the methylated extract to 3-4 hr of UV irradiation. Since the trans,trans-isomer does not occur naturally, or only in very small amounts, UV irradiation of a methylated extract leads to the establishment of an equilibrium mixture containing approximately equal amounts of the two isomers, which can be readily separated by GLC (Lenton et al., 1971). Application of this simple isomerization procedure followed by further GLC examination of the extract provides good confirmation that the peak provisionally identified as Me-ABA during the initial GLC analysis involving co-chromatography with authentic cis-Me-ABA is indeed the peak due to the presence of cis-Me-ABA in the extract. This UV irradiation procedure was first employed successfully by Lenton and coworkers in their quantitative analysis of ABA in birch shoots, lemon and yew fruits (Lenton et al., 1971) (Fig. 5), and in their examination of the ABA content of birch, maple, and sycamore plants in relation to photoperiodically induced bud dormancy (Lenton et al., 1972). At the same time, full confirmation of the identity of the presumptive Me-ABA peak in many of the extracts used in these investigations was obtained by GC-MS.

The demonstration by Wright and Hiron (1969, 1972) that there is a striking increase in ABA levels in leaves during a period of wilting stimulated many studies during the early 1970s examining the relationship between ABA metabolism and leaf water status under stress conditions. In many of these investigations the changes in ABA levels were determined by GLC analysis of leaf extracts using the very sensitive EC detector system (Mizrahi et al., 1971; Zabadal, 1974; Beardsell and Cohen, 1975; Harrison and Walton, 1975). Other more recent studies of changes in endogenous levels of ABA using both GLC and combined GC-MS for conclusive identification of the Me-ABA are those of McWha and Hillman (1974) examining the role of ABA in the regulation of lettuce seed germination, of Loveys and Kriedemann (1974) on the effect of environmental stress factors and fruit excision on the hormone physiology of grape leaf tissue (Fig. 6), of Loveys (1977) to determine the intracellular location of ABA in water-stressed and non-stressed leaf tissue (Table 3), and of Zeevaart (1977) investigating the levels of ABA synthesis and metabolism in the shoot apex and leaves of castor bean plants (Fig. 7). The most recent study on ABA analysis involving GLC is that by Quarrie (1978), who describes a rapid TLC purification of leaf extracts followed by isothermal GLC using a highly selective EC detector. Quantification of the ABA was achieved by reference

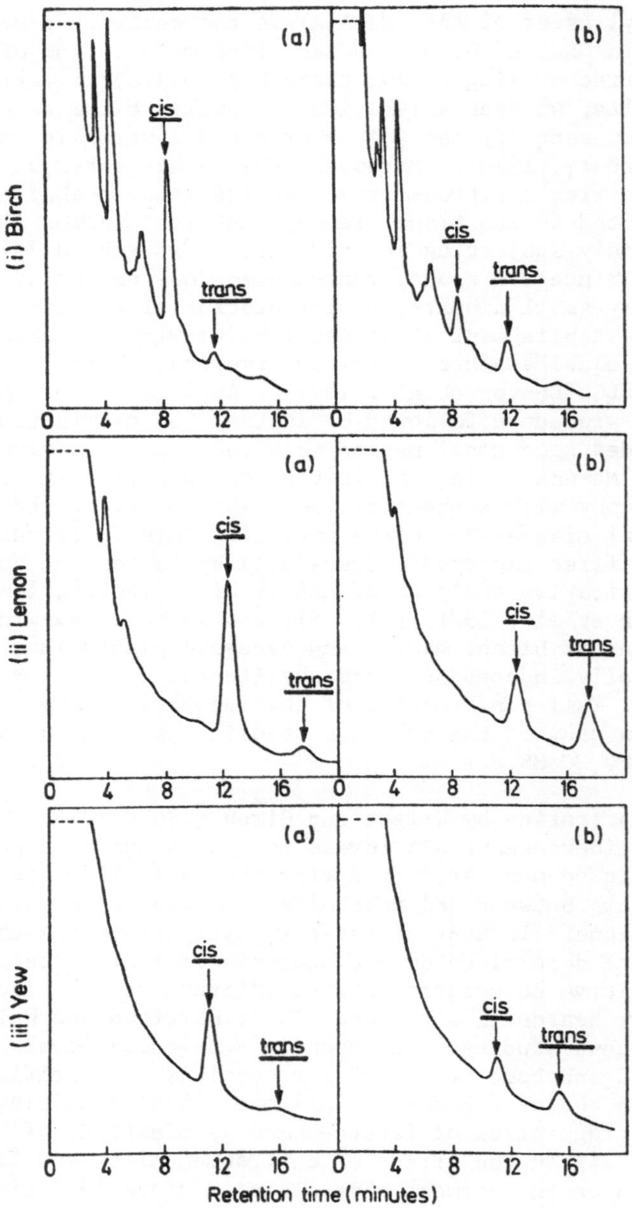

Fig. 5. Gas chromatograms of purified and methylated fractions from (i) birch shoots, (ii) lemon fruit, and (iii) yew arils. Samples were chromatographed on columns of 2% Epon 1001 at about 210°C before irradiation (a) and after irradiation (b) with UV light. Arrows indicate peaks corresponding to authentic methyl 2-cis-abscisate and methyl 2-trans-abscisate (from Lenton et al., 1971).

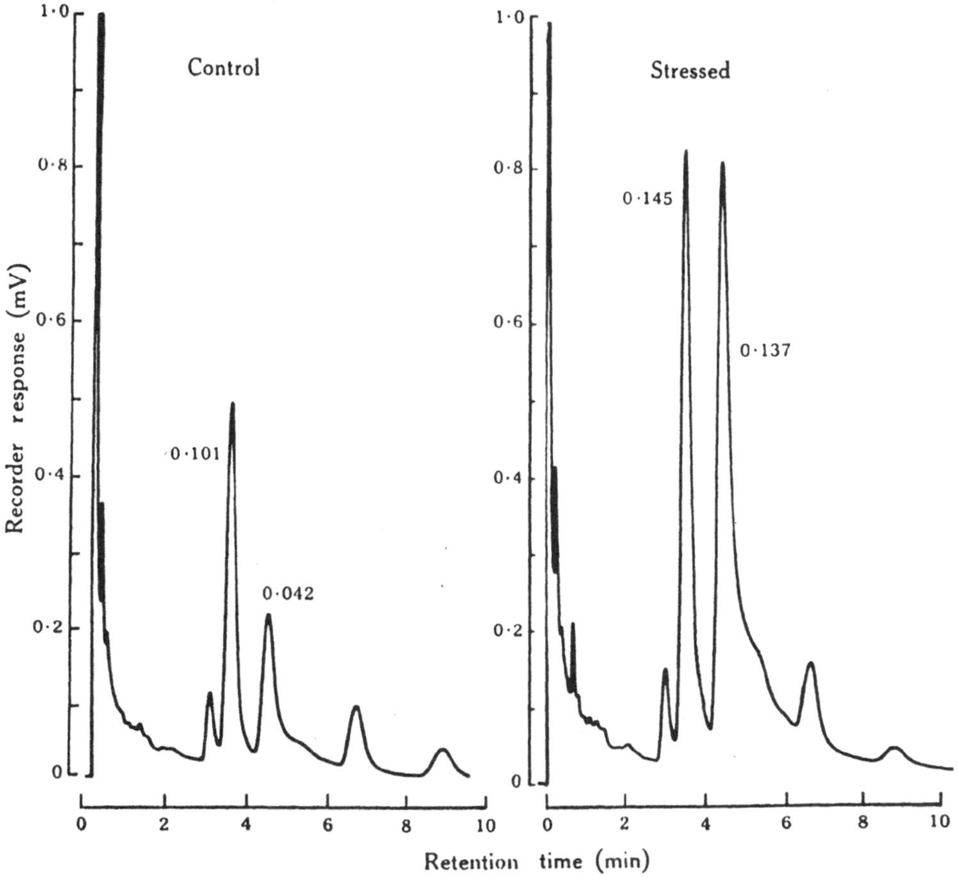

Fig. 6. Gas chromatograms of extracts from control and partly desiccated grape leaves (Vitis vinifera L.). Retention times were: methyl abscisate, 3.5 min; methyl phaseate, 4.5 min. Values alongside each peak show the calculated concentration of each compound, in mg per kg of fresh tissue; phaseic acid levels are expressed in terms of abscisic acid equivalent (from Loveys and Kriedemann, 1974).

to an internal standard of authentic ethyl abscisate added to the TLC-purified extract prior to its derivatization for GLC analysis.

The first report of the successful use of gas chromatography for the identification of cytokinins in plant extracts was made by Most et al. (1968), who showed that the TMS-derivatives of isopentyladenine (2iP), dihydrozeatin, zeatin, isopentenyladenosine (2iPA), and zeatin riboside (ZR) will separate very well on a column

Table 3. ABA Content of Intact Leaves and Chloroplasts Prepared from Stressed and Non-Stressed Spinach. The Plants Were Stressed by Exposing Their Roots to 500 mM Mannitol for 4 Hours Before Chloroplast Isolation (from Loveys, 1977)

Treatment	Intact Leaves ng/mg Chlorophyll	Chloroplasts ng/mg Chlorophyll	Chloroplasts % of ABA in Chloroplasts
Non-Stressed	*14.9 ± 1.1	*14.4 ± 1.1	96.6
Stressed	**161.5 ± 9.6	**24.6 ± 3.2	15.2

*Mean of six determinations ± SE.

**Mean of three determinations ± SE.

of 3% SE-52 using temperature programming procedures. Flame ionization detectors were used and the limit of detection was approximately 5 ng. This report was soon followed by the GLC analysis of cytokinin substances present in extracts of yeast t-RNA and of culture filtrates of *Agrobacterium tumefaciens*, when the highly active cytokinin 6-(3-methyl-2-butenylamino) purine was isolated and tentatively identified (Upper et al., 1970). Also, in 1970 at the 8th International Conference on Plant Growth Substances in Canberra, Upper and coworkers reported the development of temperature programming procedures for the GLC analysis of cytokinins using a 3% OV-17 column which gave good resolution of the TMS derivatives of several natural cytokinins (Upper et al., 1972). They carried out a preliminary study of the cytokinins in tobacco shoot extracts and tentatively identified 2iP, zeatin, and ZR by co-chromatography with the authentic TMS derivatives. They also reported preliminary experiments demonstrating the potential use of GC-MS procedures for the conclusive identification of cytokinins in plant extracts. In 1974, Taylor and coworkers investigated the cytokinin substances in fruitlets and tracheal fluid of cotton plants from extracts partially purified by TLC and then analyzed by GLC and combined GC-MS, using columns of 2% DC-11 on Gas Chrom Q (Taylor et al., 1974). Both TMS and permethyl derivatives were used in both the GLC and GC-MS determinations. A method for the rapid purification of free cytokinin bases and ribosides in ethyl acetate extracts of plant material employing analytical GLC as the final step for identification and quantification was described by Hahn (1975).

The most extensive and successful use of combined GC-MS techniques for the conclusive identification and quantification of

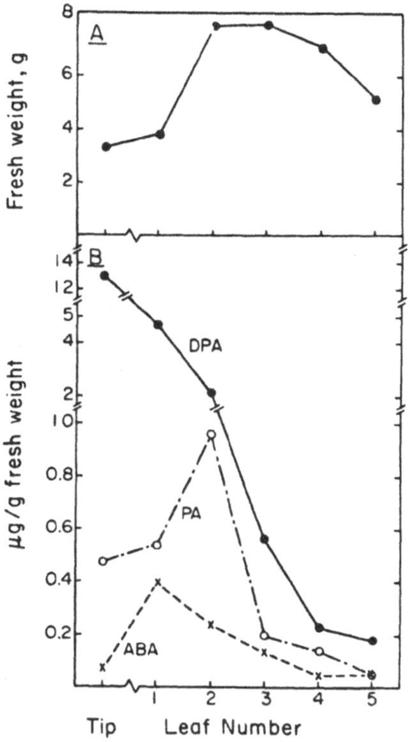

Fig. 7. Changes in endogenous levels of abscisic acid (ABA) and its two metabolites, phaseic acid (PA) and dihydrophaseic acid (DPA), in castor bean (Ricinus communis L.) shoot tip and leaves at different stages of development. A: Fresh weight of shoot tip and leaves of different ages. B: ABA, PA, and DPA content of shoot tip and leaves of different ages, expressed in μg per gm fresh weight (from Zeevaart, 1977).

natural cytokinins has been the work of Horgan and coworkers in their studies of the cytokinins present in winter and spring sap of sycamore trees (Horgan et al., 1973; Purse et al., 1976) and in buds during the winter period and immediately prior to bud burst (Lorenzi et al., 1975; Horgan et al., 1975). TMS derivatives were used in all the above investigations, since in this form all the known free cytokinin bases and ribosides have been found to separate very well on columns of SE-52 (Most et al., 1968), OV-17 (Upper et al., 1972), OV-1 (Purse et al., 1976; Horgan, 1978), and SE-33 (McRae, 1978) when temperature programming procedures are employed (Fig. 8). However, the early work of Taylor et al. (1974) and more recently of Young (1977) has shown that permethylated derivatives of the main natural cytokinins are also quite stable esters that can be well separated

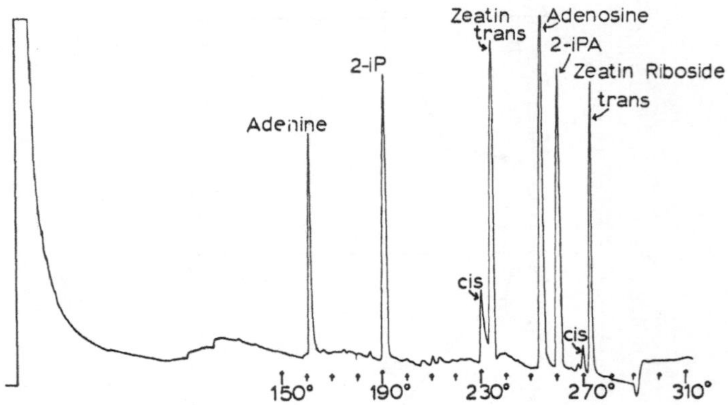

Fig. 8. Gas chromatogram of silylated mixture of authentic cytokinin compounds obtained by temperature program analysis using a 2% SE-33 column.

on columns of DC-11 or OV-22 and can be identified and quantified by GC-MS using the multiple ion detection technique.

As a final part to this section, some remarks are in order about column stationary phases that seem to have given the best results to date in the GLC analysis of plant growth regulator extracts. The choice of stationary phase and oven temperature will depend on the chemical nature of the growth regulator(s) under analysis and the type of derivative being used. For IAA analysis, using either methylated or TMS derivatives, the nonpolar silicones OV-1, OV-17, SE-30, and SE-33 at 3-5% concentration coated on Gas Chrom Q or Chromosorb W (80-100 or 100-120 mesh) have been found to give good resolution between IAA and other components in a partially purified extract when the sample is analyzed by isothermal GLC at column temperatures between 200° and 210°C (see McDougall and Hillman, 1978b). We have found that excellent resolution of IAA, and of other related indole and phenyl acids, can be obtained when either methylated or silylated ether extracts are analyzed on columns of 3% OV-17 using temperature programming procedures running from 95°C-260°C at 3° per min (Fig. 9). For the GLC analysis of gibberellins, the stationary phase usually employed has again been one of the wide range of silicones, because of their good temperature stability. The most frequently used phases, in increasing order of polarity, are SE-30, OV-1, SE-33, OV-17, OF-1, OV-210, OV-225, and XE-60 coated at 2-3% on Gas Chrom Q or Chromosorb W (80-100 or 100-120 mesh). Although good separation of the methyl and TMS esters of most gibberellins can be achieved by isothermal GLC at column temperatures around 220°C, the best separations are achieved when temperature programming procedures are used over the range 180°-300°C (Fig. 10), depending on the column stationary phase and the degree of

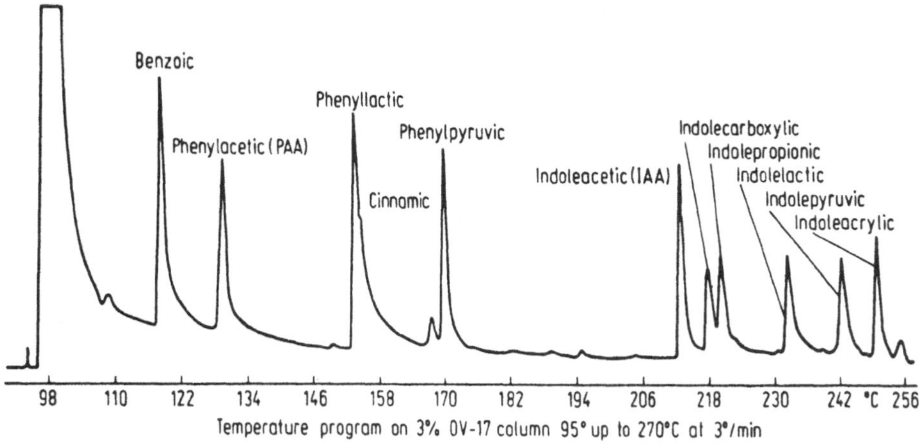

Fig. 9. Gas chromatogram of methylated mixture of authentic phenyl and indole acids obtained by temperature program analysis using a 3% OV-17 column (95°-270°C at 3°/min--attenuation: 2 X 10^2; chart speed: 0.5"/min; N_2 flow rate: 32 ml/min).

pre-purification of the plant extract (see Gaskin and MacMillan, 1978). For good resolution of ABA, a range of column stationary phases have been employed but the most frequently used phases have again been SE-30, OV-17, and XE-60, as well as Epon 1001 coated at 1-3% on Gas Chrom Q or Chromosorb W of 80-100 mesh. Most investigations have used isothermal GLC at column temperatures of around 200°C and the detector system employed has usually been ECD (see Saunders, 1978; Quarrie, 1978). The most suitable column phases for the GLC analysis of cytokinins have already been discussed in an earlier paragraph. These compounds are easily detected by FID and the best separations have been achieved by using the temperature programming technique (see Horgan, 1978).

HIGH PERFORMANCE LIQUID CHROMATOGRAPHY OF THE GROWTH REGULATORS IN PLANT EXTRACTS

In comparison to the wide use of GLC over the last ten years for the analysis of plant growth regulator extracts, the use of HPLC for analyzing similar extracts has been much less extensive and the technique is still undergoing development in several laboratories, especially with respect to the use of gradient elution procedures for determining the growth regulator content of unpurified or solvent fractionated plant extracts. As in the early development of GLC techniques for growth hormone analysis, Powell and coworkers have again played a pioneer role in the demonstration that HPLC offers great potential for the purification and provisional identification of the growth regulators in a plant extract (Powell, 1972; Pool and Powell, 1972, 1974). Brenner and coworkers (Carnes et al.,

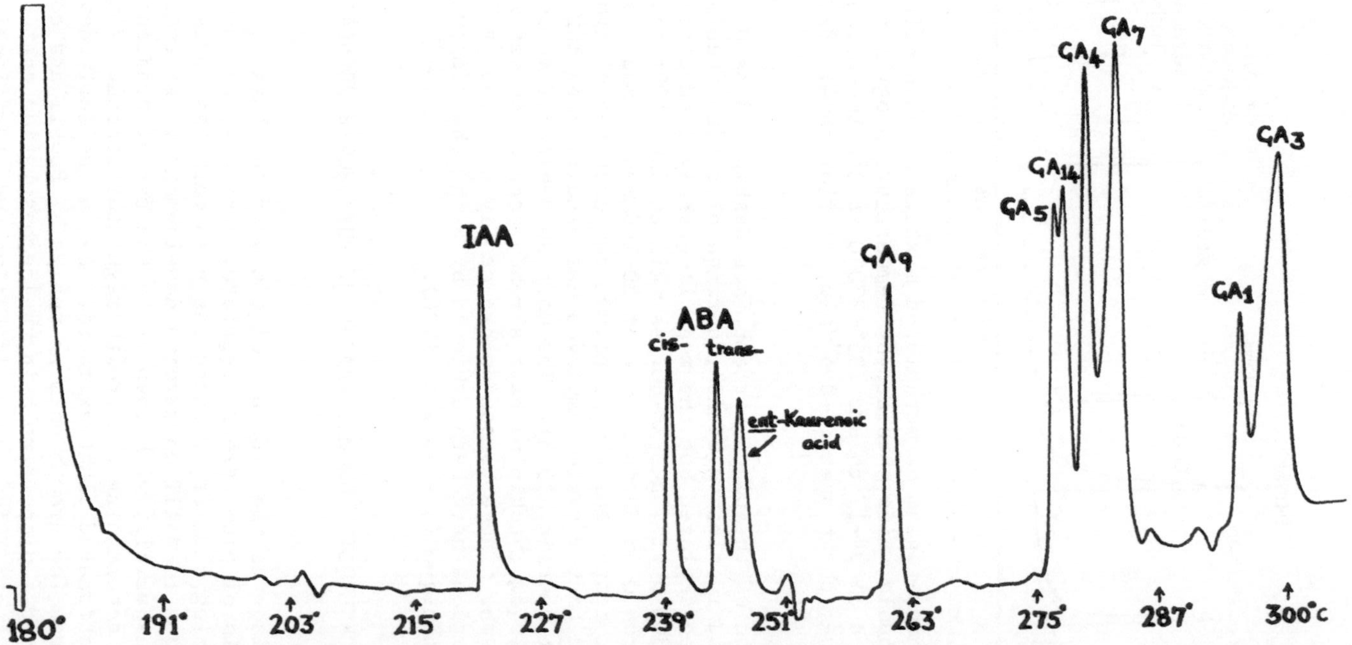

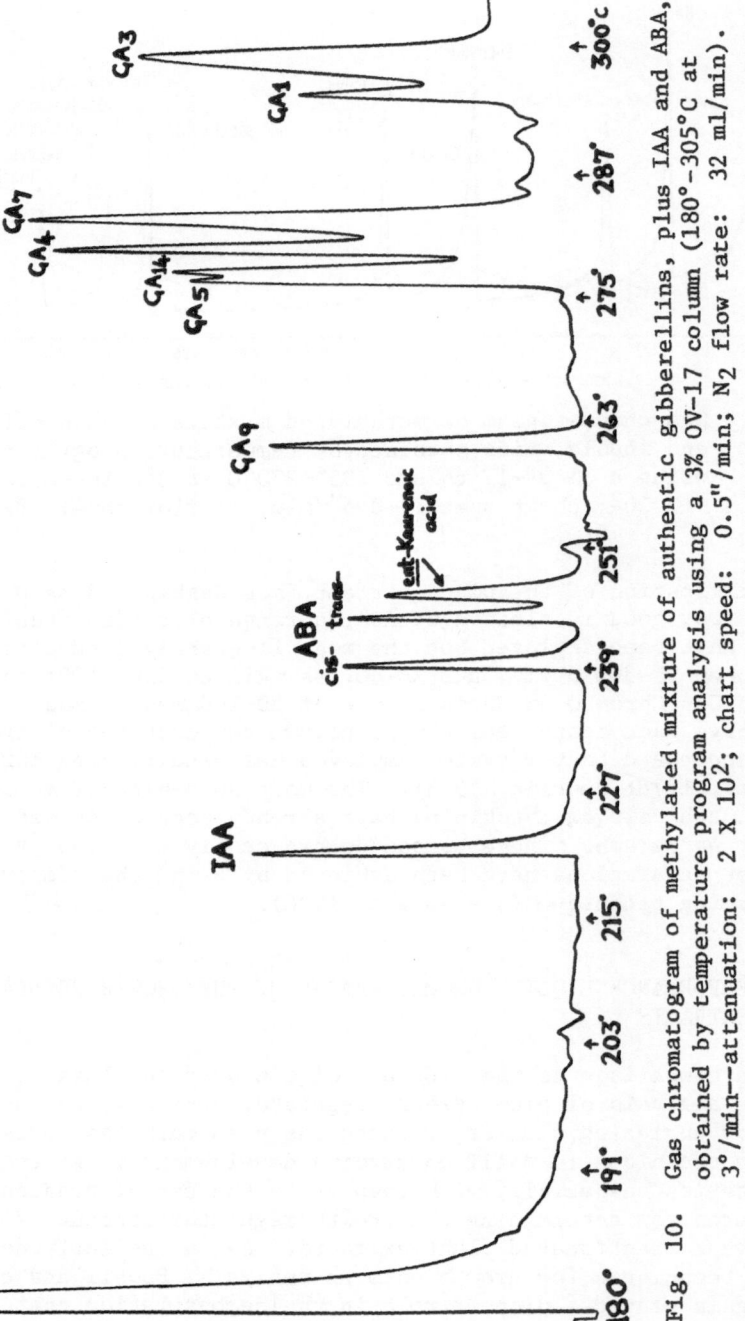

Fig. 10. Gas chromatogram of methylated mixture of authentic gibberellins, plus IAA and ABA, obtained by temperature program analysis using a 3% OV-17 column (180°-305°C at 3°/min--attenuation: 2 X 10^2; chart speed: 0.5"/min; N_2 flow rate: 32 ml/min).

1974, 1975; Ciha et al., 1977; Brenner, 1979) and Reeve and Crozier have also been extensively involved in the development of this excellent separatory technique for the analysis of growth regulator extracts (Reeve et al., 1976; Reeve and Crozier, 1977, 1978; Crozier and Reeve, 1977).

Early investigations using HPLC showed the potential use of this procedure for separating cytokinin substances in xylem exudates from grape roots (Pool and Powell, 1974) and tomato roots (Carnes et al., 1974, 1975). The special suitability of employing this separatory technique for analyzing tissue extracts where the cytokinin activity of each component substance can also be determined by standard bioassay procedures has now been demonstrated by several workers (Thomas et al., 1975; Dekhuijzen and Gevers, 1975; Hahn, 1976; Morris et al., 1976; Kannangara et al., 1978). Early workers employed columns of chemically bonded pellicular ion exchange materials, such as the anion exchange resins Bondapak AX and Vydac AX, or the cation exchange resins Bondapak CX, Vydac CX, and Zipax SCX, and used phosphate buffers of varying pH and ionic strength as the eluting solvent. These conditions, however, did not allow for the elution of all the natural cytokinins within reasonable times and an improved procedure giving better and faster separations was described by Challice (1975) using columns packed with pellicular polyamide and eluting with a phosphate buffer containing 10% v/v methanol.

Superior column efficiency in HPLC has been achieved by the development of micro-particulate silica column packings and the use of reverse phase coatings in which functional molecules, such as the octadecyl group, are chemically bonded onto a solid support material such as spherical or porous silica particles. When the silica particles are very small and uniform in size distribution, as in a micro-octadecylsilica column, the efficiency and separatory performance of the column are extremely good. The superior properties of the micro-octadecylsilica column, μBondapack/C18 (Waters Associates), for the separation of naturally occurring cytokinins when gradient elution procedures are employed, have been well demonstrated by Morris et al. (1976) and Kannangara et al. (1978) (Fig. 11).

The most widely used detector system for HPLC that is directly coupled to the outlet of the column is a fixed wavelength (254 nm), dual wavelength (254 and 280 nm), or variable wavelength UV detector. With such detectors, all the standard plant growth regulators, except the gibberellins, can be readily detected at 254 nm in a wide range of column elutants, the limit of sensitivity of most monitors being around 5 ng for cytokinins, ABA, and indole compounds. The problem of detecting gibberellins in HPLC analyses has been solved by Crozier and Reeve (1977), who developed a simple procedure for converting the carboxyl function at C-7 on all gibberellins into the corresponding benzyl ester, which will readily absorb in the

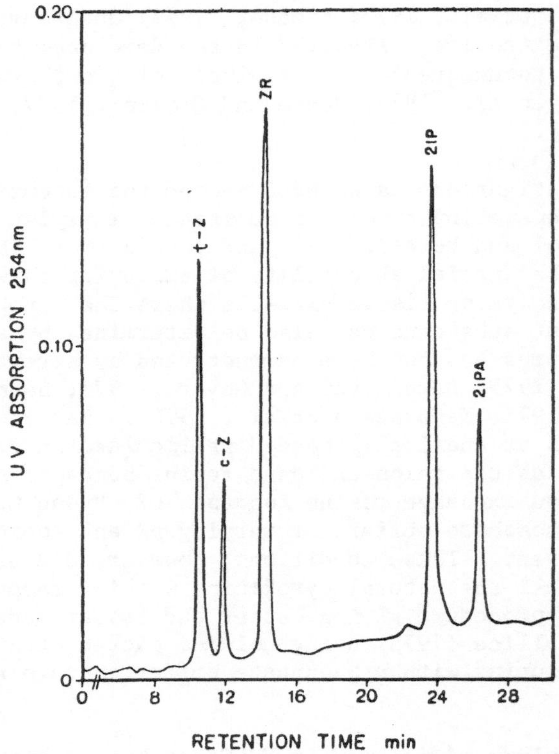

Fig. 11. HPLC scan of mixture of authentic cytokinin compounds obtained by gradient elution analysis on a μBondapack C_{18} column. Injected amounts: 50 ng for zeatin (Z), zeatin riboside (ZR), and isopentenyladenine (2iP); 25 ng for isopentenyladenosine (2iPA). Injection volume: 10 μl of methanol. Solvent A was water/methanol (90:10) and solvent B was methanol, both solvents being 0.2 M with respect to acetic acid. Elution conditions: flow rate was 0.8 ml min^{-1} with a 20 min gradient starting with 15% B (in A) and ending with 42% B (from Kannangara et al., 1978).

256 nm region of the UV spectrum. A refinement of this method was recently reported by Heftmann et al. (1978), who demonstrated the separation of pairs of closely related gibberellins in the form of their p-nitrobenzyl esters, using silver nitrate-impregnated silica columns. This form of derivatization of the six gibberellins examined not only enhanced their UV absorption, and so improved the detector sensitivity, but it also facilitated the identification of each gibberellin by mass spectroscopy. Much lower detection limits in HPLC analyses have recently been achieved by employing two

additional, highly selective detectors working in series with a standard 254 nm UV detector (Sweetser and Swartzfager, 1978). The additional detectors used by these workers were a fluorescence detector with a Corion 281 nm interference filter and a 0 to 54 cut-off emission filter (giving 85% transmittance at 340 nm), and an electrochemical detector operating in the amperometric mode. Both these systems are highly sensitive and selective for the detection of indole compounds and are therefore especially suitable for the detection and quantification of IAA. A comparison of the relative sensitivity of the UV, fluorescence, and electrochemical detector systems to ng amounts of IAA eluting off an HPLC column is shown in Fig. 12.

There are other aspects of HPLC technology that the potential user of this technique for growth regulator analysis needs to be aware of, such as the best type of high pressure solvent delivery pumps, the most suitable sample injector, and the advantages and disadvantages of gradient solvent elution compared with isochratic solvent elution, but these will not be considered here since they have been covered extensively in recent papers by Sweetser (1978) and Brenner (1979).

Although early studies on the application of HPLC to growth regulator analysis were directed mainly toward the separation of the natural cytokinin substances, much work has been done over the last five years on the development of HPLC procedures for the separation of plant gibberellins; these investigations are well summarized in a recent review by Reeve and Crozier (1978). This work was initially handicapped by the absence of a simple, sensitive detector system for gibberellin compounds as they elute off the HPLC column. The difficulty was partly overcome by the use of a sensitive on-stream radioactive monitor for analyzing mixtures of ^{3}H- and ^{14}C-labeled gibberellins (Reeve et al., 1976; Crozier and Reeve, 1977), but as indicated earlier, the problem has been solved by the benzyl esterification of these compounds to produce GA-benzyl esters which can be readily detected in a wide range of solvents using a standard UV monitor operating at 254 nm (Reeve and Crozier, 1978) (Fig. 13). This type of derivatization offers much promise for future studies on the identification and quantification of gibberellins in plant extracts since in this form, suspected gibberellins cannot only be separated by preparative or analytical HPLC, but collected fractions can then be directly injected into the GC-MS for conclusive identification.

The presence and amount of ABA in a range of plant tissues has also recently been determined by HPLC analysis. During and Bachmann (1975) used this method to follow the changes in ABA levels in buds and nodes of *Vitis vinifera* during the autumn and early winter and demonstrated that a close relationship exists between endogenous ABA levels and the degree of dormancy shown by the buds (Fig. 14).

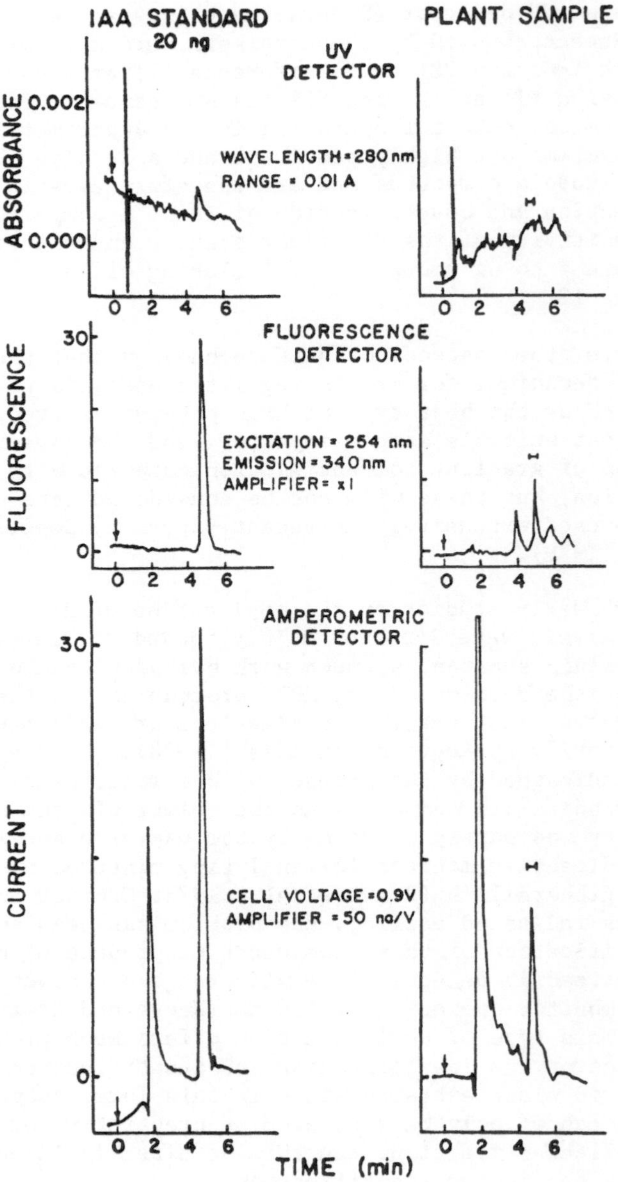

Fig. 12. Comparison of the relative sensitivity of UV, fluorescence, and electrochemical (amperometric) detector systems for HPLC analysis of 20 ng amounts of authentic IAA, and for the determination of ng amounts of IAA in comparable aliquots of a plant extract (from Sweetser, 1979).

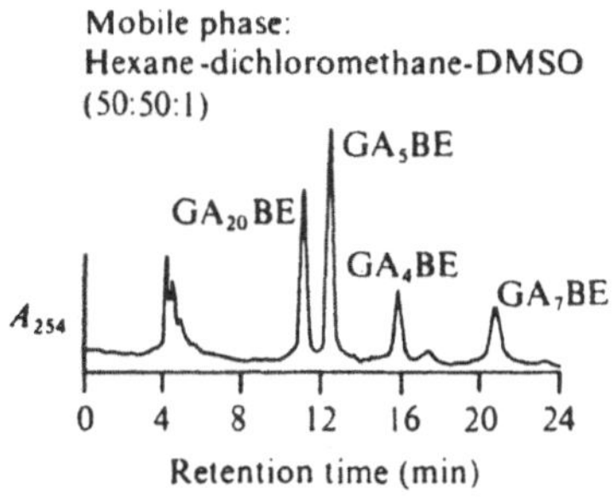

Fig. 13. The influence of DMSO modifier on the analytical HPLC retention characteristics of several authentic gibberellin benzyl esters using a 4.6 X 500 mm Partisil 10 column. The mobile phase used is indicated on the figure and the detector employed was a UV monitor operating at 254 nm (from Reeve and Crozier, 1978).

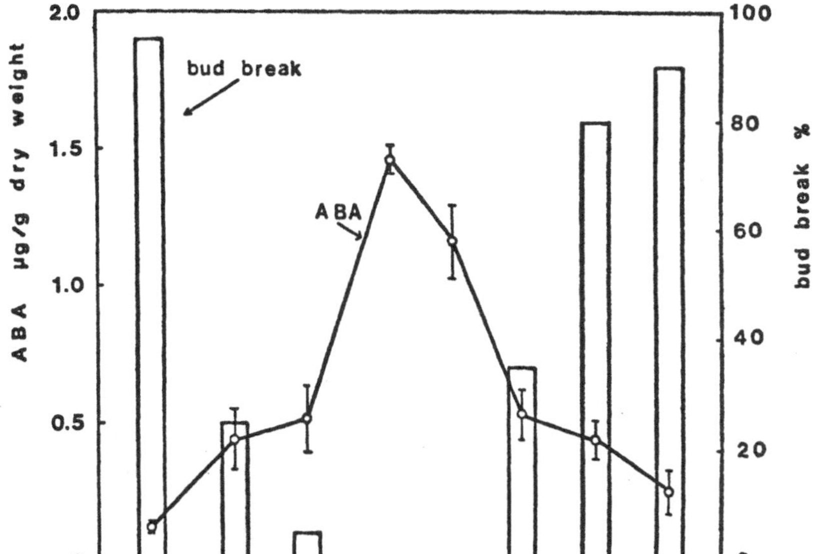

Fig. 14. Comparison of the changing rate of bud break and ABA content in buds and nodes of field-grown grape canes (*Vitis vinifera* L. cv. Riesling) during the period from early September to mid-December, 1974. ABA levels were determined by HPLC analysis of TLC-purified acidic ether extracts of bud and nodal tissue (from During and Bachmann, 1975).

Table 4. Abscisic Acid Levels in Various Plant Tissues as Determined by HPLC Analysis of Acidic Ether Extracts Partially Purified by Column Chromatography on Sephadex G-25 (from Sweetser and Vatvars, 1976)

Plant Material	ABA (ng/g fresh weight)*
Kent soybeans	
Growing tip	60-122
Expanding leaves	40-60
Mature leaves	4-7
(Wilted) mature leaves	100-175
Pinto beans	
Leaves	4-40
Wilted leaves	80-170
Roots	8-16
Roots wilted plant	25-60
Cotton	
Expanding leaves	26-400
Mature leaves	12-140
Apple seedling	
Leaves	2-5
Stems	2-28
Roots	1-30
Orange peel	
Flavedo	600-1,500
Albedo	1,600-2,400

*One reason for the range of ABA levels in some plant materials is probably the differences in environmental humidity at the time of harvest, since ABA levels are greatly affected by water stress.

Sweetser and Vatvars (1976) report on the ABA content of acidic ether fractions from a wide range of leaves, stems, and root tissues and from the peel of two orange varieties (Table 4). Prior to analysis by HPLC, using isochratic conditions, they partially purified the ether fractions by passing the fractions through a column of Sephadex G-25. Employing similar Sephadex purification and HPLC procedures, Quebedeaux et al. (1976) made a comparative study of the ABA content and growth rates of the developing seeds and pod walls of soybean reproductive structures (Fig. 15), conclusive identification of the suspected ABA being confirmed by mass spectrographic analysis of ABA fractions collected during HPLC. These workers also

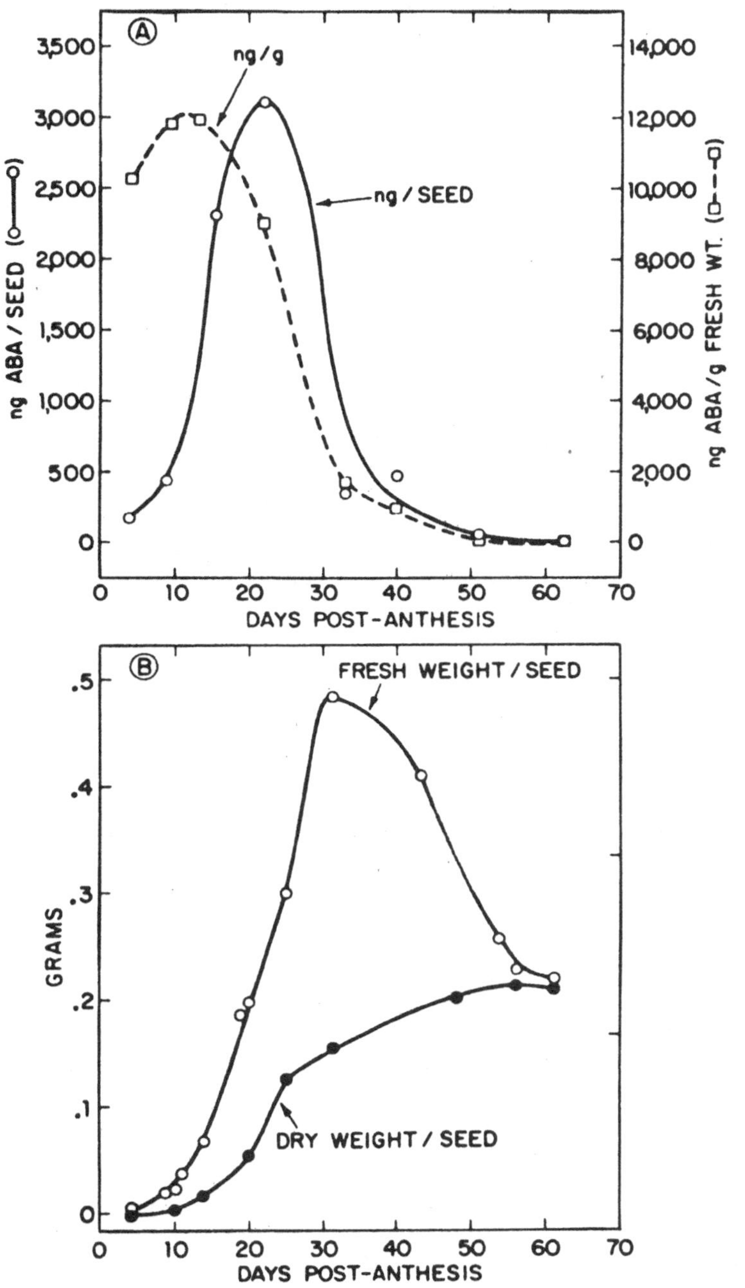

Fig. 15. Changes in fresh and dry weight (B) and in ABA content (A) of developing soybean seed from anthesis to seed maturation. ABA levels were determined by HPLC analysis of acidic ether extracts partially purified by Sephadex G-25 column chromatography (from Quebedeaux et al., 1976).

investigated the physiological significance of the initially high and then declining ABA levels in the seed by observing the ability of the root-shoot axes of the embryo to grow in liquid culture when excised from seeds at different stages of development. Their results show clearly that the length of time required for the excised embryos to commence growth in liquid culture decreased as seed development progressed and the levels of ABA in the seed declined.

Brenner and coworkers have also examined ABA levels in soybean seed extracts using a preparative HPLC separatory procedure which required no prior solvent partitioning or Sephadex chromatographic purification of the extract, and gave a 98.9% quantitative recovery of ABA as demonstrated by using an internal standard of [2-^{14}C]ABA (Ciha et al., 1977). After preparative HPLC purification of the seed extract (Fig. 16), quantification of the ABA was achieved by employing either analytical GLC with an EC detector, or analytical HPLC with a UV detector (Fig. 17). A similar approach employing preparative followed by analytical HPLC procedures has been used by Durley and coworkers (1978) to investigate the levels of ABA and its metabolites, phaseic and dihydrophaseic acids, in normal and water-stressed leaf tissue of sorghum. Unfortunately, however, the paper reports only the amounts found in normal leaf tissue.

The possible use of HPLC for the determination of IAA, or of other auxin substances in plant extracts, has so far received the least attention even though Crozier and Reeve (1977) have shown that both acidic and neutral indole compounds can be readily separated by HPLC (Fig. 18). To date, only one substantial study has been made using HPLC for the identification and quantification of IAA in a range of plant tissues (Sweetser and Swartzfager, 1978). These workers used a microparticulate strong anion exchange column (Whatman Partisil-10-SAX) to analyze partially purified acidic ether fractions and employed several column-mobile phase systems to achieve the best separations. Quantitation of the IAA was achieved by using two highly sensitive detectors, a fluorescence monitor and an electrochemical monitor operating in the amperometric mode, both connected in series with the column effluent. A typical HPLC analysis for IAA in pinto bean stem extracts using the fluorescence and electrochemical detector systems is shown in Fig. 19. Similar procedures were used to determine the levels of IAA in a range of plant tissues (Table 5) and although direct comparisons could not be made with previously published data because of differences in plant age or varieties used, nevertheless, the range of values obtained by Sweetser and Swartzfager for IAA levels in related tissues were found to be very similar to previously published results obtained mainly from the analysis of extracts by paper chromatography or GLC.

Table 5. Levels of IAA in a Range of Plant Tissues as Determined by HPLC Analysis of Acidic Ether Extracts Partially Purified by Sephadex Chromatography (from Sweetser and Swartzfager, 1978)

Species	Plant Part	IAA ng/g (fresh weight)*
Pinto bean	seeds-immature	200-336
(Phaseolus vulgaris)	trifoliates (older)	4-5
	trifoliates (younger)	14-16
	stem (lower)	22-36
	stem (upper)	50-54
	petioles (younger)	25
Soybean	seeds-immature	50-200
(Glycine max cv Wye)	primary leaves	6-10
	trifoliates	6-10
	stems	24-48
	cotyledon	18
	roots	14
Soybean	primary leaves	2-3
(Glycine max cv Kent)	trifoliates	4
	stems	12-45
	cotyledon	69
	petioles	45
	roots	14-22
Cotton	apex	17-40
(Gossypium hirsutum	leaves (younger)	18-30
cv Stoneville 213)	leaves (older)	3-10
	petiole (younger)	40-50
	petiole (older)	5-24
	stem	32-59
Wheat (Tritricum aestivum cv Selkirk)	seed-immature	150-800
Corn	stem (seedling)	10-12
(Zea mays cv Pioneer brand 3331)	leaf (seedling)	5-15

*IAA values corrected for losses during purification procedure.

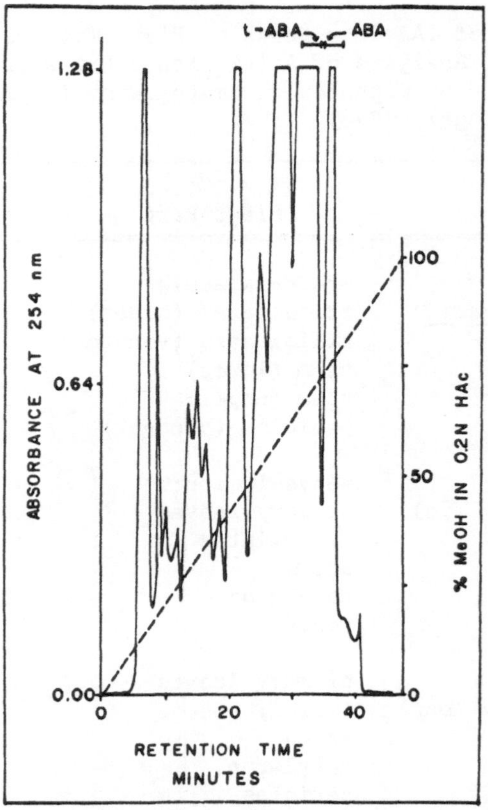

Fig. 16. Typical trace of the UV absorbance at 254 nm of an unpurified soybean seed extract analyzed by preparative HPLC. Dotted line indicates the concentration gradient of methanol in 0.2 N acetic acid used as the eluting solvent (from Ciha et al., 1977).

APPLICATION OF GAS-LIQUID CHROMATOGRAPHY TO STUDIES OF THE GROWTH REGULATOR CHANGES IN WINTER WHEAT SEEDLINGS DURING ACCLIMATION TO COLD STRESS CONDITIONS

Work in my laboratory over the last few years has been concerned with the development of solvent fractionation procedures and refined gas chromatographic techniques to allow for the extraction, separation, provisional identification, and quantitative measurement of all, or most of the known growth regulating substances present in extracts of a plant organ prepared at different stages in its growth and development. This approach to utilizing analytical GLC for the separation, provisional identification, and quantitative determination of auxin substances, ABA, and a range of gibberellins and cytokinins in a plant extract has, to date, only been attempted by

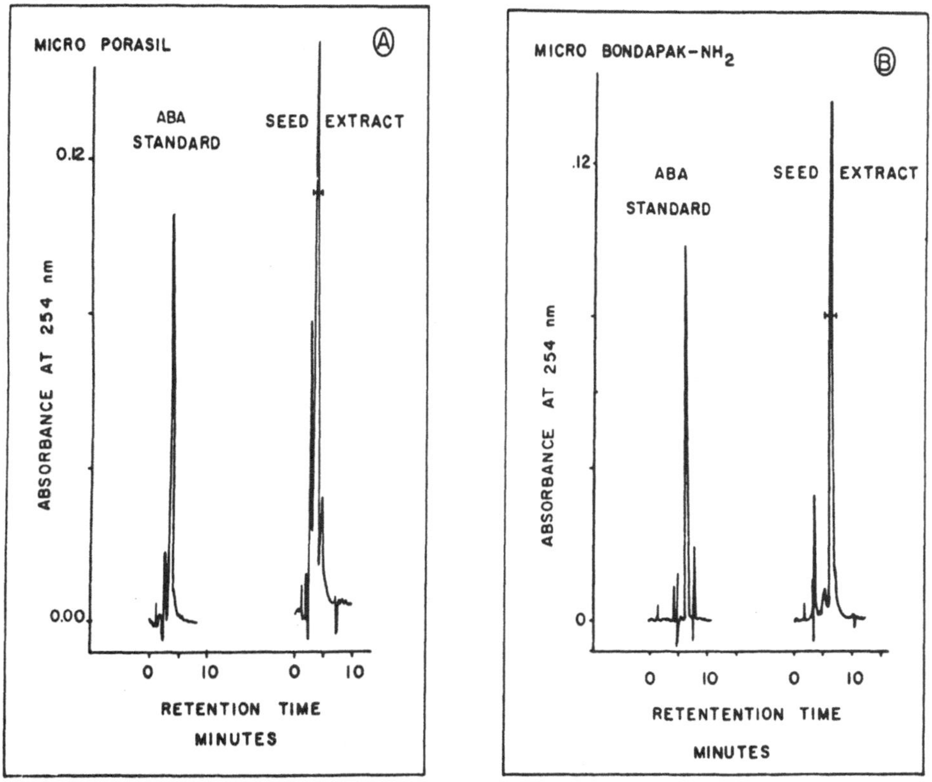

Fig. 17. Traces of the UV absorbance (254 nm) of authentic ABA (500 ng) and of the suspected ABA fraction from preparative-HPLC purified soybean seed extract re-chromatographed on μPorasil (A) and μBondapak-NH_2 (B) analytical HPLC columns (from Ciha et al., 1977).

Shindy and Smith (1975) using ethyl acetate and n-butanol extracts of the ovules from 8-day-old cotton fruits. Although these workers claimed to have verified their GLC identification of GA_1, GA_3, GA_4, and GA_7, and of IAA, ABA, and three cytokinins by combined GC-MS examination of their extracts, unfortunately no experimental data were provided to support this claim.

Our GLC studies have been concerned with the changes in endogenous growth regulators in winter wheat and tobacco plants during development of the shoot under abnormal growth conditions, such as the stress conditions imposed by the gradual reduction of air temperature to 0°C or the rapid development of a virus infection. Some of our results dealing with the changes in auxin substances, several gibberellins, and cytokinins in tobacco leaves during normal growth and development have already been reported (Wightman,

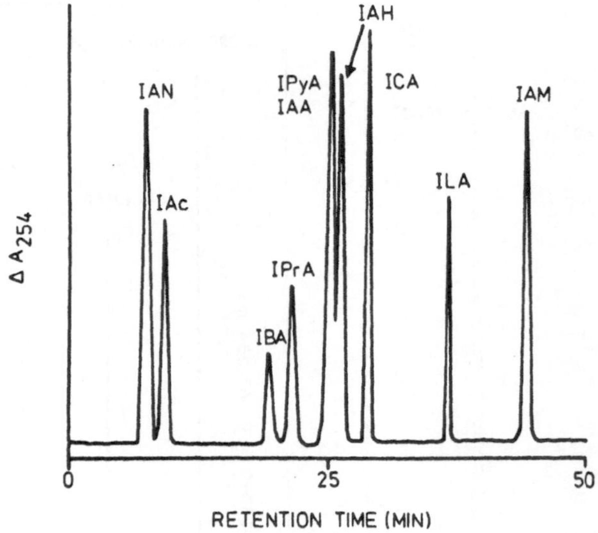

Fig. 18. Separation of neutral and acidic indole compounds by preparative HPLC using a Partisil 10 column and UV detector system. The stationary phase was 40% 0.5 M formic acid, and the mobile phase was a gradient of 30-90% ethyl acetate in hexane. Sample mixture contained 200 μg each of 3-indolylacetonitrile (IAN), 3-indolylacetone (IAc), 3-indolylacetamide (IAM), 3-indolealdehyde (IAH), 3-indolecarboxylic acid (ICA), 3-indolylacetic acid (IAA), 3-indolylpropionic acid (IPrA), 3-indolylbutyric acid (IBA), 3-indolylpyruvic acid (IPyA), and 3-indolyllactic acid (ILA) (from Crozier and Reeve, 1977).

1977; Phipps and Wightman, 1977). In this article, we wish to present some of our data showing the changes in amounts of several growth regulators in winter wheat seedlings during their acclimation to cold temperature conditions. Full details of the hormone changes observed in leaf, crown, and root tissue of cold-treated and control plants have already been published in a Master's thesis (McRae, 1978) and only the results obtained from crown tissue of the two winter wheat varieties examined will be reported here, since it is from this tissue that new shoot growth is initiated when cold temperature conditions are removed, as in the early spring.

The two varieties chosen for study were Kharkov 22-MC and Cappelle-Desprez; the former is a well-known hardy winter wheat whereas the latter shows only moderate cold hardiness. Plants were grown from seed in controlled-environment chambers at 25°C under 16 hour photoperiods, and after one week half the population was transferred to another chamber to undergo gradual cold-temperature

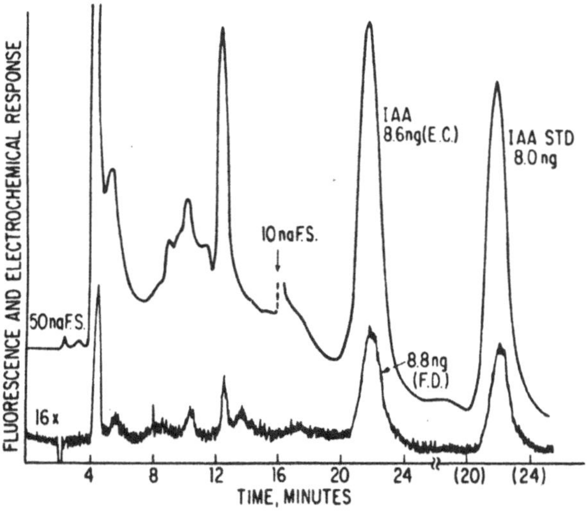

Fig. 19. HPLC determination of IAA in pinto bean stem extracts using a Partisil-SAX column and employing fluorescence (FD) and electrochemical (EC) detectors. Column mobile phase was 0.01 M KH_2PO_4 plus 0.05 M $NaClO_4$, at 500 psi and 0.8 ml/min flow rate. The 40 µl plant sample injected represented 0.5 g fresh weight of shoot tissue. An 8 ng sample of authentic IAA was also injected 8 min after injection of the plant sample to provide an IAA peak for calculating the response of both the EC and fluorescence detectors (from Sweetser and Swartzfager, 1978).

treatment and a decrease in daily photoperiod, as indicated in Fig. 20. Sampling of control and cold-treated plants was carried out at the end of each week for a period of five weeks and at each time interval the two batches of plants were divided into samples of leaf, crown, and root tissue. All three samples of tissue from each type of plant were analyzed for fresh and dry weight changes, chlorophyll and soluble protein content, and for changes in the levels of several growth regulating substances.

Only the crown tissue was examined each week to determine its developing degree of cold hardiness, using a standard procedure employed in this type of plant research work (McRae, 1978) involving fairly rapid cold treatment of the tissue at the rate of 1°C decrease in temperature per hour down to -22°C. During this chilling procedure, samples of the crown tissue were removed at each 2 hour interval, allowed to thaw out slowly to 2°C, and then replanted in trays of soil and placed in the greenhouse at 25°C to determine the tissue's potential for regrowth. After 3 weeks, each sample of crown tissue was visually scored for regrowth capacity and the level of cold temperature treatment at which 50% survival occurred

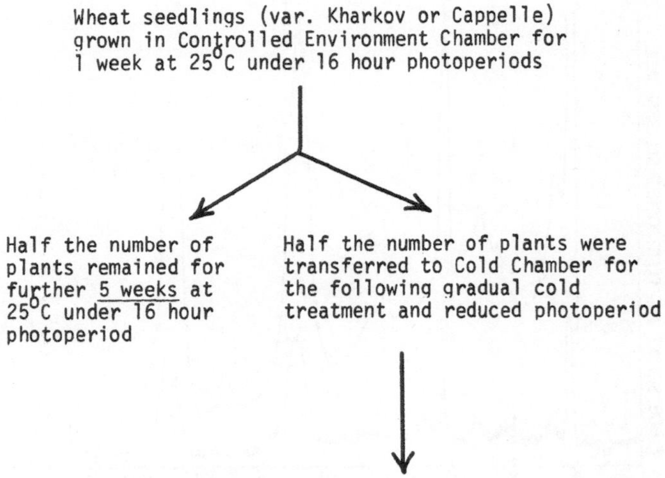
Wheat seedlings (var. Kharkov or Cappelle) grown in Controlled Environment Chamber for 1 week at 25°C under 16 hour photoperiods
Half the number of plants remained for further 5 weeks at 25°C under 16 hour photoperiod
Half the number of plants were transferred to Cold Chamber for the following gradual cold treatment and reduced photoperiod

Weeks of treatment	Day/night temp.	Daily photoperiod
First:	15°C/10°C	14 hour
Second:	10°C/5°C	12 hour
Third:	5°C/2°C	10 hour
Fourth:	2°C/0°C	8 hour
Fifth:	2°C/0°C	8 hour

Fig. 20. Design of experiment for gradual cold-treatment of winter wheat seedlings (var. Kharkov or Capelle-Desprez).

was taken as a measure of the tissue's cold hardiness and referred to as its LT_{50} value. As seen in Fig. 21, the results from such freeze tests showed that Kharkov crown tissue attained a maximum level of hardiness of about -19°C, whereas the corresponding Capelle tissue reached its maximum hardiness around -9°C.

Analysis of the growth parameters for the two varieties showed that during cold acclimation there was a reduction in both the fresh and dry weights of the leaf and root tissue but an increase in the corresponding weights for crown tissue (Fig. 22). Soluble protein levels increased considerably in all cold-treated tissues of both varieties, and showed the greatest increase in crown tissue (Fig. 23).

Changes in the endogenous amounts of growth regulating substances in the weekly samples of crown tissue from both varieties was determined by acetone extraction of the tissue and solvent fractionation of the concentrated extract, as outlined in Fig. 24,

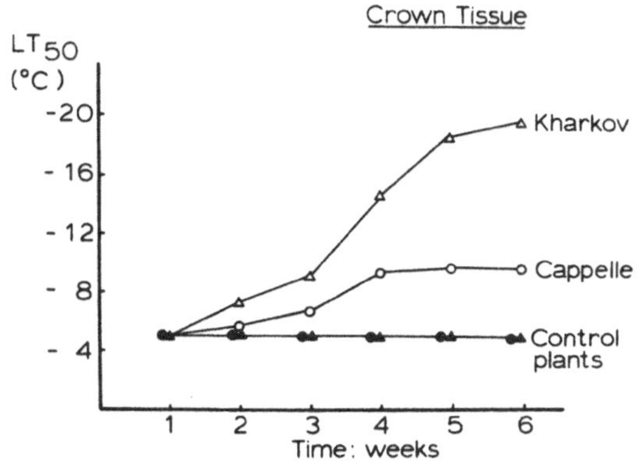

Fig. 21. Comparison of the level of cold hardiness developed by the crown tissue of Kharkov and Cappelle wheat seedlings growing under control or cold temperature conditions.

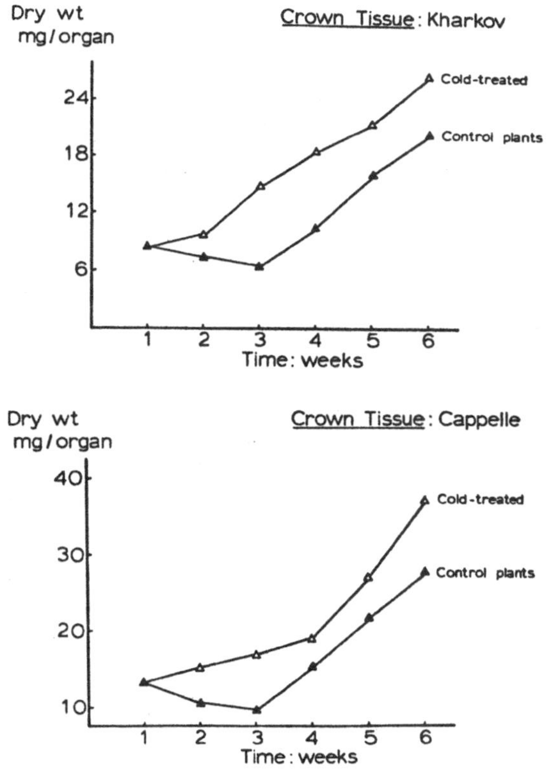

Fig. 22. Dry weight changes in crown tissue from Kharkov and Cappelle seedlings growing under control or cold temperature conditions.

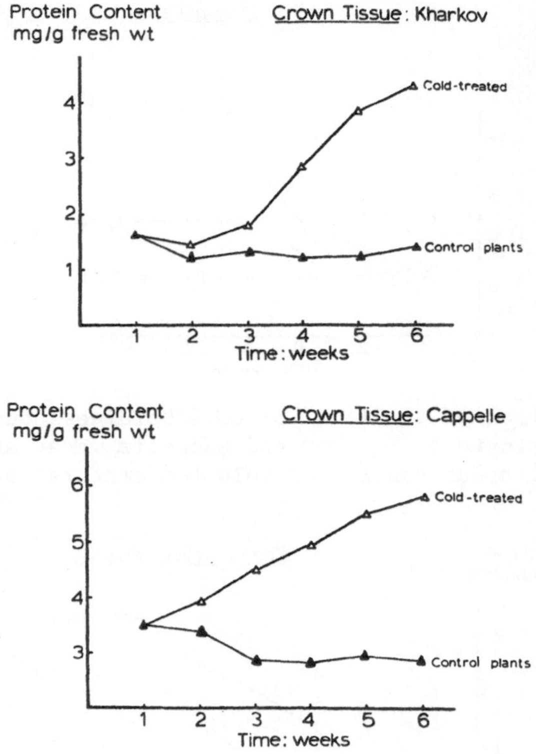

Fig. 23. Changes in soluble protein in crown tissue from Kharkov and Cappelle seedlings growing under control or cold temperature conditions.

followed by detailed examination of the acidic ether and neutral butanol fractions by analytical gas chromatography using temperature programming procedures. For analysis of the methylated acidic ether fractions, dual glass columns packed with 3% OV-17 on Chromosorb W (100-120 mesh) were employed and the temperature program begun at 70°C was increased linearly at the rate of 3° per min up to 310°C. For examination of the silylated neutral butanol fractions, columns packed with 2% SE-33 on Chromosorb W (80-100 mesh) were used and the temperature program begun at 120°C, with a 7 min isothermal period, was increased linearly at the rate of 3° per min up to 300°C. By employing such temperature programming procedures, a wide range of authentic phenyl, indole, and gibberellin methyl esters can be well separated by GLC, as shown in Fig. 25, and typical scans obtained when acidic ether fractions of crown tissue were analyzed on columns of 3% OV-17 are shown in Fig. 26. The method of using internal authentic standards was employed for provisional identification of the different growth regulators in each fraction and for constructing

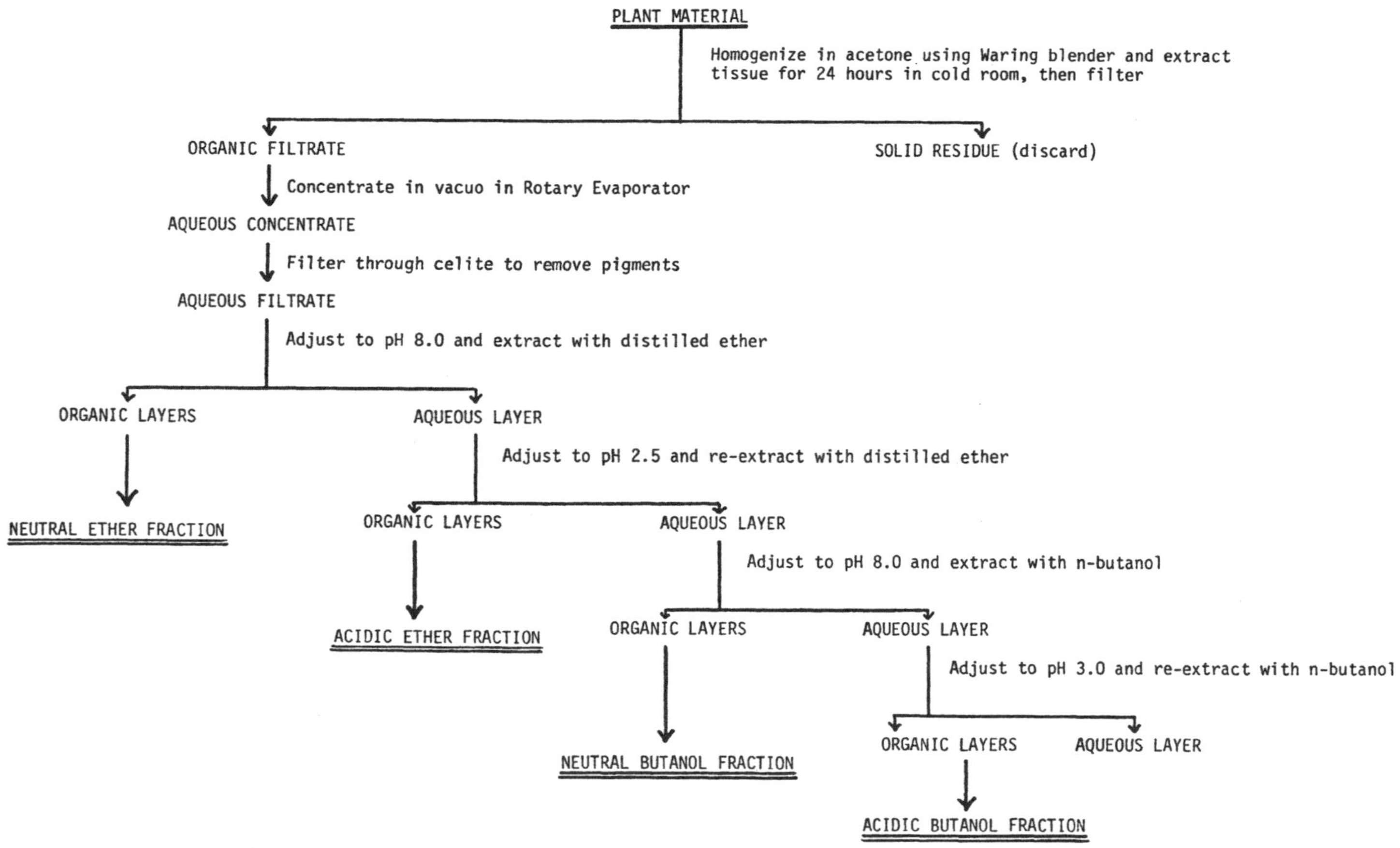

Fig. 24. Procedure for the extraction and solvent fractionation of growth regulating substances occurring in plants.

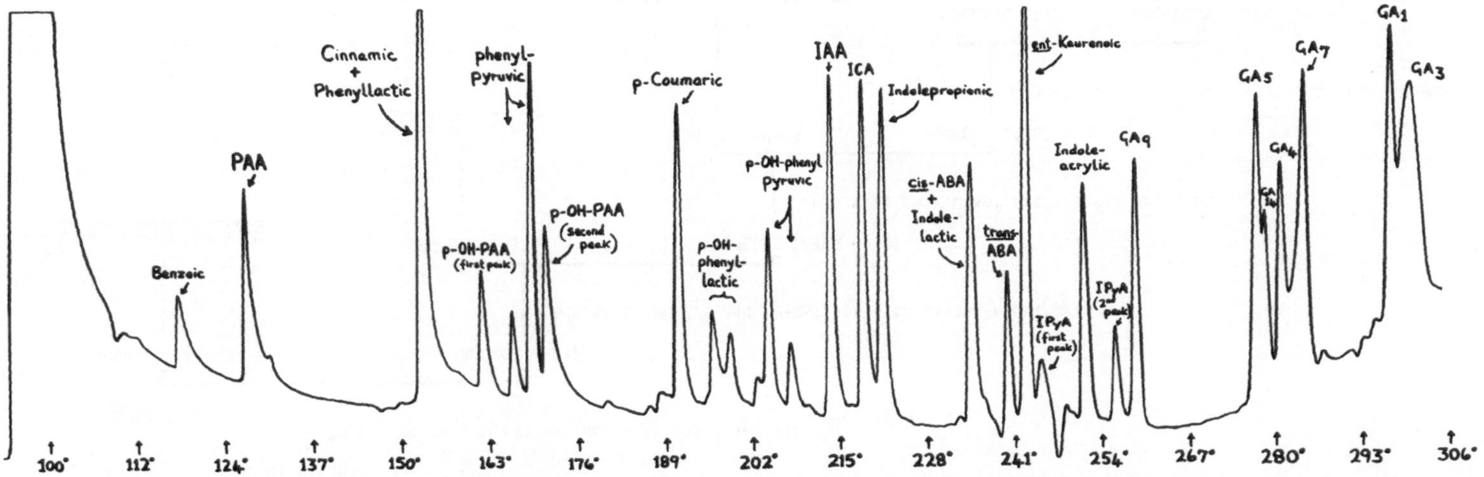

Fig. 25. Resolution of methylated mixture of authentic phenyl-, p-hydroxyphenyl-, and indolyl-acids plus several gibberellins by analytical GLC, using a 3% OV-17 column and temperature programming procedures (95°-310°C at 3°/min--attenuation: 2 X 10^2; chart speed: 0.5"/min; N_2 flow rate: 32 ml/min).

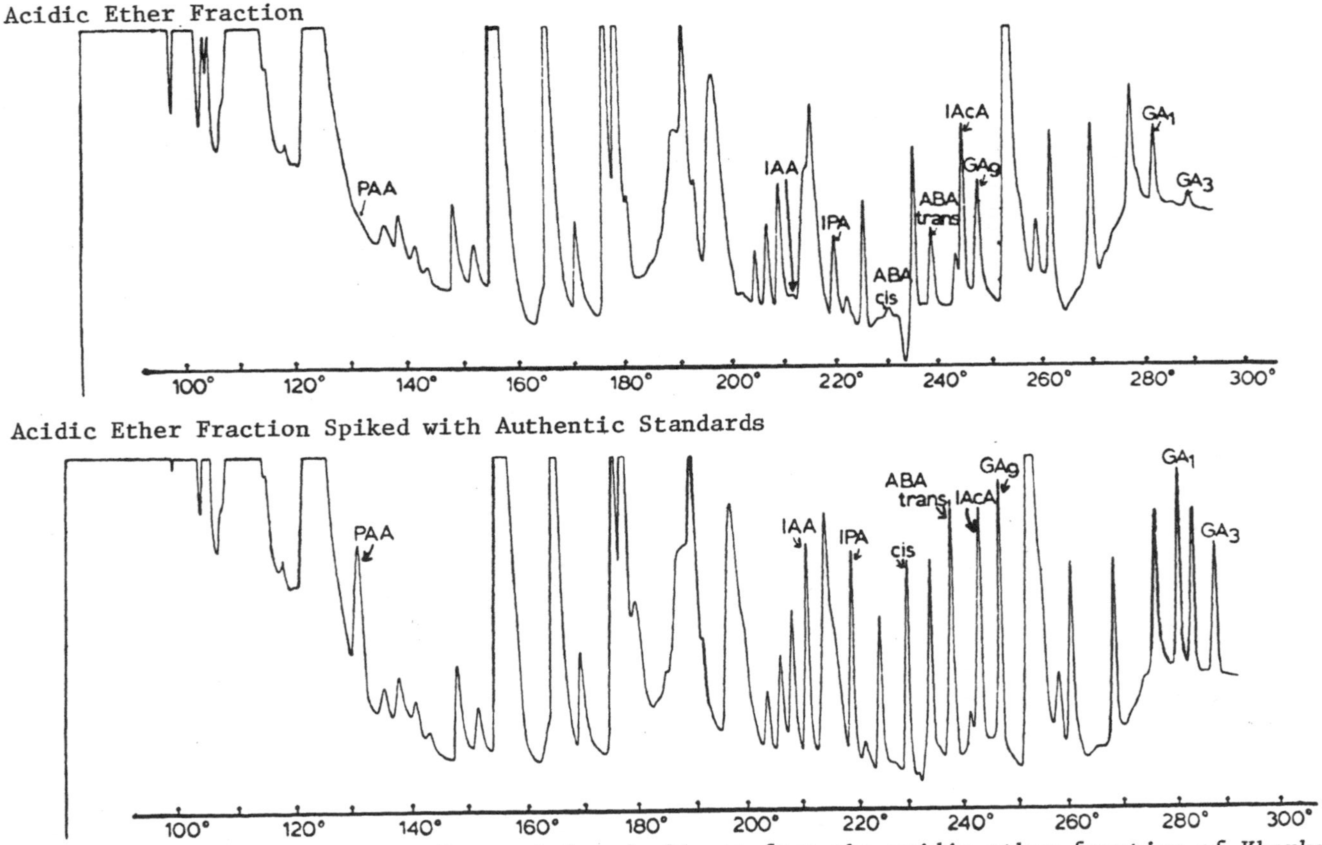

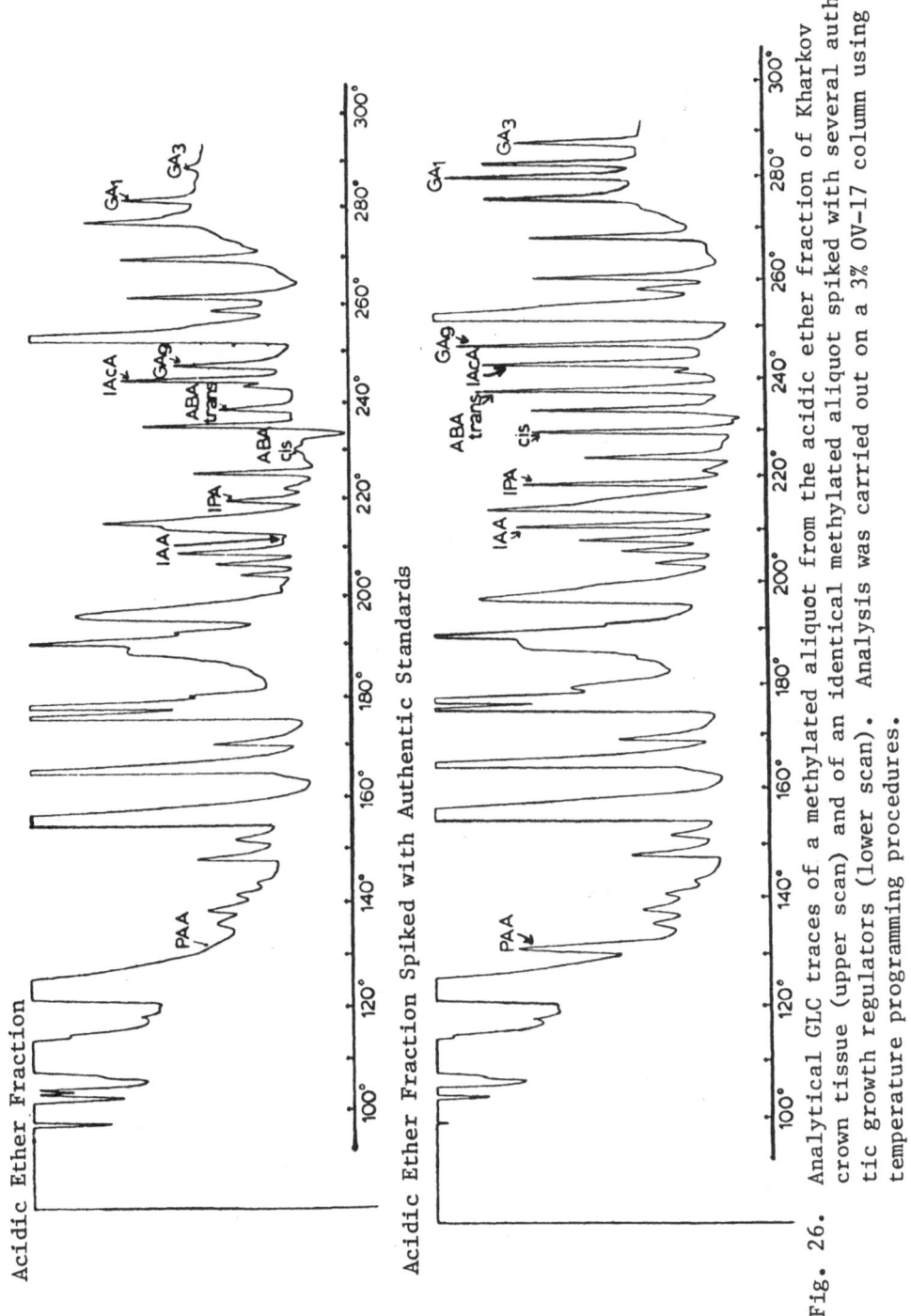

Fig. 26. Analytical GLC traces of a methylated aliquot from the acidic ether fraction of Kharkov crown tissue (upper scan) and of an identical methylated aliquot spiked with several authentic growth regulators (lower scan). Analysis was carried out on a 3% OV-17 column using temperature programming procedures.

standard curves for quantitative determinations. An estimate of the losses of each type of growth regulator at the various steps in the solvent purification procedure prior to GLC analysis was obtained in a preliminary experiment in which an appropriate amount (usually 2 μc) of ^{14}C-IAA, ^{14}C-ABA, ^{14}C-GA_3, or ^{14}C-adenine was added to separate portions of an acetone extract of Kharkov crown tissue taken from 2-week-old plants. Each radioactive acetone extract was then taken through the concentration and solvent purification procedure outlined in Fig. 24 and an estimate of the loss in radioactivity at each step was made by liquid scintillation spectrometry. Recoveries of 82% and 85% of ^{14}C-IAA and ^{14}C-ABA, respectively, were obtained in the acidic ether fraction, but only 60% of the ^{14}C-adenine was recovered in the neutral butanol fraction. The recovery values for ^{14}C-IAA are close to those reported by McDougall and Hillman (1978a) employing a similar ether fractionation procedure with methanolic extracts of bean shoots.

Although identification of all the growth regulators observed in this study is based on co-chromatography with authentic standards in the analytical GLC, and is therefore only provisional, the conclusive identification of IAA, ABA, and IAcA in the acidic ether fraction has recently been obtained by preparative GLC analysis of this fraction followed by combined GC-MS examination of collected fractions. We are presently awaiting GC-MS confirmation of the presence of the other growth regulators provisionally identified in the acidic ether fraction of crown tissue, and of the presence of zeatin and zeatin riboside in the neutral butanol fraction.

As seen from the data presented in Figs. 27, 28, and 29, the endogenous levels of several auxin, gibberellin, and cytokinin substances did not change significantly in crown tissue from either variety during acclimation of the plants to cold temperature conditions. The only exception to this general conclusion on the levels of the main types of growth promoting substances is the appreciable rise in zeatin riboside observed in the cold-treated crown tissue from Capelle plants (Fig. 29), although why such increased levels of zeatin riboside should occur in Capelle, but not in Kharkov crown tissue, is not yet understood. However, the most consistent and significant rise in the endogenous level of a growth regulator during cold acclimation of crown tissue is seen in the changes in amounts of ABA in both varieties during the 5-week treatment period (Fig. 30). Clearly, the levels of this inhibitor substance increased strikingly in the crown tissue of both varieties during cold treatment, at rates which correlate well with the rate at which each tissue was found to develop cold hardiness (Fig. 21). This finding clearly suggests that at least in crown tissue of winter wheat, ABA plays a significant metabolic role, either directly or indirectly, in promoting cold hardiness of the tissue.

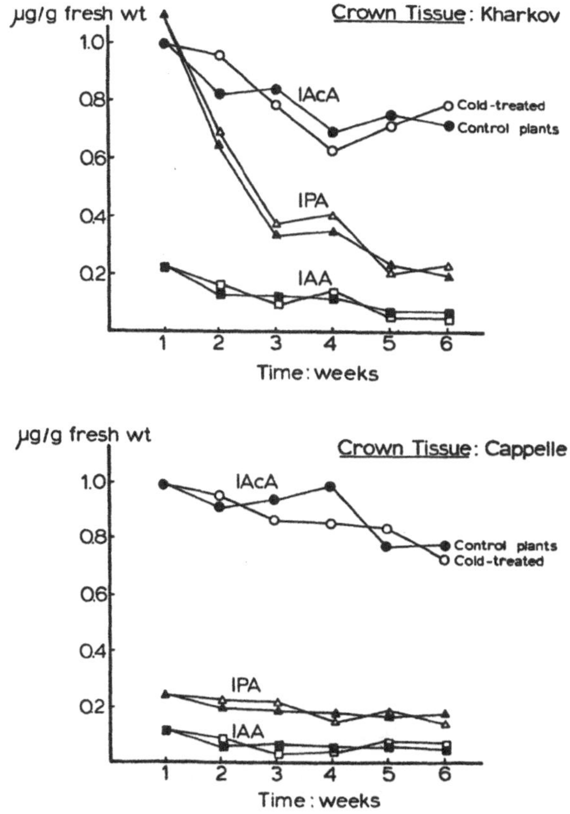

Fig. 27. Changes in the endogenous levels of three auxin substances (3-indolylacetic, propionic, and acrylic acids) in crown tissue from Kharkov and Cappelle seedlings growing under control or cold temperature conditions.

In conclusion, it is interesting to observe that winter wheat tissue subjected to cold stress behaves similarly to many other plant tissues subjected to drought stress conditions; namely, the tissues appear to synthesize abnormally high levels of ABA. We have also observed a similar large increase in endogenous ABA in young tobacco leaf tissue reacting to the stress conditions imposed by the rapid development of tobacco mosaic virus (TMV) infection. The full significance of these similar reactions of plant tissue to stress physiological conditions is not yet understood and

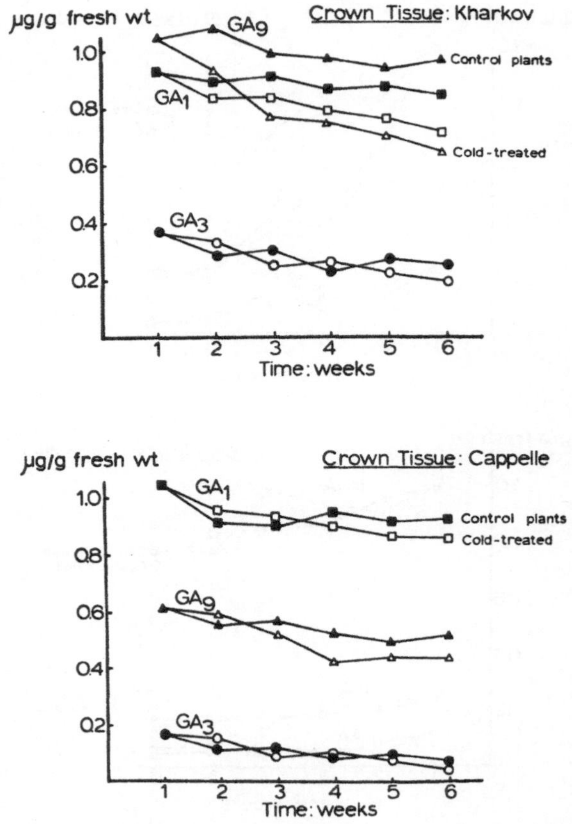

Fig. 28. Changes in the endogenous levels of three gibberellins (GA_1, GA_3, and GA_9) in crown tissue from Kharkov and Cappelle seedlings growing under control or cold temperature conditions.

investigation of the role of ABA on the biochemistry of plant tissues reacting to stress situations is certainly a promising area of study for future research.

ACKNOWLEDGMENTS

The author would like to acknowledge the appreciable contribution of Donald McRae to the work presented in the last section of this paper. Thanks are also due to my research associates, Drs. Jenny Phipps and Elnora A. Schneider, for their help and advice during the preparation of this paper. The National Research Council of Canada kindly provided funds as a Grant-in-aid of Research to the author to support this work.

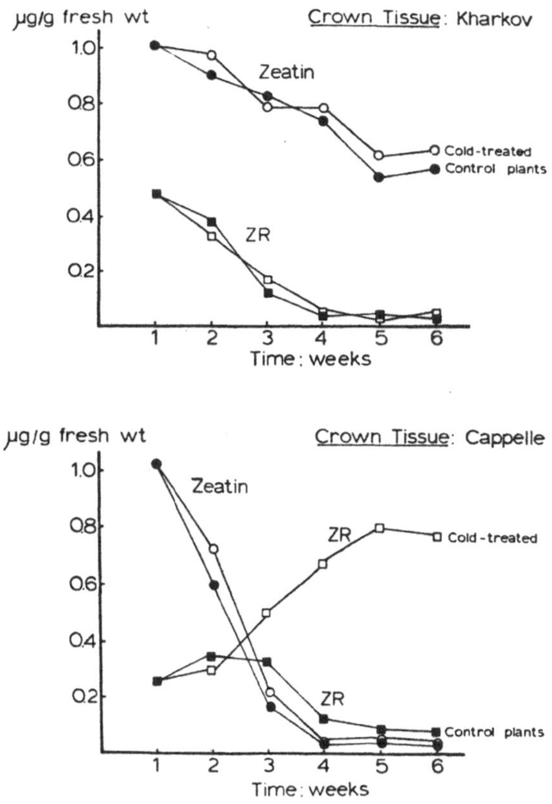

Fig. 29. Changes in the endogenous levels of two cytokinin substances, zeatin and zeatin riboside (ZR), in crown tissue from Kharkov and Cappelle seedlings growing under control or cold temperature conditions.

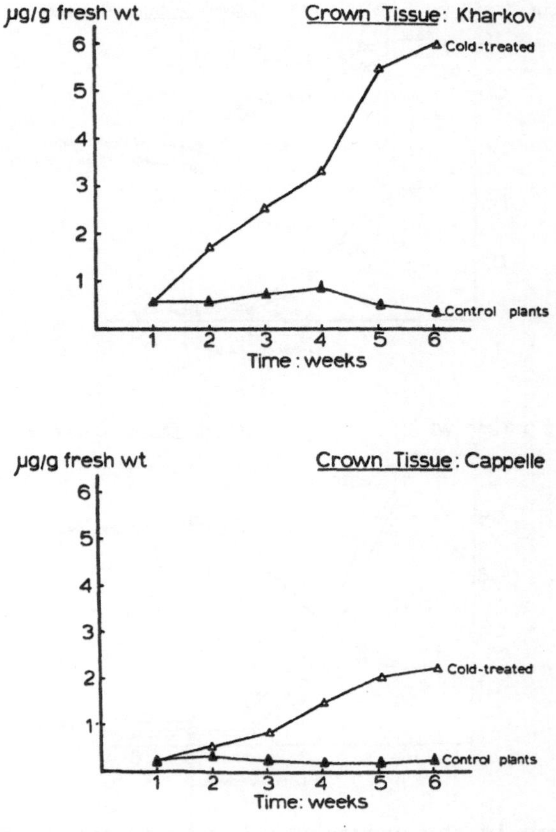

Fig. 30. Changes in the endogenous levels of abscisic acid in crown tissue from Kharkov and Cappelle seedlings growing under control or cold temperature conditions.

REFERENCES

Bandurski, R. S., and Schulze, A., 1974, Concentrations of indole-3-acetic acid and its esters in Avena and Zea, Plant Physiol., 54:257-262.

Bandurski, R. S., and Schulze, A., 1977, Concentrations of indole-3-acetic acid and its derivatives in plants, Plant Physiol., 60: 211-213.

Bayer, M. H., 1969, Gas chromatographic analysis of acidic indole auxins in Nicotiana, Plant Physiol., 44:267-271.

Beardsell, M. R., and Cohen, D., 1975, Relationships between leaf water status, abscisic acid levels, and stomatal resistance in maize and sorghum, Plant Physiol., 56:207-212.

Berger, J., and Avery, G. S., 1944, Isolation of an auxin precursor and an auxin; indoleacetic acid, from maize, Amer. J. Bot., 31:199-203.

Bowen, D. H., Crozier, A., MacMillan, J., and Reid, D. M., 1973, Characterization of gibberellins from light-grown Phaseolus coccineus seedlings by combined GC-MS, Phytochemistry, 12: 2935-2941.

Brenner, M. L., 1979, Use of modern forms of chromatography for plant growth substance analysis, in: "Techniques for Growth Regulator Assay," Vol. II, American Association of Plant Physiologists/Plant Growth Regulator Working Group Symposium, in press.

Bridges, I. G., Hillman, J. R., and Wilkins, M. B., 1973, Identification and localisation of auxin in primary roots of Zea mays by mass spectrometry, Planta, 115:189-192.

Browning, G., and Saunders, P. F., 1977, Membrane localised gibberellins A_2 and A_4 in wheat chloroplasts, Nature, 265: 375-377.

Carnes, M. G., Brenner, M. L., and Andersen, C. R., 1974, Rapid separation and identification of plant growth substances using high pressure liquid chromatography, in: "Plant Growth Substances 1973," S. Tamura, ed., Hirokawa Publishing Company, Tokyo.

Carnes, M. G., Brenner, M. L., and Anderson, C. R., 1975, Comparison of reverse-phase high pressure liquid chromatography with Sephadex LH-20 for cytokinin analysis of tomato root pressure exudate, J. Chromatogr., 108:95-106.

Cavell, B. D., MacMillan, J., Pryce, R. J., and Sheppard, A. C., 1967, Thin-layer and gas-liquid chromatography of the gibberellins; direct identification of the gibberellins in a crude plant extract by gas-liquid chromatography, Phytochemistry, 6:867-874.

Challice, J. S., 1975, Separation of cytokinins by high pressure liquid chromatography, Planta, 122:203-207.

Ciha, A. J., Brenner, M. L., and Brun, W. A., 1977, Rapid separation and quantification of abscisic acid from plant tissues using high performance liquid chromatography, Plant Physiol., 59: 821-826.

Crozier, A., Bowen, D. H., MacMillan, J., Reid, D. M., and Most, B. H., 1971, Characterization of gibberellins from dark-grown Phaseolus coccineus seedlings by gas-liquid chromatography and combined gas chromatography-mass spectrometry, Planta, 97: 142-154.

Crozier, A., and Reeve, D. R., 1977, The application of high performance liquid chromatography to the analysis of plant hormones, in: "Plant Growth Regulation," P. E. Pilet, ed., Springer-Verlag, Berlin.

Davis, L. A., Heinz, D. E., and Addicott, F. T., 1968, Gas-liquid chromatography of trimethylsilyl derivatives of abscisic acid and other plant hormones, Plant Physiol., 43:1389-1394.

Dekhuijzen, H. M., and Gevers, E. C. T., 1975, The recovery of cytokinins during extraction and purification of club root tissue, Physiol. Plant., 35:297-302.

DeYoe, D. R., and Zaerr, J. B., 1976, Indole-3-acetic acid in Douglas fir. Analysis of gas-liquid chromatography and mass spectrometry, Plant Physiol., 58:299-303.

During, H., and Bachmann, O., 1975, Abscisic acid analysis in Vitis vinifera in the period of endogenous bud dormancy by high pressure liquid chromatography, Physiol. Plant., 34:201-203.

Durley, R. C., Kannangara, T., and Simpson, G. M., 1978, Analysis of abscisins and 3-indolylacetic acid in leaves of Sorghum bicolor by high performance liquid chromatography, Can. J. Bot., 56:157-161.

Edelbluth, E., and Kaldewey, H., 1976, Auxins in scapes, flower buds, flowers and fruits of daffodil (Narcissus pseudonarcissus L.), Planta, 131:285-291.

Elliott, M. C., and Greenwood, M. S., 1974, Indole-3-yl-acetic acid in roots of Zea mays, Phytochemistry, 11:345-351.

Engvild, K. C., Egsgaard, H., and Larsen, E., 1978, Gas chromatographic-mass spectrometric identification of 4-chlorindolyl-3-acetic acid methyl ester in immature green peas, Physiol. Plant., 42:365-368.

Frydman, V. M., Gaskin, P., and MacMillan, J., 1974, Qualitative and quantitative analyses of gibberellins throughout seed maturation in Pisum sativum cv Progress No. 9, Planta, 118: 123-132.

Gaskin, P., and MacMillan, J., 1968, Plant hormones VII. Identification and estimation of abscisic acid in a crude plant extract by combined gas chromatography-mass spectrometry, Phytochemistry, 7:1699-1701.

Gaskin, P., and MacMillan, J., 1978, GC and GC-MS techniques for gibberellins, in: "Isolation of Plant Growth Substances," J. R. Hillman, ed., Cambridge Univ. Press, Cambridge.

Gaskin, P., MacMillan, J., and Zeevaart, J. A. D., 1973, Identification of gibberellin A_{20}, abscisic acid and phaseic acid from flowering Bryophyllum diagremontianum by combined gas chromatography-mass spectrometry, Planta, 111:347-352.

Grunwald, C., Mendez, J., and Stowe, B. B., 1968, Substrates for the optimum gas chromatographic separation of indolic methyl esters and the resolution of components of methyl-3-indolepyruvate solutions, in: "Biochemistry and Physiology of Plant Growth Substances," F. Wightman and G. Setterfield, eds., Runge Press Ltd., Ottawa.

Grunwald, C., Vendrell, M., and Stowe, B. B., 1967, Evaluation of gas and other chromatographic separations of indolic methyl esters, Anal. Biochem., 20:484-496.

Hahn, H., 1975, Cytokinins; a rapid extraction and purification method, Physiol. Plant., 34:204-207.

Hahn, H., 1976, High-performance liquid chromatography and its use in cytokinin determination in Agrobacterium tumefaciens B6, Plant and Cell Physiol., 17:1053-1058.

Hall, S. M., and Medlow, G. C., 1974, Identification of IAA in phloem and root pressure saps of Ricinus communis L. by mass spectrometry, Planta, 119:257-261.

Harrison, M. A., and Saunders, P. F., 1975, The abscisic acid content of dormant birch buds, Planta, 123:291-298.

Harrison, M. A., and Walton, D. C., 1975, Abscisic acid metabolism in water-stressed bean leaves, Plant Physiol., 56:250-254.

Heftmann, E., Saunders, G. A., and Haddon, W. F., 1978, Argentation high-pressure liquid chromatography and mass spectrometry of gibberellin esters, J. Chromatog., 156:71-77.

Hillman, J. R., Math, V. B., and Medlow, G. C., 1977, Apical dominance and the levels of indole acetic acid in Phaseolus lateral buds, Planta, 134:191-193.

Hopping, M. E., and Bukovac, M. J., 1975, Endogenous plant growth substances in developing fruit of Prunus cerasus L. III. Isolation of indole-3-acetic acid from the seed, J. Amer. Soc. Hort. Sci., 100:384-386.

Horgan, R., 1978, Analytical procedures for cytokinins, in: "Isolation of Plant Growth Substances," J. R. Hillman, ed., Cambridge Univ. Press, Cambridge.

Horgan, R., Hewett, E. W., Horgan, J. M., Purse, J., and Wareing, P. F., 1975, A new cytokinin from Populus x Robusta, Phytochemistry, 14:1005-1008.

Horgan, R., Hewett, E. W., Purse, J. G., Horgan, J. M., and Wareing, P. F., 1973, Identification of a cytokinin in sycamore sap by gas chromatography-mass spectrometry, Plant Sci. Lett., 1: 321-324.

Jones, E. R. H., Henbest, B., Smith, G. F., and Bentley, J. A., 1952, 3-indolylacetonitrile: A naturally occurring plant growth hormone, Nature, 169:485-487.

Kannangara, T., Durley, R. C., and Simpson, G. M., 1978, High performance liquid chromatographic analysis of cytokinins in Sorghum bicolor leaves, Physiol. Plant., 44:295-299.

Lenton, J. R., Bowen, M. R., and Saunders, P. F., 1968, Detection of abscisic acid in the xylem sap of willow (Salix viminalis L.) by gas-liquid chromatography, Nature, 220:86-87.

Lenton, J. R., Perry, V. M., and Saunders, P. F., 1971, The identification and quantitative analysis of abscisic acid in plant extracts by gas-liquid chromatography, Planta, 96: 271-280.
Lenton, J. R., Perry, V. M., and Saunders, P. F., 1972, Endogenous abscisic acid in relation to photoperiodically induced bud dormancy, Planta, 106:13-22.
Lorenzi, R., Horgan, R., and Wareing, P. F., 1975, Cytokinins in Picea sitchensis Carriere: Identification and relation to growth, Biochem. Physiol. Pflanzen, 168:333-339.
Loveys, B. R., 1977, The intracellular location of abscisic acid in stressed and non-stressed leaf tissue, Physiol. Plant., 40: 6-10.
Loveys, B. R., and Kriedemann, P. E., 1974, Internal control of stomatal physiology and photosynthesis. I. Stomatal regulation and associated changes in endogenous levels of abscisic and phaseic acids, Aust. J. Plant Physiol., 1:407-415.
Loveys, B. R., Leopold, A. C., and Kriedemann, P. E., 1974, Abscisic acid metabolism and stomatal physiology in Betula lutea following alteration of photoperiod, Ann. Bot., 38:85-92.
MacMillan, J., 1968, Direct identification of gibberellins in plant extracts by gas chromatography-mass spectrometry, in: "Biochemistry and Physiology of Plant Growth Substances," F. Wightman and G. Setterfield, eds., Runge Press Ltd., Ottawa.
MacMillan, J., 1972, A system for the characterization of plant growth substances based upon the direct coupling of a gas chromatograph, a mass spectrometer, and a small computer--Recent examples of its applications, in: "Plant Growth Substances 1970," D. J. Carr, ed., Springer-Verlag, Berlin.
Marumo, S., Abe, H., Hattori, H., and Munakata, K., 1968a, Isolation of a novel auxin, methyl 4-chloroindoleacetate, from immature seeds of Pisum sativum, Agric. Biol. Chem., 32:117-118.
Marumo, S., Hattori, H., and Abe, H., 1971, Chromatography of a new natural auxin, 4-chloroindolyl-3-acetic acid and related chloro derivatives, Anal. Biochem., 40:488-490.
Marumo, S., Hattori, H., Abe, H., and Munakata, K., 1968b, Isolation of 4-chloroindolyl-3-acetic acid from immature seeds of Pisum sativum, Nature, 219:959-960.
McDougall, J., and Hillman, J. R., 1978a, Purification of IAA from shoot tissues of Phaseolus vulgaris and its analysis by GC-MS, J. Exp. Bot., 29:375-386.
McDougall, J., and Hillman, J. R., 1978b, Analysis of indole-3-acetic acid using GC-MS techniques, in: "Isolation of Plant Growth Substances," J. R. Hillman, ed., Cambridge Univ. Press, Cambridge.
McRae, D. G., 1978, Changes in the growth-regulating substances of winter wheat during cold acclimation, Master's Thesis, Carleton University, Ottawa.
McWha, J. A., and Hillman, J. R., 1974, Endogenous abscisic acid in lettuce fruit, Z. Pflanzenphysiol., 74:292-297.

Mizrahi, Y., Blumenfield, A., Bittner, S., and Richmond, A. E., 1971, Abscisic acid and cytokinin contents of leaves in relation to salinity and relative humidity, Plant Physiol., 48: 752-755.
Morris, R. O., Zaerr, J. B., and Chapman, R. W., 1976, Trace enrichment of cytokinins from Douglas fir xylem exudate, Planta, 131:271-274.
Most, B. H., Williams, J. C., and Parker, K. J., 1968, Gas chromatography of cytokinin, J. Chromatog., 38:136-138.
Phipps, J., and Wightman, F., 1977, Chromatographic procedures for the total growth substance analysis of developing plant organs, Plant Physiol., 59:11.
Pool, R. M., and Powell, L. E., 1972, The use of pellicular ion-exchange resins to separate plant cytokinins by high pressure liquid chromatography, HortScience, 7:330.
Pool, R. M., and Powell, L. E., 1974, Cytokinin analysis by high pressure liquid chromatography, in: "Plant Growth Substances 1973," S. Tamura, ed., Hirokawa Publishing Company, Tokyo.
Powell, L. E., 1964, Preparation of indole extracts from plants for gas chromatography and spectrophotofluorometry, Plant Physiol., 39:836-842.
Powell, L. E., 1972, The evolution of plant hormone analysis, HortScience, 7:236-238.
Purse, J. G., Horgan, R., Horgan, J. M., and Wareing, P. F., 1976, Cytokinins of sycamore spring sap, Planta, 132:1-8.
Quarrie, S. A., 1978, A rapid and sensitive assay for abscisic acid using ethyl abscisate as an internal standard, Anal. Biochem., 87:148-156.
Quebedeaux, B., Sweetser, P. B., and Rowell, J. C., 1976, Abscisic acid levels in soybean reproductive structures during development, Plant Physiol., 58:363-366.
Reeve, D. R., and Crozier, A., 1977, Radioactivity monitor for high performance liquid chromatography, J. Chromatogr., 137:271-282.
Reeve, D. R., and Crozier, A., 1978, The analysis of gibberellins by high performance liquid chromatography, in: "Isolation of Plant Growth Substances," J. R. Hillman, ed., Cambridge Univ. Press, Cambridge.
Reeve, D. R., Yokota, T., Nash, L. J., and Crozier, A., 1976, The development of a high performance liquid chromatograph with a sensitive onstream radioactivity monitor for the analysis of ^{3}H and ^{14}C-labelled gibberellins, J. Exp. Bot., 21:1243-1258.
Rivier, L., Milon, H., and Pilet, P. E., 1977, Gas chromatography-mass spectrometric determinations of abscisic acid levels in the cap and the apex of maize roots, Planta, 134:23-37.
Rivier, L., and Pilet, P. E., 1974, Indolyl-3-acetic acid in cap and apex of maize roots; identification and quantification of mass fragmentography, Planta, 120:107-112.
Robertson, J., Hillman, J. R., and Berrie, A. M. M., 1976, The involvement of indole acetic acid in the thermodormancy of lettuce fruits, Lactuca sativa cv Grant Rapids, Planta, 131: 309-313.

Saunders, P. F., 1978, The identification and quantitative analysis of abscisic acid in plant extracts, in: "Isolation of Plant Growth Substances," J. R. Hillman, ed., Cambridge Univ. Press, Cambridge.

Schlenk, H., and Gellerman, J. L., 1960, Esterification of fatty acids with diazomethane on a small scale, Anal. Chem., 32: 1412-1414.

Seeley, S.D., and Powell, L.E., 1970, Electron capture-gas chromatography for sensitive assay of abscisic acid, Anal. Biochem., 35:530-532.

Seeley, S. D., and Powell, L. E., 1974, Gas chromatography and detection of microquantities of gibberellins and indole acetic acid as their fluorinated derivatives, Anal. Biochem., 58: 39-46.

Shindy, W. W., and Smith, O. E., 1975, Identification of plant hormones from cotton ovules, Plant Physiol., 55:550-554.

Stowe, B. B., and Schilke, J. F., 1964, Submicrogram identification and analysis of indole auxins by gas chromatography and spectrophotofluorometry, in: "Regulateurs Natureles de la Croissance Vegetale," J. P. Nitsch, ed., C.N.R.S., Paris, No. 123.

Sweetser, P. B., 1979, Use of modern forms of chromatography for plant growth substance analysis, in: "Techniques for Growth Regulator Assay," Vol. I, American Society of Plant Physiologists/Plant Growth Regulator Working Group Symposium, in press.

Sweetser, P. B., and Swartzfager, D. G., 1978, Indole-3-acetic acid levels of plant tissue as determined by a new high performance liquid chromatographic method, Plant Physiol., 61:254-258.

Sweetser, P. B., and Vatvars, A., 1976, High-performance liquid chromatographic analysis of abscisic acid in plant extracts, Anal. Biochem., 71:68-78.

Takahashi, N., Yamaguchi, I., Kono, T., Igoshi, M., Hirose, K., and Suzuki, K., 1975, Characterization of plant growth substances in Citrus unshiu and their changes in fruit development, Plant and Cell Physiol., 16:1101-1111.

Taylor, P. A., Kosuge, T., and DeVay, J. E., 1974, Compounds associated with cytokinin activity in fruitlets and tracheal fluid of Gossypium hirsutum, Physiol. Plant., 30:119-124.

Thomas, T. H., Carrol, J. E., Isenberg, F. M. R., Pendergrass, A., and Howell, L., 1975, A simple, inexpensive, high pressure liquid chromatographic method for separating cytokinins in plant extracts, Plant Physiol., 56:410-414.

Upper, C. D., Helgeson, J. P., Kemp, J. D., and Schmidt, C. J., 1970, Gas-liquid chromatographic isolation of cytokinins from natural sources, Plant Physiol., 45:543-547.

Upper, C. D., Helgeson, J. P., and Schmidt, C. J., 1972, Identification of cytokinins by gas-liquid chromatography and gas-liquid chromatography-mass spectrometry, in: "Plant Growth Substances 1970," D. J. Carr, ed., Springer-Verlag, Berlin.

White, J. C., Medlow, G. C., Hillman, J. R., and Wilkins, M. B., 1975, Correlative inhibition of lateral bud growth in

Phaseolus vulgaris L. Isolation of indoleacetic acid from the inhibitory region, J. Exptl. Bot., 26:419-424.

Wightman, F., 1973, Biosynthesis of auxins in tomato shoots, in: "Nitrogen Metabolism in Plants," T. W. Goodwin and R. M. S. Smellie, eds., Biochem. Soc. Symp., 38:247-275.

Wightman, F., 1977, Gas chromatographic identification and quantitative estimation of natural auxins in developing plant organs, in: "Plant Growth Regulation," P. E. Pilet, ed., Springer-Verlag, Berlin.

Wightman, F., and Rauthan, B. S., 1974, Evidence for the biosynthesis and natural occurrence of the auxin, phenylacetic acid, in shoots of higher plants, in: "Plant Growth Substances 1973," S. Tamura, ed., Hirokawa Publishing Company, Tokyo.

Wright, S. T. C., and Hiron, R. W. P., 1969, (+) Abscisic acid, the growth inhibitor induced in detached wheat leaves by a period of wilting, Nature, 224:719-720.

Wright, S. T. C., and Hiron, R. W. P., 1972, The accumulation of abscisic acid in plants during wilting and under other stress conditions, in: "Plant Growth Substances 1970," D. J. Carr, ed., Springer-Verlag, Berlin.

Young, H., 1977, Identification of cytokinins from natural sources by gas-liquid chromatography-mass spectrometry, Anal. Biochem., 79:226-233.

Zabadal, T. J., 1974, A water potential threshold for the increase of abscisic acid in leaves, Plant Physiol., 53:125-127.

Zeevaart, J. A. D., 1977, Sites of abscisic acid synthesis and metabolism in Ricinus communis L., Plant Physiol., 59:788-791.

20

A PROPOSAL FOR THE APPLICATION OF GROWTH REGULATORS IN TURKEY IN RELATION TO AGRICULTURAL POTENTIAL

Yusuf Vardar[1]

Karsiyaka
Izmir, Turkey

It is well known that a worldwide application of plant growth regulators to increase yield has not been made to a large extent before now. We can say that we are actually only at the beginning of the commercial exploitation of plant growth substances in the production, harvesting, and storage of food (Barrass, 1974).

Today there is general agreement among scientists that all scientific and technical possibilities and strategies should be tried in determining the agricultural strategy for the year 2000 and that not even a trivial alternative should be neglected (Wise and Fell, 1978).

In all probability, accelerating the development of crop plants to maturity by shortening the periods between sowing and harvesting, flowering and maturation, and also reducing stem growth without reducing fruit, tuber, or top root production will be practiced widely in the very near future. It may be possible to increase production by completing more growing cycles in one growing season. Also, the nutritional quality of the product may be improved by influencing the direction of plant metabolism with regulators (Wareing, 1977; Kefeli, 1978). Actually, Vlitos (1970) has shown an excellent and realistic model of the latter in sugarcane cultivation.

Therefore, it is my opinion that significant improvements could be made in the world's agricultural production by the worldwide application of plant growth regulators. In view of this, to design

[1]Formerly Professor of Botany at the Ege University, Izmir, Turkey (now retired).

an agricultural strategy for the year 2000, it is necessary to develop and employ a regulatory agricultural plan, "RAP," that parallels the green plan being presently applied in the world at national and international levels with the support of the Food and Agricultural Organization (FAO) and other international organizations. A large scale application of such a plan should contribute immensely to the improvement of the world's agricultural production. Turkey, like other countries, must determine goals and devise an agricultural regulatory plan at the national level and find out ways of employing it effectively.

Undoubtedly, there are various possibilities of increasing crop yield in Turkey and these could be exploited by other means. Thus, projects emphasizing plant breeding and genetic manipulation, the improvement and conservation of soil, the gaining of new cultivation areas, mechanization and modernization of agriculture, and also irrigation, fertilization, and pest control have been already put forth in the plans extending to the year 2000. As a matter of fact, the project to irrigate 8.5 billion hectares of land included in the current plan extending to the year 2000 by itself promises a big explosion in our national agricultural production. Similarly, the project for breeding wheat to get more productive crops has given very promising results and two new types of wheat have been obtained (Cumhuriyet 75 and Gediz 75). An increase of 20-25% in annual wheat production is expected by the year 2000 merely by introducing these new varieties on a large scale in the presently cultivated areas in Turkey (Şölen and Dutlu, personal communication). Furthermore, Turkey has other arable areas, one of which, Çukurova, has been reported in the statistics of 1977 as one of the three regions in the world giving the highest yield per hectare.

On the other hand, Turkey is one of the 9 countries out of 149 in the world that do not need to import food presently. There is also a high percentage of arable land that is not being used effectively and which could feed twice our present population if it were exploited effectively and scientifically. However, we should not overlook the fact that the Turkish people have one of the highest rates of bread consumption per head in the world (Davit, 1977).

In spite of all these hopeful factors, if we take into consideration our high population growth rate (2.6%), (Tayşi, 1976) and also the possible reflection of a world food crisis, Turkey undoubtedly has to take some precautions. These could be accomplished by encouraging the application of plant growth regulators for achieving a higher production in addition to utilizing other possibilities mentioned previously for increasing agricultural productivity. We need a national plan which includes the application of regulators. Of course, such a national plan should take into consideration the agricultural structure and characteristics of the country, together with the country's agricultural potential and its future goals, and it should determine the details of application carefully. Therefore, before outlining the basic aims of such a national regulatory agricultural plan, we should look briefly at the ecological and agricultural structure and characteristics of Turkey, taking into consideration the close relationship of such a plan to the agricultural structure.

Turkey is considered to be in the Mediterranean agricultural belt and possesses Mediterranean ecological conditions. Therefore, it is necessary to examine briefly the conditions determining and limiting the agricultural structure and potential of the region.

The Mediterranean region is a characteristic area of the world with its typical ecology, economy, and demography. The maximum spread of this area is approximately between 30-45°N and the general east-west trend is 10°W to 50°E longitude. There are certain general climatic and ecological factors that are considered specific to the region and these determine the agricultural structure of the region. Actually, the term Mediterranean is defined as a climatic term (Aschmann, 1973). The rough specifications of these general climatic and ecological factors are as Vlitos (1976) reports:

(1) Lack of fresh water,
(2) Abundant solar energy,
(3) Generally poor fertility and difficult soil structure, and
(4) Ill-defined, frost-free areas.

In the Mediterranean ecosystem where these basic climatic and ecological factors are dominant, the environmentally imposed conditions of summer drought provide severe physiological stress on plant life. At least 65% of the year's precipitation occurs in the winter half-year. Winter rainfall is more effective in sustaining plant growth than is warm season precipitation because of lower evaporation. Effective precipitation as reported by Aschmann (1973) falls between values of 3.4 m/yr and 8.7 m/yr in the Mediterranean climate.

These distinctive patterns of hydrology and drought play an extremely important role in determining plant community (Rundel, 1978) and agricultural structure. The moisture content limits the plant growth in the region, especially during the summer months when favorable air temperatures for high-rate photosynthetic activity occur. High agricultural production thus is hindered.

Nevertheless, the long summers, bright sunshine, and the remarkable heterogeneity of soil produce typical micro-ecological variations. This creates a potential for a diversified, high quality, and high quantity agricultural productivity. So, it seems that:

(1) Cultivating crops in each season throughout the year,
(2) Having two or three harvests in a year, and/or,
(3) Realizing multiple cropping,

are the main possible ways for getting a higher total yield in the Mediterranean region.

Actually, the fact that out of 115 fruits cultivated in the world, 95 can be grown in the Mediterranean region, can be considered a good example supporting this point of view. Therefore, it can roughly be concluded that, if the ecological and climatic conditions and the limiting factors mentioned above can be regulated wisely and effectively, the role of the Mediterranean belt in world agriculture will gain an undeniable significance.

As pointed out above, Turkey is situated in the Mediterranean region, lying between 26-45°E longitude and between 36-42°N latitude. It stands like a bridge between Asia and Europe. The major part of the country lies in Asia and is known as Anatolia or Asia Minor. This is divided into five districts, namely, East, West, North, South, and Central Anatolia (Vardar, 1965). The total area, excluding the lakes, is 780,576 km^2. Approximately 3% of this, 23,623 km^2, lies in Europe and the remaining 97% in Asia. The land surface of Turkey is very much folded. For example, there are steep mountain chains on the Black Sea coast, Tauros mountains on the Mediterranean coast, a high plateau in eastern Anatolia.

Actually, it could be said that the term "The Anatolian Plateau" is misleading, since only 12% of the area has a slope of less than 1%. Also, two-thirds of the country suffers from some form of soil erosion, and about 80% of the country lies 500 m above sea level. In short, Anatolia is above all a land of conspicious extreme geographical, geological, climatic, ecological, and other contrasts.

As pointed out above, crudely speaking, we can say that Turkey has a Mediterranean climate, but with a monsoonal tendency. In summer, the rainfall is very low due to feeble cyclonic activity of the air masses, a tendency that is strengthened by the development of a high pressure area in the Mediterranean. Thus extreme summer dryness affects the agricultural structure and vegetation. However, in winter, the tropical and continental air masses cause instability with heavy rainfall. The rains cause variable climatic conditions in the country. Thus, it is possible to find different climatic conditions from subtropical and semitropical to continental Boreal in the country.

Similarly, it is possible to see frost as early as in August (Kars, Kütahya) and as late as in May (Kars, Erzurum).

According to De Martonno's drought index calculations, approximately 4.5% of the arable land has droughty and arid and approximately 29.3% has semidroughty land characteristics (drought index 0-15). Only 21.7% of the arable land has less than 100 summer days (when the air temperature is above 25°C). In the remaining 78.3%, the number of summer days in one year is above 100.

Presently, in planning its agricultural activities, the Ministry of Agriculture has divided the country into four different climatic districts--central, east, and southeast Anatolia, and inland-coast transition districts--taking into consideration the varying characteristics and agricultural conditions (Baade, 1959).

Together with climatic variations, there are ecological variations in the country. In addition to these variations, the fact that Anatolia has the features of a basin being surrounded by high mountains on all four sides induces some further agricultural difficulties. On the other hand, it exhibits some agricultural and structural pecularities that provide a wide agricultural potential and numerous alternatives. Therefore, it is obvious that the country's potential is huge, whether for new crops or for expanding existing crops including everything from tea to asparagus. It has the third largest cultivable area in Europe, after France and the Soviet Union (Davit, 1977).

According to our best information regarding national statistics, the arable land in Turkey covers 59,226 km^2, which is 20.4% of the total area (İmar ve İskan Bakanligi, 1969).

Within the limits of the agricultural structure defined by the above-mentioned characteristics, the cultivation area for agricultural crops lies basically from 0-500 m above sea level. As we proceed inland from the coast the favorable conditions during the growing period diminish, causing a reduction in the number of crop varieties that can be cultivated. As a matter of fact, near 500 m above sea level the agriculture remains restricted only to some cereals and vegetables.

The agricultural structure and characteristics summarized above determine the present productivity of Turkey and at the same time define its future agricultural productivity potential. However, the future goals need to be specified very carefully and painstakingly and serious scientific plans need to be made (West, 1958). Undoubtedly, irrigation, plant breeding, soil conservation and management, fertilization, perfection of disease control, and the predomination of agricultural mechanization and modernization are the most important factors included in these plans. However, we have also to look to the methods which have given satisfactory and successful results in other countries (Wain, 1977)--intercropping, increasing the number of crop varieties, intensive agriculture, emphasizing the cultivation of industrial plants and fruits, abolishing monoculture in irrigated cropping especially by introducing rotation between cotton and other plants, and making it possible to have two or three harvests in a year. These should be the basic principles of the agricultural strategy of Turkey up to the year 2000.

At this point, we can now turn to the question of the application of plant regulators for increasing yield within the limits of the sketch drawn above. Undoubtedly, as emphasized before, these applications have to be planned in detail and in harmony with the agricultural structure and potential of the country.

However, we could consider the following proposals as the basic points of such a plan:

(1) Enlarging and renewing the orchards are among the essentials of our agricultural activity. There is an utter need for large nurseries. It would be possible to obtain good and homogeneous nurslings from these nurseries in a short time and to obtain nurslings of agriculturally significant plants such as vines, olives, and figs (Kaldewey, 1970) by a wide scope application of plant growth regulators and to produce an indirect increase in the agricultural yield.

(2) It has been stated that there is a 15-20% loss in yield, especially in cereals, as a result of improper control of tillering. According to the results reported (Leopold, 1949; Wünshe, 1977), it seems that it will be possible to prevent this loss and have an indirect increase in the yield by using growth regulators in controlling tillering in cereal agriculture. Similar possibilities could be experimented with in Turkey by practicing a weed control program based on scientific principles (Häfliger and Brun-Holl, 1975).

(3) In the case of pomology, which has a specific importance in Turkish agriculture, it is clear that the application of plant growth regulators in controlling flower and fruit development can produce promising results.

Similarly, it is possible to prevent loss in the yield of olive trees, which are specific and important in the agriculture of Turkey and especially of this region, by applying Alsol 2-chloroethyl-tris (2-methoxy-ethoxy)-silan (Ciba-Geigy, cod. no. 13586) as reported by Rufener and Green (1977). Furthermore, according to the results reported for other plants (Crane, 1965), an application aimed at obtaining a parthenocarpic fruit in olives may result in a reasonable increase in the edible part of the fruit (approximately 40% of the olive fruit consists of hard seed).

(4) Another case of special attention for Turkey could be the control of flower and fruit development in poppy (Papaver somniferum). As is commonly known, the axial growth of poppy is characteristically uniaxial. The main axis generally ends with a single flower. According to Sladky and Konecma (1977) the differentiation of single and double flowers in poppy is a process regulated with growth substances.

The change of this uniaxial behavior by the application of regulators in poppy agriculture will thus clearly mean getting the same yield from a smaller field and simplifying the problems of efficient inspection.

Similarly, a large scale application of growth regulators in the cotton crop, again one of the important crops in Turkey, on the lines reported by Dimitrova (1977) seems a promising way to speed ripening and to increase the number of bolls, resulting in higher yield.

(5) Under the extreme and varying climatic conditions, we encounter big losses in Turkish agricultural products due to frost every year. Keeping this in mind, if the growth of major crops can be controlled by shortening (or lengthening) their periods of development with the use of growth regulators, we can prevent this now inevitable loss and consequently increase the total yield. Moreover, a temporary drought resistance that can be developed with the application of antitranspirants and other synthetic growth substances (Henckel and Postovoitova, 1977) could create excellent possibilities of gaining the crops normally lost during the long drought periods in each summer.

(6) Turkey is also known for having favorable environmental conditions for numerous wild, medicinally significant plants as well as industrially important ones.

It is known that the accumulation of secondary metabolic plant products are stimulated by growth substances (Constabel et al., 1971; Scott, 1972). On the other hand, as has been reported by Zenk and his coworkers (Zenk et al., 1975; Zenk et al., 1977), the production of the medicinally important substances, which are also considered as typical secondary metabolic products of plants, could be increased by 20-30% as a result of treatment by growth regulators in a liquid cell culture medium of the plants.

Similarly, field experiments were carried out with Mentha piperita (Iliev et al., 1977), and the treatment of root stocks with growth regulators has shown an obvious increase in growth, in the yield of green mass, and in the yield of essential oil.

Consequently, the treatment of essential-oil bearing plants and other medicinally important plants that could be cultivated in Turkey by plant growth regulators could result in a remarkable increase in total yield.

(7) Finally, in addition to all that has been discussed above, one further point should be taken into consideration with respect to the basic problem of increase in general productivity. It is known that the solar energy incident on the earth's surface is about 2×10^{24} J per annum. The global annual productivity of photosynthesis equals 3×10^{21} J of stored solar energy. This represents an overall efficiency of solar energy conversion of 0.15%. On the other hand, it is also known that the maximum short-term growth rates of high yielding land crops represent solar energy conversion efficiencies of 2.7-4.6%, but productivities are considerably lower (0.16-1.6%). I believe there are numerous promising possibilities which can result in increasing this low annual productivity. With an increase in productivity, growth regulators might well be employed on a larger scale to motivate new and different possible applications. The aims of the growth regulator applications pointed out above could, in my opinion, easily be extended and generalized for the whole Mediterranean agricultural belt.

Therefore, in conclusion we can say that the large scale application of growth regulators in this direction can contribute a great deal to the future of mankind by producing an increase in the agricultural productivity at national and international levels. However, as stated by Vlitos (in press): To attain this, the auxinologists must be successful in achieving a more dynamic and interdisciplinary cooperation among themselves.

REFERENCES

Aschmann, H., 1973, Distribution and peculiarity of Mediterranean Ecosystems, quoted in: "Ecological Studies 7," F. D. Castri and H. A. Mooney, eds., Springer-Verlag, Berlin.

Baade, F., 1959, "Report for Turkey," United Nations Food and Agriculture Organization, Rome.

Barrass, R., 1974, "Biology, Food and People," Unibooks, English Univ. Press, Ltd., London.

Constabel, F., Shyluk, J., and Gamborg, O., 1971, The effect of hormones on authocyanin accumulation in cell culture of Happlopappus gracilis, Planta, 96:306-316.

Crane, J. C., 1965, The chemical induction of parthenocarpy in the Calimyrna fig and its physiological significance, Plant Physiol., 40:606-610.

Davit, T., 1977, Turkey VII, Agricultural yields improve, Financial Times, Nov. 23, London.

Dimitrova, L. N., 1977, Effect of some plant growth regulators on fruiting characteristics of cotton, quoted in: "Proceedings of International Symposium on Plant Growth Regulators," T. Kudrew, I. Ivanova, and E. Karanov, eds., Sofia.
Häfliger, E., and Brun-Holl, J., 1975, "Ciba-Geigy Weed Tables, A Synoptic Presentation of the Flora Accompanying Agricultural Crops," Basel.
Henckel, P. A., and Postovoitova, T. H., 1977, The role of growth inhibitors in adaptive modifications of plants under drought conditions, quoted in: "Proceedings of International Symposium on Plant Growth Regulators," T. Kudrew, I. Ivanova, and E. Karanov, eds., Sofia.
Iliev, I., Zlatev, S., and Zlateva, M., 1977, Influence of some synthetic growth regulators on growth and development of mint, quoted in: "Proceedings of International Symposium on Plant Growth Regulators, T. Kudrew, I. Ivanova, and E. Karanov, eds., Sofia.
Imar ve Iskan Bakanligi, 1969, Türkiye'de Tabiî ve Beserî Kaynaklarin Bölgelere Göre Dagilimi, Bölge Plânlama Dairesi, Ankara.
Kaldewey, H., 1970, "Agricultural Research in Turkey with Special Reference to Plant Physiology," Organization for Economic Cooperation and Development consultant's report.
Kefeli, V. I., 1978, "Natural Plant Growth Inhibitors and Phytohormones," Dr. W. Junk, The Hague, Boston.
Leopold, A. C., 1949, The control of tillering in grasses by auxin, Amer. J. Bot., 36:437-440.
Rufener, J., and Green, D. H., 1977, A new chemical harvest-aid for olives, quoted in: "Proceedings of International Symposium on Plant Growth Regulators," T. Kudrew, I. Ivanova, and E. Karanov, eds., Sofia.
Rundel, P. W., 1978, Water balance in Mediterranean sclerophyll ecosystems, quoted in: "Proceedings of the Symposium on the Invir. Cons. of Fire and Fuel Management in Mediterranean Ecosystems," U.S. Department of Agriculture, Washington, D.C.
Scott, T. K., 1972, Auxins and roots, Ann. Rev. Plant Physiol., 23:125-140.
Sladky, Z., and Konecma, 1977, Endogenous regulators in flower differentiation of Papaver sommniferum, quoted in: "Proceedings of International Symposium on Plant Growth Regulators," T. Kudrew, I. Ivanova, and E. Karanov, eds., Sofia.
Taysi, V., 1976, Agriculture in Turkey, quoted in: "Fertilizer Use and Plant Health," International Photosynthesis Institute, Bern.
Vardar, Y., 1965, Outline of the vegetation of West Anatolia, Schweiz Naturforsch. Gesel.
Vlitos, A. J., 1970, "A Review of Plant Growth Regulating Chemicals in Sugarcane Cultivation," Tate and Lyle Ltd. Research Center Seminar, Keston, Kent, Private circulation.
Vlitos, A. J., 1976, Some problems of Mediterranean agriculture and likely future trends, quoted in: "Proceedings of the Third

Mediterranean Plant Physiology Meeting," Y. Vardar, K. H. Sheikh, and M. A. Öztürk, eds., Izmir.

Vlitos, A. J., in press, Food, energy and the environment. A review and summary of the theme, in: "Proceedings of the British Association for the Advancement of Science (sec. k.) Conference," Bath, 1978.

Wain, R. L. 1977, Science and practice in China's agriculture, Span, 20:3.

Wareing, P. F., 1977, Growth substances and integration in the whole plant, quoted in: "Integration of Plant Activity in Higher Plants," D. H. Jennings, ed., Symposium XXXI, Society for Experimental Biology, Cambridge Univ. Press, Cambridge.

West, Q. M., 1958, "Agriculture Development in Turkey: Effect on Products Competitive with U.S. Farm Exports," Foreign Agriculture Report 106, U.S. Department of Agriculture, Washington, D.C.

Wise, W. S., and Fell, E., 1978, United Kingdom agricultural productivity and the land budget, J. Agric. Econ., 29:1.

Wünshe, U., 1977, Effects of growth retardants on tillering of cereals, quoted in: "Proceedings of International Symposium on Plant Growth Regulators," T. Kudrew, I. Ivanova, and E. Karanov, eds., Sofia.

Zenk, M. H., El-Shagi, H., and Schulte, V., 1975, Anthaquinove production by cell suspension culture of Morinda citrifolia, Planta Medica, Supplement.

Zenk, M. H., El-Shagi, H., and Ulbrich, B., 1977, Production of rosmarinic acid by cell suspension culture of Coleus blumei, Naturwiss., 64:585.

21

CREATIVE BOTANY: ITS ROLE IN MEETING THE MAJOR TEMPERATE AND TROPICAL AGRICULTURAL PROBLEMS OF THE FUTURE

A. J. Vlitos

Tate & Lyle, Limited
Philip Lyle Memorial Research Laboratory
The University, Whiteknights
Reading, England

INTRODUCTION

Three themes are likely to dominate and challenge the next generation of botanists: food, energy, and the environment. Without doubt, the challenge to increase food production, to improve the distribution of food, to rationalize energy resources, and to protect the environment will require multidisciplinary approaches. These approaches need not be inhibited nor polarized by scientific lines of demarcation nor by geographical boundaries. There is also a universality in the three themes which requires an international approach. It may require as well a reexamination of the definition of botany.

Most laymen, and indeed many scientists who are not botanists, tend to regard botany as a descriptive science, concerned primarily with taxonomy and morphology. In fact, botany is already very much an interdisciplinary science, and it is unique in its breadth. Not only does it include in its domain two classical branches (taxonomy and morphology), but it also includes plant genetics, physiology and biochemistry, mycology, plant pathology, and microbiology. It is the combination of the classical descriptive branches with the dynamic ones which eminently qualifies botanists to make creative contributions in assisting to solve some of the food, energy, and environmental problems of the future.

Creative botany is, in a sense, synonymous with interdisciplinary botany. It is also "relevant" botany--relevant to the major problems facing us all whether we happen to live in Europe, North America, Bangladesh, or the Sudan. In this short paper it is possible to present only a few illustrations of the impact which creative botany can make on solving some problems of fundamental and universal importance.

FOOD AND ENERGY

Increasingly, the key factor in agriculture is the balance of the amount of energy going into the production of a crop and the amount of energy recoverable from the crop at harvest. Most, if not all, of the world's major crops consume more energy, especially if their production relies more on mechanical devices than on hand labor, than is recovered at harvest. Even in crops such as rice, which are traditionally labor intensive, the energy balance is not favorable mainly because of the increasing costs of nitrogenous fertilizers. One of the keys to achieving more favorable energy balances in crop production is to find more effective means of fixing atmospheric nitrogen.

This is of particular importance in the tropics where traditionally mono-cultures of carbohydrate crops such as rice, sugarcane, and cassava require relatively heavy applications of nitrogenous fertilizers, at increasing cost, to achieve economical yields. Botanical contributions to alleviating the nitrogen problem could come in two ways: First, through the identification of leguminous species which are more efficient in fixing atmospheric nitrogen and which could be grown in rotation with the traditional cash crops. Second, a better understanding of the nitrogen fixation process itself could lead to the selection of more effective strains of bacteria for inoculating crops and enhancing nodulation. The inoculation of soils with nonsymbiotic nitrogen fixing bacteria has not proved very effective in the past, but this does not necessarily eliminate this approach, especially if the techniques could be improved.

It is probably worth mentioning here the interesting studies underway with the "winged-bean" (Psophocarpus tetragonolobus (L.) DC). Undoubtedly we shall hear a great deal more about this plant in the future. It offers interesting potential for rotation with certain carbohydrate crops because of its nitrogen fixing ability, and might reduce the cost of nitrogenous fertilization in such crops.

Another botanical aspect of agriculture linked intimately with the energy theme is the identification of species which mature rapidly enough to provide alternative sources of fuel. Rapidly maturing trees, such as leucaena, are already being experimented with in the Philippines and elsewhere. The long-term plan there is to grow such species in three to five years (from seedling to maturity, and to utilize the wood as fuel (for home cooking) and the foliage as animal feed. This approach to reducing the dependence on fossil fuels makes some sense in the tropics--for there is no better way of collecting solar energy, converting it to latent chemical energy, storing it, and then utilizing the stored energy than to grow rapidly maturing trees or some of the more conventional carbohydrate crops such as sugarcane and cassava.

The jargon for growing crops as sources of energy is the term "biomass." Unfortunately the term has led to some misconceptions. Most discussions of the energy problem tend to become polarized. There are those who maintain that there are sufficient stores of coal to be liquified in the future as an alternative fuel to make up for any deficiency in petroleum. There are those who believe that nuclear energy is the only hope for providing a feasible alternative for oil. There are those who believe firmly in geothermal sources, and there are, of course, the solar energy adherents. The most likely energy "scenario" is that in most nations <u>all</u> sources of energy will have to be exploited in the future, and it is most likely that electricity and power generation will depend on nuclear sources, while the replacement of petrochemical "feedstocks" for the chemical industry will have to come from regenerable agricultural sources (i.e., "solar" energy). The most likely uses of "biomass" will be in the area of chemical usage rather than as a provider of power and electrical supplies. One of the roles of the creative botanist in the future will be to evaluate the potential of various plants as sources of specific chemicals which might replace chemical derivatives presently dependent upon petrochemicals. Solar energy research at present is more heavily concentrated on <u>mechanical</u> devices for collecting, converting, storing, and releasing the sun's energy when required. It seems equally important to consider the other route to utilizing solar energy; that is, to evaluate the agricultural potential for producing the substitutes for petrochemicals without which most of the necessities for the life we have become accustomed to would be in jeopardy.

The pivotal compound in industrial chemistry today is ethylene. Ethylene is derived mainly by the so-called "cracking" of naptha, a petroleum derivative. In fifteen to twenty years the supplies of ethylene from petroleum are likely to diminish. It will become a very expensive compound indeed. Another source of ethylene is ethanol, but today it is more economical to convert ethylene to "industrial" ethanol rather than the other way around. We shall most likely witness over the next fifteen years a reversal of the process. Fermentation alcohol is likely to become the pivotal compound in industrial chemistry. By the year 1995 most ethylene will probably be derived from ethanol produced by fermentation of carbohydrate crops. Agriculture will have to become the major supplier of chemical "feedstocks." It is this aspect of "solar energy" which today requires the attention of the creative botanist and which seems the most amenable to an interdisciplinary approach. There is an exciting potential for utilizing carbohydrates and fats as substitutes for petrochemicals in the chemical industry.

Although most of the 100 million tons of sucrose produced in the world is used as a sweetener, recent progress in sucrochemistry indicates that sucrose and starches are viable economical alternatives to certain petrochemicals as industrial "feedstocks"-- ranging from alcohol via fermentation to surfactants via straightforward reactions of the sucrose with either animal fats or vegetable oils. Britain will probably take an early lead in this new field now that a chemical complex is under construction near Liverpool which will use natural products to produce surfactants and sugars to produce microbial polysaccharides (alginates and xanthan gum) via fermentation. The increased prices for petroleum and for certain petrochemicals offer unique opportunities <u>even today</u> for substituting "regenerable" energy sources such as sugars, starches, and vegetable oils more extensively in the chemical industry. Some may ask whether all this is relevant to botany. It is relevant if we accept that the interdisciplinary approach is a more effective means of achieving the objectives.

Sugarcane and cassava represent two of the most efficient devices for collecting and converting solar to chemical energy via photosynthesis. Although yields of sugarcane have been improved over the past fifty years there is still substantial room for improvement. If more sugar is to be channeled into the chemical and fermentation industries in the future, there will be increasing pressures to improve the yields of sugarcane (and of sugar beet in temperate zones). In the tropics, which include most of the areas of the world in which total calorie intake in the diet is often insufficient, sugar still represents one of the least expensive and most desirable forms of food. This situation is in contrast to the industrialized societies of Western Europe and North America where nutritional arguments have tended to hold down the level of sucrose in the diet.

The type of research needed to ensure more economical yields of carbohydrate crops, if they are to be employed both as sources of chemical substrate <u>and</u> as food, will probably take the form of (a) more efficient plant breeding and (b) specific treatments to enhance CO_2 fixation and/or to prevent the utilization and breakdown of the carbohydrate in the plant after it has been formed. Most carbohydrate crops are characterized by their ability to store the carbohydrate efficiently, but they are equally notorious for mobilizing their energy reserves and using them for their own growth under adverse conditions. This characteristic has been controlled in sugarcane by the application of a so-called "ripening" agent which ensures that the sucrose stored in the stalks will not be metabolized before the crop is harvested. Techniques of this type are highly desirable provided of course that the cost of the treatment does not exceed the value of the resultant sugar.

Another tropical species which is capable of providing substantial substrate for fermentation is the cassava. The starch produced by cassava can be converted to ethanol--but most of the world's supply of cassava is consumed as food, either for animals or for humans. The attraction of the cassava is its ability to grow on marginal land where very few other crops would survive. Its yield of starch per hectare exceeds that of maize by a factor of three to four. The potential for improving yields of cassava is probably greater than it is for sugarcane. In addition to sugarcane and cassava, recent studies with leucaena (as mentioned above) indicate that this leguminous tropical tree can reach maturity within three to five years of planting. The foliage of the shrub forms are used as animal feeds, while the wood in the tree forms is a cheap source of fuel. Obviously, biomass production makes good economic sense in those areas of the world which are blessed with solar energy and with agricultural potential.

The evolution of a biomass strategy for Europe and North America is likely to take an alternative route. Urban and agricultural wastes, salt water algae, industrial potatoes, sugar beets, and wood products are likely to be the preferred substrates in the temperate zones, while sugarcane, cassava, freshwater algae, and tropical species of trees would have obvious advantages in the tropics.

Undoubtedly, alcohol produced by fermentation will find attractive markets as an alternative fuel as the price of petroleum continues to increase. Brazil, for example, has begun to produce larger quantities of fermentation alcohol as a natural extension of its sugar and molasses industry. A direct spin-off of the resurgence of fermentation alcohol as an economical alternative to petroleum is the development of the new "Totem" engine by Fiat which can utilize 80% raw alcohol as a fuel. The new engine, which is still in the development phase, offers a number of attractive applications. One of these is a system combining the engine with fermentation as a means of recycling agricultural wastes. The heat produced by the system is used to activate distillation to produce ethanol which, in turn, is utilized as the fuel to run the engine--a truly cyclic system. There is a good chance that fermentation alcohol in the future could represent the "pivotal" compound in organic chemical syntheses, somewhat analogous to the position now held by ethylene in the petrochemical industry. Curiously, even though a technical development of this sort may seem rather far removed from botany it is not. The ultimate success of a chemical industry which is based on natural products or on fermentation alcohol will depend on the more efficient use of solar energy by crops and on finding effective means of increasing yields economically. At present, the two major sugar crops, cane and beet, and their molasses by-product, meet the economical criteria. Also, there is an extensive infrastructure for growing, harvesting, extracting, shipping, and storing the commodities which does not exist for other possible substrates such as cellulose, cassava, or the algae. However, algae, in particular, could in the future prove to be attractive substrates for fermentation.

In general, the algae offer some interesting prospects. They have already been shown to be excellent sources of protein (i.e., *Spirulina*), to be useful as food supplements both in humans and in livestock, and to be effective as nitrogenous fertilizers and soil conditioners. Species of algae are known to produce specific sugars such as glucose and fructose. They also produce specific polysaccharides such as alginates. These are exploited commercially and are used in foods, textiles, and in several other industries. More recently strains of algae have been isolated which produce glycerol and a number of hydrocarbons. A potential exists for producing algal hydrocarbons ranging in chain lengths from C_7 to C_{28} and above. Once the pathways of synthesis have been elucidated, it might be economically feasible to manufacture specific products utilizing immobilized algal cells or their enzymes. For this to become a reality will require considerable research, applying to the algae those botanical skills which have been so effective in developing the newer varieties of higher plants which today represent the viable commodities in agriculture (maize, wheat, rice, cotton, sugar, etc.). A less sophisticated exploitation of the algae is already underway in some developing nations, where certain strains are grown in mass either for use as fertilizers or in animal feeding. These are by no means novel applications. However, uses of algae such as for soil conditioners, as partial replacements for inorganic nitrogen fertilizers, or as a potential source of fuel are certainly worth further consideration.

THE ENVIRONMENT

Although thus far in this discussion only brief mention has been made of botany's likely contributions to protecting the environment (i.e., recycling urban wastes and effluents to produce fuels), the classical branches of botany are likely to play an increasingly important role. In a world in which small factories may dominate the landscape--recycling, wastes, utilizing biomass to produce gases and fuels, cultivating algae, fungi, and bacteria either for use as food or to produce alcohol and other chemicals--who would argue with the proposition that botany's role in providing the public and private botanical garden, the tree-lined streets, the green lawns and sculptured hedges will be as important as assisting in producing food and fuels? For it is the quality of life which is at risk in the future just as much as the quantity of products which will be at our disposal. "Creative botany" obviously provides a host of challenges for the next generation of botanists, not the least of which will be related to food, energy, *and* the environment.

22

PRECONDITIONING OF SEEDS TO IMPROVE PERFORMANCE

A. A. Khan,* C. M. Karssen,* E. F. Leue,* and C. H. Roe†

*New York State Agricultural Experiment Station
Cornell University
Geneva, New York

†Agricultural University
Wageningen
The Netherlands

INTRODUCTION

The extent to which a seed will perform is governed by its genetic makeup and the biochemical and physiological characteristics of the component parts, all of which are subject to control by environmental factors. High germinability in a seed lot is not always a measure of good seed quality or high vigor. It is not uncommon to find a seed lot with high germinability in the laboratory perform poorly in the field. Various laboratory tests, including stress tests simulating field conditions, are available and others are being designed to predict accurately the performance of a seed lot in the field. Progress, however, is extremely slow in this direction.

Aside from predicting seed performance, efforts are continually being made to improve seed performance in the field. A seed lot is considered to perform well when it is able to withstand the adverse effects of environment reasonably well. Some of the adverse environmental factors decreasing seed performance have been tabulated (see Table 1). Improved performance can mean one or a combination of things: (a) advancement of germination time, (b) decrease in the spread of germination in a seed population, (c) uniformity of seedling size or seedling stand, (d) alleviation of environmental and biotic stress, (e) invigoration of seeds as measured by increased rate of growth in emerging root and shoot, and (f) increased yield.

Various types of seed pretreatments or preconditioning are used to improve seed performance. These can be broadly classified as chemical, physical, and/or physiological (see Heydecker, 1973/1974;

Table 1. Some Environmental Factors Affecting Seed Performance in Soil

Physical Factors
Supra- and suboptimal temperatures
Unfavorable light conditions
Drought
Flooding
Unfavorable gaseous environment
Mechanical Factors
Soil texture and composition
Depth of sowing
Crusting of soil surface
Compaction of soil and inadequate soil-seed contact
Chemical Factors
Colloidal content
Salinity
Pesticides and herbicides and their residues
Toxic gases
Soil pH
Fertilizers
Biotic Factors
Insects
Fungi, bacteria
Rodents, birds
Weeds

Khan et al., 1976 for details). In this report we will discuss methods of seed preconditioning that have proved effective in improving seed performance under various environmental conditions. An assessment of the physiological and biochemical changes induced by growth regulators and by osmotic treatment will be made in an attempt to find the bases for increased seed performance.

METHODS OF PRECONDITIONING TO IMPROVE SEED PERFORMANCE

Improving Seed Performance by Infusion of Biologically Active Chemicals

Organic solvent (acetone, dichloromethane, etc.) infusion of chemicals as a means to improve seed performance has proved highly effective in recent years. The method consists of immersing seeds in the solvent containing one or more dissolved chemicals for 1-4 hr followed by removal of the solvent and drying the seeds in air or by vacuum desiccation (Milborrow, 1963; Meyer and Mayer, 1971; Khan et al., 1973). The kinetics of penetration using ^{14}C-IAA and ^{3}H-GA_3 showed the extent of penetration to be dependent upon the penetration time, the type of seed, the concentration of solute used, and the type of chemical (Tao and Khan, 1974). Autoradiographs of excised lettuce and squash embryos made following infusion of radioisotopes into intact seeds revealed the radioactivity in the peripheral regions only (Tao and Khan, 1974).

Organic solvent infusion technique was first exploited to study the effects of growth regulators (Fig. 1) in improving germination or seedling emergence in lettuce and celery seeds under various conditions (Joshua and Heydecker, 1971; Thomas et al., 1972; Khan et al., 1973). Since then a number of studies have shown that the method can be effectively used to increase seed performance under a variety of stress conditions. Lettuce seeds (both light requiring and dark germinating) infused with a combination of kinetin, ethephon, and GA_3 (K+E+G) via acetone were shown to resist the adverse effects of supraoptimal soil temperatures (e.g., 25 or 30°C night and 35°C day), high level of soil salinity (0.1 M NaCl), and water stress, induced artificially on filter paper by polyethylene glycol-6000 (-3 bars) or in two different types of soil by decreasing the moisture content (Braun and Khan, 1976; Khan et al., 1976; Khan, 1977). When regulators were applied singly or in paired combinations, they were not as effective. In celery seed the infusion of a mixture of GA_4 and GA_7 with 6-benzylaminopurine or K was also effective in alleviating the effects of supraoptimal temperatures (Palevitch and Thomas, 1974).

In recent years studies have been conducted with a fungal toxin, fusicoccin (FC), isolated from Fusicoccum amygdali (Ballio et al., 1968), and a group of compounds called cotylenins; e.g., cotylenin E (CN) and its aglycone, cotylenol, isolated from Cladosporium sp. (Sassa et al., 1975) (Fig. 1). When these compounds were infused into lettuce seeds via acetone they were as or more active than the combination K+E+G in alleviating high temperature, salinity, and water stresses (Braun and Khan, 1976; Khan, 1977, 1978a, and unpublished data). These compounds were especially active against osmotic stress caused by NaCl (0.1 M) and polyethylene glycol-6000 (15 g/100 ml).

Aqueous seed soaks have also been found to be effective in infusing growth regulators into seeds to improve their performance. A 3-min to 1-hr seed soak in solutions of FC, CN, K, or K+E+G proved as effective as 1-hr infusion of these chemicals via acetone in alleviating the high temperature stress in lettuce seeds (Khan, 1977, 1978a, and unpublished data). Aqueous soak of celery seeds with growth regulators, such as combinations of GA_4+GA_7, E, and daminozide, also proved effective in removing the temperature stress (Thomas et al., 1978). Aqueous seed soak, though effective for growth regulators

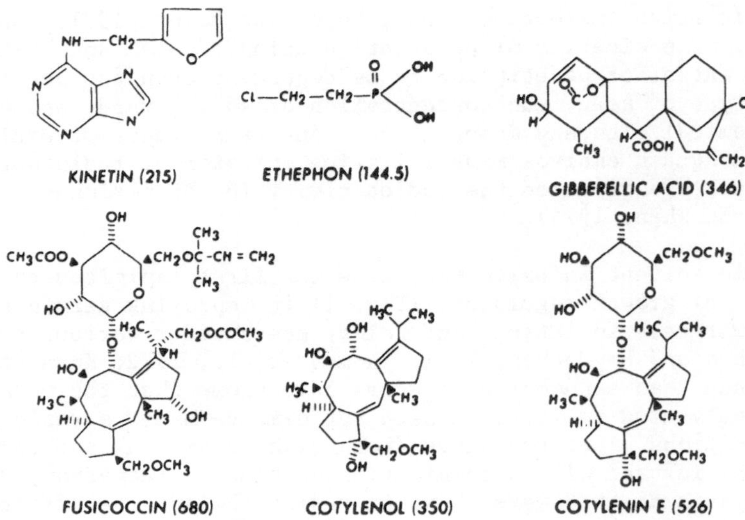

Fig. 1. Growth regulators that have been successfully infused into seeds via an organic solvent or water to improve seed performance. Numbers in parentheses are molecular weights.

and perhaps other water soluble compounds, is a time consuming procedure and requires extreme caution. The prolonged period of drying of lettuce seeds following an aqueous soak had an adverse effect on seed performance (Joshua and Heydecker, 1971; Khan, 1977).

Recent studies show that the organic solvent infusion method is particularly suitable for treating seeds with pesticides and antibiotics to combat the adverse effects of biotic factors on seed performance. A beginning was made with the demonstration that solvents, such as acetone and dichloromethane, can be used to infuse the fungicide pentachloronitrobenzene into pea seeds to control Aspergillus ruber, a storage fungus, and the insecticde chlorpyrifos into lima bean seeds to reduce the damage by the seedcorn maggot, Hylemya platura (Khan and Tao, 1973; Eckenrode et al., 1974; Tao et al., 1974). Among other successful uses are the reduction of internally borne Phomopsis spp. and Penicillium expansum in soybeans infused with methyl 2-benzimidazole carbamate and thiabendazole via dichloromethane (Ellis et al., 1976), the control of pre-emergence and post-emergence damping off and root rot by soil-borne Phytophthora megasperma var. Sojae in soybeans infused with pyroxychlor via acetone (Papavizas and Lewis, 1976), reduction of cotton root rot via acetone infusion of carboxin (Papavizas and Lewis, 1977), and reduction of Phythium blight on snapbeans by infusions of ethazol and other fungicides via acetone or ethanol (Papavizas et al., 1977). Other studies indicate that bacterial proliferation can also be checked by infusion of antibiotics via an organic solvent (Tao et al., 1974; Royse et al., 1975).

Other possible uses of the organic solvent infusion method and its advantages over other known methods of seed treatment have been discussed elsewhere (Khan et al., 1976; Khan, 1977, 1978a).

Improving Seed Performance by Osmoconditioning

In recent years a great deal of interest has centered around improving seed performance by osmotic means. Osmotic pretreatment or osmoconditioning (OC) of seeds can be regarded as a physiological method together with other physiological pretreatments, such as stratification, wetting and drying, and fluid drilling (see Heydecker, 1973/1974 for a review of this area). The aims of OC are (1) to shorten the time required for germination and seedling emergence in soil, (2) to decrease the spread of germination in a seed population, (3) to alleviate environmental stress, and (4) to invigorate the seed so that the rate of germination and/or growth is enhanced. Osmotic seed treatment with inorganic salts with the aim of improving seed performance was first attempted in tomato seeds (Ells, 1963; Oyer and Koehler, 1966; Koehler, 1967). While some success was evident from these studies, other early studies indicated that small salt molecules were often toxic to seeds. It was left to Heydecker and his associates to fully exploit the merits of this method. These workers used the chemically inert polymer of polyethylene glycol, PEG-6000 (Carbowax), to condition the seeds (Heydecker, 1973/1974).

The method as it is generally used now consists of treating seeds under aerobic condition at relatively low temperatures (e.g., 5-15°C) with PEG solution of a concentration high enough (usually 20-35 g per 100 ml of water) to prevent germination. Other parameters which affect OC include the duration of treatment, size of treatment chamber, whether conditioning is carried out in light or in darkness, the manner of seed handling following the treatment, and the characteristics of the seed. The method has been used extensively to treat small flower and vegetable seeds (Heydecker et al., 1975; Heydecker, 1977). Recent studies show that even large seeds of legumes and cereals, such as soybeans, peas, and sweet corn, can be conditioned by this method (Khan, 1977; Khan et al., 1978). Among the small vegetable seeds that have shown beneficial effects of OC are tomato, beet, onion, lettuce, celery, carrot, cabbage, brussels sprouts, parsnip, and parsley (Heydecker et al., 1975; Heydecker, 1977; Khan, 1977; Khan et al., 1978).

In studies conducted in the phytotron and in the field with seeds of lettuce, cabbage, brussels sprouts, and others it was found that OC, although effective in increasing seedling emergence at suboptimal temperatures (usually 8-15°C), had little or no effect when the soil temperatures increased (Khan, 1977 and unpublished data). Furthermore, OC had little effect in lettuce seeds in alleviating the adverse effects of drought and salinity (Khan, 1977). The results obtained in field trials at Geneva, New York with a number of crops in the spring of 1978 indicate that osmotic treatment should be combined with other treatments to take full advantage of the benefits of OC (see below for further discussion).

Improving Seed Performance by Combining Growth Regulator Infusion and Seed Pelleting

The main purpose of seed pelleting is to achieve precision planting. Pelleting or coating gives spherical shape to otherwise small, irregularly shaped vegetable seeds. Nutrients and seed protectants can also be incorporated in the pellet to improve seed performance. In a study conducted at Geneva lettuce seeds infused with various growth regulators (FC, K+E, K+E+G) via acetone were then pelleted by a procedure of Millier and Bensin (1974) using fine quartz sand and 5% Gelvatol as a binder. Although pelleting had some adverse effect, it reduced only slightly the stress-alleviating capabilities of the infused regulators. For example, there was little difference between the pelleted and unpelleted lettuce seeds, previously infused with regulators, in alleviating water stress (Khan et al., 1976; Khan, 1977). Pelleted or unpelleted seeds not infused with growth regulators performed poorly. Growth regulators had little effect when they were incorporated directly in the pellet during the pelleting procedure. Evidently the regulators in this case were not available to the seed embryo to affect its performance (Khan et al., 1976).

A detailed field study with Grand Rapids lettuce seeds, subjected to pre-pelleting infusion with 0.5 mM FC or 0.5 mM CN via acetone, was conducted in the summer of 1978 at three locations, one in the United States (Geneva, New York) and two in the Netherlands (Wageningen and Enkhuizen). Regulator infused seeds were kindly pelleted by the Royal Sluis, Holland, to produce "Splitkote" pellets designed for direct sowing in the field. In laboratory tests with the untreated-pelleted seeds, dark germination was impeded (13% at 18°C). In seeds subjected to pre-pelleting infusion with FC or CN germination was 67-70% at this temperature. Poor germination in untreated-pelleted seeds was shown to be due to restriction of oxygen. Thus, infused regulators which are readily available to the embryo on soaking can remove the adverse effect of anaerobiosis on germination. In soil planting (9 replicates of 100 seeds each) at Enkhuizen in July 1978 untreated pelleted seeds gave 53% emergence compared to 66% for seeds subjected to pre-pelleting infusion with CN or FC. The promotive effects of FC and CN were shown with or without pelleting at all three locations. Details of this study will be published elsewhere.

Studies conducted by Thomas et al. (1978) showed that pelleting of celery seeds retained the advantages of the previously infused growth regulators, such as combinations of GA_4+GA_7, E, and daminozide. As in the case of lettuce seed the regulators reduced the adverse effect of pelleting. This study further showed that seeds could be successfully pelleted following infusion of growth regulators via an aqueous soak.

Improving Seed Performance by Combining Osmoconditioning and Chemical Treatment

Highly encouraging results have been obtained by combining OC with infusion of bioactive chemicals into seeds. This was achieved in one of two ways: (1) infusion of chemical(s) via an organic solvent, such as acetone, followed by osmotic treatment in PEG, and (2) addition of chemical(s) directly to the osmoticum during osmotic treatment (Khan, 1977; Khan et al., 1978). Lettuce seeds subjected both to OC and FC treatments in either of the two ways combined the ability to resist the adverse effects of both supraoptimal and suboptimal temperatures on seedling emergence (Fig. 2). In this way it should also be possible to deal with the adverse effects of suboptimal temperatures and soil salinity or water stress.

Another interesting area which has shown definite promise is the treatment of seeds with fungicides and antibiotics during OC. By including fungicides, such as thiram (0.2%), in PEG solution during osmotic treatment of soybeans (cvs. Traverse and Altona), peas (cv. Alaska), and sweet corn (cv. Tendersweet), it has been possible to reduce markedly the proliferation of seed-borne fungi (Khan, 1977; Khan et al., 1978). In the absence of fungicide it was not possible to observe the advantages of OC in soybeans. Osmotic treatment of soybeans and peas in 25-35% PEG at 15°C for 4-10 days in the presence of 0.2% thiram caused an advancement of germination and an invigoration of seedling growth as measured by the increased rate of root and shoot growth (Fig. 3 and Khan et al., 1978).

An extensive field trial involving seeds of several crops was conducted in April of 1978 at the Vegetable Research Station of the New York State Agricultural Experiment Station at Geneva to determine the combined effects of OC and chemicals, such as fungicides, antibiotics, and growth regulators. Six treatments were evaluated for each crop and each treatment was replicated with six 5-meter plots (100 seeds per plot) arranged in the field in a 6 X 6 Latin Square. Soil temperatures stayed in the range of 5-15°C for the first 3.5 weeks after planting. Positive effects of the treatments

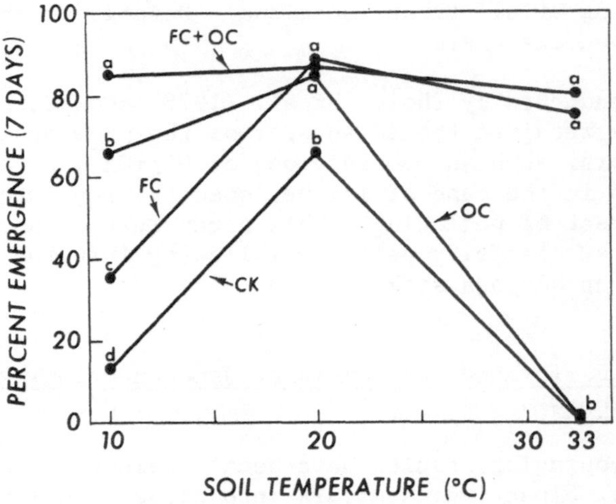

Fig. 2. Increased performance of lettuce seeds at nonoptimal temperatures by infusion of fusicoccin (FC), osmoconditioning (OC), and a combination of the two methods (FC + OC). In combination treatment FC (0.5 mM) was infused into lettuce seeds via acetone, air-dried for 1 hr at 25°C, and then osmotically treated in 25% PEG-6000 at 15°C for 14 days. Seeds were then dried by air for 1 hr at 25°C before planting in the soil (Khan et al., 1978).

were shown in soybeans, peas, brussels sprouts, and cabbage. In cabbage and brussels sprouts OC in the presence of 0.2% thiram proved most effective. Seven weeks after planting, stands obtained from treated brussels sprouts seeds showed 43 plants per row versus 35 plants in the untreated controls and gave 32% higher fresh weight. In soybeans the best treatment consisted of OC in presence of 0.2% thiram and 1 mM GA_3 (Fig. 4). Results in peas were similar to those of soybeans. Although the emergence time was enhanced in both soybeans and peas by the presence of GA_3, the final stand counts made after six weeks decreased somewhat compared to the untreated controls. Thus, additional steps may be needed to improve seedling survival.

In a recent study Hepperly and Sinclair (1977) successfully incorporated antibiotics during osmotic treatment with PEG to control seed-borne bacteria in soybeans.

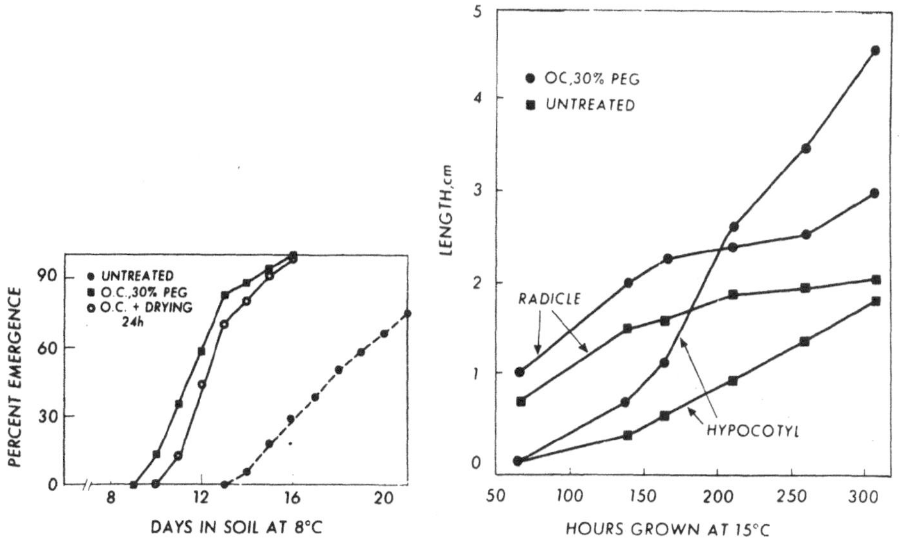

Fig. 3. Invigoration of soybean (cv. Traverse) seeds by OC in 30% PEG-6000 containing 0.2% thiram at 15°C for 8 days. Left: Conditioned seeds were rinsed, air-dried at 25°C for 2 and 24 hr, and then sown in soil (1:1 sandy loam:peat moss; soil water content, 23% of dry soil weight) in plastic boxes in growth chambers programmed for 8°C temperature and 12 hr photoperiod (Knypl and Khan, unpublished data). Right: Conditioned seeds rinsed, air-dried for 2 hr at 25°C, and then sown in glass dishes lined with filter papers. Each point on the curves is a mean of 20 seedling lengths (Khan, unpublished data).

PHYSIOLOGICAL AND BIOCHEMICAL ASPECTS OF IMPROVED PERFORMANCE BY GROWTH REGULATORS

The performance of a seed can vary profoundly depending upon the environment is finds itself in. Of immediate importance to a germinating seed are such factors as texture and composition of the soil, composition of gases in the immediate vicinity, water potential differences between the seed and the soil, solute content and ionic composition, temperature and light condition, and of course the characteristics of the seed itself. It is obvious from recent studies that gibberellins, cytokinins, and ethylene (or ethephon which decomposes to ethylene at pH 4.0 or above) act rather selectively to effect germination. This is suggested, for example, in studies with lettuce seed on the alleviation of high temperature (25-35°C or 30-35°C) effect on germination by a combination of K+E+G, and not by any of the components or paired combinations (Khan, 1977). Thus,

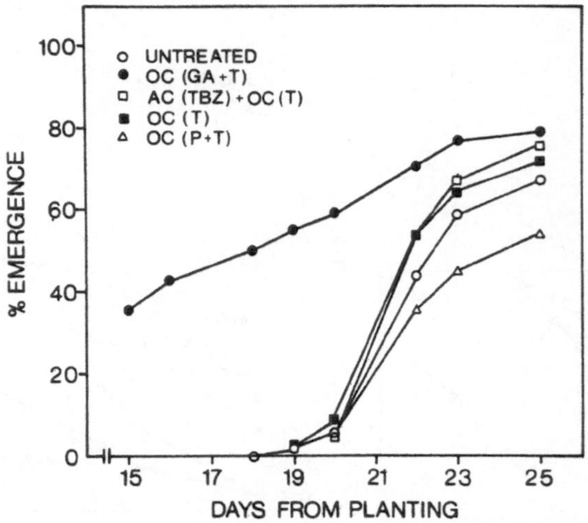

Fig. 4. Performance of soybean (cv. Altona) seeds preconditioned by combining OC and chemical treatment. OC was as in Fig. 3. The chemicals added to PEG solution during OC and shown in parentheses are 1 mM GA_3 (GA), 0.2% each of thiram (T) and thiabendazole (TBZ), and 1000 units/ml of penicillin G (P). In one case TBZ was infused via acetone (Ac) followed by OC in presence of T (Khan et al., unpublished data).

germination or emergence under stress may be a result of various physiological and biochemical events all of which have to be satisfied before a seedling will emerge.

It is now well known that profound changes in the levels of endogenous hormones occur in a variety of plant tissues when they are subjected to drought, supraoptimal temperatures, and changes in osmotic environment. These conditions lead to water potential differences and permeability changes and often cause an increase in the content of abscisic acid (ABA) and a decrease in that of cytokinins (see Khan, 1977 for a review). Other studies show that cytokinins and several inhibitors including ABA have opposite effects on a wide variety of plant processes, including those of seeds (Khan, 1971, 1975). Furthermore, when ABA or other inhibitors are supplied exogenously, they block the promotive effect of GA in many seeds including those of lettuce and barley. Under these conditions only the presence of cytokinins effectively removes the block (Khan, 1971). Thus, GA, though present, may be rendered ineffective under conditions of stress when the levels of ABA and perhaps other inhibitors rise.

Recent studies reveal the relative importance of various gases such as oxygen, carbon dioxide, and ethylene in lettuce seed germination. The presence of all these gases in the ambient atmosphere, at least in low concentrations, appears to be essential for the efficient working of GA and K in improving lettuce seed germination (Keys et al., 1975; Rudnicki et al., 1978). Conversely, it can be suggested that a combination of these gases could increase seed germination in the presence of suboptimal levels of endogenous hormones. In the same context the action of FC or CN, which is as great or greater than the regulator combination K+E+G in alleviating temperature, salinity, and water stresses, may be examined. FC and CN through their effects on H^+/K^+ ion exchange, changes in membrane permeability, and related cellular processes might improve the efficiency of endogenous hormones which may be at suboptimal levels, at least with regard to their functions or ability to reach the active centers (see Marré, 1977). It has been shown that FC (20 μM) induced germination in Mesa 659 seed at 35°C and enhanced it at 25°C (germination at both temperatures occurred in 6-7 hr compared to 12 hr in untreated seeds at 25°C). At the same time, FC enhanced the rate of disappearance of ABA at these temperatures (Borkowska et al., 1978).

PHYSIOLOGICAL AND BIOCHEMICAL CHANGES DURING AND FOLLOWING SEED OSMOCONDITIONING

Physiological Changes

Studies of Khan (1960) showed that a treatment of photosensitive lettuce seeds with an osmoticum, such as mannitol, inhibited germination and the inhibition was abolished by red light (R). Furthermore, prolonged exposure to the osmoticum in the dark induced dark osmotic inhibition or secondary dormancy as the seeds failed to germinate on subsequent transfer to water. The ability of R to reduce the dark osmotic inhibition by mannitol was also shown in *Chenopodium album* by Karssen (1970). In experiments with lettuce seeds using PEG-6000 (250 g/liter) at 15°C it was confirmed that prolonged dark osmotic treatment (2-14 days) induced secondary dormancy as determined by subsequent germination in water at 25°C. However, the induction of secondary dormancy was not limited to the photosensitive Grand Rapids lettuce seeds but was found also in a photoinsensitive cultivar of lettuce, Mesa 659. It was further revealed that brief R exposures given daily during osmotic treatment at 15°C not only prevented the induction of secondary dormancy but actually advanced the time and rate of germination when the seeds were transferred to water at 25°C in light or in the dark (Khan, 1978b; see also Fig. 5).

A more recent study with *Chenopodium bonus-henricus* L., a weed species, gave similar results. These seeds have to be chilled for 30-40 days to remove the light requirement for germination (Karssen, unpublished data). One-year-old seeds give 40-50% germination in the dark compared to nearly 100% in the light. Osmotic treatment of

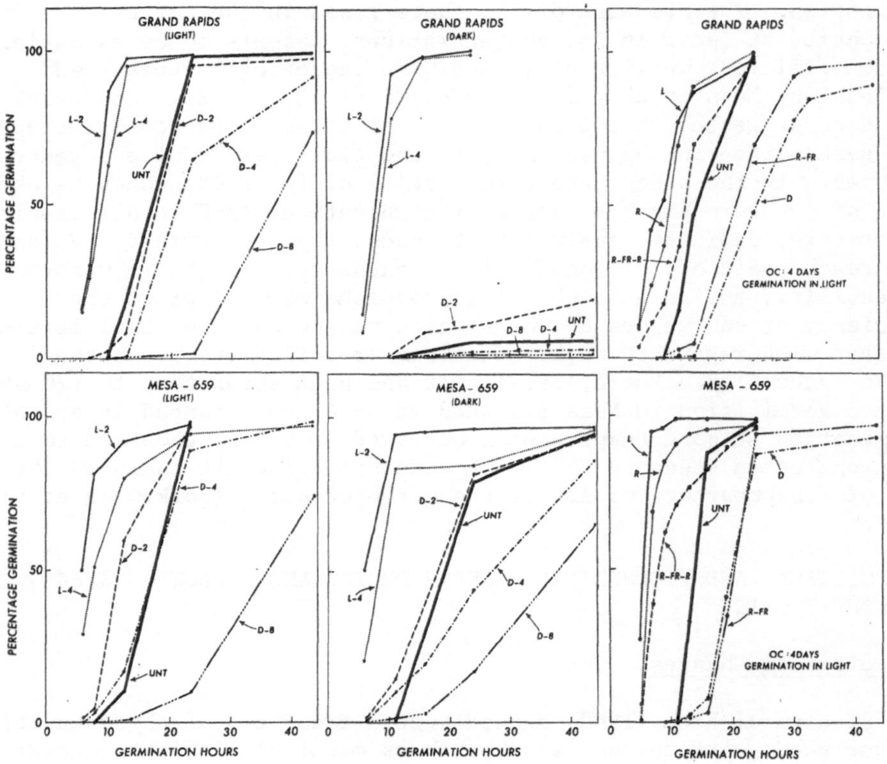

Fig. 5. Light osmotic promotion and dark osmotic inhibition of germination of light sensitive (cv. Grand Rapids) and dark germinating (cv. Mesa 659) lettuce seeds. Osmotic treatment (25% PEG-6000, 15°C) was in continuous light (L), darkness (D), or in darkness interrupted daily with 5 min red (R), 5 min red plus 5 min far-red (R+FR), or 5 min red plus 5 min far-red plus 5 min red (R+FR+R). Energy level was kept at 1500 µW/cm^2 for both R and FR. Following osmotic treatment seeds were germinated in water at 25°C in both light and darkness (indicated in parentheses). Numbers following letters refer to days of osmotic treatment. UNT, untreated seeds (Khan, unpublished data).

chilled seeds with PEG (250 g/liter) at 15°C in combination with brief R or red plus far-red plus red (R+FR+R) exposures, every day for 7 days, advanced the germination time in water in both light and darkness at 22:12°C when compared to the chilled seeds not exposed to the osmoticum (Khan and Karssen, unpublished data). Similar enhancement in germination was noted when a combination of K+E+G was added to the PEG solution during dark osmotic treatment of chilled seeds (Khan and Karssen, unpublished data). In the dark or in R+FR, a secondary dormancy was induced (Fig. 6). After 21 days in the osmoticum in the dark, the seeds failed to germinate in the dark at 22:12°C. Seeds kept in the dark during osmotic treatment germinated in the light but showed no enhancement effect. This suggests that light and/or hormone-dependent changes are required during the prolonged osmotic treatment at 15°C to produce an enhancement effect in light or darkness on subsequent transfer to water at 22:12°C. As dark osmotic treatment induces secondary dormancy and simulates conditions in the soil, it may be possible to release secondary dormancy of light sensitive weed seeds by application of appropriate growth regulators.

The osmotic treatment of unchilled seeds of C. bonus-henricus in light caused similar enhancement in germination at 22:12°C to that in chilled seeds. Unlike chilled seeds, however, these seeds still germinated in the dark (22%) following osmotic treatment in the dark for up to 28 days. A 7-14 days dark osmotic treatment actually enhanced the rate and number of seeds that germinated. Thus the mechanism of induction of secondary dormancy by osmotic treatment may be controlled by factors which differ in the chilled and unchilled seeds. One possible cause of the difference could be the differences in the levels of promotive and inhibitory hormones.

It was interesting to note that seeds such as soybeans germinated equally well following osmotic treatment in light or darkness. Presumably these seeds lack phytochrome control.

Biochemical Changes

In an attempt to determine the underlying causes of the enhancement effect of OC and the increased performance of osmotically treated lettuce seeds, studies were conducted to determine changes both during OC at 15°C and during incubation at 25°C.

An analysis of total proteins in conditioned (25% PEG, 14 days at 15°C) and untreated lettuce seeds was made in precipitates of 30,000 g supernatant of seed homogenate following dialyses (Fraction I, precipitate settling in the dialysis bag) and after 0-50 and 50-100% ammonium sulfate saturation cuts (Fractions II and III). Proteins were resolved on polyacrylamide gels. Profound quantitative differences with respect to number and intensity of individual bands were found in all three protein fractions (Khan et al., 1978).

Activities of a number of enzymes implicated in germination were studied at the conclusion of 14 day osmotic treatment of lettuce seeds at 15°C in light. Enzymes were isolated from 30,000 g supernatant of seed homogenate. Increases in activity of acid

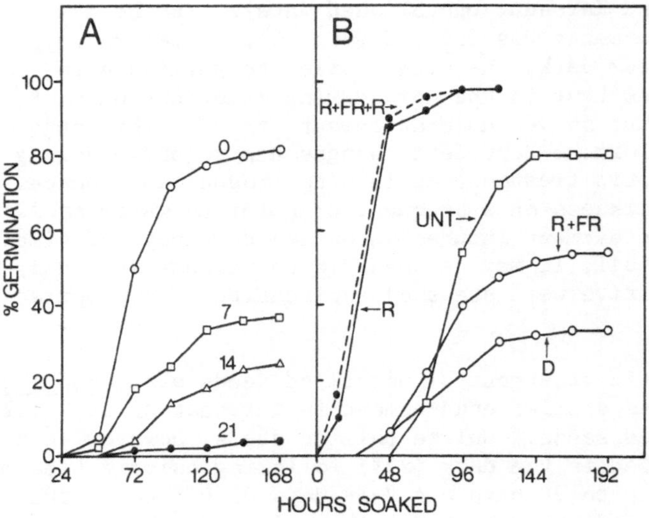

Fig. 6. Light osmotic promotion and dark osmotic inhibition of germination of C. bonus-henricus L. seeds. A: Osmotic treatment (25% PEG-6000, 15°C) in darkness for 0, 7, 14, and 21 days was followed by germination of seeds in water in darkness at 22:12°C (12 hr:12 hr). B: Osmotic treatment in the dark with daily interruptions of R, R+FR, and R+FR+R as in Fig. 5. D, seeds kept continuously in darkness. UNT, untreated seeds (Khan and Karssen, unpublished data).

phosphatase (160% of untreated seeds) and esterase (382% of untreated seeds) were shown while no significant changes were noted in the activities of alkaline phosphatase, peroxidase, aminoacyl t-RNA synthetase, malate dehydrogenase, and 3-phosphoglyceraldehyde dehydrogenase (Khan et al., 1978). The presence of 50 μM GA_3, 50 μM FC, or 50 μM K added to the PEG solution further increased the activity of acid phosphatase and esterase. Polyacrylamide gel electrophoresis profiles of the enzymes showed increases in activities of some isozymes of acid phosphatase and esterase and decreases in others. The presence of GA_3, FC, or K during OC increased the number of acid phosphatases and esterases (Khan et al., 1978). Inhibitor studies showed that ImM cordycepin (CP) had no effect on total esterase activity. Cycloheximide (20 μM) effect on esterases and acid phosphatases, on the other hand, ranged from a complete inhibition of the activities of some isozymes to partial inhibition of others to no inhibition in still others (Khan et al., 1978).

A 14 days osmotic treatment of lettuce seeds (Mesa 659) in light led to a complete disappearance of both free and bound forms of ABA. The levels of free and bound forms of ABA in the dry seeds were 24 and 3 ng per 100 seeds respectively (Khan et al., 1978). A more recent study showed very little ABA in these seeds after as little as 8 hr of osmotic treatment at 15°C and a complete disappearance after 24 hr of treatment (Borkowska et al., 1978).

To determine the nature of changes during osmotic treatment affecting the germination process of lettuce and C. bonus-henricus seeds, studies were conducted on RNA and protein metabolism during early hours of incubation at 25°and 22:12°C, respectively, following the osmotic treatment. A time course of ^{14}C-leucine incorporation into TCA-precipitable fraction from Grand Rapids lettuce seeds showed the rate and the quantity of protein synthesized in the conditioned seeds to be higher than in the untreated seeds (Khan et al., 1978). These results were consistent with the more rapid formation of polyribosomes in the conditioned seeds (Khan et al., 1978). The time course of ^{3}H-uridine incorporation into RNA of lettuce seeds during soaking at 25°C prior to radicle protrusion also showed RNA synthesis to begin earlier in the conditioned seeds and the amount of radioactivity incorporated into RNA was also higher than in the untreated seeds (Khan et al., 1978).

Preliminary results have been obtained in studies conducted on the qualitative and quantitative changes in RNA of chilled (28 days) C. bonus-henricus seeds. These seeds were osmotically treated in PEG (25%, 15°C) for 7 days either in light or in darkness. Following osmotic treatment the seeds were soaked at 22:12°C in 1 ml solution of ^{3}H-adenosine (20 μCi) and 50 μg/ml of chloramphenicol for 24 hr in the dark. The incorporation of ^{3}H-adenosine into RNA was inhibited by about 42% when the osmotic treatment was in the dark. Germination in the seeds was 23% compared to 96% in those given light during osmotic treatment. More important, the content of poly A(+) RNA synthesized as resolved by oligo (dt)-cellulose chromatography was higher in the seeds conditioned in the light (1.3% of the total RNA synthesized) than those conditioned in the dark (0.8% of total RNA synthesized). These data suggest that poly A(+) RNA synthesis might be related to light-induced processes affecting germination. Further work is in progress on the RNA metabolism of these seeds in relation to induction and release of secondary dormancy.

Biochemical studies indicate that osmotic treatment of seeds causes mobilization of storage materials, thus making available to seeds precursors utilized for enhanced macromolecular synthesis required for rapid germination and growth. Disappearance of ABA during osmotic treatment may be a part of the overall changes related to improved mobilization of storage products in preparation for germination.

SUMMARY

From the data presented here it can be seen that preconditioning of seeds by growth regulator infusion and by osmotic treatment can be highly effective in improving seed performance, especially under less than ideal conditions prevailing in the field. These methods can be combined with other seed treatment methods to further increase seed survival and performance. It is also necessary to understand the physiological and biochemical basis of high and low performance in a seed lot to modify the existing methods of seed treatments and to design new ones. Often seeds are thrown into induced or secondary dormancy in the complex environment of the soil. An understanding of the factors inducing and removing secondary dormancy may be of paramount importance in improving seed performance.

ACKNOWLEDGMENTS

The senior author is grateful to the Department of Plant Physiology of the Agricultural University, Wageningen, for providing a senior research fellowship which enabled him to conduct studies in the field of seed performance.

The authors are grateful to Professor A. Ballio and Dr. T. Sassa for making available generous amounts of fusicoccin and cotylenins used in these studies. Without the cooperation of Mr. J. de Boer of the Royal Sluis, Holland it would not have been possible to conduct a detailed and a meaningful study of the effects of seed pelleting. We are thankful to several chemical companies for generous amounts of chemicals, to Boehringer Mannheim GmbH for α-amanitin, to Sigma for penicillin G, and to Merck for thiabendazole.

REFERENCES

Ballio, A., Brufani, M., Casinovi, C. G., Gerrini, S., Fedeli, W., Pelliciari, B., Santurbano, B., and Vaciago, A., 1968, The structure of Fusicoccin A., Experientia, 24:631-635.

Borkowska, B., Singha, S., and Khan, A. A., 1978, Changes in abscisic acid content of lettuce seeds by osmotic fusicoccin and other treatments, Plant Physiol., 61: s-94.

Braun, J. W., and Khan, A. A., 1976, Alleviation of salinity and high temperature stress by plant growth regulators permeated into lettuce seeds via acetone, J. Amer. Soc. Hort. Sci., 101:716-721.

Eckenrode, C. J., Kuhr, R. J., and Khan, A. A., 1974, Treatment of seeds by solvent infusion for control of the seedcorn maggot, J. Econ. Entomol., 67:284-286.

Ellis, M. A., Foor, S. R., and Sinclair, J. B., 1976, Dichloromethane: Nonaqueous vehicle for systemic fungicides in soybean seeds, Phytopathology, 66:1249-1251.

Ells, J. E., 1963, The influence of treating tomato seed with nutrient solutions on emergence rate and seedling growth, Proc. Amer. Soc. Hort. Sci., 83:684-687.

Hepperly, P. R., and Sinclair, J. B., 1977, Aqueous polyethylene glycol solutions for treating soybean seeds with antibiotics, Seed Sci. & Technol., 5:727-734.

Heydecker, W., 1973/1974, University of Nottingham School of Agricultural Science Report, 50:67.

Heydecker, W., 1977, Stress and seed germination: An agronomic view, in: "Physiology and Biochemistry of Seed Dormancy and Germination," A. A. Khan, ed., Elsevier/North-Holland Biomedical Press, Amsterdam.

Heydecker, W., Higgins, J., and Turner, Y. T., 1975, Invigoration of seeds?, Seed Sci. & Technol., 3:881-888.

Joshua, A., and Heydecker, W., 1971, Chemicals may aid lettuce germination at high temperature, The Grower, 76:852.

Karssen, C. M., 1970, The light promoted germination of the seeds of Chenopodium album L. IV. Effects of red, far-red and white light on non-photoblastic seeds incubated in mannitol, Acta Bot. Neerl., 19:95-108.

Keys, R. D., Smith, O. E., Kumamoto, J., and Lyon, J. L., 1975, Effect of gibberellic acid, kinetin, and ethylene plus carbon dioxide on the thermodormancy of lettuce seed (Lactoca sativa L. cv. Mesa 659), Plant Physiol., 56:826-829.

Khan, A. A., 1960, An analysis of "dark-osmotic inhibition" of germination of lettuce seeds, Plant Physiol., 35:1-7.

Khan, A. A., 1971, Cytokinins: Permissive role in seed germination, Science, 171:853-859.

Khan, A. A., 1975, Primary, preventive and permissive role of hormones in plant systems, Bot. Rev., 41:391-420.

Khan, A. A., 1977, Preconditioning, germination and performance of seeds, in: "Physiology and Biochemistry of Seed Dormancy and Germination," A. A. Khan, ed., Elsevier/North-Holland Biomedical Press, Amsterdam.

Khan, A. A., 1978a, Incorporation of bioactive chemicals into seeds to alleviate environmental stress, Acta Hort., 83:225-234.

Khan, A. A., 1978b, Photo control and hormonal control of osmotic processes affecting lettuce seed germination, Plant Physiol., 61:s-33.

Khan, A. A., Braun, J. W., Tao, K. L., Millier, W. F., and Bensin, R. F., 1976, New methods for maintaining seed vigor and improving performance, J. Seed Technol., 1:33-57.

Khan, A. A., and Tao, K. L., 1973, Novel chemical treatment protects seeds from deterioration, N.Y. Food & Life Sci. Quart., 6:3-5.

Khan, A. A., Tao, K. L., Knypl, J. S., Borkowska, B., and Powell, L. E., 1978, Osmotic conditioning of [vegetable] seeds: Physiological and biochemical changes, Acta Hort., 83:267-278.

Khan, A. A., Tao, K. L., and Roe, C. H., 1973, Isolation and properties of nuclei from control and auxin-treated soybean hypocotyl, Plant Physiol., 52:79-81.

Koehler, D. E., 1967, Studies on a treatment hastening germination of tomato seeds (Lycopersicon esculentum Mill.), Master's Thesis, Purdue University, Lafayette, Indiana.

Marré, E., 1977, Effects of fusicoccin and hormones on plant cell membrane activities: Observations and hypotheses, in: "Regulation of Cell Membrane Activities in Plants," E. Marré and O. Ciferri, eds., Elsevier/North-Holland Biomedical Press, Amsterdam.

Meyer, H., and Mayer, A. M., 1971, Permeation of dry seeds with chemicals: Use of dichloromethane, Science, 171:583-584.

Milborrow, B. V., 1963, Penetration of seeds by acetone solutes, Nature (London), 199:716-717.

Millier, W. F., and Bensin, R. F., 1974, Tailoring pelleted seed coatings to soil moisture conditions, N.Y. Food & Life Sci. Quart., 7:20-23.

Oyer, E. B., and Koehler, D. E., 1966, A method of treating tomato seeds to hasten germination and emergence at suboptimal temperatures, 17th Int. Hort. Congr., 1: Abstract No. 626.

Palevitch, D., and Thomas, T. H., 1974, Thermodormancy release of celery seed by gibberellins, 6-benzylaminopurine, and Ethephon applied in organic solvent to dry seeds, J. Exp. Bot., 25:981-986.

Papavizas, G. C., and Lewis, J. A., 1976, Acetone infusion of pyroxychor into soybean seed for the control of Phytophthora megasperma var. Sojae, Plant Dis. Rep., 60:484-488.

Papavizas, G. C., and Lewis, J. A., 1977, Effect of cottonseed treatment with systemic fungicides on seedling disease, Plant Dis. Rep., 61:538-542.

Papavizas, G. C., Lewis, J. A., Lumsden, R. D., Adams, P. C., Ayers, W. A., and Kantzes, J. G., 1977, Control of Phythium blight on bean with ethazol and prothiocarb, Phytopathology, 67:1293-1299.

Royse, D. J., Ellis, M. A., and Sinclair, J. B., 1975, Movement of penicillin into soybean seeds using dichloromethane, Phytopathology, 65:1319-1320.

Rudnicki, R. M., Braun, J. W., and Khan, A. A., 1978, Low pressure and ethylene in lettuce seed germination, Physiol. Plant, 43:189-193.

Sassa, T., Togushi, M., and Kitaguchi, T., 1975, The structures of cotylenins A, B, C, D and E, Agr. Biol. Chem. (Japan), 39: 1735-1744.

Tao, K. L., and Khan, A. A., 1974, Penetration of dry seeds with chemicals applied to acetone, Plant Physiol., 54:956-958.

Tao, K. L., Khan, A. A., Harman, G. E., and Eckenrode, C. J., 1974, Practical significance of the application of chemicals in organic solvents to dry seeds, J. Amer. Soc. Hort. Sci., 99: 217-220.

Thomas, T. H., Biddington, N. L., and Palevitch, D., 1978, Improving the performance of pelleted celery seeds with growth regulator treatments, Acta Hort., 83:235-243.
Thomas, T. H., Palevitch, D., and Austin, R. B., 1972, Stimulation of celery seed germination with plant growth regulators, in: "Proceedings of the Eleventh British Weed Control Conference," British Crop Protection Council.

23

WATER STRESS: A CHALLENGE FOR THE FUTURE OF AGRICULTURE

A. J. Karamanos

The Agricultural College, Votanikos
Athens, Greece

INTRODUCTION

When analyzing the progress of agriculture in recent years we find a boom in farm yields after World War II until about 1970. This is mainly attributed to massive inputs of energy in agriculture by means of fertilizers, pesticides, irrigation, and mechanization, as well as to the genetic improvement of the crops. The yields per unit farm area, however, have not increased since 1970 and, accordingly, any overall increase in crop production during this period was achieved mainly by cropping more land. In fact, more land was brought under cultivation in the arid and semiarid regions by means of large irrigation projects. No doubt there is still potential for further expansion of irrigated land. Assuming that all the current and planned development projects will be achieved, Jewitt (1966) estimates that by the end of the century the world's irrigated area is very likely to expand by an additional 40 million to a total of 200 million hectares. However, despite these perspectives, it is important to consider that irrigation itself is by no means equivalent to an intensive and more productive agriculture, as the failure of many irrigation projects suggests (Arnon, 1972). The vast capital investments together with the continuously increasing costs of energy make the success of such plans ambiguous. It appears, therefore, that a change in the priorities of agricultural research is necessary. Future research has to point to a more intensive study of the factors which limit crop production as well as to ways of enabling the plants to utilize more effectively the available environmental resources. According to a recent joint report of the National Research Council and the National Academy of Sciences of the United States, the research targets in the near future must include methods of improving photosynthetic efficiency, biological nitrogen fixation, nutrient and water use efficiency, and resistance to environmental stresses (Wittwer, 1978). Obviously, the crops of the future must work more effectively than the present ones in order to meet the continuously increasing demands for food and fiber.

It is not surprising that the study of plant water relations in terms of increasing water use efficiency and improving plant resistance to desiccation is among the research priorities mentioned above. Water is a well-known limiting factor in plant growth and numerous studies have been done to understand its mode of action. It is self-evident that water deficits cause a general reduction in the size of most plants. Stanhill (1957) found that in 66 out of 80 papers dealing with crop response to different soil moisture regimes water shortage was related to a depression in plant growth and in most cases to a reduction in yield. There has also been a lot of work done on the effects of water stress on plant morphology, physiology, and biochemistry (for reviews, see Maximov, 1929; Crafts, 1968; Parker, 1968; Todd, 1972; Hsiao, 1973), which advanced considerably our knowledge. Nevertheless, a widely accepted integrated view on the water stress-induced sequence of the metabolic events leading finally to growth suppression is still lacking.

In view of the critical role of water in crop production, an effort will be made to identify and assess its effects on the various processes contributing to plant growth and yield. By knowing the sensitivity of each of these processes to water shortage, one should be able to distinguish the ones which limit crop production. Then an attempt will be made to examine the existing methods of restricting the retarding effects of water stress and the possibilities for their effective use in the future.

HOW WATER STRESS AFFECTS PLANT YIELD

A prerequisite of high yields is a high production of total dry matter (Arnon, 1972; Yoshida, 1972). At any time, plant dry matter is the result of cumulative gains and losses during the plant's life (Fig. 1). The plant accumulates dry matter mainly from photosynthesis and secondarily from mineral absorption; photosynthesis usually accounts for 80-90% of the dry matter production. The plant factors determining the effectiveness of photosynthesis are the assimilating area, which represents the capacity of the photosynthetic system, and the efficiency of this system, i.e., its productivity per unit leaf area. The losses in dry matter originate from respiration and, secondarily, from the abscission of the senescing plant organs. Finally, the proportion of the total biomass which is converted into economic yield is controlled by the translocation of assimilates from the other parts of the plant. Obviously, this statement does not

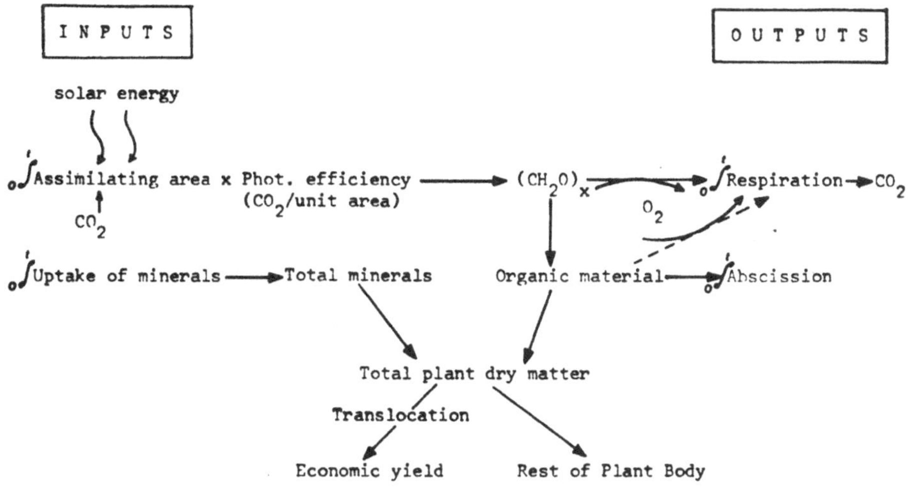

Fig. 1. Diagrammatic representation of the physiological processes determining the total plant dry matter and the economic yield after a time of t days from sowing.

refer to crops where the total of the biomass is of economic significance, as for example in forage crops.

Photosynthesis

Effects on the assimilating area. Leaf area represents to a close approximation the total assimilating area of a plant and hence its whole capacity to photosynthesize. The area of other green parts, such as stems, pods, leaf sheaths, and ears in cereals, may also be important (Asana and Mani, 1949), but only at early stages when the canopy is still open.

There is well-established experimental evidence that water shortage causes a reduction in the various expressions of plant or crop leaf area (for a review see Karamanos, 1976). In Fig. 2, for example, the total plant leaf area of field grown field beans decreased linearly with the average leaf water potential during plant growth. The origin of these reductions in plant leaf area can be detected by examining the response of the different mechanisms which determine leaf area growth, namely leaf production, leaf death, and laminar expansion. The first two determine the number of live leaves at any time, while the third one is associated with leaf size. All three mechanisms have been found to be affected by water stress but to varying extents. This is not surprising in view of the enormous differences in their physiology.

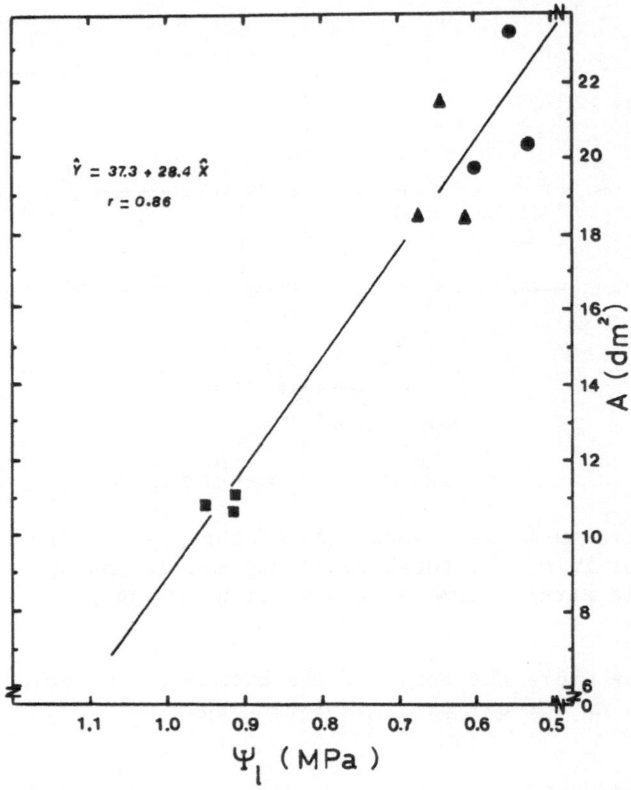

Fig. 2. The relation between the total leaf area of field bean plants after 95 days from sowing (A) and the mean leaf water potential at 1500h (Ψ_l) during the same period. The plants were grown in the field and were subjected to three irrigation treatments randomized in three replicates (● wet, ▲ medium, and ■ dry treatment). Each point is the average for each replicate (mean of 4 plants). The fitted linear regression is also shown (adapted from Karamanos, 1978a).

Leaf production was unaffected by water stress in flax (Milthorpe, 1945) and sugar beet (Morton and Watson, 1948; Milford and Lawlor, 1975). On the other hand, a considerable depression of leaf production by water stress was found in Pelargonium (Amer and Williams, 1958), tobacco (Hopkinson, 1968; Clough and Milthorpe, 1975), sunflower (Marc and Palmer, 1976), barley (Nicholls and May, 1963; Husain and Aspinall, 1970), lupin (C. T. Gates, 1968), and field beans (Karamanos, 1978a). From microscopic observations of the stem apex (Nicholls and May, 1963; Gates, 1968; Husain and Aspinall, 1970) it was concluded that primordial initiation was very sensitive to water stress. The degree of sensitivity is likely to differ among plant species and may also be affected by plant development. It is also likely that plant water potential exerts a cumulative rather than a short-term effect on leaf production (Karamanos, 1978a).

The work of Milthorpe (1945) with flax, where leaf size was unaffected by water stress, is rather exceptional. In contrast to leaf production, there is little doubt concerning the sensitivity of leaf expansion to water stress. Laminar expansion is difficult to express quantitatively because of the sigmoid pattern it follows. Many investigators found that the ultimate leaf size, the final result of the whole process, was smaller in stressed plants (e.g., Penfound, 1931; Martin, 1940; Morton and Watson, 1948). Others (e.g., Brouwer, 1963; Boyer, 1968; Acevedo et al., 1971; Gandar and Tanner, 1976; Bunce, 1977a) found the rates of leaf expansion considerably reduced by water stress. An integrated picture of the whole process of leaf expansion can be obtained by a parametrization of the sigmoid curves fitted to the actual measurements of leaf area against time (Richards, 1959). In such a treatment, the ultimate leaf size (A) is considered to result from three parameters, namely average growth rate (F), the duration of growth (τ), and the area at the initial measurement (a_o) as follows (see also Fig. 3):

$$A = a_o + \tau F. \tag{1}$$

It was found in field beans that both a_o and F were positively and well correlated with the mean leaf water potential (Ψ_1) which prevailed six days before unfolding and during expansion respectively (Fig. 4a,b), while the duration of growth was unaffected by water stress (Fig. 4c; cf. also McCree and Davis, 1974). Finally, the ultimate leaf size was also positively and well correlated with Ψ_1 (Fig. 4d). Leaf expansion proceeds first by means of cell divisions which are followed by cell enlargement. The different sensitivity of these two processes to water stress could explain the differences in the correlation coefficients between each of the parameters and Ψ_1 (Fig. 4). Cell divisions are relatively unaffected at moderate stresses while leaf enlargement is suppressed to a considerable extent (Meyer and Boyer, 1972; Clough and Milthorpe, 1975; Kleinendorst, 1975). a_o, the area at which field bean leaves unfold, is mainly determined by cell divisions (Sunderland, 1960; Milthorpe and Newton, 1963; Dale, 1964; Wilson, 1966) and hence its correlation with Ψ_1 was weaker than that of the growth rate F, which refers to the period after unfolding, namely to cell enlargement (Karamanos, 1976).

The sensitivity of leaf enlargement to water stress has long ago (Pfeffer, 1877) been attributed to cell turgor. Nowadays, the dependence of growth on turgor is rather well documented both theoretically and experimentally. The theoretical treatment of the plant cell as a cylinder with walls having viscoelastic properties

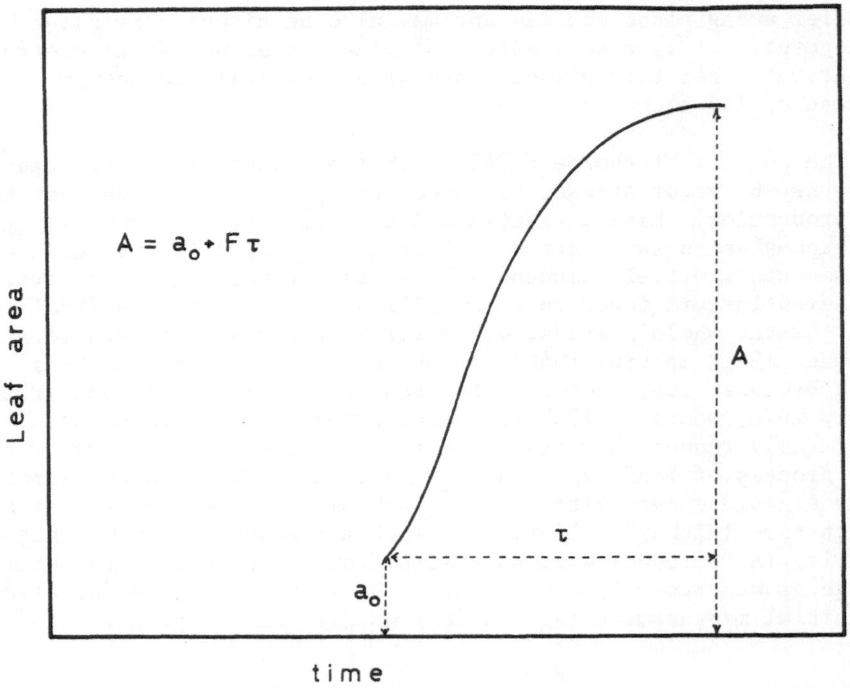

Fig. 3. The parametrization of the generalized logistic curve used for the description of laminar growth in field beans (Karamanos, 1976). The final area of a leaf (A) is the sum of the area at leaf unfolding (a_o) plus the product of mean growth rate during expansion (F) and the duration of growth (τ).

(Lockhart, 1965) and the implications arising from such a treatment seem to agree with the experimental results. An extreme sensitivity of cell growth to transient changes in cell pressure potential (ϕ_p) was found using sophisticated apparatus such as linear transducers, auxanometers, etc. (Acevedo et al., 1971; Green and Cummins, 1974). The presence of a threshold value of ϕ_p necessary for cell enlargement has also been confirmed (Boyer, 1970a; Green et al., 1971; Green and Cummins, 1974; Hsiao et al., 1976).

Effects on photosynthetic efficiency. The efficiency of the photosynthetic apparatus, usually expressed as amount of CO_2 uptake per unit leaf area and time, is also seriously affected by water stress. From the existing experimental evidence it appears that the sensitivity of photosynthesis to water stress varies enormously between plant species (Boyer, 1976). In most mesophytes photosynthesis is first reduced at leaf water potentials between -0.3 to -1.5 MPa and declines more or less linearly with cell turgor becoming

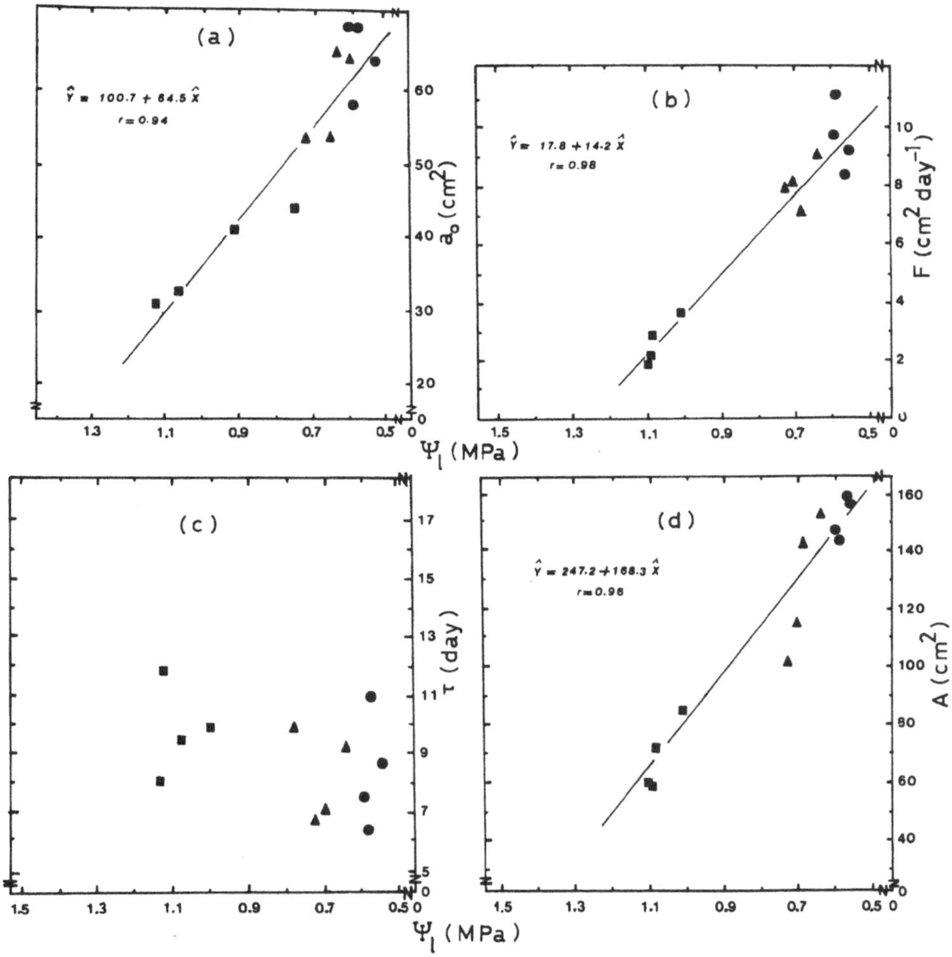

Fig. 4. The relations between the average leaf water potential at 1500h during laminar expansion (Ψ_1) and the average growth rate (b), the duration of growth (c), and the final area (d) for four different leaf insertion levels in field-grown field beans. The area at leaf unfolding (a_o) was correlated with the average Ψ_1 for six days before unfolding (a). Results are from three irrigation treatments (for symbols, see Fig. 2). Each point is the mean of four determinations. The fitted linear regressions in (a), (b), and (d) are also shown. No relation was apparent in (c) (Karamanos, unpublished data).

zero at approximately $\phi_p = 0$ (Slatyer, 1967). On the other hand, plants adapted to xerophytism are able to photosynthesize at Ψ_1 as low as -3.0 to -6.0 MPa. The sensitivity of photosynthesis to water stress is also affected by plant development, especially in wheat and maize (Boyer and McPherson, 1975).

Pfeffer (1900) attributed the inhibition of photosynthesis by desiccation to the closure of stomata, "which will render the absorption of carbon dioxide extremely difficult." Nowadays, such an explanation does not appear to be absolutely right because there is adequate evidence about nonstomatal inhibition of photosynthesis. Gaastra (1959) expressed the rate of photosynthesis in terms of a driving force and a number of resistances:

$$P = \frac{[CO_2]_a - [CO_2]_{chl}}{r'_a + r'_l + r'_m} \quad (g\ cm^{-2}\ s^{-1}), \qquad (2)$$

where $[CO_2]_a$ and $[CO_2]_{chl}$ are the CO_2 concentrations in the bulk air and the chloroplasts respectively ($g\ cm^{-3}$), and r'_a, r'_l, r'_m the resistances to the diffusion of CO_2 in the boundary layer, leaf air space, and mesophyll respectively ($s\ cm^{-1}$). The resistance r'_l is composed by the stomatal (r'_s), cuticular (r'_c), and intercellular space resistance (r'_i). Nonetheless, the variations in r'_l can be attributed with great approximation to changes in r'_s. r'_m is related to the biochemistry of photosynthesis and represents the nonstomatal factors controlling the photosynthetic rate. Although there is little doubt that water stress restricts the entry of CO_2 into the leaf by means of stomatal closure, there is ample evidence that r'_m also increases with increasing stress (Boyer, 1965, 1970b; Gale et al., 1966; Troughton, 1969). The relative contribution of the resistances r'_l and r'_m to the water stress induced inhibition of photosynthesis appears to vary with plant species. Slatyer (1973) reported that a reduction in photosynthesis in wheat and millet was achieved exclusively by stomatal closure since r'_m was unaffected even at very low relative water contents, while this did not happen in maize and cotton. The response of r'_m to desiccation is related to the drought sensitivity of the examined species (Slatyer, 1973; Bunce, 1977b). In general, it appears that the observed reductions in photosynthesis with increasing water stress can be mainly attributed to stomatal closure until quite severe stress exists (Slatyer, 1973).

In view of the in vivo evidence for the increase in r'_m at low leaf water potentials, attempts have been made to detect the origin of this behavior in chloroplast activity. A suppression in chloroplast Hill activity in both severely (Nir and Poljakoff-Mayber, 1967; Santarius and Heber, 1967; Fry, 1970) and moderately desiccated leaf tissue (Boyer and Bowen, 1970; see also Fig. 5) has been observed. Keck and Boyer (1974) found that the activity of the photosystem II was affected more than that of the photosystem I and suggested that electron transport was inhibited during early

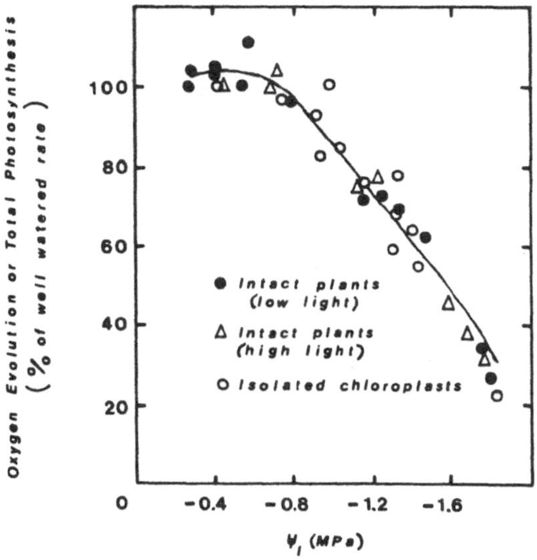

Fig. 5. Oxygen evolution by sunflower chloroplasts and total photosynthesis by sunflower leaves at various leaf water potentials (Ψ_1). The chloroplast assays and some of the measurements with intact leaves were conducted at saturating irradiances, whereas others with intact leaves were carried out at limiting irradiances (from Boyer, 1976).

desiccation while photophosphorylation was affected at more severe water stress. As regards the "dark" reactions of photosynthesis, a reduction in the ribulose-1,5-diphosphocarboxylase activity in desiccated leaves was reported, although the effect was not considered to be large enough as to account for the inhibition of photosynthesis in the intact leaf (Jones, 1973). Attempts to associate these alterations in chloroplast activity with ultrastructural deformations led to contradicting results. Boyer (1976) found that the lamellar system appeared normal in cells exhibiting considerable reduction in photosystem II activity and was affected only in irreversibly dehydrated tissue. On the other hand, Kurkova and Motorina (1974) and Kurkova (1975) reported a fragmentation of the lamellae and an increase in the volume of stroma in bean leaves dehydrated only 4% more than the controls. Ultrastructural changes were also reported in works where water stress was induced by using osmotic substances (Plaut, 1971; Plaut and Bravdo, 1973; Vieira da Silva et al., 1974), but there is no adequate evidence about possible effects of the solutes on the various chloroplast systems.

Mineral Absorption

The contribution of minerals to the increase in total plant dry matter is much less than that of photosynthesis, ranging among different plant species from 2-20% of the total dry weight (Evans, 1972; Milthorpe and Moorby, 1974). The movement of water in the rhizosphere facilitates the supply of nutrients to the roots. When the movement of soil water ceases because of soil dryness, nutrient uptake occurs only by diffusion close to the root. This sort of supply becomes limiting in a very short time since the nutrient reserves are very quickly depleted (Crafts, 1968). Consequently, increasing water shortage should be associated with a decreasing rate of mineral absorption. However, despite the close relationship between soil water and nutrient availability, a sharp distinction between direct effects of water stress on mineral absorption and more general effects on root growth and differentiation is difficult, in view of the effects of water stress on roots and their physiological processes (Viets, 1972; Kramer, 1969; Slatyer, 1969).

Barber et al. (1963) suggested that mass flow could account for most of the transport of Ca, Mg, and N, while P and K moved mainly by diffusion, which is a very sensitive process to soil water content. It is not, therefore, surprising that plants subjected to water stress had a lower content in P and K than the controls (Jenne et al., 1958; Mederski and Wilson, 1960; Greenway et al., 1969; Marais and Wiersma, 1975). Regarding the nutrients moving mainly by mass flow, the accumulation of Mg was reduced by soil water stress while that of Ca was unaffected (Jenne et al., 1958; Mederski and Wilson, 1960). Finally, the evidence for N is rather contradictory. The increase in the N-content of the tissues with increasing water stress mentioned by Richards and Wadleigh (1952) is likely to be associated with effects on the nitrate reductase enzyme system (Viets, 1972). On the other hand, there is evidence that the total accumulation of N in plant tissues is reduced by water stress (Jenne et al., 1958). In any case, the decrease in the microbiological activity of the soil with increasing dryness (Kramer, 1969) causes a reduction in the rate of the decomposition of organic matter. This results in a decrease in the rates of both ammonification and nitrification of organic matter (Reichmann et al., 1966), and hence in a decrease in the nitrogen availability of the soil.

Respiration

Since the process of respiration is a series of enzymatic reactions, and given that both the function and structure of the enzymes are affected by plant water status (Todd, 1972), it follows that respiration should be affected in some way by the hydration of tissues (Crafts, 1968). Generally, the effect of water stress on respiration is less clear than that on photosynthesis. The results reported by Brix (1962) are indicative of the confusion that existed some years ago. Respiration rate, expressed as a fraction of that of well-hydrated plants, decreased steadily with decreasing diffusion pressure deficit (DPD) in tomato plants (Fig. 6a). This was not true in loblolly pine seedlings where respiration followed an S-shaped rather than a linear pattern against DPD (Fig. 6b). This different response of respiration to low and moderate water stress may be a characteristic of the examined species (Boyer, 1976) but may also arise from the adopted experimental technique for imposing water stress (Slatyer, 1967). Regardless of the response at low and moderate stress, the ultimate effect of a severe desiccation is usually a decrease in dark respiration (Flowers and Hanson, 1969; Boyer, 1970a; Wesselius and Brouwer, 1972; Lawlor, 1976; Ludlow and Ng, 1976). There is also evidence that photorespiration also declines with decreasing Ψ_1 (Boyer, 1971; Lawlor, 1976). Boyer (1971) suggested that the decrease in photorespiration was steeper than that in dark respiration.

There is little doubt that both dark and photorespiration are less sensitive to water stress than photosynthesis (Schneider and Childers, 1941; Brix, 1962; Boyer, 1970a). The relative sensitivities of photosynthesis and respiration to water stress can be evaluated by following the course of the CO_2-compensation concentration (Γ) with decreasing Ψ_1. With only a few exceptions (e.g., Troughton and Slayter, 1969), Γ was found to increase substantially with increasing water stress (Heath and Meidner, 1961; Meidner, 1967; Glinka and Katchansky, 1970; Lawlor, 1976). Such an increase implies that respiration increases in relation to assimilation with increasing water stress. It is suggested (Boyer, 1976; Lawlor, 1976) that dark respiration, the process that is most insensitive to desiccation, is responsible for the observed rise in Γ with water stress.

Leaf Shedding

Leaf shedding constitutes both a loss in dry matter and a reduction in the assimilating area of the plant.

Premature leaf shedding is associated with water stress in many plant species (Milthorpe, 1945; Boyer and McPherson, 1975; Finch-Savage and Elston, 1977; Karamonos, 1978a). Usually, older or shaded leaves are the first to die under water stress. In some species, as for instance in cotton, leaf shedding does not occur until after rehydration of the stressed plants (Bruce and Romkens, 1965; McMichael et al., 1972; Jordan et al., 1972). This may imply that abscission is initiated during the stress period and requires water to complete the hydrolytic reactions in the abscission zone (Kozlowski, 1976).

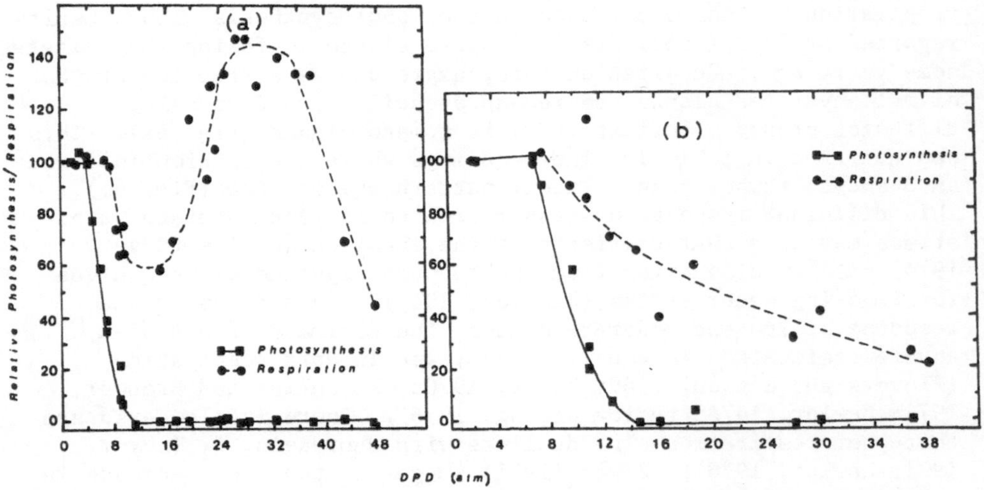

Fig. 6. The effects of water stress, expressed as diffusion pressure deficit (DPD), on photosynthesis and respiration in loblolly pine seedlings (a) and tomato plants (b). Photosynthesis and respiration are expressed as percentage of rates of controls kept at field capacity. Note the different response of respiration in the two species (from Brix, 1962).

It is suggested (Brady et al., 1974; Kozlowski, 1976) that water stress alters the hormonal balance of the leaves, thus promoting both an overall senescence and a hydrolysis of the middle lamellae between cells in the abscission layer. Water stress is associated with an increase in the concentration of abscisic acid (ABA) (Wright and Hiron, 1969; Mizrahi et al., 1970), as well as with a reduced supply of cytokinins to leaves (Livné and Vaadia, 1965; Ben-Zioni et al., 1967). An increase in the ABA concentration induces preabscission changes in the tissue near the abscission zone (Addicott, 1970), while a reduced level of cytokinins accelerates leaf senescence by means of an increased proteolysis (Itai and Vaadia, 1971). Thus, it appears that a change in the ABA/cytokinin balance might be responsible for the enhancement of leaf senescence and abscission by water stress (Brady et al., 1974).

Translocation of Assimilates

There is substantial evidence that the translocation of assimilates is suppressed by water stress (for a review, see Crafts, 1968). Roberts (1964) found in yellow poplar seedlings that many parameters of translocation, namely velocity, distance, and amount of transport, were lowered by leaf water deficits of more than 5%.

Wiebe and Wihrheim (1962) found that the translocation of photosynthates out of sunflower leaves was reduced by about one-third as Ψ_1 fell to about -10 bar. Nevertheless, Wardlaw (1967, 1969) found that the velocity of assimilate movement in the conducting system of stressed wheat was little affected in comparison with controls.

The translocation of assimilates is a mass flow through the sieve tube elements determined on the basis of a source-to-sink relationship. Consequently, the observed reductions in the rates of translocation could result either from a reduction in the amount of photosynthate available for transport or from an inhibition of the translocation process per se. By manipulating the relative magnitudes of source and sink in wheat, Wardlaw (1969) found that the translocation mechanism was relatively unaffected by desiccation and that the effects of water shortage on the source and sink accounted for most of the changes observed. Water stress reduces both source strength by reducing photosynthesis and sink strength by inhibiting growth. A further conclusion from Wardlaw's work is that translocation is less sensitive than photosynthesis to water stress. Boyer and McPherson (1975) reached a similar conclusion working with maize.

Conclusions

Water stress reduces plant yield by considerably suppressing photosynthesis and, to some extent, mineral absorption. In addition, water shortage promotes an irreversible loss in dry matter and assimilating surface by accelerating leaf senescence and death. Although respiration is also reduced by water stress, this reduction occurs at very low leaf water potentials where photosynthesis has already been completely impaired (Slatyer, 1967). The adverse effects on the translocation of assimilates to the economically important parts of the plant complete the picture of the disturbances caused by water stress on the main physiological processes determining plant yield.

The process of photosynthesis has received much attention as the main determinant of plant yield. Of the two components of photosynthesis, leaf area was considered in early works (e.g., Heath and Gregory, 1938; Watson, 1947) as exclusively contributing to the variations in dry matter yield, while some other investigators (Thorne, 1966; Wallace and Munger, 1966) ascribed also a role to photosynthetic efficiency. Irrespective of the relative significance of the two components under non-stress conditions, it has already been shown that a significant ecological factor such as water supply affects drastically both the size and the efficiency of the system. Apart from some exceptions (e.g., Ludlow and Ng, 1976), there are many indications that, in a number of species, leaf area growth is more sensitive to water stress than the photosynthetic process itself (Wardlaw, 1969; Boyer, 1970a; Wesselius and Brouwer, 1972; Hsiao and Acevedo, 1974; Lawlor and Milford, 1973). Accordingly, water shortage affects yield mainly by reducing the assimilating area. Both seed and dry matter yields of field beans were strongly correlated with the plant leaf area integrated over the whole period of growth (Fig. 7a,b). When the average net assimilation rate (NAR) over the same period was plotted against yields, the correlations were weaker (Fig. 7c,d). This emphasizes the importance of leaf area for agronomic purposes. The correlation coefficients between the yields and both integrated leaf area and mean net assimilation rate reported here are much higher than those found by other investigators in field beans (Ishag, 1969; Rajaratnam, 1969). In their experiments, the differences in crop leaf area were produced by different crop densities, while those reported here were induced by subjecting the plants to different degrees of water stress. This implies that the great differences in crop yields reported here are unlikely to be caused exclusively by differences in leaf area, in view of the impact of water stress on many other physiological processes.

When evaluating the relative sensitivities of the capacity and the efficiency of the photosynthetic system to water shortage and their significance to final yield, one should also take into account the stage of crop growth at which water stress occurs. If the stress is imposed when leaf area is already well developed and the canopy closed, i.e., when there is no limitation of light interception and gas exchange, then a reduction in leaf area growth does not decisively affect dry matter production and a reduction in the rate of photosynthesis is more important. Alternatively, if the stress occurs when the canopy is still open, then a reduction in the development of the assimilating area is more important than any suppression of the photosynthetic rate in view of the greater sensitivity of the former to water deficits (cf. Hsiao and Acevedo, 1974).

POSSIBILITIES OF MEETING THE CHALLENGE

To evaluate the possibilities of diminishing the detrimental effects of water stress on plant growth and yield in the future, it is necessary to understand how plants respond to brief or long periods of water shortage. It is very likely we may detect some techniques of increasing crop drought resistance among the many adaptive mechanisms developed by different plant species.

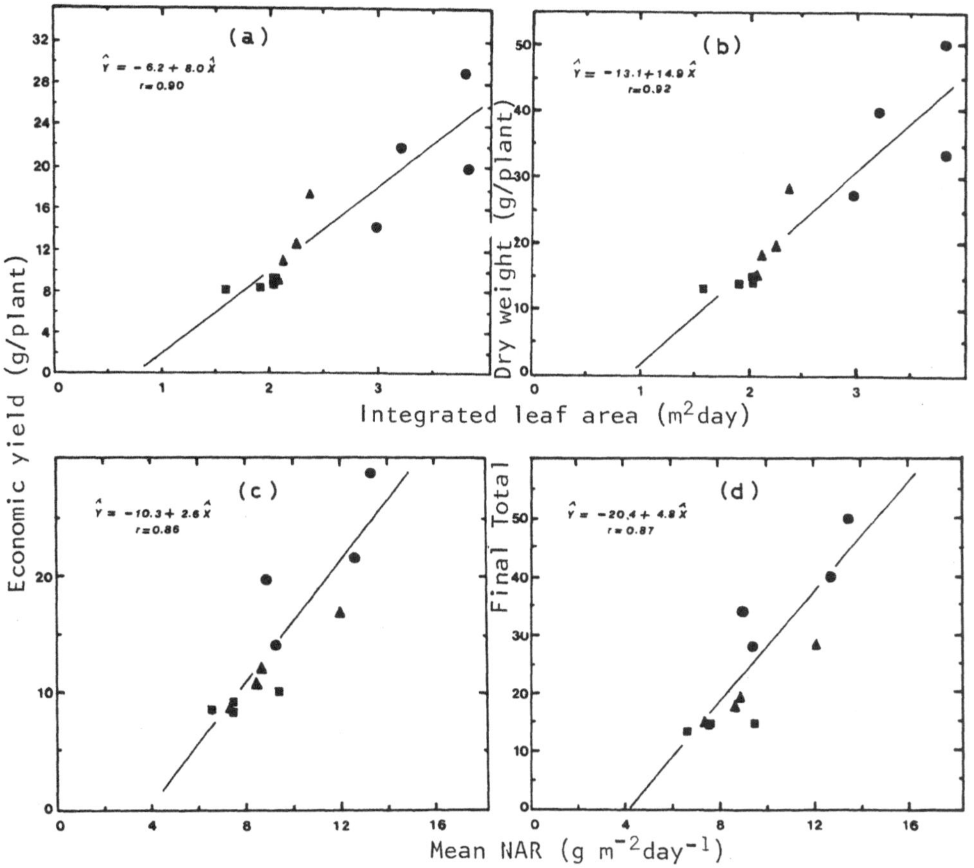

Fig. 7. The relations of the economic [(a) and (c)] and the final total dry matter [(b) and (d)] yields with the integrated leaf area and the mean net assimilation rate during the growth of field bean crops subjected to three irrigation treatments (symbols are the same as in Fig. 2). The mean NAR was calculated by dividing the final yields by the integrated leaf area. The fitted linear regressions are also shown. Note that the correlation coefficients are higher in (a) and (b) than in (c) and (d) (Karamanos, unpublished data).

The Adaptations to Water Stress

Some of the drought resistance mechanisms developed by xerophytes are also encountered in crop plants. Using Levitt's (1972) terminology these mechanisms are divided into two groups (Fig. 8):

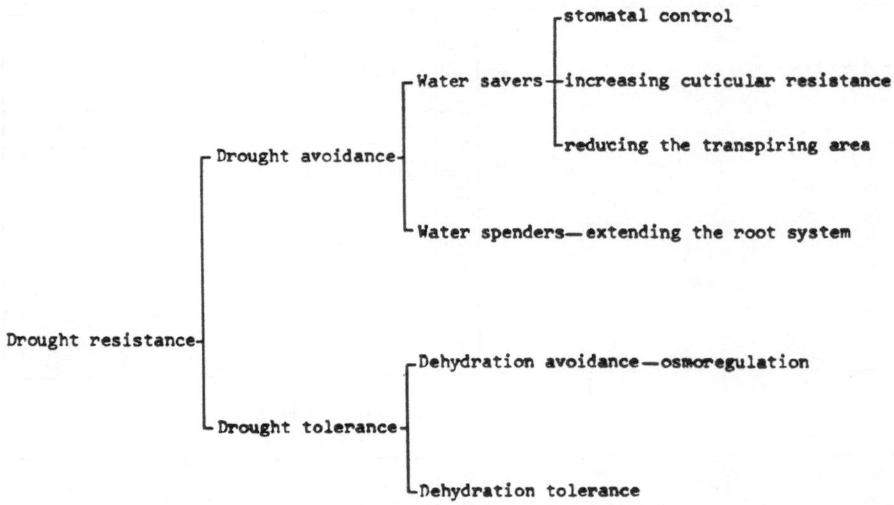

Fig. 8. Diagrammatic representation of the main adapted mechanisms developed by crop plants. For an analysis, see text (adapted from Levitt, 1972).

(1) Drought avoidance. By definition, the plants avoiding drought must maintain a high water potential when exposed to stress. There are two distinct groups of drought avoiders, the water savers that conserve water and the water spenders which absorb water so rapidly as to meet transpirational loss.

Water savers conserve their water supply (a) by controlling stomatal aperture so as to prevent any excessive water loss; (b) by diminishing cuticular transpiration by means of thicker cuticles enriched with hydrophobic substances; and (c) by reducing the transpiring area by means of leaf shedding, rolling, or folding.

The basic adaptation characterizing water spenders is the development of an extended and physiologically active root system which permits the plant not to suffer from water stress.

(2) Drought tolerance or "true xerophytism" (Maximov, 1929) is the adaptive mechanism that enables plants to survive under severe water stress without conserving water. In contrast to the largely morphological and anatomical nature of drought avoidance, drought tolerance is associated with the ability of the various physiological processes to proceed uninhibited even at high levels of dehydration. Drought tolerance can be further distinguished into dehydration avoidance and dehydration tolerance. In the former case protoplasmic activity is not seriously affected since cells maintain their turgor above zero by increasing the osmotic value of their sap in relation to the water potential of their environment. Dehydration

tolerance usually refers to the behavior of the kinetics of specific metabolic reactions under water stress.

This classification offers a picture of the basic drought adaptations developed by plants. In practice, the reactions of most plants to water shortage usually extend to more than one of the categories mentioned above. It is important to note that drought avoidance is an adaptation usually encountered in mesophytes while drought tolerance is exclusively found in xerophytes and microorganisms (Levitt, 1972). By avoiding water stress, plants maintain their water potential and turgor at high levels in spite of the low water potential of the environment. Thus, growth, metabolism, and development progress unimpaired. On the other hand, tolerance aims at the survival rather than the growth of the plant during the stress period since tolerant plants, with the exception of the dehydration avoiders, have no positive ϕ_p when subjected to water stress. It appears, therefore, that the avoidance adaptations are of greater value than those of tolerance for the cultivated plants where a promotion in growth and yield is the main target. There are, however, some techniques of increasing crop production by improving drought tolerance.

Methods of Increasing the Productivity of Water Stressed Plants

An attempt will be made to describe and evaluate the various techniques used to increase crop yield by improving plant water status. The techniques inducing drought avoidance will be divided into those reducing transpiration and those increasing water absorption. Reference will also be made to some techniques aiming at increasing drought tolerance.

Reducing transpiration. It is self-evident that among the water saving mechanisms mentioned above (Fig. 8) only those reducing transpiration are of practical importance. A reduction in the transpiring area is undesirable for the reasons already mentioned above.

There is still some confusion about the role of transpiration in plant physiology. Thus, transpiration is regarded either as a necessary or as an unavoidable evil (Arnon, 1972). It appears that the beneficial role of transpiration is restricted to mineral uptake and distribution and leaf cooling (Poljakoff-Mayber and Gale, 1972). Therefore, when attempting to reduce transpiration one should also consider the physiological disturbances which are likely to arise.

Mineral transport does not seem to be a cause of trouble in view of the existing evidence that solute movement is adequate even at very low transpiration rates (Scott-Russell and Barber, 1960; Gale and Hagan, 1966).

Considerable progress has been made toward the understanding of the cooling effect of transpiration after the comprehensive works of D. M. Gates (1964, 1968). The net incoming radiation intercepted by a leaf surface (R_n) is dissipated in three ways according to the leaf energy balance equation (Raschke, 1960; D. M. Gates, 1968):

$$R_n = R_L + H + \lambda E. \tag{3}$$

R_L represents the long wave reradiation which, according to the law of Stephan-Boltzmann, is related to the fourth power of leaf temperature. Leaves are considered to behave as completely black bodies in the wave range of 300 to 25000 nm (Knoerr and Gay, 1965). H is the convective heat transfer due to the temperature difference between leaf and air. Finally, λE is the energy dissipation by latent heat flux (λ is the heat of vaporization of water) which is identical to transpiration. The transpiration rate (T) is given by the equation:

$$T = \frac{[H_2O]_l - [H_2O]_a}{r_l + r_a} \quad (g\ cm^{-2}\ s^{-1}), \tag{4}$$

where $[H_2O]_l - [H_2O]_a$ is the difference in vapor concentration between leaf and air ($g\ cm^{-3}$), and r_l and r_a the leaf and boundary layer resistances to water vapor transport ($s\ cm^{-1}$). Since $[H_2O]_l$ is exponentially dependent on leaf temperature, it appears that all three dissipation components of Equation (3) depend on leaf temperature. Therefore, there is no simple and unique effect of a reduction in transpiration on leaf temperature. All three components interact continuously and dynamically to give their instantaneous relative magnitude, and leaf temperature is the passive result of these interactions (Gates, 1964; Slatyer, 1967). In view of the strong dependence of R_L on leaf temperature, much more energy is dissipated by reradiation than by convection or transpiration at low windspeeds (Idso and Baker, 1967; Hoffman and Gates, 1971). As windspeed increases a considerable amount of energy is also dissipated by advection. Consequently, any reduction in transpiration under windy conditions will result in a smaller increase in leaf temperature than in still air. Both theoretical and experimental results have shown that, except for conditions of high insolation and humidity, leaf temperatures are very close to air temperatures (Gale et al., 1965; D. M. Gates, 1968). Poljakoff-Mayber and Gale (1972) report that even under conditions of still air a reduction in transpiration by 40-50% produces at the most a 2-2.5°C rise in leaf temperature. In conclusion, the older theories considering transpiration as the unique way of leaf cooling (e.g., Thorntwaite and Mather, 1954) do not appear to be valid anymore. However, one should remember that a rise in leaf temperature even by

3-4°C may considerably reduce net photosynthesis by increasing the rate of photorespiration in some species.

In addition to the factors mentioned above, the fact that both water loss and CO_2 uptake occur through the same pathway complicates considerably the problem of reducing transpiration. Stomatal closure effectively confers drought avoidance but it simultaneously inhibits photosynthesis. Nevertheless, both theoretical and practical considerations of the problem (Slatyer and Bierhuizen, 1964; Cowan and Troughton, 1971; Raschke, 1976) have shown that partial stomatal closure increases the ratio of assimilation over transpiration, or assimilation ratio (Fig. 9). This is because the rate of photosynthesis, in addition to its dependence on stomatal conductance, follows saturation kinetics as regards the intercellular CO_2 concentration. A further evidence for an increase in the assimilation ratio by stomatal closure is apparent when comparing Equations (2) and (4). If r_m' is of the same order of magnitude as r_a and r_l, a closure of stomata will bring about a larger percentage reduction in transpiration than in photosynthesis.

Antitranspirants. Antitranspirants are substances applied to decrease transpiration rates. They can be divided into film-forming materials and chemicals inducing stomatal closure.

The method of decreasing water loss by coating leaf surface with materials impervious to water vapor traces its origin from Theophrastus (c. 300 B.C.) according to Poljakoff-Mayber and Gale (1972). These materials act on the leaf surface as physical barriers to vapor diffusion. There are usually polymers such as polyvinyl waxes, polyethylene, and vinyl-acrylate as well as higher alcohols such as hexadecanol. In order to be effective, a film-forming antitranspirant must be nontoxic, easy to spread and stick onto surfaces, stable under solar radiation, elastic and durable, and, of course, impermeable to water vapor (Gale and Hagan, 1966). The main shortcoming of the currently used materials is that their permeability to CO_2 is several times smaller than that to water vapor (Waggoner, 1966; Woolley, 1967). The possibilities of inventing a material with selective permeability to CO_2 are very small in view of the smaller molecular weight and dimensions of the water molecule. Thus, the existing materials impair photosynthesis more effectively than transpiration if the coating extends over the whole leaf surface. In practice, with an average coating of about 50%, transpiration is reduced by 30-50% (Poljakoff-Mayber and Gale, 1972) and photosynthesis proceeds unimpaired through the uncovered leaf area. According to Poljakoff-Mayber and Gale (1972), the use of an impervious antitranspirant under hot Mediterranean conditions causes a small increase in leaf temperature (1.2°C on the average) and a considerable water saving. Only when air is almost still would there be a possibly harmful rise of 3-4°C in leaf temperature.

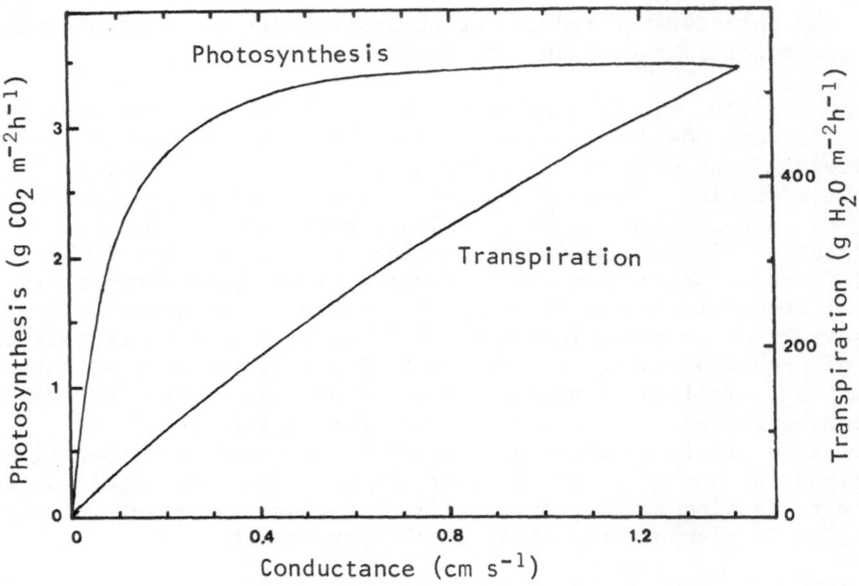

Fig. 9. The computed dependence of CO_2 assimilation and transpiration on stomatal conductance (k_s) using parameters obtained from measurements on leaves of Xanthium strumarium. At $k_s > 0.5$ cm s^{-1} changes in stomatal aperture affect transpiration but hardly change photosynthesis. At $k_s < 0.2$ cm s^{-1} CO_2 uptake is greatly reduced by any further reduction in stomatal aperture (from Raschke, 1976).

The use of chemical antitranspirants appears to be more promising because they induce partial stomatal closure which increases the assimilation ratio (see above and Fig. 9). However, several precautions must be taken when considering a certain chemical as an antitranspirant. First, the substance must not be toxic to the plant. Second, the closure of stomata must not be induced by increasing the CO_2 concentration of the mesophyll since the concentration gradient of CO_2 between air and mesophyll is also reduced. This results in a proportionally greater inhibition of photosynthesis in comparison to water vapor loss (Mansfield, 1976; see also Equation (2)). Third, the effects of the antitranspirant must be restricted to the guard cells without affecting the other cells of the leaf. To avoid major metabolic disturbances, the best solution would be to invent a substance interfering only with the mechanisms which produce the turgor changes in the guard cells.

Various compounds have been used for the chemical control of stomatal opening (for a review, see Gale and Hagan, 1966). However, only a few of them fill the requirements mentioned above. Metabolic inhibitors such as sodium azide and potassium cyanide induce overall toxic effects (Waggoner, 1966). Decenylsuccinic acid, a substance which increases guard cell permeability (Zelitch, 1964), was harmful to both roots and shoots of some species (Newman and Kramer, 1966; Kozlowski and Clausen, 1970). Hydroxysulphonates and synthetic auxins decreased the assimilation ratio by increasing the internal CO_2 concentration, the former by inhibiting photosynthesis, the latter by stimulating respiration (Mansfield, 1976). Phenylmercuric acetate (PMA) gave encouraging results by increasing the assimilation ratio on many occasions (Zelitch and Waggoner, 1962; Shimshi, 1963; Slatyer and Bierhuizen, 1964; Davenport, 1967). PMA is supposed to act solely on the guard cells by inhibiting photophosphorylation without entering the mesophyll. Nevertheless, in some cases it was also detected in the mesophyll cells (Squire and Jones, 1971) and caused phytotoxic symptoms (Keller, 1966). A further shortcoming of PMA is its human and animal toxicity, which restricts its use to nonedible plants. More promising results are expected from the growth retardant abscisic acid (ABA), which seems to possess all the properties of an ideal antitranspirant. This naturally occurring substance was first used as an antitranspirant by Jones and Mansfield (1970) with encouraging results. ABA was found to increase considerably the assimilation ratio by inducing partial stomatal closure (Jones and Mansfield, 1972; Mizrahi et al., 1974, Raschke, 1974). It acts by reducing the solute content and hence the turgor of the guard cells without affecting the other epidermal cells (Mansfield and Jones, 1971). Its effects on plant growth were not considered as significant in the concentrations used for exogenous applications (10^{-4} to 10^{-5}M) (Jones and Mansfield, 1972; Mizrahi et al., 1974). Other natural substances with chemical structure similar to that of ABA, for instance all-trans-farnesol, are also being studied for their suitability as antitranspirants (Mansfield, 1976).

Enclosures. Covered enclosures reduce the transpiration of the growing plants by means of the high air vapor concentration which reduces the gradient for the movement of water vapor out of the leaf (Equation (4)). In addition there is a further possibility of decreasing transpiration with a concurrent increase in the assimilation ratio by adding CO_2 in the enclosure (Moss et al., 1961; Wittwer and Robb, 1964). The increased CO_2 concentration induces partial stomatal closure and thus decreases water loss. At the same time, despite the increased resistance of the epidermis, photosynthesis is maintained at quite high levels because of the steeper gradient in CO_2 concentration between mesophyll and air (Equation (2)). Although CO_2 itself is considered as an ideal antitranspirant (Kramer, 1969), its application is limited only to restricted areas under covers (Pallas, 1970).

Reflecting materials. The use of reflective materials sprayed onto transpiring plant surfaces aims at modifying their energy balance. One approach is to use reflective materials to decrease the net radiation of the surface. Such a reduction in R_n also results in a decrease in the latent heat dissipation component λE (Equation (3)). It should also be possible to use a selective pigment transmitting the radiation between 400 and 700 nm and reflecting all other parts of the spectrum (Poljakoff-Mayber and Gale, 1972). In this way plants would avoid about 60% of the total incoming radiation, which is mainly restricted to the long-wave band (Gates, 1962). This second alternative is a future objective given that selective pigments of this sort do not exist at present. Whatever method is finally adopted, the use of reflective materials must be restricted in areas where insolation is high because leaf coating reduces the absorption of solar radiation by about 25% (Moreshet et al., 1968).

Theoretical considerations of the problem were promising. Seginer (1969) calculated that the use of simple reflective materials should bring about a saving in irrigation water of 30% by increasing the natural albedo from 0.25 to 0.4. Abou Khaled et al. (1970) found in controlled environments that the use of kaolin suspension sprays caused a reduction in transpiration by 22-28% without any corresponding reduction in the CO_2 fixation rate. Fuchs et al. (1976), Stanhill et al. (1976), and Moreshet et al. (1977) found that the situation was more complicated in a field experiment with sorghum plants. Grain yield was increased in the treated plants in spite of a reduction in CO_2 fixation rate of 23%, while neither the total seasonal water use nor the rate of soil water depletion was significantly affected by the treatment. Furthermore, kaolin coating was found to enhance leaf senescence. In relation to water use, Stanhill et al. (1976) pointed out that their results were not in conflict with the expected improvement in plant water status since the potential water loss in their experiments was much greater than the amount of available soil water. It seems therefore that considerable experimental work is still necessary in order to understand the impact of reflective materials in plant physiology. Fuchs (1972) has shown that there are considerable interactions between the effects of changing the reflectivity of the foliage and the absorptivity of the crop canopy.

Windbreaks. A beneficial effect of windbreaks on the assimilation ratio is expected only when advective heat increases considerably the energy balance of the leaf ("oasis-effect"). In that case, the lowering of wind speed decreases the amount of advective heat conveyed to leaves and increases the water vapor content of the air near the leaves (Poljakoff-Mayber and Gale, 1972).

Breeding techniques. It is possible to select for some morphological and physiological characteristics which enable plants to reduce water loss and to introduce them in breeding programs aimed at increasing crop productivity.

The relationship between stomatal resistance (r_s) and Ψ_l appears to be a parameter which to a great extent determines the ability of a plant to avoid drought (Hurd, 1976). Several investigators have found that Ψ_l can vary over a considerable range above a critical value without having any effect on r_s. When the critical value is reached, stomata tend to close either rapidly or more gradually, depending on the manner by which drought was imposed (Fig. 10) (Begg et al., 1964; Kanemasu and Tanner, 1969; Jordan and Ritchie, 1971; Biscoe, 1972). This critical Ψ_l is of great value in breeding programs. It was found to differ among plant species with varying drought resistance (for a review, see Kozlowski, 1972). Significant differences have also been found between varieties in sorghum (Blum, 1974; Henzell et al., 1975, 1976), wheat (Dedio, 1975), corn (Dubé et al., 1974), and potato (Kozlowski, 1972). It must be emphasized, however, that the relationship between r_s and Ψ_l depends also on leaf age (Doley, 1967; Gee and Federer, 1972), the size of stomata (Waisel et al., 1969; Gindel, 1969), and preconditioning (see below). The aims of breeding for stomatal control of transpiration are not straightforward. One could select genotypes where the critical Ψ_l is either high or low according to the other drought resistance characteristics of the plant. A low critical value of Ψ_l will enable CO_2 diffusion across the epidermis to proceed at higher stresses than a higher value. This will enable plants to photosynthesize at low water potentials if the mesophyll resistance of photosynthesis r_m' is not significantly increased at these levels of Ψ_l. In addition, the increased water loss by the closing of stomata at lower Ψ_l must be accompanied by plant characteristics which increase the water supply to leaves. A high value of critical Ψ_l is more preferable whenever these requirements are not met.

Stomatal frequency is among the useful morphological characteristics for improving drought resistance. A low stomatal frequency was associated with an increase in the assimilation ratio in barley (Miskin et al., 1972), *Phaseolus* (Izhar and Wallace, 1967), and *Panicum* (Dobrenz et al., 1969), mainly by reducing transpiration. Stomatal frequency was found to differ significantly among cultivars of some species and to be relatively consistent in different environments (Izhar and Wallace, 1967; Miskin and Rasmusson, 1970; Shearman and Beard, 1972).

It may also be possible to improve leaf energy balance by genetic means. Increasing leaf hairiness brings about a relief of the leaf from excessive radiative load (Eller, 1977) and thus reduces its temperature (Eslick and Hackett, 1975). Isogenic lines of barley cultivars have been developed with light-green and golden leaves, which reflect more light than darker-colored ones (Hurd, 1976). Despite their light colors, these isogenic lines exhibited

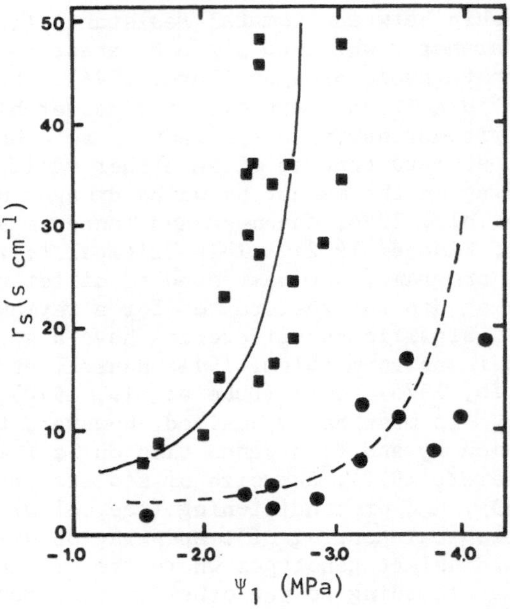

Fig. 10. The dependence of stomatal resistance (r_s) on leaf water potential (Ψ_1) for the lower surface of leaf number 10 of control (■——■) and stress-preconditioned (●---●) cotton plants (from Brown et al., 1976).

photosynthetic rates per unit leaf surface which were equivalent to or even higher than those of the darker colored lines (Ferguson, 1974).

A further means of reducing water loss is by reducing cuticular transpiration. The overall leaf resistance to water vapor movement (r_l, Equation (4)) is thought to consist of the stomatal (r_s) and cuticular (r_c) resistances connected in parallel:

$$r_l = \frac{r_s r_c}{r_s + r_c} \, . \tag{5}$$

The cuticular resistance in mesophytes lies in the range 20-80 s cm^{-1} while that of xerophytes is much higher (> 200 s cm^{-1}) (Slatyer, 1967). A high r_c increases the assimilation ratio, since little CO_2 transfer is expected via the cuticle (Jones, 1976). Although there is some evidence about varietal differences in r_c in some species (e.g., Dubé et al., 1975), it has not been yet clarified which morphological characteristics are responsible. It is not certain whether the thickness of the cuticle and r_c are necessarily correlated (Kamp, 1930; Parker, 1968). The structure and chemical composition of cuticle seem to play an equally important role in the rate of cuticular transpiration (Parker, 1968).

Increasing water absorption. An extended, well-established, and physiologically active root system is necessary to maintain an adequate water supply. Deep-rooted plants show greater drought avoidance than shallow-rooted ones when ground water is available at the deeper soil layers.

Root growth can be introduced as an important parameter for drought resistance in breeding programs, since there is ample evidence for intervarietal differences (for reviews, see Troughton and Whittington, 1969; Zobel, 1975). Intervarietal differences in root systems have been demonstrated in maize (Spencer, 1940), wheat (Hurd, 1968; Devera et al., 1969), barley (Engledow and Wardlaw, 1923; Hackett, 1968), tomatoes and beans (Zobel, 1975), soybeans (Raper and Barber, 1970), and other crop plants. However, breeding for varieties with deeper root systems does not always ensure a greater water supply. Soil factors such as the availability and distribution of nutrients, the gradients in soil water potential, and soil structure may so decisively affect rooting patterns as to completely mask the genetically controlled variability (Scott-Russell, 1977). Hence, soil must be always considered seriously when introducing deep-rooted varieties.

Inducing Drought Tolerance

The methods used to induce drought tolerance in crop species can be broadly divided into those involving the procedure of hardening and those based on plant breeding.

Hardening. Drought hardening is the procedure whereby plants are subjected to a degree of stress for a given period in order to improve their drought resistance thereafter (Levitt, 1972).

It might be possible to increase drought resistance by pretreating seeds before sowing ("presowing hardening"; see Henckel, 1964; Salim and Todd, 1968). The pretreatment consists of a number of cycles of soaking and drying of seeds. Such treatments were found to be related in some cases to higher yields (Levitt, 1972). There are, however, some doubts concerning the association of the increased yields with an increase in drought resistance (Keller and Black, 1968). Presowing hardiness is still supported by Soviet investigators as a means of increasing drought resistance; they maintain that both DNA and RNA contents were significantly raised in treated plants (Levitt, 1972).

Hardening after emergence is induced by withholding water from plants for some days so as to allow them to undergo water stress down to temporary wilting. As a result, treated plants are more capable of withstanding drought than untreated ones. Several factors may be responsible for this drought tolerance. A decrease in the osmotic potential (ϕ_s) of the prestressed plants has been reported on many occasions (Levitt, 1956; Goode and Higgs, 1973; Simmelsgaard, 1976). There is evidence that this reduction in ϕ_s does not result from a simple dehydration of plant cells, but is merely related to an increase in the solute content of the cells (Hsiao et al., 1976; Karamanos, 1976, 1978b; Kassam and Elston, 1976; Cutler and Rains, 1977; Morgan, 1977; see also Fig. 11). A decrease in ϕ_s by osmoregulatory mechanisms increases the absorbing potential of the plant by maintaining the necessary potential gradient between plant and soil at low soil water potentials.

Apart from the osmoregulatory dehydration avoidance, the preconditioning to drought causes the stomata to stay open at more negative water potentials (Stocker, 1960; Jordan and Ritchie, 1971; McCree, 1974; Brown et al., 1976; see also Fig. 10). Such a behavior was ascribed either to an osmotic adjustment of the guard cells (Millar et al., 1971; Turner and Begg, 1973) or to alterations in the elasticity of the guard cell walls (Demichele and Sharpe, 1973). It is possible that all these changes are induced by alterations in the concentration of ABA (Zabadal, 1974). The conditions under which such behavior of the stomata is beneficial for crop production have already been mentioned above.

Another useful alteration caused by preconditioning stress is related to the structure of the cuticle. It has been found that prestressed soybean plants have a greater proportion of hydrophobic substances in their cuticle, such as lipids (Clark and Levitt, 1956) and waxes (Skoss, 1955). These materials increase considerably the r_c. This may be partly responsible for the reduction in the rates of cuticular transpiration with increasing stress observed on several occasions (Slavik, 1958; Oppenheimer, 1961).

Plant breeding. The inducing of desiccation tolerance by plant breeding appears to be a promising perspective. Among the various characteristics the ability of the photosynthetic mechanism to proceed unimpaired at low water potentials is of great importance. Slatyer (1973) reported differences among plant species in the response of their mesophyll resistance to different levels of desiccation. There is also evidence for intervarietal differences in wheat regarding the desiccation tolerance of their photosynthetic mechanisms (Kaul, 1974). Though interesting, this field of research is still relatively unexplored.

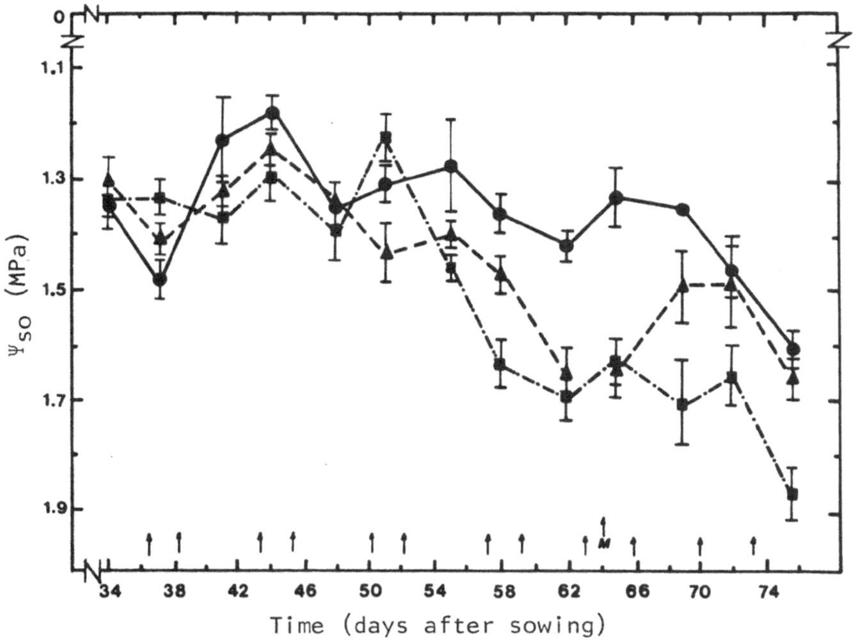

Fig. 11. The time course of the solute potential at zero turgor (ϕ_{so}) of the youngest fully expanded leaf in field beans grown in the field under three different irrigation regimes (●——● wet, ▲---▲ medium, and ■-·-■ dry treatment). The wet treatment was irrigated 12 times (see the lower array of arrows) and the medium once (M). The dry treatment was not irrigated. Each point is the mean of 4 determinations with the vertical bars representing the standard errors of the means. The ϕ_{so} in the dry treatment was systematically lower than that in the wet during the second half of the observations. After the irrigation on day 64, the ϕ_{so} in the medium treatment was raised to less negative values but with a log which indicates that the mechanism is not easily reversible.

CONCLUSIONS

It appears that there are many possibilities, some of them still unexplored, for increasing crop drought resistance (Fig. 12). However, the problem of selecting the most appropriate method or combination of methods is complicated and must be considered in relation to environmental, economic, social, and other factors prevailing in a certain region. The introduction of crops and varieties endowed with desirable drought resistance characteristics is not always the best and cheapest solution. A more extended root

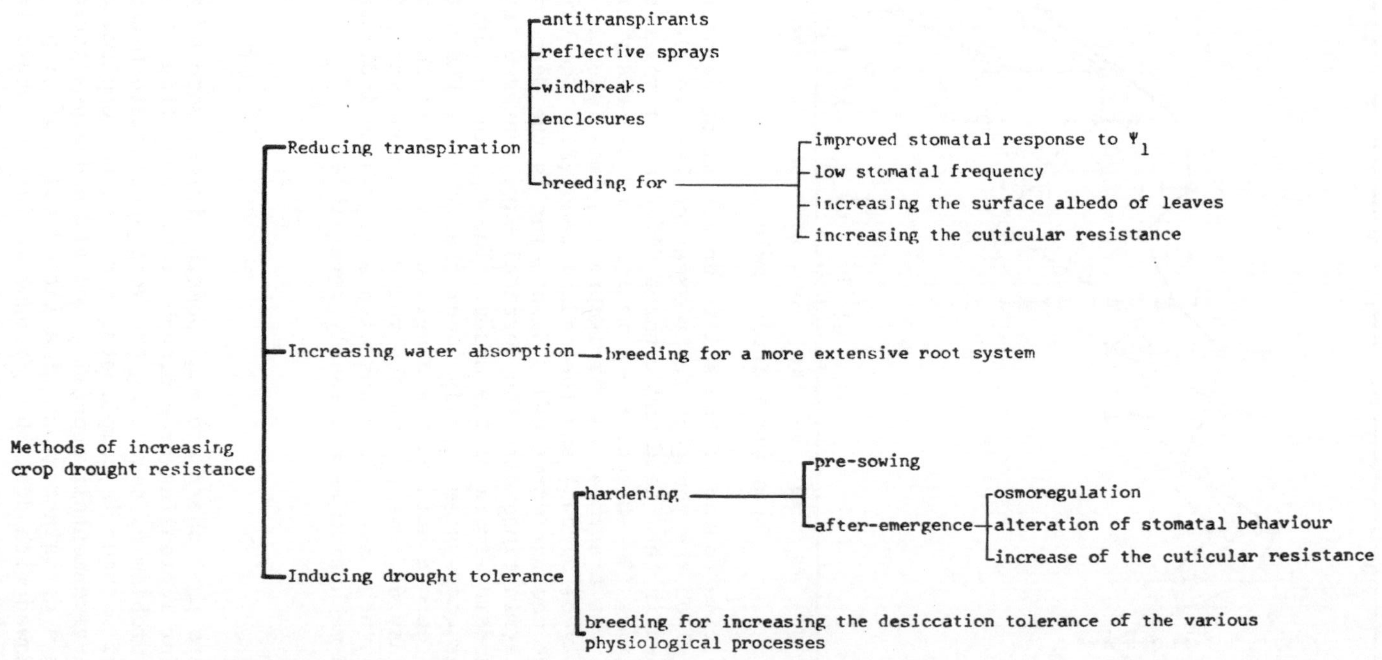

Fig. 12. Diagrammatic representation of the various methods used to increase crop drought resistance.

system implies a greater diversion of metabolites to the underground part, an increase in the root/top ratio, and a reduction in the potential for high yields. Varieties with stomata closing at high Ψ_1 reduce considerably assimilation both on a daily and a seasonal basis, while those with stomata closing at low Ψ_1 must also be accompanied by other characteristics. A high protoplasmic resistance to desiccation may well enable plants to survive under stress but it does not necessarily imply a satisfactory production efficiency under non-stress conditions. It seems that drought resistant crops and varieties must be used in climates where drought is a regular characteristic of the growing season.

In more temperate climates, where temporary droughts at critical growth stages can also reduce considerably crop yields, there is no need to replace high-yielding crop species and varieties with less productive drought resistant ones. The use of antitranspirants during the drought period would be of considerable value, provided that the cost from their use is at least compensated for by the benefits obtained (i.e., increased productivity plus the saving of irrigation). Physiological disturbances arising from increasing leaf temperatures are more unlikely to occur in temperate climates because of the lower insolation.

Regarding the other methods, reflective sprays must be used cautiously until their effects on crop physiology are fully elucidated. In any case, their use must be restricted in regions where solar irradiance is not a limiting factor in crop production. Windshelters and enclosures are of much more limited use. Finally, the various techniques of inducing hardiness are cheap and attractive but they still need much research in order to be fully understood and standardized. In contrast to the existing confusion about the effectiveness of presowing hardening, drought preconditioning of the plants during the noncritical periods of their development is an effective technique for inducing hardiness and increasing production.

REFERENCES

Abu Khaled, A., Hagan, R. M., and Davenport, D. C., 1970, Effects of kaolinite as a reflective antitranspirant on leaf temperature, transpiration, photosynthesis and water use efficiency, Water Resour. Res., 6:280-282.

Acevedo, E., Hsiao, T. C., and Henderson, D. W., 1971, Immediate and subsequent growth responses of maize leaves to changes in water status, Pl. Physiol., 48:631-636.

Addicott, F. T., 1970, Plant hormones in the control of abscission, Biol. Rev. Cambridge Phil. Soc., 45:485-524.

Amer, F. A., and Williams, W. T., 1958, Drought resistance in Pelargonium zonale, Ann. Bot., 22:369-378.

Arnon, I., 1972, "Crop Production in Dry Regions. I. Background and

Principles," Leonard Hill, London.
Asana, R. D., and Mani, V. S., 1949, Photosynthesis in the ears of five varieties of wheat, Nature, 163:450-451.
Barber, S. A., Walker, J. M., and Vasey, E. H., 1963, Mechanisms for the movement of plant nutrients from the soil and fertilizer to the plant root, J. Agr. Food Chem., 11:204-207.
Begg, J. E., Bierhuizen, J. F., Lemon, E. R., Misra, D. K., Slatyer, R. O., and Stern, W. R., 1964, Diurnal energy and water exchanges in bulrush millet in an area of high solar radiation, Agric. Meteorol., 1:294-312.
Ben-Zioni, A., Itai, C., and Vaadia, Y., 1967, Water and salt stresses, kinetin and protein synthesis in tobacco leaves, Pl. Physiol., 42:361-365.
Biscoe, P. V., 1972, The diffusion resistance and water status of leaves of Beta vulgaris, J. Exp. Bot., 23:930-940.
Blum, A., 1974, Genotypic responses in sorghum to drought stress. I. Response to soil moisture stress, Crop Sci., 14:361-365.
Boyer, J. S., 1965, Effects of osmotic water stress on metabolic rates of cotton plants with open stomata, Pl. Physiol., 40:229-234.
Boyer, J. S., 1968, Relationship of water potential to growth of leaves, Pl. Physiol., 43:1056-1062.
Boyer, J. S., 1970a, Leaf enlargement and metabolic rates in corn, soybean and sunflower at various leaf water potentials, Pl. Physiol., 46:233-235.
Boyer, J. S., 1970b, Differing sensitivity of photosynthesis to low leaf water potentials in corn and soybean, Pl. Physiol., 46: 236-239.
Boyer, J. S., 1971, Nonstomatal inhibition of photosynthesis in sunflower at low leaf water potentials and high light intensities, Pl. Physiol., 48:532-536.
Boyer, J. S., 1976, Water deficits and photosynthesis, in: "Water Deficits and Plant Growth," T. T. Kozlowski, ed., Vol. IV, Academic Press, New York, San Francisco, London.
Boyer, J. S., and Bowen, B. L., 1970, Inhibition of O_2-evolution by chloroplasts isolated from leaves with low water potentials, Pl. Physiol., 45:612-615.
Boyer, J. S., and McPherson, H. G., 1975, Physiology of water deficits in cereal crops, Adv. Agron., 27:1-23.
Brady, C. J., Scott, N. S., and Munns, R., 1974, The interaction of water stress with the senescence pattern of leaves, R. Soc. NZ Bull., 12:403-409.
Brix, H., 1962, The effect of water stress on the rates of photosynthesis and respiration in tomato plants and loblolly pine seedlings, Physiologia Pl., 15:10-20.
Brouwer, R., 1963, The influence of the suction tension of the nutrient solutions on growth, transpiration and diffusion pressure deficit of bean leaves (Phaseolus vulgaris), Acta Bot. Neerl., 12:248-261.
Brown, K. W., Jordan, W. R., and Thomas, J. C., 1976, Water stress induced alterations of the stomatal response to decreases in

leaf water potential, Physiologia Pl., 37:1-5.
Bruce, R. R., and Romkens, M. J. M., 1965, Fruiting and growth characteristics of cotton in relation to soil moisture tension, Agron. J., 57:135-140.
Bunce, J. A., 1977a, Leaf elongation in relation to leaf water potential in soybean, J. Exp. Bot., 28:156-161.
Bunce, J. A., 1977b, Nonstomatal inhibition of photosynthesis at low water potentials in intact leaves of species from a variety of habitats, Pl. Physiol., 59:348-350.
Clark, J. A., and Levitt, J., 1956, The basis of drought resistance in the soybean plant, Physiologia Pl., 9:598-606.
Clough, B. F., and Milthorpe, F. L., 1975, Effects of water deficit on leaf development in tobacco, Aust. J. Pl. Physiol., 2:291-300.
Cowan, I. R., and Troughton, J. H., 1971, The relative role of stomata in transpiration and assimilation, Planta, 97:325-336.
Crafts, A. S., 1968, Water deficits and physiological processes, in: "Water Deficits and Plant Growth," T. T. Kozlowski, ed., Vol. II, Academic Press, New York and London.
Cutler, J. M., and Rains, D. W., 1977, Effects of irrigation history on responses of cotton to subsequent water stress, Crop Sci., 17:329-335.
Dale, J. E., 1964, Leaf growth in Phaseolus vulgaris. I. Growth of the first pair of leaves under constant conditions, Ann. Bot., 28:579-590.
Davenport, D. C., 1967, Effects of chemical antitranspirants on transpiration and growth of grass, J. Exp. Bot., 18:332-347.
Dedio, W., 1975, Water relations in wheat leaves as screening tests for drought resistance, Can. J. Pl. Sci., 55:369-378.
Demichele, D. W., and Sharpe, P. J. H., 1973, An analysis of the mechanics of guard cell motion, J. Theor. Biol., 41:77-96.
Devera, N. F., Marshall, D. R., and Balaam, L. N., 1969, Genetic variability in root development in relation to drought tolerance in spring wheats, Expl. Agric., 5:327-337.
Dobrenz, A. K., Wright, L. N., Massengale, M. A., and Kneebone, W. R., 1969, Water use efficiency and its association with several characteristics of blue panicgrass (Panicum antidotale Retz.), Crop Sci., 9:213-215.
Doley, D., 1967, Water relations of Eucalyptus marginata SM. under natural conditions, J. Ecol., 55:597.
Dubé, P. A., Stevenson, K. R., and Thurtell, G., 1974, Comparison between two inbred corn lines for diffusion resistances, photosynthesis, and transpiration as a function of leaf water potential, Can. J. Pl. Sci., 54:765-770.
Dubé, P. A., Stevenson, K. R., Thurtell, G., and Hunter, R. B., 1975, Effects of water stress on leaf respiration, transpiration rates in the dark and cuticular resistance to water vapour diffusion of two corn inbreds, Can. J. Pl. Sci., 55:565-572.
Eller, B. M., 1977, Leaf pubescence: The significance of lower surface hairs for the spectral properties of the upper surface, J. Exp. Bot., 28:1054-1059.

Engledow, F. L., and Wardlaw, S., 1923, Investigation on yield in cereals, J. Agric. Sci., 13:390-439.
Eslick, F. R., and Hackett, E. A., 1975, Genetic engineering as a key to water use efficiency, Agric. Meteorol., 14:13-22.
Evans, C. G., 1972, "The Quantitative Analysis of Plant Growth," Blackwell Scientific Publications, Oxford and London.
Ferguson, H., 1974, Use of variety isogenes in plant-water use efficiency studies, Agric. Meteorol., 14:25-29.
Finch-Savage, W. E., and Elston, J., 1977, The death of leaves in crops of field beans, Ann. Appl. Biol., 85:463-465.
Flowers, T. J., and Hanson, J. B., 1969, The effect of reduced water potential on soybean mitochondria, Pl. Physiol., 44:939-945.
Fry, K. E., 1970, Some factors affecting the Hill reaction activity in cotton chloroplasts, Pl. Physiol., 45:465-469.
Fuchs, M., 1972, The control of the radiation climate of plant communities, in: "Optimizing the Soil and Physical Environment Toward Greater Crop Yields," D. Hillel, ed., Academic Press, New York.
Fuchs, M., Stanhill, G., and Moreshet, S., 1976, Effect of increasing foliage and soil reflectivity on the solar radiation balance of wide-row grain sorghum, Agron. J., 68:865-871.
Gaastra, P., 1959, Photosynthesis of crop plants as influenced by light, carbon dioxide, temperature and stomatal diffusion resistance, Meded. Landbouwhogesch. Wageningen, 59:1-68.
Gale, J., and Hagan, R. M., 1966, Plant antitranspirants, A. Rev. Pl. Physiol., 17:269-282.
Gale, J., Kohl, H. C., and Hagan, R. M., 1966, Mesophyll and stomatal resistances affecting photosynthesis under varying conditions of soil water and evaporation demand, Isr. J. Bot., 15:64-71.
Gale, J., Poljakoff-Mayber, A., Nir, I., and Kahane, I., 1965, Effect of antitranspirant treatment on leaf temperatures, Pl. Cell Physiol., 6:111.
Gandar, P. W., and Tanner, C. B., 1976, Leaf growth, tuber growth, and water potential in potatoes, Crop Sci., 16:534-538.
Gates, C. T., 1968, Water deficits and growth of herbaceous plants, in: "Water Deficits and Plant Growth," T. T. Kozlowski, ed., Vol. II, Academic Press, New York and London.
Gates, D. M., 1962, "Energy Exchange in the Biosphere," Harper, New York.
Gates, D. M., 1964, Leaf temperature and transpiration, Agron. J., 56:273-277.
Gates, D. M., 1968, Transpiration and leaf temperature, A. Rev. Pl. Physiol., 19:211-238.
Gee, G. W., and Federer, C. A., 1972, Stomatal resistance during senescence of hardwood leaves, Water Resour. Res., 8:1456-1460.
Gindel, I., 1969, Stomatal constellation in the leaves of cotton, maize and wheat plants as a function of soil moisture environment, Physiologia Pl., 22:1143-1151.
Glinka, Z., and Katchansky, M. Y., 1970, The effect of water potential on the CO_2-compensation point of maize and sunflower leaf tissue, Isr. J. Bot., 19:533-541.

Goode, J. E., and Higgs, K. H., 1973, Water, osmotic, and pressure potential relationships in apple leaves, J. Hort. Sci., 48: 203-215.
Green, P. B., and Cummins, W. R., 1974, Growth rate and turgor pressure. Auxin effect studies with an automated apparatus for single coleoptiles, Pl. Physiol., 54:863-869.
Green, P. B., Erickson, R. O., and Buggy, J., 1971, Metabolic and physical control of cell elongation rate. In vivo studies with Nitella, Pl. Physiol., 47:423-430.
Greenway, H., Hughes, P. G., and Klepper, B., 1969, Effects of water deficit on phosphorus nutrition in tomato plants, Physiologia Pl., 22:199-207.
Hackett, C., 1968, A study of the root system of barley. I. Effects of nutrition on two varieties, New Phytol., 67:287-300.
Heath, O. V. S., and Gregory, F. G., 1938, The constancy of the mean assimilation rate and its ecological importance, Ann. Bot., 2:25-36.
Heath, O. V. S., and Meidner, H., 1961, The influence of water strain on the minimum intercellular space, CO_2 concentration, Γ, and stomatal movements in wheat leaves, J. Exp. Bot., 12: 226-242.
Henckel, P. A., 1964, Physiology of plants under drought, A. Rev. Pl. Physiol., 15:363-386.
Henzell, R. G., McCree, K. J., van Bavel, C. H. M., and Schertz, K. P., 1975, Method for screening sorghum genotypes for stomatal sensitivity to water deficits, Crop Sci., 15:516-518.
Henzell, R. G., McCree, K. J., van Bavel, C. H. M., and Schertz, K. P., 1976, Sorghum genotype variation in stomatal sensitivity to leaf water deficits, Crop Sci., 16:660-662.
Hoffman, G. R., and Gates, D. M., 1971, Transpirational water loss and energy budgets of selected plant species, Oecol. Plant., 6:115-131.
Hopkinson, J. M., 1968, Effects of early drought and transplanting on the subsequent development of the tobacco plant, Aust. J. Agric. Res., 19:47-57.
Hsiao, T. C., 1973, Plant responses to water stress, A. Rev. Pl. Physiol., 24:519-570.
Hsiao, T. C., and Acevedo, E., 1974, Plant responses of water deficits, water use efficiency and drought resistance, Agric. Meteorol., 14:59-84.
Hsiao, T. C., Acevedo, E., Fereres, E., and Henderson, D. W., 1976, Water stress, growth and osmotic adjustment, Phil. Trans. R. Soc. Lond. B, 273:479-500.
Hurd, E. A., 1968, Growth of roots of seven varieties of spring wheat at high and low moisture levels, Agron. J., 60:201-205.
Hurd, E. A., 1976, Plant breeding for drought resistance, in: "Water Deficits and Plant Growth," T. T. Kozlowski, ed., Vol. IV, Academic Press, New York, San Francisco, London.
Husain, I., and Aspinall, D., 1970, Water stress and apical morphogenesis in barley, Ann. Bot., 34:393-407.

Idso, S. B., and Baker, D. G., 1967, Relative importance of reradiation, convection and transpiration in heat transfer from plants, Pl. Physiol., 42:631-640.
Ishag, H. M. H., 1969, Physiology of seed yield in Vicia faba L., Ph.D. Thesis, Univ. of Reading, England.
Itai, C., and Vaadia, Y., 1971, Cytokinin activity in water stressed plants, Pl. Physiol., 47:87-90.
Izhar, S., and Wallace, D. A., 1967, Studies of the physiological basis for yield differences. III. Genetic variation in photosynthetic efficiency of Phaseolus vulgaris L., Crop Sci., 7:457-460.
Jenne, E. A., Rhoades, H. F., Yien, C. H., and Howe, O. W., 1958, Change in nutrient element accumulation by corn with depletion of soil moisture, Agron. J., 50:71-74.
Jewitt, T. N., 1966, Soils of arid lands, in: "Arid Lands: A Geographical Appraisal," E. S. Hall, ed., UNESCO, Paris.
Jones, H. G., 1973, Moderate-term water stresses and associated changes in some photosynthetic parameters in cotton, New Phytol., 72:1095-1105.
Jones, H. G., 1976, Crop characteristics and the ratio between assimilation and transpiration, J. Appl. Ecol., 13:605-622.
Jones, R. J., and Mansfield, T. A., 1970, Suppression of stomatal opening in leaves treated with abscisic acid, J. Exp. Bot., 21:714-719.
Jones, R. J., and Mansfield, T. A., 1972, Effects of abscisic acid and its esters on stomatal aperture and the transpiration ratio, Physiologia Pl., 26:321-327.
Jordan, W. R., Morgan, P. W., and Davenport, T. L., 1972, Water stress enhances ethylene-mediated leaf abscission in cotton, Pl. Physiol., 50:756-758.
Jordan, W. R., and Ritchie, J. T., 1971, Influence of soil water stress on evaporation, root absorption and internal water status of cotton, Pl. Physiol., 48:783-788.
Kamp, H., 1930, Untersuchungen über Kutikularbau und Kutikulare Transpiration von Blättern, Jb. Wiss. Bot., 72:403-465.
Kanemasu, E. T., and Tanner, C. B., 1969, Stomatal diffusion resistance of snap beans. I. Influence of leaf water potential, Pl. Physiol., 44:1542-1552.
Karamanos, A. J., 1976, An analysis of the effect of water stress on leaf area growth in Vicia faba L. in the field, Ph.D. Thesis, Univ. of Reading, England.
Karamanos, A. J., 1978a, Water stress and leaf growth of field beans (Vicia faba L.) in the field: Leaf number and total leaf area, Ann. Bot., 42 (in press).
Karamanos, A. J., 1978b, Understanding the origin of the responses of plants to water stress by means of an equilibrium model, Praktika Acad. Athens, 53 (in press).
Kassam, A. H., and Elston, J. F., 1976, Changes with age in the status of water and tissue characteristics in individual leaves of Vicia faba L., Ann. Bot., 40:669-679.

Kaul, R., 1974, Potential net photosynthesis in flag leaves of severely drought-stressed wheat cultivars and its relationship to grain yield, Can. J. Pl. Sci., 54:811-815.
Keck, R. W., and Boyer, J. S., 1974, Chloroplast response to low leaf water potentials. III. Differing inhibition of electron transport and photophosphorylation, Pl. Physiol., 53:474-479.
Keller, T., 1966, Über den Einfluss von transpirationhemmenden Chemikalien (Antitranspirantien) auf Transpiration, CO_2-Aufnahme und Wurzel, Forstw. Cbl., 85:65-79.
Keller, W., and Black, A. T., 1968, Preplanting treatment to hasten germination and emergence of grass seed, J. Range Management, 21:213-216.
Kleinendorst, A., 1975, An explosion of leaf growth after stress conditions, Neth. J. Agric. Sci., 23:139-144.
Knoerr, K. R., and Gay, L. W., 1965, The leaf energy balance, Ecology, 46:17-24.
Kozlowski, T. T., 1972, Shrinking and swelling of plant tissues, in: "Water Deficits and Plant Growth," T. T. Kozlowski, ed., Vol. III, Academic Press, New York and London.
Kozlowski, T. T., 1976, Water supply and leaf shedding, in: "Water Deficits and Plant Growth," T. T. Kozlowski, ed., Vol. IV, Academic Press, New York, San Francisco, London.
Kozlowski, T. T., and Clausen, J. J., 1970, Effect of decenylsuccinic acid on needle moisture content and shoot growth of Pinus resinosa, Can. J. Pl. Sci., 50:355.
Kramer, P. J., 1969, "Plant and Soil Water Relationships. A Modern Synthesis," McGraw-Hill, New York.
Kurkova, E. B., 1975, Structural changes in the chloroplasts in connection with changes in the rate of photosynthesis as a result of dehydration of the leaf, Soviet Pl. Physiol., 22: 981-986.
Kurkova, E. B., and Motorina, M. V., 1974, Chloroplast ultrastructure and photosynthesis at different rates of dehydration, Soviet Pl. Physiol., 21:28-31.
Lawlor, D. W., 1976, Water stress induced changes in photosynthesis, photorespiration, respiration and CO_2 compensation concentration in wheat, Photosynthetica, 10:378-387.
Lawlor, D. W., and Milford, G. F. J., 1973, The effect of sodium on growth of water stressed sugar beet, Ann. Bot., 37:597-604.
Levitt, J., 1956, "The Hardiness of Plants," Academic Press, New York.
Levitt, J., 1972, "Responses of Plants to Environmental Stresses," Academic Press, New York and London.
Livné, A., and Vaadia, Y., 1965, Stimulation of transpiration rate in barley leaves by kinetin and gibberellic acid, Physiologia Plant., 28:658-664.
Lockhart, J. A., 1965, An analysis of irreversible plant cell elongation, J. Theor. Biol., 8:264-276.
Ludlow, M. M., and Ng, T. T., 1976, Effect of water deficit on CO_2-exchange and leaf elongation rate of Panicum maximum v. trichoglume, Aust. J. Pl. Physiol., 3:401-414.

McCree, K. J., 1974, Changes in the stomatal response characteristics of grain sorghum produced by water stress during growth, Crop Sci., 14:273-278.
McCree, K. J., and Davis, S. D., 1974, Effect of water stress and temperature on leaf size and on size and number of epidermal cells in grain sorghum, Crop Sci., 14:751-755.
McMichael, B. L., Jordan, W. R., and Powell, R. D., 1972, An effect of water stress on ethylene production by intact cotton petioles, Pl. Physiol., 49:658-660.
Mansfield, T. A., 1976, Chemical control of stomatal movements, Phil. Trans. R. Soc. Lond. B, 273:541-550.
Mansfield, T. A., and Jones, R. J., 1971, Effects of abscisic acid on potassium uptake and starch content of stomatal guard cells, Planta, 101:147-158.
Marais, J. N., and Wiersma, D., 1975, Phosphorus uptake by soybeans as influenced by moisture stress in the fertilized zone, Agron. J., 67:777-781.
Marc, J., and Palmer, J. H., 1976, Relationship between water potential and leaf and inflorescence initiation in Helianthus annuus, Physiologia Pl., 36:101-104.
Martin, E. V., 1940, Effect of soil moisture on growth and transpiration in Helianthus annuus., Pl. Physiol., 15:449-466.
Maximov, N. A., 1929, in: "The Plant in Relation to Water," R. H. Yapp, ed., Allen and Unwin, London.
Mederski, H. J., and Wilson, J. H., 1960, Relation of soil moisture to ion absorption by corn plants, Soil Sci. Soc. Am. Proc., 24: 149-152.
Meidner, H., 1967, Further observations on the minimum intercellular space CO_2 concentration (Γ) of maize leaves and the postulated roles of photorespiration and glycolate metabolism, J. Exp. Bot., 17:177-186.
Meyer, R. F., and Boyer, J. S., 1972, Sensitivity of cell division and cell elongation to low water potentials in soybean hypocotyls, Planta, 108:77-87.
Milford, G. F. J., and Lawlor, D. W., 1975, Effects of varying air and soil moisture on the water relations and growth of sugar beet, Ann. Appl. Biol., 80:93-102.
Millar, A. A., Gardner, W. R., and Goltz, S. M., 1971, Internal water status and water transport in seed onion plants, Agron. J., 63:770-784.
Milthorpe, F. L., 1945, Fibre development of flax in relation to water supply and light intensity, Ann. Bot., 9:31-53.
Milthorpe, F. L., and Moorby, J., 1974, "An Introduction to Crop Physiology," Cambridge Univ. Press, London.
Milthorpe, F. L., and Newton, P., 1963, Studies on the expansion of leaf surface. III. The influence of radiation on cell division and leaf expansion, J. Exp. Bot., 14:483-495.
Miskin, K. E., and Rasmusson, D. C., 1970, Frequency and distribution of stomata in barley, Crop Sci., 10:575-578.
Miskin, K. E., Rasmusson, D. C., and Moss, D. N., 1972, Inheritance

and physiological effects of stomatal frequency in barley, Crop Sci., 12:780-783.
Mizrahi, Y., Blumenfeld, A., and Richmond, A., 1970, Abscisic acid and transpiration in leaves in relation to osmotic root stress, Pl. Physiol., 46:169-171.
Mizrahi, Y., Scherings, S. G., Malis Arad, S., and Richmond, A., 1974, Aspects of the effects of ABA on the water status of barley and wheat seedlings, Physiologia Pl., 31:44-50.
Moreshet, S., Koller, D., and Stanhill, G., 1968, The partitioning of resistances to gaseous diffusion in the leaf epidermis and the boundary layer, Ann. Bot., 32:695-702.
Moreshet, S., Stanhill, G., and Fuchs, M., 1977, Effect of increasing foliage reflectance on the CO_2 uptake and transpiration resistance of a grain sorghum crop, Agron. J., 69:246-250.
Morgan, J. M., 1977, Differences in osmoregulation between wheat genotypes, Nature, 270:234-235.
Morton, A. G., and Watson, D. J., 1948, A physiological study of leaf growth, Ann. Bot., 12:281-310.
Moss, D. N., Musgrave, R. B., and Lemon, E. R., 1961, Photosynthesis under field conditions. III. Some effects of light, CO_2, temperature and soil moisture on photosynthesis, respiration and transpiration of corn, Crop Sci., 1:83.
Newman, E. I., and Kramer, P. J., 1966, Effect of decenylsuccinic acid on the permeability and growth of bean roots, Pl. Physiol., 41:606-609.
Nicholls, P. B., and May, L. H., 1963, Studies on the growth of the barley apex. I. Interrelationships between primordium formation, apex length, and spikelet development, Aust. J. Biol. Sci., 16:561-571.
Nir, I., and Poljakoff-Mayber, A., 1967, Effect of water stress on the photochemical activity of chloroplasts, Nature, 213:418-419.
Oppenheimer, H. R., 1961, L' adaptation á la secheresse: la xerophytisme, in: "Exchanges Hydriques des Plantes en Milieu Aride ou Semiaride," F. E. Eckardt, ed., Rechérche sur la Zone Aride, Vol. 15, UNESCO, Paris.
Pallas, J. E., 1970, Theoretical aspects of CO_2 enrichment, Trans. Am. Soc. Agr. Eng., 13:240.
Parker, J., 1968, Drought resistance mechanisms, in: "Water Deficits and Plant Growth," T. E. Kozlowski, ed., Vol. I, Academic Press, New York and London.
Penfound, W. T., 1931, Plant anatomy as conditioned by light intensity and soil moisture, Am. J. Bot., 18:558-572.
Pfeffer, W., 1877, "Osmotische Untersuchungen," W. Engelmann, Leipzig.
Pfeffer, W., 1900, "The Physiology of Plants," Vol. 1, Oxford Univ. Press, London and New York (English translation).
Plaut, Z., 1971, Inhibition of photosynthetic CO_2-fixation in isolated spinach chloroplasts exposed to reduced osmotic potentials, Pl. Physiol., 48:591-595.
Plaut, Z., and Bravdo, B., 1973, Response of CO_2 to water stress, Pl. Physiol., 52:28-32.

Poljakoff-Mayber, A., and Gale, J., 1972, Physiological basis and practical problems of reducing transpiration, in: "Water Deficits and Plant Growth," T. T. Kozlowski, ed., Vol. III, Academic Press, New York and London.

Rajaratnam, N., 1969, Density studies in field beans, Ph.D. Thesis, Univ. of Reading, England.

Raper, C. O., and Barber, S. A., 1970, Rooting systems of soybeans. I. Differences in root morphology among varieties, Agron. J., 62:581-584.

Raschke, K., 1960, Heat transfer between the plant and the environment, A. Rev. Pl. Physiol., 11:111-126.

Raschke, K., 1974, Simultaneous requirement of ABA and CO_2 for the modulation of stomatal conductance in *Xanthium strumarium*, Pl. Physiol., 53:S 55.

Raschke, K., 1976, How stomata resolve the dilemma of opposing priorities, Phil. Trans. R. Soc. Lond. B, 273:551-560.

Reichmann, G. A., Crunes, D. L., and Viets, F. G., Jr., 1966, Effects of soil moisture on ammonification and nitrification in two Northern Plains soils, Soil Sci. Soc. Am. Proc., 30: 363-366.

Richards, F. J., 1959, A flexible growth function for empirical use, J. Exp. Bot., 10:290-300.

Richards, L. A., and Wadleigh, C. H., 1952, Soil water and plant growth, in: "Soil Physical Conditions and Plant Growth," B. T. Shaw, ed., Academic Press, New York.

Roberts, B. R., 1964, Effect of water stress on the translocation of photosynthetically assimilated ^{14}C in yellow poplar, in: "The Formation of Wood in Forest Trees," M. H. Zimmerman, ed., Academic Press, New York.

Salim, M. H., and Todd, G. W., 1968, Seed soaking as a pre-sowing drought hardening treatment in wheat and barley seedlings, Agron. J., 60:179-182.

Santarius, K. A., and Heber, U., 1967, Das Verhalten von Hill-Reaktion und Photophosphorylierung isolierter Chloroplasten in abhängigkeit vom Wassergehalt. I. Wasserentzug mittels konzentrierter Lösungen, Planta, 73:91-108.

Schneider, W. G., and Childers, N. F., 1941, Influence of soil moisture on photosynthesis, respiration and transpiration of apple leaves, Pl. Physiol., 16:565-583.

Scott-Russell, R., 1977, "Plant Root Systems: Their Function and Interaction with the Soil," McGraw-Hill, London.

Scott-Russell, R., and Barber, D. A., 1960, The relationship between salt uptake and the absorption of water by intact plants, A. Rev. Pl. Physiol., 11:127-140.

Seginer, I., 1969, The effect of albedo on the evapotranspiration rate, Agric. Meteorol., 6:5-10.

Shearman, R. C., and Beard, J. B., 1972, Stomatal density and distribution in *Agrostis* as influenced by species, cultivar and leaf blade surface and position, Crop Sci., 12:822-823.

Shimshi, D., 1963, Effect of soil moisture and phenylmercuric acetate upon stomatal aperture, transpiration and photosynthesis, Pl. Physiol., 38:713-721.
Simmelsgaard, S. E., 1976, Adaptation to water stress in wheat, Physiologia Pl., 37:167-174.
Skoss, J. D., 1955, Structure and composition of plant cuticle in relation to environmental factors and permeability, Bot. Gaz., 117:55-72.
Slatyer, R. O., 1967, "Plant Water Relationships," Academic Press, London and New York.
Slatyer, R. O., 1969, Physiological significance of internal water relations in crop yield, in: "Physiological Aspects of Crop Yield," J. D. Eastin et al., eds., American Society of Agronomy, Madison, Wisconsin.
Slatyer, R. O., 1973, The effect of internal water status on plant growth, development and yield, in: "Plant Response to Climatic Factors," R. O. Slatyer, ed., Uppsala Symp. Proc., UNESCO, Paris.
Slatyer, R. O., and Bierhuizen, J. F., 1964, The influence of several transpiration suppressants on transpiration, photosynthesis and water-use efficiency of cotton leaves, Aust. J. Biol. Sci., 17:131-146.
Slavik, B., 1958, The influence of water deficit on transpiration, Physiologia Pl., 11:524-536.
Spencer, J. T., 1940, A comparative study of the seasonal root development of some inbred lines and hybrids of maize, J. Agric. Res., 61:521-538.
Squire, G. R., and Jones, M. B., 1971, Studies on the mechanism of action of the antitranspirant phenylmercuric acetate and its penetration into the mesophyll, J. Exp. Bot., 22:980-991.
Stanhill, G., 1957, The effect of difference in soil moisture status on plant growth: A review and analysis of soil moisture regime experiments, Soil Sci., 84:205-214.
Stanhill, G., Moreshet, S., and Fuchs, M., 1976, Effect of increasing foliage and soil reflectivity on the yield and water use efficiency of grain sorghum, Agron. J., 68:329-332.
Stocker, O., 1960, Physiological and morphological changes in plants due to water deficiency, in: "Plant Water Relationships in Arid and Semiarid Conditions," UNESCO, Paris.
Sunderland, N., 1960, Cell division and expansion in the growth of the leaf, J. Exp. Bot., 11:68-80.
Thorne, G. N., 1966, Physiological aspects of grain yield in cereals, in: "The Growth of Cereals and Grasses," F. L. Milthorpe and J. D. Ivins, eds., Butterworths, London.
Thorntwaite, C. W., and Mather, J. R., 1954, Climate in relation to crops, Am. Met. Soc. Meteorological Monographs, 2:1-10.
Todd, G. W., 1972, Water deficits and enzymatic activity, in: "Water Deficits and Plant Growth," T. T. Kozlowski, ed., Vol. III, Academic Press, New York and London.

Troughton, A., and Whittington, W. J., 1969, The significance of genetic variation in root systems, in: "Root Growth," W. J. Whittington, ed., Butterworths, London.
Troughton, J. H., 1969, Plant water status and CO_2-exchange of cotton leaves, Aust. J. Biol. Sci., 22:289-302.
Troughton, J. H., and Slatyer, R. O., 1969, Plant water status, leaf temperature and the calculated mesophyll resistance to CO_2 of cotton leaves, Aust. J. Biol. Sci., 22:815-828.
Turner, N. C., and Begg, J. E., 1973, Stomatal behaviour and water status of maize, sorghum and tobacco under field conditions. I. At high soil water potential, Pl. Physiol., 51:31-36.
Vieira da Silva, J., Naylor, A. W., and Kramer, P. J., 1974, Some ultrastructural and enzymatic effects of water stress in cotton (Gossypium hirsutum L.) leaves, Proc. Natl. Acad. Sci. USA, 71:3243-3247.
Viets, F. G., Jr., 1972, Water deficits and nutrient availability, in: "Water Deficits and Plant Growth," T. T. Kozlowski, ed., Vol. III, Academic Press, New York and London.
Waggoner, P. E., 1966, Decreasing transpiration and the effect upon growth, in: "Plant Environment and Efficient Water Use," W. H. Pierre et al., eds., American Society of Agronomy, Madison, Wisconsin.
Waisel, Y., Borger, G. A., and Kozlowski, T. T., 1969, Effects of PMA on stomatal movements and transpiration of excised Betula papyrifera Marsh. leaves, Pl. Physiol., 44:685-690.
Wallace, D. H., and Munger, H. M., 1966, Studies of the physiological basis for yield differences, Crop Sci., 6:503-507.
Wardlaw, I. F., 1967, The effect of water stress on translocation in relation to photosynthesis and growth. I. Effect during grain development in wheat, Aust. J. Biol. Sci., 20:25-36.
Wardlaw, I. F., 1969, The effect of water stress on translocation in relation to photosynthesis and growth. II. Effect during leaf development in Lolium temulentum, Aust. J. Biol. Sci., 22:1-16.
Watson, D. J., 1947, Comparative physiological studies on the growth of field crops. I. Variation in net assimilation rate and leaf area between species and varieties and within and between years, Ann. Bot., 11:41-76.
Wesselius, J. C., and Brouwer, R., 1972, Influence of water stress on photosynthesis, respiration and growth of Zea mays L., Meded. Landbouwhogesch. Wageningen, 72:1-15.
Wiebe, H. H., and Wihrheim, S. E., 1962, The influence of internal moisture deficit on translocation, Pl. Physiol., 37:1-11.
Wilson, G. L., 1966, Studies on the expansion of the leaf surface. V. Cell division and expansion in a developing leaf as influenced by light and upper leaves, J. Exp. Bot., 17:440-451.
Wittwer, S. H., 1978, The next generation of agricultural research, Science, 199:1.
Wittwer, S. H., and Robb, W., 1964, Carbon dioxide enrichment of greenhouse atmospheres for crop production, Econ. Bot., 18:34-56.

Woolley, J. T., 1967, Relative permeabilities of plastic films to water and carbon dioxide, Pl. Physiol., 42:641-643.
Wright, S. T. C., and Hiron, R. W. P., 1969, (+) - ABA. The growth inhibitor induced in detached wheat leaves by a period of wilting, Nature, 224:719-720.
Yoshida, S., 1972, Physiological aspects of grain yield, A. Rev. Pl. Physiol., 23:437-464.
Zabadal, T. J., 1974, A water potential threshold for the increase of ABA in leaves, Pl. Physiol., 53:125-127.
Zelitch, I., 1964, Reduction of transpiration of leaves through stomatal closure induced by alkenylsuccinic acids, Science, 143:692-693.
Zelitch, I., and Waggoner, P. E., 1962, Effect of chemical control of stomata on transpiration and photosynthesis, Proc. Natl. Acad. Sci. USA, 48:1101-1108.
Zobel, R. W., 1975, The genetics of root development, in: "The Development and Function of Roots," J. G. Torrey and D. C. Clarkson, eds., Academic Press, London and New York.

24

WATER STRESS AND ITS IMPLICATIONS (IRRIGATION) IN THE FUTURE OF AGRICULTURE

Osman Tekinel

University of Cukurova
Adana, Turkey

INTRODUCTION

The demand for agricultural production is getting larger everyday with the increasing population of the world. Therefore, it is our responsibility as plant physiologists, crop and soil scientists, and agricultural engineers to create an environment for plants that will result in the maximum production from the available land and water resources.

One of the basic ingredients of plant production is the availability of water. Plants use enormous amounts of water during their lifetime. A single mature plant weighing 1 kg excluding roots may contain 8 kg water. The same plant may have transpired 50 kg of water during its growing period. Studies have revealed that to produce 1 kg of dry grain requires roughly 1 ton of water, and 2 tons of water are needed to yield 1 kg of dry timber. In order to obtain maximum production, required amounts of water must be supplied to plants either naturally (i.e., by precipitation) or artificially (i.e., by irrigation), or a combination of the two.

Although the earth is known as the planet of water, freshwater supplies for domestic and agricultural use are extremely limited. Eagleson (1970) indicates that about 97% of the earth's total water resources is contained in oceans, 2% is frozen in icecaps, and .31% is in storage as deep groundwater. Approximately .37% of the remainder, which is on the order of 4.12 cubic million kms, has a potential of being used by man as the "fresh" water resource. This includes water of freshwater lakes, stream channels, shallow groundwater, soil moisture, and atmospheric moisture. Precipitation is the only source which replenishes the depleted freshwater supplies within the dynamic nature of the hydrologic cycle.

According to Budyko et al. (1962), global annual average precipitation over land area of the earth is 72 cm. Forty-one cm of this amount (i.e., 57%) is lost back to the atmosphere by evaporation and transpiration. The remainder, 31 cm of water, may replenish the freshwater supplies or reach to oceans or may be retained in plants. This percentage varies locally and seasonally. Although some parts of the world get sufficient precipitation for plant consumption during the growing season, most parts do not receive enough water. In these regions, water deficiency becomes a limiting factor for plant growth, and the water needs of plants should be fulfilled artificially for optimum production. This is where irrigation and engineering are required to provide the necessary water to plants. Therefore, irrigation and drainage engineers must know the atmospheric and soil environment of plants and understand the development and significance of water stress in plant production.

THE DEVELOPMENT AND SIGNIFICANCE OF WATER STRESS

In order to understand the development and significance of water stress in plant production, one should review the factors controlling plant production, the environment and growth process of a plant, and the mechanism of water transfer through the soil-plant-atmosphere continuum.

Factors Controlling Plant Production

A study of plant physiology shows that plants are extremely complex organisms as are all forms of life. The growth and productivity of plants, therefore, depend on a great variety of factors. None of the factors can be ignored because production is limited by the weakest link in the chain of variables controlling growth.

Among the variables most often limiting production are:

(1) supply of H_2O in the root environment,
(2) supply of O_2 in the root environment,
(3) supply of various minerals in the root environment,
(4) other chemical factors of the root environment,
(5) competing and parasitic organisms,
(6) genetic properties of plants,
(7) temperature,
(8) radiant energy.

Of the variables listed, all are within the control of man except that the last two usually cannot be controlled economically for large scale agricultural production.

Plant Environments and Growth Process

As we all know, a plant is made of three main components, leaves, stem, and roots. Living leaves contain a variety of cells and membranes in which complex biological processes such as photosynthesis, respiration, and transpiration take place. The stem provides a connection between the leaves and the root system for the transportation of water, nutrients, and carbohydrates. The roots of a plant grow downward into the soil and serve to anchor the plant as well as absorb water and nutrients from the soil. The three parts are interrelated into a complex organization with control over one another as shown in Fig. 1.

Plant growth is a function of the two major energy converting processes, photosynthesis and respiration. The energy input to the plant system is the light energy absorbed by the chlorophyll and utilized in the photosynthetic process. Hence, the rate of photosynthesis is a function of the light intensity, temperature, and the availability of carbon dioxide and water supply. Carbohydrates are produced as a result of the photosynthetic process. Part of the carbohydrates are used during respiration, which is essentially the reverse process of photosynthesis. The constituents required for respiration are oxidizable carbohydrates and oxygen. Carbohydrates are transformed through the respiration process into an appropriate form for use in assimilation, which is interrelated with the translocation of carbohydrates and the availability of oxygen.

The Soil Environment

Water, minerals, and free oxygen must enter the plants through the roots. The supply of these depends on:

(1) The volume of soil occupied by roots and
(2) the concentration of supplies in the soil.

These two factors, however, are interrelated because the penetration of roots into soil material depends on a suitable soil environment. Requirements for a suitable soil environment are:

(1) A soil solution of favorable chemical composition (e.g., not too high a concentration of solutes, which cause plasmolysis, a favorable pH range, say 5.5-7.5, and an absence of other toxic substances).

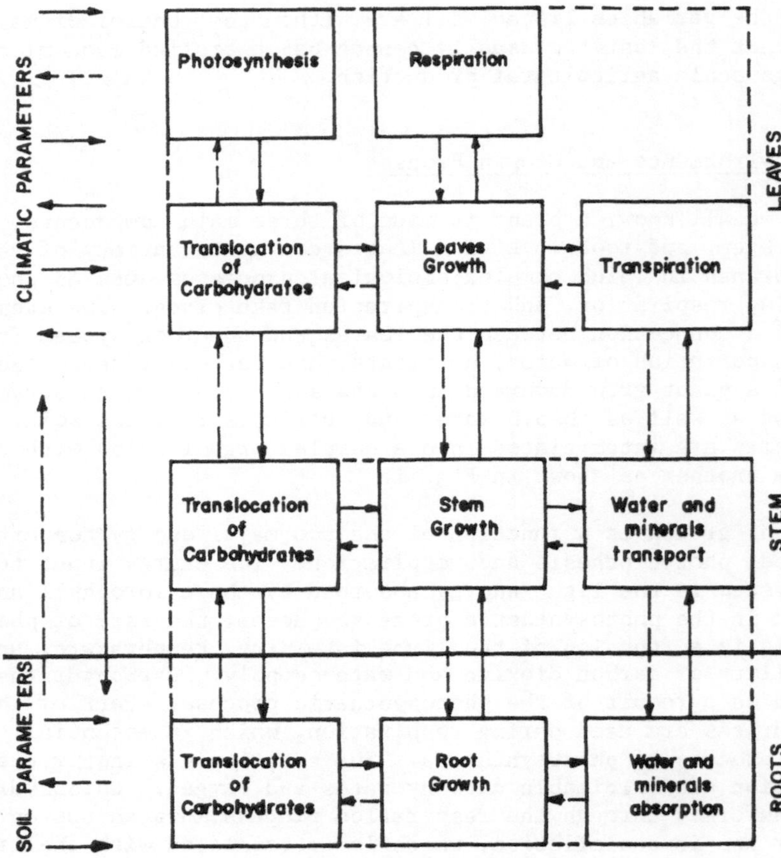

Fig. 1. Block diagram of soil-plant-atmosphere system.

(2) Presence of O_2 and not too much CO_2. Oxygen must diffuse from the atmosphere. This requires a continuous network of air-filled pores either through the soil or through plant tissues.

(3) A soil mechanically suitable for root penetration.

Water Transfer Through the Soil-Plant-Atmosphere Continuum

In nature, plant leaves lose water vapor to the air when their stomates are open to admit sufficient carbon dioxide for photosynthesis. This process is called transpiration. The rate of transpiration is proportional to the difference between the water potential inside and outside the leaf as well as to degree of stomatal opening. The stomatal openings are controlled by guard cells which are sensitive to environmental parameters such as sunlight and operate in response to turgor pressure of the cells. Sunlight not only affects stomatal opening, but also exerts strong physical effects on the transpiration rate. This combined influence of sunlight causes daily fluctuations in the rate of transpiration. The water loss from leaf cells will be absorbed from the xylem of the leaves. The removal of water reduces the water potential of xylem. Thus, a potential gradient will exist between the leaf and root xylem--to transfer water from the root system to the leaves of the plant. The amount of water transferred has to be provided by the absorbtion of water from the soil.

Gardner (1960) and Cowan (1965) reported that the rate of water flow toward the root surface is controlled by the hydraulic conductivities of the soil, and the only water available is that occurring within a few centimeters of the root. Kilic (1973) reported that the rate of water uptake reaches to a limiting value as the potential gradient increases between soil and root xylem. Therefore, an equilibrium condition may exist between total transpiration and root surface with a minimum root potential and optimum water uptake under a normal environment.

The Development of Water Stress

As was shown in the previous section, water flow through the soil-plant system tends to occur along the gradient of decreasing water potential. This means that plant water potential has to be lower than soil water potential in order to accomplish the flow of water.

Assume that the internal gradients within the plant and soil have been eliminated by the overnight equilibration period, even though the actual levels of soil and plant water potential decline each day. In addition to the decline in plant and soil water potential due to drying of soil profile, there is also a diurnal rhythm in plant water potential caused by the relative rate of daily transpiration. At the beginning of each day transpiration initially removes water from the leaves and reduces the water potential of the leaves. Absorption commences as soon as potential gradients extend down to and across the soil-root interface, and thus a quantitative lag of absorption exists. Consequently, the magnitude of the internal water deficit continues to increase until the rate of absorption equals the rate of transpiration. The interrelationships between these two phenomena are illustrated schematically in Fig. 2. The upper curve shows the progressive decline in the water potential of the soil mass, as the soil dries due to evaporation and transpiration. The other curves show the

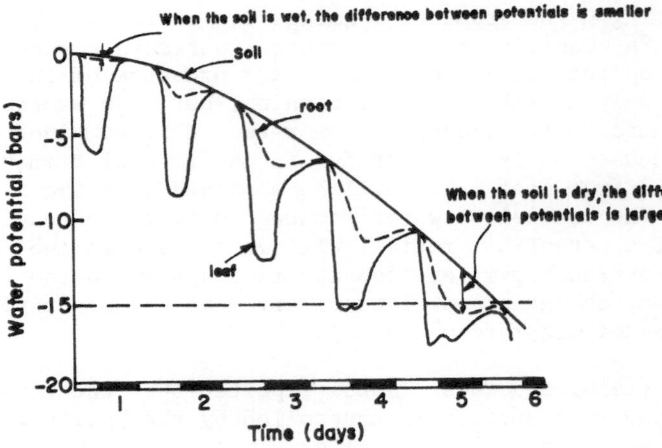

Fig. 2. Schematic representation of changes in leaf water potential (leaf), root surface water potential (root), and soil mass water potential (soil) as transpiration proceeds from a plant rooted in initially wet (root ≈ 0) soil (Slatyer, 1967).

water potential at the root surface and in the leaves by assuming that transpiration proceeds for 12 hr and then ceases for 12 hr.

When the soil is wet, the difference between the soil and root water potential is small. However, when the soil is dry, the difference between the soil and root water potential is increasing in order to maintain the water flow at the desired level. By the fourth day, water potential of leaves falls below the -15 bar line for several hours. This is the diurnal wilting which may occur, even in water culture, under the conditions of high evaporative demand. At this point, partial stomatal closure may retard the demand for water absorption. However, by the fifth day, the soil water potential has also fallen below the line of -15 bars. It is then impossible for leaf water potential to recover. The plant would be permanently wilted and recovery may be possible only with soil water recharge.

Although this is only schematic, it is of interest that actual data obtained by Gardner and Nieman (1964) and Kilic (1973) provide very good experimental confirmation. Hence, it appears that real water stress may develop in two ways. First, the partial closure of stomata take place temporarily during the daytime in order to retard the transpiration demand. This is called "midday closure" of stomata and commonly occurs under field conditions of evaporative demand. During midday closure transpiration rate is sharply reduced and turgor recovery occurs. As long as adequate soil water is available the deficits are eliminated each night. The second way is the permanent water stress which occurs when the soil is dry.

Significance of Water Stress

Water deficits interfere with plant growth and if severe cause the death of plants. The integrity of specific protein-water structure and the entire cytoplasm is essential for the continuance of most physiological processes at maximum rates. Most processes are probably not unduly suppressed by the degree of stress which exists diurnally in well-watered plants, but as soil water stress increases, key processes will become progressively inactivated.

Although any factor which affects cell metabolism must affect cell enlargement and plant growth, some effects of water deficits on plants appear to be more directly mediated by turgor pressure. The guard cell turgor directly regulates stomatal aperture which ultimately influences both transpiration and photosynthesis. Complete or partial closure can reduce both processes and so ultimately reduce growth. The stomatal closure may also increase the temperature of leaves to a damaging level. A number of workers have observed that leaf enlargement and elongation, the development of root tips, and root elongation are affected by water stress. It appears that turgor pressure does not control the rate of enlargement but direct hydration effects are operative in cell enlargement and cell division.

Two main modes of action of water deficits on photosynthesis can be recognized. In the first place, stomatal closure and reduced rates of CO_2 exchange can influence the supply of CO_2. Second, there is a direct effect of water deficits on the biochemical processes involved in photosynthesis.

As water stress is imposed, an increase in respiration rate may first be observed, followed by a reduction in rate as the plant adapts to stress. If stress is imposed gradually the first phase may not become apparent, but rather a progressive decline in respiration rate with increasing stress has been observed.

In a typical plant, growing with adequate water and nutrient supply and normal transpiration rates, only small diurnal water deficits will arise. Under these conditions, it seems probable that the only observable effects of water stress will be a reduced rate of cell division and elongation. Growth of the whole plant could usually proceed unimpeded, since both the degree and duration of the water deficit will be restricted to a few hours.

As the soil dries, however, and base level of stress is imposed by the soil water potential in addition to the superimposed diurnal lag of absorption behind transpiration, there will be an accelerated breakdown of photosynthesis, respiration, and other biological activities. Initially, there will be a tendency for suppression of metabolism to occur only during the diurnal period of maximum water deficit, but this period will retard transpiration and increase leaf temperature, and may cause a reduction in photosynthesis through its effect on CO_2 exchange. All these factors will cause a gradual falling off in growth rates.

As desiccation continues, cell division and elongation also cease and there will be a progressive loss of dry weight through continued respiration, overall growth rates becoming negative. If stress is imposed slowly, death occurs first in the older leaves, but if stress is rapid the youngest leaves with lowest potential values may die first. Root hairs also appear to die at relatively low stress levels and marked root suberization develops as desiccation proceeds. In some species the tops die out completely before the roots but in other cases there is evidence that most of the roots die before the shoots.

If the water supply is renewed before death occurs, the recovery to normal metabolic behavior appears to take several days. In many cases, recovery never appears to be complete. There is evidence that recovery is delayed first by the marked reduction in rates of water absorption caused by death of root hairs, or roots, and increased suberization of the root system which reduces the permeability of the root to water and nutrients. Brix (1962) observed that in wilted tomato plants full recovery did not occur, even though turgor was regained.

The stage of growth at which water stress occurs can exert an important influence on the final yield of some crop plants, particularly in annual cereals. With corn, for example, Robins and Domingo (1953) found that maximum yield was reduced by water stress at the tasseling stage and Denmead and Shaw (1960) found that a reduction in yield of about 50% was caused by water stress at the silking stage. For wheat and cotton, somewhat similar results have been observed. However, each crop has a different period when it exhibits pronounced sensitivity to stress. In summary, water stress appears to cause significant and progressive decrements in most processes concerned with plant growth and plant production.

IRRIGATION

Irrigation has been practiced over the world since ancient civilizations. Many countries with large arid and semiarid regions have owed their survival to the knowledge of irrigation practices throughout the centuries. Presently, much of the food production in China, Pakistan, India, Egypt, Israel, Iraq, large sections of Latin America and the Far East, and many other parts of the world depends on irrigation. The International Commission on Drainage and Irrigation indicates that an area of 201 million hectares are irrigated in 103 countries presently and this area can be expanded to 458 million hectares. Moen and Beek (1974) have given nearly the same information and have found the potentially irrigable land area for the whole world to be 470 million hectares. Continental distribution of potentially irrigable land is shown in Table 1.

The predominant irrigation method practiced over the world since the beginning of civilization involves diverting water from a source and allowing it to flow downgrade by gravity. It is astonishing that no basic change has taken place in these surface or gravity irrigation practices despite the fact that tremendous advances of civilization have taken place in the past centuries. Modern irrigation schemes currently applied in many parts of the world differ only slightly from the ancient irrigation schemes if such minor improvements as the use of concrete instead of masonry, or the introduction of sophisticated measuring devices and gates, or better canal linings, or advancements in engineering practices, are disregarded.

An ideal method of irrigation is one that applies water evenly over a field at a rate which results in no surface runoff, deep percolation, and in the meantime provides a continuous supply of water for plant consumption by making the fullest use of the available stream of water. All of this should be accomplished with a minimum investment for equipment, labor, and maintenance and a minimum wastage of land in water conveyance systems.

The Soil Environment as Influenced by Irrigation

The objectives of irrigation and drainage are to produce a root zone (as deep as practical) containing continuous air-filled pores, and, at the same time, containing a sufficient amount of available

Table 1. Distribution of Potentially Irrigable Land

Continent	Area of Irrigable Land (in millions of hectares)
South America	17.9
Australia	5.3
Africa	19.7
Asia	314.1
North America	37.1
Europe	75.9
Total	470.0

water of proper chemical composition. The above objective cannot be accomplished in a sufficient soil depth if we have either (a) not enough water or (b) too much water. Not enough water leads to the following:

(1) Water will not move into plants fast enough to keep the plant cells in a turgid condition (particularly the leaf cells). This may force the guard cells to close, thus reducing the rate at which CO_2 is trapped and thereby decreasing the rate of photosynthesis. In fact, if the soil becomes too dry, water might move out of the plant into the soil through the roots.

(2) Salt in the soil solution may become too concentrated and cause plasmolysis, in which case the plant will be desiccated.

(3) Roots will not develop in dry regions, so that when water is added plants cannot immediately make use of it and mechanical support for the plant is limited.

Too much water leads to the following:

(1) The gas phase is eliminated or at least becomes discontinuous. Oxygen will not diffuse downward from the atmosphere at a rate sufficient to supply respiration needs of the root system. Carbon dioxide and other products of metabolism will not diffuse upward as fast as they are produced by microorganisms and the plant roots. Carbon dioxide may accumulate to toxic concentrations. The rhizosphere may become anaerobic and lead to decomposition, which in turn could give rise to the production of methane and other toxic gases, aldhydes and sulfides, and other toxic substances. Certain necessary minerals may become insoluble and unavailable to plants.

(2) The water table may rise, thus greatly accelerating evaporation from the soil surface, preventing the soil from warming normally in the spring, allowing salts to accumulate at the surface, and creating unstable soil which is difficult to cultivate.

(3) Roots will not penetrate, so plants lack mechanical support and ability to gather materials, even water.

(4) Excessive leaching may remove soil minerals too fast, leading to poor fertility and also to poor physical condition.

Good agriculture, therefore, often involves both the application of water and improving the drainage of excess water from the soil profile.

When irrigation water is added, the objective is to add enough that the total water added plus precipitation and dew is slightly greater than evapotranspiration. The rate of application should not allow too much water to infiltrate below the possible root zone, nor keep the root zone too saturated for too long a period of time or produce runoff from the surface.

The frequency should be sufficient so that the root zone always contains enough water for the best growth consistent with economic considerations. The application should be as even as possible so that not too much is applied in one place nor too little in another.

It often happens, especially in irrigated regions, that water applied at the surface causes water to rise in the subsoil, forming a high water table. When this occurs, there is a need to improve the natural drainage to avoid damaging conditions. The function of subsoil drainage is, therefore, to control the water table elevation, or at least to maintain it at an elevation not dangerous for plant growth.

Water Stress in Relation to Irrigation

Intensive research has been carried out by plant physiologists, agronomists, and to some extent by engineers on soil-plant-water relations during the last forty years. Many previously unknown points concerning the movement of water deficiency effects on biochemical, morphological, and anatomical features of plants have come to light. For agronomists, as summarized by Goldberg et al. (1976), it is not important how the water is supplied to the rooting environment, just so long as the soil water content is optimal for the plant. The less the water available to the root zone, the more the plant is liable to suffer from water stress. This phenomenon may be worsened if irrigation water contains a high concentration of salts and the evaporation rate is high. A state of water stress develops when water uptake by roots is less than the amount of water demanded by transpiration. Growth is retarded even when water stress is moderate, and high yield drops are common. When water stress becomes more severe or exists for longer periods, most biochemical activities in the plant come to a halt, causing weathering and death of the plant.

There has not yet been complete agreement among scientists studying soil-plant-water relations whether there is a sharp drop in plant physiological activity at a certain point between the field capacity and the permanant wilting point. However, many authors of previously released publications on the subject indicate that the longer soil moisture is maintained at the field capacity, the more vigorous is plant growth and thus the greater the yield. These observations encouraged irrigation engineers to devise a method which can supply water to plants at any predetermined quantities and intervals with the aim of keeping the soil moisture tension around the field capacity. In recent years a new development on application of irrigation water has created widespread attention around the world. This new method of water application is known as drip or trickle irrigation. In the following sections various irrigation methods will be evaluated.

Gravity Irrigation

In the traditional gravity irrigation methods, water infiltrates the soil profile as the sheet of water advances in furrow, border, or basin. Soil moisture is increased to its full capacity by subsequent ponding and lateral movement of water. Generally less than half of the water released from a source reaches the plant under open ditch conveyance in surface irrigation methods. This low efficiency is mostly attributed to losses due to conveyance seepage, evaporation, deep percolation, inadequate land preparation, and surface runoff resulting from excess water application. In addition, this low efficiency results in the use of larger quantities of water per unit area, requirement of larger storage facilities, erosion, salinity, and waterlogging, the latter requiring costly drainage works. By the gravity method water is applied at relatively large intervals to the plant. When irrigation is completed, soil moisture reaches field capacity. At this point water stress on the plants is non-existent. However, depending upon the nature of the plants and soil and climatic conditions, water stress begins to develop shortly after the cessation of irrigation. Stress keeps increasing until the next irrigation begins. When soil moisture reaches the field capacity, stress drops to zero again. This periodic rise and decline of water stress affects the physiologic growth of the plant adversely. Consequently, yield drops are substantial.

Sprinkler Irrigation

Although traditional gravity irrigation methods are still used widely in many regions of the world, advancements in the science of hydraulics along with progress in industry have brought new ideas for irrigation and resulted in new methods of water application at the beginning of the twentieth century. One of the developments, which is considered a major breakthrough in irrigation concepts, is sprinkler irrigation. The sprinkler method is simulation of rain, with an exception that its intensity and duration can be controlled, which has great importance for plant-soil-water relations. Sprinkler irrigation has been practiced on a rather small scale for the last fifty years, but new advancements in sprinkler products have boosted usage of sprinklers all over the world recently. The sprinkler method has many advantages over conventional gravity irrigation methods. Control of water application minimizes creation of water stress between irrigation intervals and land preparation work, reduces the need for drainage, and prevents potential salinity problems. As a result, the sprinkler provides considerable water saving and increase in crop yields.

Drip Irrigation

The drip irrigation method is defined as slow, precision application of water on and under the surface of the soil through orifices placed at suitable intervals on plastic tubing. The modern concept of drip irrigation was originated in Israel during the early sixties. Experiments conducted under field conditions showed that drip irrigation is the most advantageous method under certain circumstances that are marginal for other irrigation methods. Drip irrigation has the property that water can be applied to plants in any quantities and at any interval with convenience. This means that the matric tension may not be allowed to exceed levels much beyond the field capacity, which, if expressed in terms of water stress, corresponds to 30 to 50 centibars. Such low tensions are extremely hard to achieve by any other irrigation methods simply because irrigation at such short intervals is impractical for both sprinkler and gravity irrigation since it requires a very high use of labor. Also, from the technical standpoint, it is impossible to irrigate with the conventional methods at such short intervals since such an attempt would result in consumption of large amounts of water and requirement of extraordinary drainage facilities.

A series of experiments carried out by Goldberg (1971) showed that a direct relationship exists between crop response and water stress. In one experiment comparing drip and sprinkler irrigation on response of tomatoes, cucumbers, and muskmelons to irrigation intervals, he found that, with the same amount of water given, yield increased markedly as the intervals between water applications were reduced. Further, he has shown that under desert conditions where transpiration is high and the soils coarse with low water holding capacity, daily irrigation, or even more than one irrigation per day, produced the highest yields.

In another experiment when comparing irrigation applications and yields of tomatoes, cucumbers, muskmelons, peppers, and sweet corn under drip and sprinkler irrigation methods, Goldberg observed that in all cases yields under drip irrigation far exceeded sprinkler irrigation and in some cases, yields were more than doubled despite the fact the quantities of water applied to any particular crop were identical or less for drip irrigation.

Similar phenological observations were carried out by Goldberg on pepper plants. After 110 days of growth, the rate of growth under drip irrigation was considerably greater than under sprinkler irrigation. Total number of leaves, number of plant embranchments,

Table 2. Yields of Crops with Trickle, Sprinkler, and Furrow Irrigation

Crop	Period of Growth	Irrigation Water Applied (in cm)	Yields Trickle	Sprinkler	Furrow
			(tons/hectare)		
Tomatoes	September to March	98.3	65.0	39.0	-
Cucumbers	September to December	67.1	49.0	no yield	-
Muskmelons	August to December	65.5	43.0	24.0	24.0
Peppers	September to March	141.7	9.5	4.8	-
Sweet corn	February to May	67.6	12.9	5.3	-

Table 3. Vegetative Growth of Pepper Plants After 110 Days of Growth Under Trickle and Sprinkler Irrigation (Goldberg, 1974)

Item	Trickle Irrigation	Sprinkler Irrigation	Significance Percentages
Total number of leaves	65	47	5.0
Number of plant embranchments	3	2	0.1
Plant height (cm)	30.0	16.8	0.1
Depth of tap root (cm)	21.6	15.2	1.0
Diameter of root stem (cm)	1.17	0.71	1.0

plant height, depth of tap root, and diameter of root stem were superior under drip irrigation. This accelerated rate of growth led to two important results; it led to earlier, as well as larger, yields and consequently to higher product value.

In another experiment, using waters of an area which had an electrical conductivity of 3000 micromhos/cm, and another with good quality water of an electrical conductivity of 400 micromhos/cm, Goldberg found that drip irrigation gave yields higher than for sprinkler irrigation, irrespective of the water quality. Furthermore, there was practically no difference in yields for the low and high quality water under drip irrigation. This was due to the effect of keeping soil moisture tension low with drip irrigation. Hence, the crop was able to withstand the higher osmotic tensions inherent in waters of high salinity.

Experiments comparing hand watering with drip irrigation on Gloxinia, Saintpaulia ionantha, Chrysanthemum, and Euphorbia pulcherrima resulted in bigger plants, bigger flowers, earlier flowering, and more flowers under drip irrigation except in the case of E. pulcherrima (Wolff, 1974).

Substantial research has been conducted on comparing drip irrigation with conventional and sprinkler methods using saline and nonsaline water. The crops were observed in terms of germination, growth pattern, total yield, exportable yield, early cropping, and quality of product. Publications by Cole (1971), Goldberg and Shmueli (1970, 1971), Gustafson (1972, 1973), Larkman (1971), Milligen (1973), and Viziri (1973) are among the important ones. All these publications indicate that drip irrigation surpasses the other conventional irrigation methods.

Drip irrigation is by no means the perfect irrigation method. It has its own drawbacks and problems. Problems associated with engineering design more than likely will be solved as time goes by. However, many points concerning the effects on soil-plant-water

Table 4. Tomato Yields Under Trickle and Sprinkler Irrigation with Good and Poor Quality Water (ton/hectare) (Goldberg, 1974)

Irrigation Method	High Quality Water E.C.--400 micromhos/cm	Saline Water E.C.--3000 micromhos/cm
Trickle	66.7	65.0
Sprinkler	52.0	39.2

relations are not presently known. Once questions regarding soil-plant-water relations are answered, drip irrigation probably will be modified accordingly, or a new water application method might be devised which would serve the plants better than drip irrigation.

CONCLUSION

Water stress in crops is poorly defined and poorly understood. Stress is an omnibus word. Different variables will depress the rates of different processes. Therefore, the definition and measurement of water stress is still to be determined.

Also, the development and significance of water stress at different stages of growth in various crops has remained as one of the most challenging problems of our time.

Our objective should be the development and implementation of a reasonably priced irrigation system which will produce a root zone containing air-filled pores with a sufficient amount of water and nutrients.

REFERENCES

Brix, H., 1962, The effect of water stress on the rates of photosynthesis and respiration in tomato plant and loblolly pine seedlings, Physiologia Plant., 15:10-20.

Budyko, M. I., Efimova, N. A., Zubenok, L. T., and Stronika, L. A., 1962, "The Heat Balance of the Earth's Surface," Akad. Nauk, USSR, Izv. Ser. Georgr., No. 1.

Cole, T. D., 1971, "Sub-surface and Trickle Irrigation--A Survey of Potentials and Problems," Reprint ORNL-NDIC-9, Oak Ridge National Laboratory, Oak Ridge, Tenn.

Cowan, I. R., 1965, Transport of water in the soil-plant-atmosphere system, J. Appl. Ecol., 2:221-239.

Denmead, O. T., and Shaw, R. H., 1960, The effects of soil moisture stress at different stages of growth on the development of yield of corn, Agron. J., 52:272-274.

Eagleson, P. S., 1970, "Dynamic Hydrology," McGraw-Hill, New York.

Gardner, W. R., 1960, Dynamic aspects of water availability to plants, Soil Sci., 89:63-73.

Gardner, W. R., and Nieman, R. H., 1964, Lower limit of water availability to plants, Science, 143:1460-1462.

Goldberg, D., 1971, "Modern Concepts of Irrigation," The Israel National Committee of the International Commission on Drainage and Irrigation, Rehovot, Israel.

Goldberg, D., 1974, "Techniques and Methods for Efficient Use of Water in Agriculture, Pressure Irrigation Principles and Practices," The Hebrew University, Jerusalem, Israel.

Goldberg, D., Gornat, B., and Rimon, D., 1976, "Drip Irrigation, Principles, Design, and Agricultural Practices," Drip Irrigation Scientific Publications, Kfar Shmaryahu, Israel.

Goldberg, D., and Shmueli, M., 1970, Drip Irrigation Method Used Under Arid and Desert Conditions of High Water and Soil Salinity, ASAE Trans., 13:38-41.

Goldberg, D., and Shmueli, M., 1971, The effect of distance from the tricklers on soil salinity and growth and yield of sweet corn in an arid zone, HortScience, 6:565-567.

Gustafson, C. D., ed., 1972, "Proceedings of 3rd Annual Drip Irrigation Seminar," Univ. of California.

Gustafson, C. D., ed., 1973, "Proceedings of 4th Annual Drip Irrigation Seminar," Univ. of California.

Kilic, N. K., 1973, The analysis and simulation of water transfer through the soil-root domain. Ph.D. thesis, Michigan State Univ., East Lansing.

Larkman, E., ed., 1971, "Trickle Irrigation," ICI, Australia.

Milligen, T., ed., 1973, Trickle irrigation. Special Issue, Irrigation Age, 7: No. 11.

Moen, H. J., and Beek, K. J., 1974, "Literature Study on the Potential Irrigated Acreage in the World," ILRI, Wageningen, The Netherlands.

Robins, J. S., and Domingo, C. E., 1953, Some effects of severe soil moisture deficits at specific growth stages on corn, Agron. J., 45:618-621.

Slatyer, R. O., 1967, "Plant-Water Relationships," Academic Press, London and New York.

Viziri, C. M., 1973, "Proceedings of Sub-Surface and Drip Irrigation," Univ. of Hawaii.

Wolff, P., 1974, "Use of Drip Irrigation in Germany," Proceedings of Second International Drip Irrigation Congress, San Diego, California.

25

BIOMASS, PRESENT AND FUTURE

J. Shen-Miller

National Science Foundation
Washington, D.C.

Normally agriculture means the production of food and fiber. Today's agriculture is not only the manufacturing of food and fiber, but also the production of fuel; the three F's of food, fiber, and fuel make up agriculture. I would like to discuss the potential uses of biomass as fuel. We are all aware that our natural resources are not infinite. According to one estimate (Klass, 1974), the average depletion rate of global coal, oil, and natural gas is between 50 and 150 years. In the United States the fossil fuel reserve is about 500 years (Fisher, 1974). Other energy sources, such as nuclear, geothermal, and wind, will probably be the major fuels of the future, but their development will take time. Therefore, alternate approaches are essential for supplementing the overall energy need. Tapping solar energy for fuel from biomass is just such an alternate. It is particularly reasonable in regions where the supply is high and the fuel demand is low.

The annual radiation that reaches the earth's surface is 3×10^{21} kJ, which is 10,000 times the total global energy consumption in 1970 (Hall, 1976). Green plants can fix this light energy into chemical energy by such processes as the production of cellulose, which is the most abundant organic compound on earth: 10^{11} tons of cellulose are produced annually (Hall, 1976). Cellulose is a clean fuel and is renewable. The major sources of cellulose are agriculture, forest, and aquatic production. The contribution of individual sources is seemingly minute, a fraction of a percent of the total energy demand; however adding them together could amount to 8% of the total estimated United States energy demand for year 2000, with monetary value of $48.3 billion (Shen-Miller, 1977).

The total land of the United States covers an area of 786 million hectares, of which one-fifth is used for agriculture, and one-fourth could become available for fuel farming, or the production of cellulose. This potential land, if planted with corn crops, would produce enough that the above ground residue alone would yield 10^{16} kJ of energy, which would be a supplement of 4.8% of the fuel demand for the year 2000 (Shen-Miller, 1977). Animal waste would produce another 0.15%, forest waste, 0.06%, and industrial and municipal waste, 3%. Aquatic production is not included in this estimation, but its contribution could be substantial. Ocean covers 71% of the earth's surface, and offers five to ten times more arable area than the terrestrial land. Algae can fix solar energy much more efficiently than higher plants, varying from 1-5% efficiency under poor conditions to 20-30% under ideal environment (Golueke and Oswald, 1963). The average efficiency for higher plants is only 0.3%.

By the processes of pyrolysis, hydrogasification, and anaerobic fermentation, cellulose can be converted to ethanol, methanol, hydrogen, methane and oil, or heat from direct burning (Shen-Miller, 1977). In fermentation, cellulose can first be converted to glucose via high temperature hydrolysis. Glucose can then be fermented to ethyl alcohol. In 1974, Brazil produced 9 million tons of raw sugar from sugarcane and cassava, 740 million liters of alcohol were produced from fermentation (Shen-Miller, 1977). The alcohol provided a 2% supplement to gasoline consumption. In 1978, 635 million gallons of ethanol were used either as a gasoline substitute or as a supplement. The fuel mixture, called gasohol, contains 80% gasoline and 20% alcohol (Rohter, 1978). Automotive dealers are now selling kits to convert gasoline engines to run on pure alcohol.

Anaerobic fermentation to natural gas has been known for over one hundred years, but it has not been popular. In the People's Republic of China, however, biogas production was first attempted on a wide scale in 1958, and became successful in the early 1970s. Essentially, the process consists of the conversion of insoluble organics to ones which are soluble, then to acetate, carbon dioxide, and hydrogen, and finally to methane and some carbon dioxide, all by microorganisms. Under ideal conditions the gas contains 70% methane and 30% carbon dioxide and traces of hydrogen, nitrogen, and hydrogen sulfide (Smil, 1977), with a fuel value of 36 kJ per gram. The fuel value for methane is 50 kJ per gram. In China the number of biogas digesters had reached 4.3 million in 1977, ranging in size from a few cubic meters to the communal tank size of 100 cubic meters (Anonymous, 1977). When properly managed, a 10 cubic meter digester can provide all the energy needed for cooking and lighting in the summer and fall months for a Chinese peasant family (Smil, 1977).

Closed-loop intensive agriculture in China is rather remarkable. The rice crop is intercropped with ducks and eels in flooded fields and with vegetables and fruit trees on dry banks. Blue-green algae (mostly Anabaena) are inoculated as nitrogen fertilizer in the rice paddies. Weeds from the field are collected by hand and carefully packed and transported to the barnyard as feed for livestock, or are used for biogas fermentation. Animal and human excrement, grasses, reeds, leaves, stalks, straws, vines, and city and industrial sewage are other raw materials for fermentation. A delegation of the Botanical Society of America visited an experimental marsh gas electrical power station near Canton during the summer of 1978. This station used human waste collected from a commune. A daily input of 60 cubic meters of raw material yielded 420 cubic meters of gas which was converted to 50 kW of electricity. We learned that the electricity was transmitted to the central pool in Canton. There are many problems with fermentation and much research is needed. First, there is no one microorganism that can carry out the entire process to completion. Second, control of the carbon to nitrogen ratio is essential, and the pH level is critical. Encouragingly, a recent news release announced that the State of New Jersey had pledged $20 million toward initiation of the construction of the nation's first large commercial plant for methane production from municipal garbage and sewage. The plant will use the anaerobic fermentation process for methane production (Resource Report, 1975).[1] In China, the residue from fermentation is continually removed and becomes fertilizer high in nitrogen which is returned to the land. This practice of conservation is efficient and admirable and could well be emphasized by other countries.

One consideration which must be evaluated is the expenditure of energy in the production of biomass. The green revolution aimed at high yield and overlooked the high energy input required for this yield. Fertilizer, particularly nitrogen, is one major source of energy in modern agriculture. Hence efforts to maximize yield and to minimize energy utilization will become the mission of plant biologists today. And this is the time for an all-out effort.

REFERENCES

Anonymous, 1977, "Marsh Gas Production and Utilization," Compiled by the Szechuan Province, Mian County Science 7 Technology Commission, Agriculture Publishing Co., Peking (in Chinese).

---

[1]After the completion of this article, BioScience (1978, 28: 669-670) printed news about a loan from the United States Department of Agriculture of $14 million to the Lamar Utility Board in Colorado to build the nation's largest animal waste bioconversion facility. The plant will produce 280,000 cubic meters of methane daily from 350 tons of animal waste. In Guymon, Oklahoma, the Caloric Recovery Anaerobic Process Inc. (CRAP) generates methane from feedlot waste of the area and pipes it into existing natural gas lines.

Fisher, J. C., 1974, "Energy Crisis in Perspective," John Wiley & Sons, New York.

Golueke, C. G., and Oswald, W. J., 1963, Power from solar energy: Via algal-produced methane, Solar Energy, 7:86-92.

Hall, D. O., 1976, Photobiological energy conversion, FEBS Letters, 64:6-16.

Klass, D. L., 1974, A perpetual methane economy, is it possible?, Chemtech (March):161-168.

Resource Report, 1975, New Jersey contracts for Nation's first methane plant, Energy, 3:415.

Rohter, L., 1978, Gas guzzlers becoming alcoholics in Brazil, Washington Post, August 30, A17.

Shen-Miller, J., 1977, Harvesting the sun: A biological approach, Perspectives Biology and Medicine, 21:77-88.

Smil, V., 1977, Energy solution in China, putting nature to work. Environment, 19:27-31.

26

REFLECTIONS ON C_4 PHOTOSYNTHESIS AND PLANT PRODUCTIVITY

W. M. Laetsch

Department of Botany
University of California
Berkeley, California 94720

Food and agricultural productivity have been fashionable subjects since increases in oil prices forced recognition of the relationship between energy expenditure and intensive agriculture, and several years of failure of the monsoons in Southeast Asia revealed the fragility of balances between food surplus and food deficits. A prominent theme in all discussions of increased plant productivity is the importance of increasing or preventing inhibition of photosynthetic efficiency. It is important, therefore, to examine relationships between growth regulators and photosynthesis and to place in perspective claims being made on connections between photosynthesis research and crop yields.

Plant growth regulators and their effects upon photosynthesis and chloroplast development were reviewed in the last NATO Advanced Study Institute in Izmir (Laetsch and Boasson, 1971). Very little additional information on this topic has accumulated since then. At least one exception to this somewhat discouraging scene is the work on sugarcane ripening. Dr. Vlitos (see Chapter 21) referred to the development of the chemical compound polaris, which inhibits growth of sugarcane but does not inhibit photosynthesis. This results in sucrose production in leaves and storage in the stem. Polaris is being widely used in Hawaii and can stimulate up to 10% increases in sugar yields. Thus it is economical (Nickell, 1977). Additional work on inhibiting sugarcane flowering in Hawaii with herbicides has shown promise (Nickell, 1976). The effect of this treatment is to inhibit senescence, which decreases photosynthesis and sugar storage. The control of senescence by growth regulators is a prime area of research with respect to photosynthesis, because the photosynthetic apparatus is affected very early in senescence (Goldthwaite and Laetsch, 1968; Kennedy and Laetsch, 1973). This is not surprising since ribulose diphosphate carboxylase in chloroplasts can constitute up to 50% of leaf soluble protein. In addition to its role in photosynthesis, this enzyme appears to serve an important role as a storage protein.

It is an article of faith that basic research is vital to agricultural progress and examples of this relationship are abundant in genetics, plant nutrition, and soil science. The direct benefits of fundamental research in photosynthesis are not so clear. A vigorous argument can be presented that improvements in agriculture have benefited little, if at all, from photosynthesis research. Possible exceptions are the use of CO_2 enrichment to increase plant growth and the breeding of plants with a morphology more suitable for intercepting radiation. It has been known for a very long time that CO_2 was required for photosynthesis, so CO_2 enrichment and improvements in plant architecture could easily be a product of strictly empirical research. Past studies in photosynthesis have not only failed to provide practical effects for agriculture, but the outlook for the future is not promising. It is difficult to see how a more complete understanding of photosynthetic mechanisms will result in rapid payoffs in crop yields. If we could solve the riddle of the light reaction and produce abundant hydrogen, the practical results for society would be great, but unless a major conceptual breakthrough is lurking about in well-disguised form, it is not apparent that research in this field will produce such results very soon. The paucity of practical results from photosynthesis research stands in contrast to major practical contributions resulting from basic research on growth regulators. The outlook for future contributions from the growth regulator field is also more encouraging than that for photosynthesis research. It is curious, then, that government agencies with competitive research grant programs, such as the United States Department of Agriculture, should give high priority to photosynthesis research and low priority to plant growth regulation.

It is clear that photosynthesis enjoys a good press, and a subset of photosynthesis research, C_4 photosynthesis, has had considerable publicity in recent years. Much of this attention has been engendered because of reported high growth rates of C_4 plants and their ability to fix greater amounts of CO_2 per unit time than C_3 plants. This has led to claims that C_4 plants have a higher photosynthetic efficiency than C_3 plants. The implications for agriculture were apparently clear.

Studies of C_4 photosynthesis turned a new page in the field of plant carbon metabolism, enlivening a somewhat drowsy discipline. It is not generally appreciated that the original basic research in C_4 photosynthesis was performed in laboratories of sugarcane companies and that the academic world was resistant to these new discoveries. Kortschak discovered the phenomenon in 1954 while working with the

Hawaiian Sugar Planters' Association, and his work inspired the efforts of Hatch, Slack, and others at the Colonial Sugar Refiners in Australia in the mid 1960s. I began work on sugarcane chloroplasts in the Tate & Lyle, Ltd. Agricultural Research Centre in Trinidad in 1964, and they supported subsequent work at Berkeley, as well as establishing an active program in photosynthesis research in their research center in England. The sequence of these research reports was reviewed previously (Laetsch, 1974). This scenerio is described because developments in agriculture cannot be hampered because of fake stereotypes. More of the academic world must realize that advancements in basic research can follow from mission-oriented endeavors.

As stated previously, the high growth rates of C_4 plants have caught the fancy of many plant scientists. The C_4 plants exhibit little photorespiration, and this plus structural features of leaves and high levels of PEP carboxylase in leaf cell cytoplasm means that C_4 plants are effective CO_2 trappers (Laetsch, 1974). As a result a large number of grant proposals and articles routinely cite the desirability of breeding C_4 characters into C_3 plants. It has even been suggested that C_4 plant chloroplasts be transplanted into C_3 plants (Mosaic, 1975). A frequent suggestion is to introduce nitrogen fixing genes into C_4 crops like sugarcane, corn, and sorghum (Calvin, 1976; Hardy et al., 1978). If all of this seriously proposed genetic engineering could be accomplished by the year 2000, the super plant depicted in Fig. 1 would result. This cross of maize and soybean (with a few sugarcane genes in to sweeten the stem) would have large root nodules and a single large ear to simplify harvesting. The production of "gasoline" directly from the plant has been a topic of much current interest (Calvin, 1976), and indeed alcohol is being used in Brazil as fuel for motor vehicles (da Silva et al., 1978).

The basis for the desire to make C_3 crops into C_4 crops is the CO_2 fixation rates displayed by single leaves and leaf parts of C_4 plants. Bull (1969), however, has shown that the high productivity of sugarcane is due to its long growing season and perennial habit. He stated that C_3 plants can grow just as fast when measured for particular parts of the life cycle and over short time periods. The difference between CO_2 incorporation and retention for C_4 and C_3 species at the leaf, single plant, and crop levels has been analyzed by Gifford (1974). The literature reveals that some C_3 plants grow as rapidly on a daily basis as do rapidly growing C_4 plants. This is in spite of the presumed disadvantage of having photorespiration. Gifford concludes that the higher crop yields of C_4 plants are due to duration of growth and not to differences in rate of growth. Proposals for creation of the super plant ignore the fact that C_3 and C_4 plants are adapted to specific conditions and if a hybrid could be produced, it could lose specific advantages of either or both parents. It is too often forgotten that C_4 plants do not grow

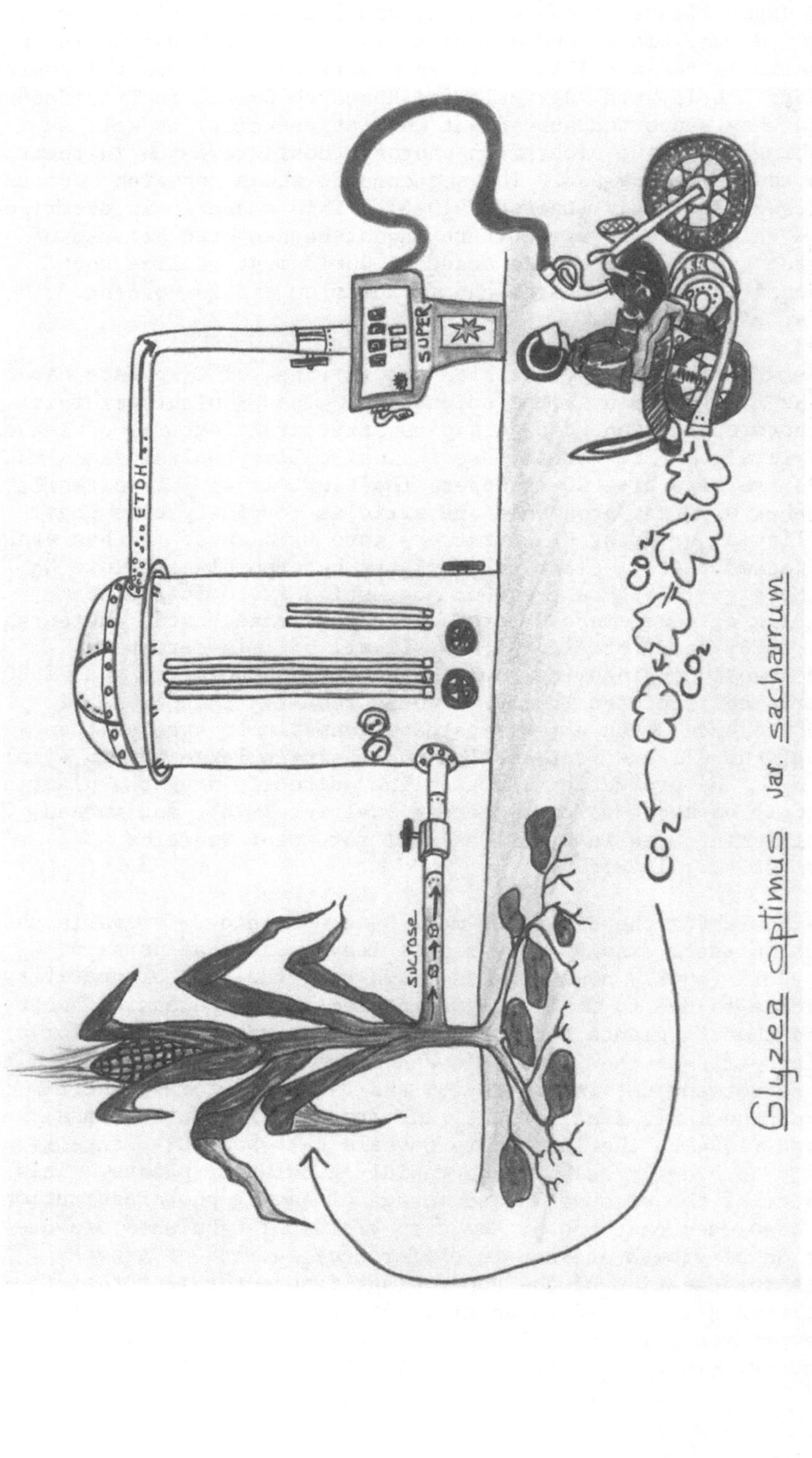

Fig. 1. A frequently proposed wonder plant for the year 2000. The potato-like clumps on the roots are nitrogen fixing nodules.

well, if at all, in cool climates with low light intensities. Many C_3 plants grow rapidly under such conditions, so why are C_3 plants often accused of having inefficient photosynthesis?

The proposal to somehow introduce genes into C_4 and other plants which would result in an ability to fix nitrogen is attractive, but it is often made on the assumption that the grain crops would continue to produce high yields. Nitrogen fixation is a high energy partitioning, this proposal assumes that the "nif" gene would photosynthate in the grain. In addition to its naiveté on resultant energy partitioning, this proposal assumes that the "n.f" gene would function independently of the extremely complex structural and functional correlates associated with root nodule initiation, development, and maintenance. It can be argued that other packages for the nitrogenase are possible, but plant evolution has provided a well-appointed laboratory for experimentation and during the many millions of years available for such experimentation only a small number of green plant taxa have evolved nitrogen fixing systems, and those with root nodules have basically similar packaging.

It has become an article of faith that photorespiration wastes energy (Zelitch, 1971; Chollet and Ogren, 1975; Bassham, 1977; Hardy et al., 1978; Ogren, 1978; Nasyrov, 1978). This light-stimulated loss of CO_2 in C_3 plants results in 30-50% loss of fixed carbon, and can be inhibited by low oxygen or high CO_2 concentrations. The C_4 plants have the cellular machinery for photorespiration, but exhibit very low rates. Enhanced CO_2 greatly stimulates growth of C_3 plants, but C_4 plant growth is also stimulated. As stated earlier, it is curious that in spite of photorespiration, some C_3 plants grow as rapidly as C_4 plants. Obviously photorespiration is but one element in the growth equation. Frankly, the multitudinous statements that photorespiration is useless and an obvious waste of energy which must be set to rights are disturbing, because they are so outrageously anthropomorphic. Providing food for people is not the driving force for plant evolution. Because our understanding of photorespiration is limited, we should not conclude that it is of no use to the plant. The major expenditure of energy represented by photorespiration must be a product of selective forces over the aeons of plant evolution. To consider it a neutral factor from the standpoint of evolution is to fly in the face of what is known about evolutionary mechanisms.

Plants have had a very long time to experiment with photorespiration, and the C_4 syndrome is one facet of such evolutionary experimentation. Most plants are not C_4 plants and no C_4 plants have originated in temperate zones. There is also evidence that plants grown under low oxygen will not complete their life cycle (Hardy, see Chapter 11). The evangelistic fervor to stamp out photorespiration is a better reflection of human hubris than it is of a general understanding of plant biology. Interventions which lead to increases in plant productivity must be based upon exhibited potential of the plants themselves.

As stated above, photosynthesis has had little effect upon agricultural practice. The same is true of C_4 photosynthesis research. Enhanced CO_2 environments have been used for many years and rapid growth rates and high water use efficiency of C_4 plants have been a part of agriculture lore and knowledge for centuries. An explanation for these and other agricultural practices has been provided by research in C_4 photosynthesis, but this knowledge has yet to provide a practical aid to the farmer.

Increased understanding of C_4 plants should lead us to exploitation of their basic adaptations. They evolved in warm regions with intermittant aridity (Laetsch, 1974) and they are xerophytes and halophytes. Rather than design the super plant of Fig. 1 for the fields of Iowa and then spread it around the world, we should use more C_4 plants for what they are basically good at and improve them for that use. This has been a longstanding practice for some C_4 plants. Sorghum is grown when it is too dry for maize, and millets are grown when it is too dry for sorghum. Unfortunately, both these crops have not received the plant breeding efforts bestowed upon maize.

Finding better uses by better plants for arid zones has to be a major goal for world agriculture, and it is here that C_4 plants can contribute. Arid zones cover one-fifth of the earth's surface and desertification is on the march around the globe. Tunisia, for example, has lost a significant amount of its arable land. Irrigation has a Faustian bargain in the form of salinization. The Punjab has lost millions of acres of irrigated land to salt and the loss continues at a high rate. Salinization is a major problem in irrigated areas of Turkey. History reveals that irrigation in arid regions has never been successful over long periods of time. Most attention has been devoted to C_4 grasses and particularly the crop grasses, sugarcane, maize, and sorghum, but many C_4 plants are successful weeds. In addition to prospering on rich cultivated soil, these weeds also grow on very dry and saline soils. Many of these weeds are also palatable for animals and humans. Why not use these characteristics to develop strains of C_4 weeds and minor crop plants for use as food and forage and in reclamation of saline soils?

Amaranthus is both a noxious weed and a food crop. The inflorescence produces a compact seed head and the seeds of *A. edulis* and other species are widely consumed in the Andes and in Southeast Asia. The seeds are rich in protein which has a high lysine content (National Academy of Sciences, 1975). *A. gangetreus* is used widely as a vegetable in India and Southeast Asia. The common name, pigweed, indicates the appeal of *Amaranthus* to livestock. *Amaranthus* is drought-resistant and grows well in saline conditions. Very little plant breeding has been done with Amaranthus and increased ploidy levels and hybridization could possibly produce spectacular increases in seed production. This genus appears ripe for development (Bourlaug, personal comm., National Academy of Sciences, 1975).

Echinochloa turnerana is another C_4 plant with potential as a food crop. It completes its life with one deep watering and bears abundant seed (National Academy of Sciences, 1975). Many C_4 plants tolerant to water stress and to salts provide excellent forage for animals. McKell (1975) has stressed the advantages of using C_4 shrubs like Atriplex, Kochia, and Suaeda for forage. The leaves are high in good quality protein and the plants produce yields similar to conventional forage crops. These shrubs also regenerate rapidly after browsing by goats and sheep, a vitally important characteristic in many regions.

The C_4 plants have the unique requirement for sodium (Brownell and Crossland, 1972) and many grow well in soils with high salinity. Portulaca oleracea, for example, shows a dry weight increase of 17% when grown in a nutrient solution with 0.05 M NaCl and it even grows in 0.1 M NaCl although it suffers a 22% decrease in dry weight (unpublished data). Portulaca is also a traditional pot herb and table green. Their tolerance of and even stimulation by salt make C_4 plants attractive candidates for reclamation of saline soils. Atriplex and Kochia have been used for this purpose in Australia, and in the Punjab Cynodon has been planted following scraping of the hardpan characteristic of saline soils in northern India. Having plants mine salts and then removing the plants for food, forage, fuel, or biomass source deserves greater consideration. Possible C_4 plant species suitable for this purpose, in addition to those mentioned, are Paspalum vaginatum, Distlichis, and Chloris gayana. Israeli workers have found that a number of C_4 grasses not generally considered to be halophytes actually grow well on high salt and actively excrete salt (Liphschitz et al., 1974). This suggests that selection of salt resistant varieties of maize, sugarcane, sorghum, and millets should be pursued. Small, two-celled salt glands are found on leaves of maize, sugarcane, and sorghum (unpublished data). Saccharum sponteneum grows abundantly on the saline soils of northern India, and it is possible that the "manufacture" of high yielding commercial varieties of maize, sugarcane, and sorghum resulted in selection against salt tolerance. Literally returning to the genetic "roots" of these crops could result in varieties which could be grown with profit on saline soils.

Many of the dicot C_4 species are members of families belonging to the Caryophyllales. This taxon has C_3, C_4, and CAM species, and it provides a natural hunting ground for species with potential in the above uses.

A primary theme of this article is to take advantage of the natural abilities of C_4 plants. The emphasis on photosynthesis and its relationship to crop yield has obscured the adaptations of C_4 plants to aridity and salinity. The C_4 plants provide greater yields for the amount of water used than most C_3 plants and this efficient use of water makes them very interesting to agriculture in arid lands. Their adaptation to aridity suggests that roots of C_4 plants and other halophytes merit further investigation. Little is known about growth regulators in halophyte roots and more information about them might have both theoretical and practical interest.

This case for the forgotten C_4 plants should not make us forget that some of them are also very good at producing biomass. Many years before that term became popular, annual reports of Tate & Lyle, Ltd. discussed the possibility that the time would come when sugarcane would be too valuable for use just for sugar production. As a year-long high speed carbon-reducing machine grown on a grand scale and with a sophisticated harvesting and transport infrastructure it possesses admirable features for a renewable source of reduced carbon. Commercial sugarcane varieties are selected to fit requirements for sugar production. As sugarcane is grown for total biomass, new varieties will be developed (or old ones brought back into cultivation) which will be more suitable for new uses. The same is true for other species with potential for large scale biomass production such as sweet sorghum, napier grass, and even maize.

My own bias concerning an area of photosynthesis research where more basic knowledge might in time lead to practical effects is the chloroplast envelope. Most work on chloroplast membranes has been devoted to chlorophyll-containing thylakoid membranes. The envelope membranes control the flow of metabolites in and out of the chloroplast and thylakoid membranes originate from the inner membrane of the envelope. In spite of the obvious significance of this membrane system, it was essentially ignored until the last few years. A number of laboratories have now isolated envelope enriched fractions and the protein and lipid composition of these fractions has been described, as well as the submembrane morphology of the inner and outer envelope membranes (Sprey and Laetsch, 1975, 1976a,b). Chloroplasts of C_4 plants have a unique structural feature which sets them apart from all chloroplasts of C_3 plants except for guard cell chloroplasts of some species (Laetsch, 1974). This peripheral reticulum is an anastamosing set of tubules contiguous with the inner membrane of the chloroplast envelope. Envelope membranes of C_4 plants have the same structure as C_3 plant chloroplasts, and the peripheral reticulum has a membrane structure identical to the inner membrane of the envelope (Sprey and Laetsch, 1978). The envelope of C_4 plant chloroplasts has now been isolated and the levels of membrane-bound, Mg^{2+}-dependent ATPase in the inner membrane and by the higher levels in C_4 plant chloroplasts. All models of C_4

photosynthesis presume a rapid interchange of metabolites between cytoplasm and chloroplasts, so it is possible that a study of this phenomenon in C_4 plant chloroplasts will lead to a better understanding of transport across the chloroplast envelopes of all plants. Since regulation of this transport is so important in photosynthesis, it is possible that ways can be found to induce changes in configurations of chloroplast envelope membranes. If the peripheral reticulum of C_4 plant chloroplasts is advantageous in terms of CO_2 fixation or maintaining chloroplast integrity during water stress, it is possible that it can be induced in C_3 plant chloroplasts. The fact that some guard cell chloroplasts have what appears to be a peripheral reticulum indicates that C_3 plants have the necessary genetic machinery.

I feel strongly that we must capitalize on what the plant can already do to some degree if we are to improve productivity. Perhaps a yet unknown growth regulator will intervene in the photosynthetic apparatus in such a manner that my gloomy predictions made earlier in this article will appear shortsighted.

ACKNOWLEDGMENT

The artist for Fig. 1 was Dr. Jenifer White of the University of California, Berkeley.

REFERENCES

Bassham, J. A., 1977, Increasing crop production through more controlled photosynthesis, Science, 197:630-638.

Brownell, P. F., and Crossland, C. J., 1972, The requirement for sodium as a micronutrient by species having the C_4 dicarboxylic photosynthetic pathway, Plant Physiol., 49:794-797.

Bull, T. A., 1969, Photosynthetic efficiencies and photorespiration in Calvin cycle and C_4-dicarboxylic acid plants, Crop Sci., 9:726-729.

Calvin, M., 1976, Photosynthesis as a resource for energy and materials, Amer. Sci., 64:270-278.

Chollet, R., and Ogren, W. L., 1975, Regulation of photorespiration in C_3 and C_4 species, Bot. Rev., 41:137-179.

da Silva, J. G., Serra, G. E., Moreira, J. R., Concalves, J. C., and Goldemberg, J., 1978, Energy balance for ethyl alcohol production from crops, Science, 201:903-906.

Gifford, R. M., 1974, A comparison of potential photosynthesis, productivity, and yield of plant species with differing photosynthetic metabolism, Aust. J. Plant Physiol., 1:107-117.

Goldthwaite, J. J., and Laetsch, W. M., 1968, Control of senescence in Rumex leaf discs by gibberellic acid, Plant Physiol., 43:1855-1858.

Hardy, R. W. F., Havelka, U. D., and Quebedeaux, B., 1978, Increasing crop productivity: The problem, strategies, approach, and selected rate-limitations related to photosynthesis, in: "Proceedings Fourth International Congress on Photosynthesis," D. O. Hall, J. Coombs, and T. W. Goodwin, eds., The Biochemical Society, London.

Kennedy, R., and Laetsch, W. M., 1973, Relationship between leaf development and primary photosynthetic products in the C_4 plant Portulaca oleracea L., Planta, 15:113-124.

Laetsch, W. M., 1974, The C_4 syndrome: A structural analysis, Ann. Rev. Plant Physiol., 25:27-52.

Laetsch, W. M., and Boasson, R., 1971, Effect of growth regulators on organelle development, in: "Hormonal Regulation in Growth and Development," H. Kaldewey and Y. Vardar, eds., Verlag Chemie, Weinheim.

Liphschitz, N., Adiva-Shomer, I., Eshul, A., and Waisel, Y., 1974, Salt glands on leaves of Rhodes grass (Chloris gayana Kth), Ann. Bot., 38:459-462.

McKell, C. M., 1975, Shrubs--A neglected resource of arid lands, Science, 187:803-809.

Mosaic (National Science Foundation Publication), 1975, A Mosaic special: Food, 6:29-35.

Nasyrov, Y. S., 1978, Genetic control of photosynthesis and improving crop productivity, Ann. Rev. Plant Physiol., 29:215-276.

National Academy of Sciences, 1975, "Underexploited Tropical Plants with Promising Economic Value," Washington, D.C.

Nickell, L. G., 1976, Chemical growth regulation in sugar cane, Outlook on Agric., 9:57-61.

Nickell, L. G., 1977, Chemical enhancement of sucrose accumulation in sugar cane, in: "Advances in Chemistry, Series No. 159, Plant Growth Regulators," C. A. Stutte, ed., American Chemical Society, Washington, D.C.

Ogren, W. L., 1978, Increasing carbon fixation by crop plants, in: "Proceedings Fourth International Congress on Photosynthesis," D. O. Hall, J. Coombs, and T. W. Goodwin, eds., The Biochemical Society, London.

Sprey, B., and Laetsch, W. M., 1975, Chloroplast envelopes of Spinacia oleracea L. I. Polypeptides of chloroplast envelopes and lamellae, Z. Pflanzenphysiol., 75:38-52.

Sprey, B., and Laetsch, W. M., 1976a, Chloroplast envelopes of Spinacia oleracea L. II. Ultrastructure of chloroplast envelopes and lamellae, Z. Pflanzenphysiol., 78:146-163.

Sprey, B., and Laetsch, W. M., 1976b, Chloroplast envelopes of Spinacia oleracea L. III. Freeze-fracturing and chloroplast envelopes, Z. Pflanzenphysiol., 78:360-371.

Sprey, B., and Laetsch, W. M., 1977, Structural studies of the peripheral reticulum and membrane-bound ATPase activity of C_4 plant chloroplast membrane fractions, Abstract, in: "Proceedings Fourth International Conference on Photosynthesis," D. O. Hall,

J. Coombs, and T. W. Goodwin, eds., The Biochemical Society, London.

Sprey, B., and Laetsch, W. M., 1978, Structural studies of peripheral reticulum in C_4 plant chloroplasts of Portulaca oleracea L., Z. Pflanzenphysiol., 87:37-53.

Zelitch, I., 1971, "Photosynthesis, Photorespiration, and Plant Productivity," Academic Press, New York.

27

AGRICULTURE IN THE YEAR 2000: A SCRIPT FOR SURVIVAL

J. A. C. Hugill

World Sugar Research Organisation, Ltd.
London, England

INTRODUCTION

It is most fitting that we should be meeting here on the shores of the Mediterranean near some of these majestic reminders of the ancient world. For modern man this collection of interconnected inland seas is the "navel" of civilization. It was the scene of Sumerian, Egyptian, Greek, and Roman cultures. It was the home of the Phoenicians who gave the world its first alphabet and brought trade and culture as far as Britain. It was where the Arabs invented the numeral. It was the birthplace of such diverse figures as Socrates, Alexander the Great, Julius Caesar, Jesus Christ, Mohammed, Christopher Columbus, and Napoleon Bonaparte. But for our purpose today it is perhaps even more important as a continuous historical model of what has happened in the past to agriculture and the ecology and perhaps as an indication of what is to come.

The collection of present day microclimates in the area are very similar to one another and so are the topographies. Southern Spain is not unlike Morocco or southern Turkey. Provence is not unlike Sicily or Greece. To the north are the mountains whose snows feed the rivers of the area. To the south and east are the deserts, like huge unharvestable seas which dwarf mankind.

The people of the area are deeply differentiated by history, religion, politics, and level of wealth, but they have perhaps more common bonds than differences. There is a basic underlying kinship, the result of millennia of proximity, of intermingling whether voluntary or involuntary. Let us look briefly at what these relatively homogeneous people have done to the ecology over the centuries. What they have done the rest of the world has been and is now doing.

The inhabitants of this region have just been at it longer. Twenty thousand years or so ago, at the end of the Ice Age, the whole area--even much of the Sahara--was largely primeval forest. Early man was Hunting Man, and, in the pursuit of wild animals, began the process of burning trees without replacing them in order to be able to reach his prey. Between five and ten thousand years ago he began to turn into Pastoral Man, usually nomadic, and he continued to burn trees and move on, not only to clear pastures for his flocks of now domesticated animals, but also to provide himself with charcoal for fuel. He often overstocked his pasturages, and his animals--cattle, goats, sheep, and camels--damaged the soil. The pressure of their hooves compacted the cropped earth to a hard surface, so that when the rains came the water rushed off, leaving in the plains a material that later crumbled to desert sand, and in the hills became a dust which was washed away leaving bare rock. Sometimes that dust was redeposited annually as, for example, the fertile alluvium of the Nile Delta. Herodotus called this "The Gift of the Nile."

Then, at about the time of Abraham, Agricultural Man made his appearance, a more settled figure, introducing irrigation to assist the growth of cereals, cotton, and fruit trees, and planting here and there palm trees in the desert, and as Dr. Simpson (see Chapter 7) tells us, beginning the breeding of plants. But his agricultural methods were faulty. In Mesopotamia, for example, between the Tigris and the Euphrates, he irrigated but did not drain, and in consequence the soil turned sour. As Dr. Laetsch has reminded us, irrigation is almost always followed by salination. Five thousand years ago that area grew wheat and barley in equal proportions and in large enough quantities to support 25 million people. Thereafter productivity fell and by 1100 B.C. there was no wheat, only a little barley, which was more resistant to salt, and then, later, the irrigation system was abandoned. Today the region supports with difficulty a population of 10 million.

Erosion and desertification have happened elsewhere. Much of the coastal belt of North Africa was once highly cultivated--indeed it was the granary of the Roman world. But the advance of armies, Roman, Carthaginian, and later those carrying Islam to the west and north, meant also the advance of flocks of goats, which are the most implacable destroyers of vegetation; in times of drought they even climb trees for the leaves. A further spread of charcoal burning accompanied the armies, too, and armies on the march have no time to think about reforestation. So, with lots of help from man, the Mediterranean littoral became in time the bare place we now know. Gibraltar, the northern Pillar of Hercules, was for long regarded as mysterious and quite useless, until the followers of Al Tarik landed there in 711 A.D. and discovered wild animals on the wooded slopes. Twelve and a half centuries later it has only scrub vegetation and a small animal population of apes, precariously preserved for superstitious reasons by its human inhabitants. Nearby southern Spain a thousand years ago supported a population of 30 million. Today the population of the whole of Spain is 35 million. Deforestation was not always even the result of a need for food and heat. The Cedars of Lebanon are celebrated in ancient song but there are precious few left there now. The Phoenicians began cutting them over five thousand years ago. The Pharaohs used them for ships. King Nebuchadnezzar of Babylon actually left an inscription in 500 B.C. recording his pleasure at having used so many. King Solomon built his temple, and Alexander the Great his ships, from them. Hadrian, the Emperor, tried to save them by decree in 138 A.D. but failed. Those cedars are not a self-renewing species. Over the centuries, too, pine and fir, juniper, and oak went much the same way in the whole area, and were unreplaced.

In the absence of cedars we do not now build consummate palaces, but we do go on building. The French Riviera has become a concrete jungle crossed by tarmac strips along which northern peoples flock in their cars in search of a suntan. Spain's Costa Brava and Costa del Sol are similar manifestations of intermittent migration, recently spurred for recreational purposes; and the east coast of Italy is one continuous summer holiday ribbon-development from Brindisi to Rimini. In general the town dweller has taken over, and agriculture is a Cinderella whose ugly sisters, the factories, have until recently been free to release their effluents into the land-locked sea.

There is nothing new about the indifference of the town dweller or the soldier toward agriculture, which they look on as a matter of mud, manure, and the facts of life. An ambitious Roman general, two thousand years ago, would acquire a couple of towns and some land, employ landless laborers, and let the productivity of the land fall.

The Mediterranean area is not alone. It may have suffered for thousands of years from the hand of man but there are many other places where a parallel neglect has been at work--the American dust bowl, for instance. Improvement of agriculture has never been an inspiring goal, for it is politically unglamorous, unrecognized, and unrewarded. Yet until agriculture is given its proper place in the world there will always be a perilous imbalance between the number of people in the world and their food supplies.

Let us leave the Mediterranean and have a look at the global situation and try to see what agriculture may be like in the year 2000. Of course that year is not necessarily going to be the beginning of the twenty-first century. The nineteenth century began in June 1815 with the end of the Napoleonic Wars. The twentieth began in August 1914. But 2000 will do as a start.

Let me begin by saying that much as I respect neo-Malthusians like the Club of Rome, I do not believe the situation then will be greatly worse, or better, than it is now, so long as we make full use of certain advantages we possess in order to deal with the various factors governing the situation. Of course nothing worthwhile is easy. There is a sixteenth-century English phrase of which we should daily remind ourselves: "We are set in the midst of so many and great dangers that by reason of the frailty of our nature we are not always able to stand upright." The factors I refer to have already been mentioned and they are interlocking: people, land availability, climate, water, and energy.

POPULATION

It is right to start off with people since they are at once the cause of the problem and the hope of solution. Dr. Thimann (see Chapter 1) has reminded us of the population increase. We are of course only a stage in evolution. Our remote ancestors, the plants, are content merely to continue their species. We are ambitious, cruel, wasteful, greedy, and unbelievably silly. But we have one priceless asset. We are what Pascal called "The Thinking Reed."

Let me put the population figures this way. From the time when our relatively recent ancestor, the first hominoid, three million years ago first stood on his hind legs, it took until 1830 for the population to reach 1,000 million. If George Orwell's spine-chilling predictions come true in 1984, a bare century and a half later, there will be 5,000 million of us. I am reminded of a cartoon in an American paper showing a mother rabbit and a father rabbit gazing fondly at an adolescent rabbit with a smug expression on its face. The caption was: "Guess what! Junior's learned how to multiply."

Of course we may be multiplying so rapidly because subconsciously as a genus we fear either a nuclear war which will wipe out a lot of us, or the appearance of some twentieth century equivalent of the Black Death for which we may be unable to find a remedy.

It is true that recent studies by United Nations authorities detect a decline in the rate of population expansion. Yet this is like putting on the brakes when you are doing a hundred miles an hour. It takes time to have any result. Dr. Thimann was right to remind us, however, of the efforts being made in various parts of the world to stem the tide. Perhaps then we shall only be 6,000 or 7,000 million by 2000 A.D., rather than 8,000. That is still, however, a large number.

And of the million or so new mouths arriving every week on earth, the larger proportion will be in the developing countries, those least technically equipped. All sorts of authorities have pointed out the inequality which exists between the life style of the populations of the industrialized countries and that of the LDCs: Boyd Orr did so in 1950, Orville Freeman has done so more recently. The World Bank does so all the time, pointing out, for example, the hundreds of millions of farmers who function only at a subsistence level. In spite, therefore, of the activities of the Food and Agriculture Organization (FAO) and other United Nations agencies, and the billions of dollars spent on aid, most of those new mouths will be undernourished and undernourishment leads to bewilderment: "I, a stranger and afraid in a world I have not made."

We should not be too pessimistic but the problem is a major one, and to solve it we shall need land.

LAND

Strictly speaking this section should talk of land, sea, and air, because we eat the fish of the sea and the fowls of the air. But although we bridge the sea and ride the sky, we are two-dimensional beings, gravitationally confined, and agriculture applies only to the land.

The oceans are a mystery, a kind of primeval forest in which we are still at the stage of Hunting Man, squabbling about who fishes what and where. Yet perhaps the disastrous drop in catches is beginning to have an effect on our behavior. (In the North Atlantic, for example, the catch of cod fell from 2 million tons in 1968 to less than half that figure last year.) Perhaps we shall by 2000 A.D. have become at least Pastoral Man, as regards the fish. We may even, as some participants have indicated, have become Agricultural Man and be running huge fish farms.

Few of us know much about birds, including myself, but it is unlikely that we shall be like the Children of Israel who were sustained by showers of exhausted migratory quails. We shall have to depend on the domestic varieties, and these will be in competition with us for the vegetable products of the earth. So will the domestic animals.

It is difficult to be sure how much land is available to us, for, as some participants have pointed out, there is no precise definition of what constitutes arable land. And there is no doubt that a great deal of such land is disappearing. Some is lost as towns increase in size. Even more has been and is being lost by erosion and desertification. In parts of Africa, where the population has increased sixfold since 1950, more livestock has been grazed than the land can carry and the soil has been breaking down under stress. The Sahara is adding 250,000 acres a year to its size. In the Indian subcontinent deforestation in the hinterland has caused flash floods in the plains, which destroy entire areas of crop on land which was once fertile, and the food-producing system of the subcontinent, which can barely support its 850 million people, is annually impaired. In Amazonia large areas are at risk as forest is cleared, for the soil is too thin to withstand tropical rain.

The total world supply of arable land is believed to be about 3,200 million hectares. The average area in use per capita is 0.41 hectares but the variation is between 0.04 in Japan and 3.00 in Australia. Reserves of semi-arable land average about 0.76 hectares per head but the actual amounts vary enormously from .004 in Taiwan to 30 in Australia. And the soil types vary too from very fertile to marginal. In many parts of equatorical Africa there are huge areas of fertile land which is underpopulated and badly farmed.

But it seems that there should be enough land in 2000 A.D. provided we do two things. First, we must breed plants which will adapt themselves to marginal conditions--as several participants have indicated--and second, we must improve productivity per hectare. Dr. Wittwer (see Chapter 2) cited the example of wheat production in Britain. Now if that fairly homogeneous country can have wheat productivity varying from under 2 tons to over 10 per hectare and an average of only 4 1/2 tons, then there is vast room for improvement, and the same goes for all other crops and all other regions.

CLIMATE

There is little we can do about the climate but accept the major divisions of frigid, temperate, and tropical and optimize our use of it. There will continue to be few years in which there is not a bad crop somewhere in the world, say, once in four years in the USSR or a failure of the monsoon in India once in five years. We may even see another period of six consecutive droughts in the Sahel.

Dr. Andersen (see Chapter 15) mentioned the rise in carbon dioxide levels from 290 to 340 ppm. There has been talk of the "greenhouse effect" of the emission of carbon dioxide, i.e., causing a rise in the earth's surface temperature, melting polar icecaps, and raising the level of the oceans. It is a possible danger, but most of the current evidence seems to indicate that it will not be a reality by the year 2000. There is often talk, too, of a new Ice Age, particularly when the annual rain-making festival at Wimbledon is more than usually chilly. But it seems as if we are in the middle of a reasonably equable world climate period and that it will probably last until 2000 A.D. Perhaps that is another reason why we are multiplying so fast; like a bacterial inoculum in some celestial petrie dish.

WATER

Thirst is a more primal urge than hunger and almost all living organisms know it. That is why there is some alarm that population growth appears to be bringing about a shortage of water. It has been forecast that by 2000 A.D. the United States may have to ration water for farmer and ordinary consumer alike, and on a broader scale the limitations to fresh water supplies are becoming recognized. Only about 4% of the world's supplies are so far used for irrigation, and cost considerations seem to be slowing down the introduction of new schemes throughout much of the world.

On the other hand there is a great deal of work being done on desalination schemes, particularly in the oil-rich Middle East. The energy demands for this are such that even there some source of energy other than oil will have to be found, but there is no reason to suppose that one will not be found, if necessary.

ENERGY

This brings us to the question of energy, which other participants have touched on. As a race we have changed our ways a lot in recent centuries. Until five centuries ago we depended on cellulose from trees, sometimes converted by pyrolysis into charcoal. In about Shakespeare's day a novel solid fuel, prepared for us by nature millions of years before, began to be widely used. It was first called in English "seacoal" to distinguish it from charcoal.

Coal, the power behind the Industrial Revolution, began to be replaced by oil within living memory. Only two years before my birth Churchill invested £4 million of Government money in Persia, to guarantee fuel for a new generation of oil-fueled battleships. (He was criticized at the time but the investment is now the enterprise known as British Petroleum.) Natural gas came still later. Atomic power has scarcely begun to be used.

Yet there is now almost a panic about our energy resources, and some talk even of our becoming dependent once more on cellulose--clogs to clogs in twenty generations. Now it is true that we use fuel very inefficiently, and we use too much. Consumption in the United States is the equivalent of 8 tons of coal a year per head. The other industrialized countries average 5 tons, and the developing countries 0.5.

Our proven latent resources (without daily input from the sun) are estimated at 5×10^{21} kilocalories, of which 96% is mineral, 3.9% nuclear, and 0.1% hydro. It is the limitation of mineral resources, including uranium, which is causing the panic. People talk of the United States running out of oil and gas in the 1980s.

This may be an exaggeration, but there is a danger. In Britain we are spending our North Sea oil like a newly landed sailor in a rumshop. The problem exists because we have been and continue to be extravagant. We have been slow in nuclear power development for understandable reasons--partly environmental, partly from a fear of dangerous raw material getting into unreliable hands. But there are a number of solutions which we are capable of exploiting.

Nuclear fusion using deuterium from the oceans is one possibility. One per cent of the deuterium available would release 500,000 times as much energy as all the fossil fuels there have ever been. However, it is only recently that scientists have got anywhere near the critical temperature required for a controlled fusion reaction. It is true that the engineering problems are colossal. But they are not insoluble and they will, under pressure of need, I believe, be solved.

At the same time there are other possibilities. Look at France, blessed with fertile land but less blessed with fuel. A Department of New Energy is at work there, investigating water-heating, industrial equipment, desalination plants, and irrigation pumps all powered by solar energy. There is tidal energy and energy from the wind. Look at the development of mass-produced photovoltaic cells in the United States. Look at the use of ethanol from sugarcane and cassava in Brazil which Dr. Vlitos (see Chapter 21) mentioned. Look at the use of agricultural waste in India on a cottage scale as a source of methane. Look at the vast amounts of biomass in the equatorial zone, particularly in Africa, where solar energy concentration is at its highest.

There will have to be economies. Much skill will have to be exercised. But there will be energy in 2000 A.D.

OUR NEEDS

Our needs vary greatly from region to region because of tradition, temperature, environment, and custom. But whoever we are we need food and water, clothes, and shelter to a greater or lesser extent. Naked came we into the world and naked we shall leave it. But it is the period between those two traumas that concerns us for it is the time of our lives. We should not think purely of calorie intake, for we need protein and micronutrients too. In North America, supplies of protein and calories exceed demand by 15 to 20%. The United States Senate is even issuing guidelines on diet recommending people eat less. In Africa south of the Sahara, supplies are 5 to 10% less than demand and in many parts of Asia the situation is worse.

For industralized countries the FAO puts the daily kilocalorie "requirement" at 2,600, for developing countries at 2,300, but the economist Colin Clark gives a figure between 1,600 and 2,000 for Asian populations. The American eats three times as much protein of all kinds as the African. The average Englishman eats 40 times as much meat and fish as the average Indian peasant.

Industralized countries tend to produce surpluses and in an ideal world these could be fed to the hungry. But it is not an ideal world and the problems of marketing, transport, and distribution appear almost insoluble, complicated by questions of money, politics, inefficiency, sometimes corruption, and lack of infrastructure. So we must think in terms of greater regional independence. How are we going to provide all these needs?

RESEARCH

This is an institute of advanced studies and we have addressed ourselves largely to research. It is indeed fortunate for the world that 95% of the research scientists who have ever existed are alive--and I hope well--today.

It would be presumptuous to attempt to give a summary of the fascinating papers which have been presented in this Institute, but certain points bear mentioning.

Of course, this Institute has concentrated on plant growth regulators, and these are a most powerful instrument which will be of increasing value over the next two decades, even if the mystery of how they operate still remains hidden from us. We have perhaps naturally had little discussion on mechanical inputs, or fertilizer and pesticide inputs, for these are fairly standard things. But we have heard quite a lot about naturally occurring substances rather than synthetics. This is perhaps a reflection of a reaction in the industrialized world against synthetics and additives, probably stemming from Rachel Carson's book "The Silent Spring." This reaction is often irrational. If the World Health Organization had not used chlorinated hydrocarbons a generation ago, many people would have died of malaria. Perhaps their great grandchildren may die of tertiary cancer, but the evidence for such a fear is just not there. And we still need artificial fertilizers, herbicides, and pesticides.

We could, for energy reasons, however, benefit from the development of graminaceous plants which will fix nitrogen as the legumes do, or of the means to improve phosphate uptake. Crop nutrition is a dynamic, not a static affair, and therefore the use of mycorrhizae to improve phosphate uptake and rhizobia to fix nitrogen is clearly desirable, even if there are formidable difficulties. Although plant growth regulators are so promising, and offer so quick a way of improving productivity, they are only one way. There are others.

Many participants have been insistent on emphasizing genetics. In some plants this can produce rapid results, in others progress will be slower. Nevertheless, there are some 80,000 edible species of plant known to man, of which only about 100 are cultivated at all, and as Dr. Wittwer (see Chapter 2) has said, only 14 or 15 are major crop plants. It is theoretically possible to supply plants with all their needs, except only latitude and day-length. By the use of plant growth regulators it is possible even to overcome resistance to saline conditions and compacted soil. But the major limiting factor remains--the genetic circumscription of the plants themselves. As Dr. Laetsch has said, they do not evolve to feed people but to please themselves, and they need help.

So it is still to the plant breeder that we must look for major breakthroughs over the next generation, although this work cannot go on in isolation; hence the value of this Institute. Many possibilities have been mentioned: new varieties which will tolerate salt or dry conditions, others which will delay flowering until it is safe, still others which will permit multiple cropping and so economize on land use, others again which will ripen early. The list is long.

What is striking, however, is how all the aspects are interlinked with the five interlocking factors. Considerations of energy demand that we use it more effectively or find new sources. Water demand implies the need to use water more efficiently, as Drs. Tekinel (see Chapter 24) and Karamanos (see Chapter 23) have indicated. In turn this may lead to economy in fertilizers and save energy. It may also help us to be simultaneously productive. But all these efforts will contribute, and will give us hope. The light at dawn is diffuse, but it is there. Three points shall be stressed.

First, it is dangerous to concentrate on only a few high yielding hybrids, for it leaves open the possibility of a catastrophe from pests and diseases specific to single widely spread varieties. The Gros Michel banana is one of the small number of successful varieties, but it is liable to Panama Disease. The Lacatan, which is resistant, is not nearly so nice a fruit. And there was a case of near-disaster in the United States in 1970 when 90% of the corn acreage was planted to varieties with a single common source of cytoplasm and then southern corn leaf blight took hold. In the case of the corn this was fairly rapidly corrected but many plants take longer. Hopefully, we shall always get high-yielders which are pest and disease resistant; we have already made a good beginning with soya and alfalfa. In addition to treated seed, as described by

Dr. Khan (see Chapter 22), we should try to get seed that is bred to be disease-resistant. But as Dr. Vasil (see Chapter 5) and others have pointed out, not much success has been achieved as yet.

The second point is that the needs and appetites of man vary greatly. In high rainfall tropical countries people eat mainly roots, tubers, bananas, and so forth, particularly in Africa. On the tropical fringe of desert they depend on millet and sorghum. This is unlikely to change much by 2000 A.D. Therefore, although the work may be less exciting, perhaps geneticists will match their considerable successes in wheat and maize and rice with advances in oil-seeds, millet, tubers, and forage crops.

The third point is that agriculture must be accompanied by forestry. Since the United Nations Conference on Desertification much attention has been focused on this. The World Bank has been spending money and the FAO has been assisting--Forestry is one of their stronger divisions. One country, Algeria, has been planting a 10-mile wide belt of trees along the whole of its desert fringe. On the other hand, another country, Zambia, is using 2 tons of wood per head per year. The number of heads will increase fourteenfold by 2000. And the cut trees are not being replaced. Of course, there are all manner of problems, particularly in tropical forestry: root fungi, shoot-boring insects, defoliating ants. But these should be solvable. After all, two centuries ago the tropics were much deadlier to man than they are now. Remember the rhyme about "The Bight of Benin, where one comes out for twenty go in?" If the tropics are now easier for man, he should in turn make them easier for trees.

There is, above all, a need for plant breeders to find new quick-growing varieties. Gmelina arborea, for example, which grows at a meter a month in Brazil, does not do so well elsewhere.

OTHER FOOD SOURCES

This paper has concentrated largely on plants, for they are the subject of this Institute, and in any case they are less complex than animals. They are often more efficient as fixers of solar energy. To take an extreme case, it requires only 0.07 of a hectare to convert solar energy to one million kilocalories worth of food in the form of sugar. It takes 7.7 hectares to fix the same amount in the form of beef. And improvements in animal species take, in general, longer to achieve than improvements in plants.

There may be new Buffalo/Angus or Charolais/Brahmin crosses by 2000 A.D. or, alternatively, there may be new developments in the ranching of wild animals in Africa rather than farming ordinary cattle, which are a prey to the tsetse fly. There will be improvements in the pig, the sheep, and the chicken. But we must look increasingly to the plant kingdom for proteins, as well as for calories. And we must look not only along the twin routes of swiftly applied plant regulators, or slower genetics, but also at chromosome engineering and biochemistry as applied to the enzymes which occur in plants--the kind of work described by Drs. Nitsch (see Chapter 4) and Vasil with plant tissues.

CROP PRESERVATION

Dr. Wain (see Chapter 10) has indicated another field which gives cause for hope that the year 2000 will see a situation not in general worse than the present, and that is crop preservation against our competitors the rat and the insect. Locusts, borers, and the like destroy an immense amount of growing crops, and must be controlled. But it is unrealistic to expect that by the year 2000 we shall see an improvement in control better than say, 10%, because even with new "slow release" pesticides and the naturally based systemic ones, the difficulties are too great.

It is what happens to produce <u>after</u> cropping that offers the greatest chance of helping to feed the world. That between 30 and 40% of harvested grain, for example, should be lost each year to vermin, when the means of preventing this are known, is nothing short of criminal negligence. Surely it is within our capacity to reduce that figure to 15 to 20% by 2000 A.D. This is a management, not a research, problem. And we shall manage it because we shall have to.

PROBLEMS

But with all these promising possibilities, there are other considerations which are less tractable. Agriculture may be greatly assisted by research, but it is also intimately entwined with social and political activities, financial and market activities, administrative activities, infrastructive, and above all, education, training, and extension work. And due to its nature, agriculture is deeply involved in the environment, in soil conservation, water management, and avoidance of pollution. Most of these are, however important, relatively peripheral considerations. But a certain broadening of base might help.

There is one social and political aspect which will continue to affect agriculture in the year 2000, and that is land tenure. There is nothing new about this. Since before the time of the Pharaohs there has been heated and inconclusive discussion. What size should farm units be? Are landlords a good or a bad thing?

Do not men working their own land work better because they get "job satisfaction?"

There is no single or simple or ideal answer. Any solution will only be reached by political compromise since it will affect the conflicting interests of various groups of people.

Latifundia, or the ownership of land in large parcels by individuals, has a bad name. Yet it can help productivity, soil conservation, water management, and the introduction of new methods. In the West Indies for example, the productivity of a large sugar-cane estate was usually more than twice that of the small cane farmer. But latifundia involves landless labor which can be easily inflamed by demagogues. It will probably still exist in the year 2000. There will probably be minifunda too, but with a tendency for very small units to agglomerate. This has already begun in France, where the tiny farms of less than 5 hectares are disappearing, if only because the young people will not stay on the land.

The corollary of minifundia is a drift to the towns followed by unemployment and eventual upheavals. Upheavals are not inevitable and can be prevented if agricultural development is accompanied by the provision of employment by government in the shape of work on infrastructure such as roads and ports, or by the establishment of public and private industry. Agriculture on its own cannot provide the food and at the same time a limitless amount of unskilled or semi-skilled jobs. It is encouraging therefore that the World Bank is already turning its attention to what it calls "Rural Enterprise and Non-farm Employment."

There is a place, too, for the type of development called appropriate technology, which is the provision of not too capital-intensive techniques. Dr. Vlitos mentioned this.

But to sum up on land, in 2000 we shall probably still see in the industrialized countries flexible, capital-intensive, owner-operators of fairly large mixed crop and livestock systems. We shall elsewhere still see some latifundia and some minifundia, both gradually becoming less pronounced.

As to concern for the environment, that is here to stay. Not so long ago, on June 13 to be precise, the Times ran this headline: "Three inch fish blocks $116 million dam." It sounded like a bit of trouble in the drawing office, but when I read on I found that a large American hydro-development was being abandoned because it would wipe out a little known fish called the "snail darter," and this would not be permitted under the Endangered Species Act. There will be more of that to come--unless mankind becomes an endangered species.

TRANSFER OF TECHNOLOGY

Now we come to a point which several others have touched on. Dr. Wittwer, for example, said: "We keep waiting for the farmer to do all the work." Dr. Bennink (see Chapter 12) emphasized the same point. To put it another way, it is no use having a plant growth regulator which increases yields by 1000%, disobeys the Second Law of Thermodynamics, and tastes nice on bread, if it is not going to be correctly applied. The same has long been the case with fertilizers, herbicides, and pesticides.

But there is, alas, a hideous and growing gap between the output of scientific research and its application, between the scientist and the layman. It is difficult enough going from lab scale to pilot scale and then to full scale in an industrial project. It is far more difficult in agriculture, because the transfer of technology is more difficult.

In addition to innovation there is a need for political will, money, and above all the spreading of understanding. This is the key, but it is a key that is yet to be cut. Maybe this Institute could help cut it. Dr. Wain rightly pointed out that a successful research product usually finds a commercial firm to develop it, but optimism is not quite enough.

Many such firms are what have been called multinationals. These get a bad press sometimes, though as a former director of one I think this a somewhat simplistic reaction. Of course multinationals are imperfect. All human agencies are, including the United Nations and the various Churches. I see that the present term for multinational is transnational, a better word. And, since nations themselves so often make a mess of things, there may be something to be said for transnationalism.

Transnationals can be useful, particularly in the rapid transfer of technology. It is to their interest that their products be sold, and that they be used safely, economically, and successfully. Many of them have gotten together to produce guide books on this, and have organized regular symposia down to the level of the man in the field.

Some of these firms belong, or used to, to a body called the Industry Cooperative Programme, attached to one of the United Nations agencies. I know of this group because I used to be its chairman.

In order to try and provide the key mentioned, this Institute might explore with some of these firms the setting up of ways and means of bringing innovations in agriculture more rapidly to the farmers. One such way would be the setting up of systems of seminars where people could be rapidly trained in the proper use of new techniques.

Now if such an idea is to be manageable it must be kept at first to a restricted area. And here we can return to the initial topic of this talk, the Mediterranean. Could we not see if some of the governments which support NATO and this Institute and some of the private enterprises which are based within the NATO grouping can select one or two such projects in one or two countries, and make them work on a continuous scale and one large enough to produce an impact.

This is only the germ of an idea, but if it seems any good, it might sprout, given a dose of NPK and a shot of gibberellic acid.

I repeat there is no single or simple solution to our problems. It is a kind of jigsaw puzzle. The world is not a regular or calculable place. But I still remain moderately optimistic, moderately sure that agriculture in the year 2000 will still be feeding all those mouths, even if on a less than entirely satisfactory basis.

I called this paper "A Script for Survival." It is far from that. It is not even a scenario, whatever that may mean. It is an expression of hope and a recognition that because as a race we are dimly conscious of our problems we tend to overcome them. We do not know all the answers, but we <u>are</u> looking for them. I sometimes think that our human condition is subject to an overriding consideration a little like the Heisenberg Uncertainty Principle. We cannot measure simultaneously the speed and position of an atomic particle, because the act of measurement introduces a change. By analogy, the very act of looking at the problems of our species also introduces a change. The very fact that people are looking at land and water and energy and plant regulators and genetics will make a change. Whereas Heisenberg's principle is a confession of limitation, this one is more positive. It is a declaration of hope.

Well, even if we do manage to feed ourselves in the year 2000, as I believe, it will be what Wellington called Waterloo: "A damned nice thing. The nearest run thing you ever saw in your life." He went on to say: "I don't think it would have done if I hadn't been there." I am unlikely to be there in 2000 A.D. myself. Perhaps not all of you will. But our children and grandchildren certainly will. And I hope, for their sakes, that I am right.

ACKNOWLEDGMENTS

Attendance at this Advanced Study Institute was most stimulating and I learned a great deal. I am most grateful to the Director,

Professor T. K. Scott, and his colleagues for inviting me.

I should like also to thank the following for help and advice, and information in the preparation of this paper.

Mr. Lester R. Brown--World Watch Society, Washington, D.C.

Dr. C. de Clercq--Editor, Agriculture & Development, Beirut, Lebanon.

Dr. J. Coombe--Philip Lyle Memorial Research Laboratory, Reading, England.

Dr. Edward J. Cornish--World Future Society, Bethesda, Maryland.

Mr. Orville Freeman--Business International Ltd., New York.

Dr. A. G. Freidrich--Industry Cooperative Programme, FAO, Rome.

Mr. B. Gardner McTaggart--Industry Cooperative Programme, FAO, Rome.

Mr. J. I. Hendrie--formerly Head Life Science Department, Shell International, England.

Mr. Hugues de Jouvenel--Futuribles Association Internationale, Paris.

Mr. M. O. Lane--Shell International, England.

Dr. K. J. Parker--Philip Lyle Memorial Research Laboratory, Reading, England.

Mr. W. W. Simons--Industry Cooperative Programme, UNHD, New York.

Mr. J. G. R. Stevens--Editor, Span, Derby, England.

Unilever Ltd.--London.

Mr. A. van Dam--C.P.C. International, Buenos Aires, Argentina.

Dr. A. J. Vlitos--Philip Lyle Memorial Research Laboratory, Reading, England.

PUBLICATIONS AND SOURCES IN WHICH PLANT GROWTH REGULATORS AND WORLD AGRICULTURE ARE DISCUSSED

Afzel, M., 1973, Implications of the green revolution for land use patterns and relative crop profitability under domestic and international prices, Pakistan Development Review.

Braudel, F., 1972, "The Mediterranean and the Mediterranean World in the Age of Philip II," Collins, London.

British Broadcasting Company, External Services, February 7, 1978, "Discovery."

Brown, L. R., 1977, The world food prospect (a paper presented at the "Limits of Growth" conference, 1974), Long Range Planning, 10 (Feb.).

Brown, L. R., 1978, "The Twenty-ninth Day," W. W. Norton, New York.

Brown, L. R., and Eckholm, E. P., 1974, "By Bread Alone," Praeger, New York.

Close, C., 1970, "Starvation or Plenty," Secker and Warburg, London.

Delegation aux Energies Nouvelles--Ministere de l'Industries et de la Recherche, "Solar Energy for France," Paris.

Durham, K., 1976, Food in the future, Unilever Magazine (Jan./Feb.).

Eckholm, E. P., 1975, "The Other Energy Crisis: Firewood," The Worldwatch Institute, Washington, D.C.

Eckholm, E. P., 1976, "Losing Ground: Environmental Stress and World Food Prospects," W. W. Norton, New York.

Eckholm, E. P., and Brown, L. R., 1977, "Spreading Deserts--The Hand of Man," The Worldwatch Institute, Washington, D.C.

Enzer, S., Drobnick, R., and Alter, S., 1978, Neither feast nor famine, Food Policy (Feb.).

Food and Agricultural Organization (United Nations), 1976, "Production Year Book."

Food and Agricultural Organization (United Nations), 1976, "The State of Food and Agriculture."

Food Foundation, 1973, "The World Food Outlook and the Foundation's Agricultural Activities."

George, S., 1976, "How the Other Half Starves," Pelican Books, London.

Gouldenberg, J., 1978, Brazil's energy options and current outlook, Science, 200 (April 14).

Grace, Murad R., 1978, "Near East Study on Agro-Industries," Food and Agricultural Organization (United Nations), Near East Regional Offices.

Green, M. B., et al., 1977, Chemicals for crop production and pest control, Future Trends.

Handler, P., 1970, "Biology and the Future of Man," Oxford Univ. Press, New York.

Handler, P., 1976, On the state of man, Interdisciplinary Science Review, 1:189.

Hayanic, Y., and Rutton, V. W., 1972, "Agricultural Development--An International Perspective," Johns Hopkins Press, Baltimore.

Heady, E. O., and Choudhury, S. R., 1977, Food demand factors, Chemtech (July).

Hutchinson, J., ed., 1969, "Population and Food Supply: Essays on Human Needs and Agricultural Prospects," Cambridge Univ. Press, London.

Industry Cooperative Programme--Mission to Brazil, 1973, "Agro-Industrial Potential of Legal Amazonia."

Institute of Fuel (United Kingdom), 1977, "The Energy Show," Catalogue (September).

Leontieff, W., et al., 1977, "The Future of the World Economy," Oxford Univ. Press, New York.

Massachusetts Institute of Technology, 1972, "The Limits to Growth," Report for the Club of Rome's Project on the Predicament of Mankind.

Mercer, J. H., 1978, Institute of Solar Studies, Ohio State University, Nature.

Mesorovic, M., and Pestel, E., 1974, "Mankind at the Turning Point," Second Report of the Club of Rome, E. P. Dutton, Readers Digest Press, New York.

Metcalf, R. L., and McKelvrey, J. A., 1974, The future for insecticides, in: Proceedings of a Rockefeller Foundation Conference (April).

Naiken, L., and Schulte, W., 1976, Population and Labour Force Projections for Agricultural Planning, Food Policy (May).

Organization for Economic Cooperation and Development, 1968, Agriculture in developing countries, in: "The Food Problems of Developing Countries."

Organization for Economic Cooperation and Development, 1977, "Study of Trends in World Supply and Demand of Major Agricultural Commodities."

Orr, D., and Van den Hoven, H. F., 1978, Unilever and the Third World food problem, Unilever Annual General Meeting, May 17.

Orr Whyte, Robert, 1976, "Land and Land Appraisal," Dr. W. Junk, The Hague.

Pimentel, D., 1976, World food crisis: Energy and pests, Bull. Entom. Soc. Amer., 22:20.

Pyke, M., 1978, Speculation on our future food, Unilever Magazine (Jan./Feb.).

Rojko, A. S., and O'Brien, P. M., 1976, Organising agriculture in the year 2000, Food Policy (May).

Sanderson, F. H., 1975, The great food fumble, Science (May 9).

Sanderson, F. H., 1976, "World Food Prospects," World Health Organization.

Span, 1978, 21: Nos. 1 & 2.

Stare, F. J., 1975, Sugar in the diet of man, World Review of Nutrition and Diet, 22:327.

Superior Farming Company, 1977, The problem: Global hunger. Will it be solved?, Food and Population (June).

United Nations Economic and Social Council, 1977, Economic Commission for Western Asia, Short Term Possibilities for Increasing Food Production in Selected Countries of the ECWA Region.

United Nations Economic Commission for Western Africa, 1977, "1975 Food Balance Sheets for Selected Commodities in Countries of Western Asia" (March).

United Nations Economic Commission for Western Africa, 1978, "Agriculture and Development" (April).

Vlitos, A. J., 1978, Technology--88, in: "The Socio-Economic Scenario: Nutrition, Energy, and the Environment," EIRMA Workshop (Feb.).

Westlake, M., 1973, Is the green revolution foundering?, The Times (April 2).

White-Spunner, D., 1973, Food, land, and people in the modern world, Rhodesia Agric. J., 73: No. i.

World Bank, 1972, Sector Working Paper on Agriculture.

World Bank, 1975, Sector Policy on Rural Development.

World Bank, 1977, "Population, Per Capita Product, and Growth Rates."

World Bank, 1978, "Annual Review of Project Performance Audit Results."

World Bank, 1978, "Forestry."

World Bank, 1978, "Rural Enterprise and Non-farm Development."

28

AGRICULTURAL MANAGEMENT STRATEGIES, INITIATIVES, AND GOALS FOR SURVIVAL

Suzanne Appelbaum and Tom K. Scott (Editors)

Department of Botany
University of North Carolina at Chapel Hill
Chapel Hill, North Carolina 27514

During the course of the Advanced Study Institute, there was a great deal of discussion concerning many and various topics related to plant growth regulation and world agriculture. Those discussions were helpful and illuminating to the participants. However, it was agreed at the outset that only points of particular strategical significance for the future of agriculture, horticulture, and associated research imperatives be given special note in this volume. There follows, therefore, a compilation of points, arguments, comments, and philosophies which grew out of these discussions and which we have brought together under an umbrella title, AGRICULTURAL MANAGEMENT STRATEGIES, INITIATIVES, AND GOALS FOR SURVIVAL.

These topics have been grouped into the following categories: Public Policy, Biomass, Enrichment of Soil and Air, Regulation of Bud Set and Growth, Chemical and Genetic Regulation of Growth, Natural Herbicides, Temperature Effects, Drought Resistance, and Seeds. The categories are somewhat arbitrarily drawn, but the editors hope there is sufficient integrity within each so that each may stand by itself and thus be a useful focus for future initiatives. Though, in all cases, at least some editorial license has been taken in organizing the various statements, the participant responsible for bringing the ideas before the conference is identified parenthetically or otherwise.

PUBLIC POLICY

Several participants have emphasized the need for greater governmental input and cooperation among scientists/scholars, government, and industry in solving agricultural and horticultural problems.

Of particular concern is the need to develop new agricultural chemicals. As Dr. Ku has pointed out, "Due to the high cost of development of new agricultural chemicals, there will be no new commercial products in the next few years, even for experimental purposes."

Dr. Wightman carries this theme a bit further in relating it to a specific country; the host country, Turkey. "Since Turkey intends to make a major effort over the next twenty years to increase greatly the production of both agricultural and horticultural crops, it is clear that growth regulating substances, as well as pesticides and fungicides, will play important roles....A range of crops will be grown, each chosen to suit the special environmental conditions found in the different regions of Anatolia.

"The agricultural chemical requirements of such a wide range of crops for regulating certain phases of growth, controlling pests, improving disease resistance, and most important, increasing crop yield, will differ from crop to crop, but since the actual acreage of land covered by each crop will not be large, it is probable that the amounts of chemicals required annually to support these crops may not be large enough to insure that the agricultural chemical companies of the western world will be prepared to put a significant amount of their research effort into solving Turkey's special agricultural problems.

"I suggest, therefore, that this Advanced Study Institute should recommend to the Turkish Government that they establish a National Institute for Agricultural Chemical Research whose primary responsibility would be to solve the special chemical problems encountered during Turkey's agricultural and horticultural expansion. If Turkey relies on the research scientists of chemical companies in other countries, her farmers may well have to wait years before the new chemicals they need are developed and made available for widespread use."

To help stimulate fundamental and applied biological-agricultural research elsewhere (i.e., the United States), Dr. Hardy recommends joint basic/applied research proposals. He suggests "establishment of a specific research fund to which only such joint proposals could be made. The current National Science Foundation University-Industrial program is an example of such an approach in another field."

Still another way in which governments can aid in utilizing the full potential of plant growth regulators in future food, fuel, and fiber production (according to Dr. Andersen) "is to help in educating the ultimate user....The days of great strides forward, like those we have witnessed in the past with such developments as herbicides, are over. The coming revolutions will be more like evolutions and yield increases of 10% will be all we can expect from any new practice. These will require great sophistication with regard to implementation on the farm; consequently the farmer must be extremely well educated. It is not enough that we have fine universities and experiment stations staffed with people educated at the universities. It is necessary that young and older farmers alike get an education in basic chemistry, physiology, and of course, economics. In Denmark, and I am sure many other farming countries, there are a great number of schools for agri- and horticulture, where the young people come for 3- or 9-month courses. Teachers here are usually graduates (MS or Ph.D.) of the agricultural universities, and some of them have part-time jobs on experiment stations. These schools are distributed throughout the farming regions and serve also as centers for 'lifelong' education and information independent of those which are supplied with great fervor by the various chemical firms."

Finally, Dr. Vardar feels that agricultural problems and long-range planning should be addressed by means of Regulatory Agricultural Plans "at national and international levels." He goes into detail on how such a plan might be enacted in Chapter 20.

BIOMASS

● Much attention is currently being focused on biomass production to provide renewable energy resources and to maximize the use of plants as biological suntraps. Many food, feed, and fiber crops of considerable commercial importance (sugarcane, sugar beets, sorghum, cassava, potatoes) offer clear possibilities for this use. Fast-growing deciduous trees such as hybrid poplars have also been suggested.

There is considerable opportunity, backed now by experimental studies, for accelerating the growth of trees under controlled environments during the early seedling stages, resulting in enhancement of biomass production. The appropriate combination of mineral nutrients, soil moisture, temperature regimes, day-length, carbon dioxide enrichment, and treatments with gibberellin and mycorrhizal inoculum for each species will result in at least a tenfold increase in growth over a 12-month period compared with normal outdoor culture. These early induced accelerated growth responses are now known to carry over in the field. The environmental and chemical regulator package will vary for each species and locality but should be vigorously pursued. Biological nitrogen fixation could also be added to the growth package for the actinomycete-nodulated angiosperms and the tree legumes of which there are many species of each. To achieve the above objectives of accelerated growth for biomass production will require not only the input of the plant physiologist but also that of the forester, the agronomist, the agricultural engineer, the microbiologist, the plant breeder, and the systems scientist. (Wittwer)

• An important option for plant scientists to pursue in the future would be to reduce the losses of nitrogen that is already "fixed" for crop production. These losses occur from nitrification and subsequent denitrification. Nitrification encourages losses in the ground and surface water by leaching. Denitrification loses nitrogen as N_2 released back to the atmosphere. It occurs under anaerobic soil conditions and requires an energy source. Nitrification is a prerequisite for denitrification. The current global losses of fertilizer nitrogen range from 12 to 15 million tons from denitrification, with an almost equal amount lost from nitrification. These losses not only result in an enormous economic loss to the farmer but also greatly reduce potential crop productivity, create potential environmental hazards, and constitute an irreversible loss of a nonrenewable resource. Research interest in this area has lagged because until recent years fertilizer (chemically fixed) nitrogen was cheap and plentiful--but no longer.

There is currently a great surge of interest in nitrifying inhibitors due to increased cost and decreased supply of fertilizer N_2. One synthetic compound, "N-Serve" (Dow Chemical Co.), which specifically inhibits the action of Nitrosomonas bacteria, has been on the market for at least ten years. Only recently, however, has interest in it been expressed and any detailed research other than through its developer been forthcoming. Naturally occurring products have also been identified as nitrifying inhibitors. One such is the meal from the fruit of the "Num" tree in India, long known for its medicinal properties. Chemical regulation of nitrification and research in soil ecology relating to the role of living organisms in regulating the growth of agricultural crops remains almost a vacuum in our research efforts. (Wittwer)

• Also see Wittwer under REGULATION OF BUD SET AND GROWTH.

• The most useful "portable" machine for both harvesting and digesting cellulose is the ruminant animal. It can recover efficiently from extensive areas cellulose (from forage plants) that would otherwise be difficult for humans to utilize. Perhaps we should consider alternative sources of cellulose for feeding ruminants. Experiments have been going on in Canada to utilize aspen poplar as a source of cellulose for cattle. Perhaps there are many other sources that are currently being wasted or underutilized. (Simpson)

• Although starch-based fermentation systems are more attractive at the moment than lignin-cellulosics, in the longer term the abundance of lignin-cellulosics and their wealth of chemical structures will make them more important as a source of chemicals for feedstocks and other uses. The major initial barrier is to discover an economical pretreatment of the lignin-cellulosics. Collection is not a serious problem. (Hardy)

• Agriculture, present and future, is the production of food, fiber, and fuel. The first two commodities have well been recognized; the third product is just as important and should be emphasized in the future practice of agriculture. One example of fuel production from biomass is the anaerobic fermentation of cellulose generated from agriculture (i.e., weeds, grasses, reeds, aboveground stalks, crop residues, vines, fast-growing plants such as water hyacinths, and livestock excrements). The product of this fermentation consists mainly of methane, and the process is carried out by microorganisms. Essentially the system involves the digestion of insoluble organic matter to soluble organics to acetate, carbon dioxide, and hydrogen, and finally to methane and CO_2. Under ideal conditions the gas contains 70% methane, 30% CO_2, and traces of H_2, N_2, and H_2S. The residue from this fermentation is a high quality fertilizer, rich in nitrogen, which can be returned to the land.

The production of fuel such as methane, oil, methanol, ethanol, hydrogen, and heat from biomass is a reasonable approach to supplementing the future demand for energy, and now is the time to give this matter a high priority and substantial support. (Shen-Miller)

• Production of fruit tissue by continuous culture is certainly a technique which could be used to increase biomass production, either with apple or pear as has already been done and also with spinach or tomato. An important question is how we can shorten the growing cycle to be able to grow a second crop which will have a good seed set. In areas having good climatic conditions and good soil, a big increase in crop production will result if two crops are grown instead of one. The solar energy is available and should be used to a maximum. It is possible to save from two to three weeks of the growing time in the field in cases where the temperature becomes less than optimum because the second crop comes in too late in the season. The problem has been solved in China in a very efficient way which permits growing up to three crops in the same land in certain places.

The growing time in the field is reduced to the minimum by starting the seeds in nursery beds and transplanting to the field after three weeks. The seedlings grown in nursery beds take very little space. They grow while the previous crop is ripening and are transplanted into the field right after the harvest. The three-weeks-old seedling transplanted to the field will then be growing when the optimal climatic conditions are still available, and the second or third crop will be as good as the previous one. (Nitsch)

ENRICHMENT OF SOIL AND AIR

There are several logical extensions of the concept of increasing biomass production. Among the ideas put forth along these lines were a number relating to enrichment of soil and air. The focus here is twofold: (1) enrichment to produce a better yield, and (2) efficient use of water, energy, fertilizer, and land to promote conservation.

● Much has been said about the losses of nitrogen following application as a fertilizer. Substantial amounts may be lost through leaching, denitrification, and other causes.

Losses of phosphate, however, are much greater. Phosphate fertilizers applied to the soil must contain soluble phosphate--and the usual form is superphosphate obtained by treating rock phosphate $CA_3(PO_4)_2$ with sulfuric acid. But when added to soil, the phosphate becomes fixed in acid soils as unsoluble iron or aluminum phosphate and in alkaline soils as calcium phosphate.

Application of most elements needed by plants can be made by spraying a soluble salt of the element onto the plant leaves (foliar application). With phosphate this does not work effectively. If we could get soluble phosphate to be taken up by the leaves and utilized by the plant it would be a development of tremendous agricultural significance. One possibility is the use of organic phosphates which might penetrate the leaves and then hydrolyze to release phosphate at the cell level where it could be utilized in the phosphate nutrition of the plant. (Wain)

● Drip or trickle irrigation has produced phenomenal results on high-value crops as a means of water, energy, and fertilizer conservation. The water is placed where the roots are. Recent results have suggested that pesticides, especially of the systemic type, may also be applied by this method. Some plant growth regulators, such as I-chloroethyltrimethylammonium chloride (CCC), can be most effectively applied if introduced into the root system. It would appear that the drip system of irrigation should be exploited also as a possible means of applying growth regulators which might have a systemic effect on growth and/or reproductive development. The efficiency of application should be comparable to that for fertilizers and pesticides, and there would be little cost of application. Uniform treatment over large areas and precise timing of applications would also be possible. (Wittwer)

● Carbon dioxide enrichment in the field is a most useful technique to assess the limitations of some aspects of the photosynthesis system for each major crop in its major areas of production, and a system such as the open-top side-enclosed forced gas one enables the experiment to be carried out in a meaningful way. Carbon dioxide enrichment is not a practical long range solution, but a very useful tool, and should be more widely applied. (Hardy)

● According to some estimates, the CO_2 concentration of the atmosphere one hundred years ago was only 290 ppm while today it is nearly 340 ppm. If we continue to burn fossil fuel at the forecasted rate, the concentration of atmospheric CO_2 may reach 400 ppm by the end of the century. This has some grave implications for the world climate, but for plant growth it can only be beneficial. In those areas of the world where sunlight is plentiful and water not a limiting factor this added atmospheric fertilization may mean a substantial increase in biomass production and agricultural efficiency.

Still, it is clear that there may often exist deficiencies of CO_2 at the sites of consumption, i.e., the canopies of crops and forests during the day. In enclosed cultivation it is possible to utilize elevated CO_2 levels. Thus, can we envision a delivery system of CO_2 from large producers, e.g., coal-burning electricity plants, to fields through some form of "drip system"? (Andersen)

REGULATION OF BUD SET AND GROWTH

● The control of the setting of terminal buds is crucial in the production of biomass from many tree species. If terminal buds set early in the growing season, as they now do for most woody species in temperate zones, production of biomass is clearly restricted. Different lines of hybrid poplars, one of the more promising species for biomass production, will vary greatly, as do individual trees within the same line, as to whether or not and as to when terminal buds set. (Wittwer)

● Though hundreds of papers have been published on hormonal control of apical dominance, the results of such studies are without application to the solution of real world agricultural and other renewable resource production problems. (Wittwer)

● Means other than hormonal control have been sought to retard the setting and growth of terminal buds. One such technique is the retarding of budbreak by evaporative cooling, which "may be a promising technique but has its shortcomings--for example, high cost of installation of the overhead sprinkler irrigation system. Furthermore, it is not applicable in ill-drained soils. A possibility for retarding budbreak should be the spraying of trees with reflective substances which reduce bud temperature by decreasing the net radiation of the plant surface, resulting in increased surface albedo. Such a technique should be easier and much cheaper than a sprinkler system. The use of filters which reflect some parts of the spectrum installed above the canopy at the required growth stage should be another alternative." (Karamanos)

● How can we improve mineral nutrition to regulate bud set?

Certain species of woody plants (e.g., *Acer pseudoplatanus* and *Picea sitchensis*) are more liable to set buds prematurely when subjected to mineral deficiency. There is reason to think that this response is mediated via the effects of nitrogen and inorganic phosphorus levels on the hormonal balance within the plant (especially with regard to gibberellins, cytokinins, and ABA). It would seem there are good prospects that we could reduce the sensitivity of such species to mineral deficiency by selection and breeding of appropriate genotypes, so that the liability to go into "check" on root sites would be reduced. (Wareing)

● My studies on early and late breaking cultivars of *Vitis vinifera* in Turkey have shown that the nutrition and translocation capabilities of some mineral ions and soluble sugars are different and earliness is related to the day of initiation of bleeding.

The number of cell layers in the phloem tissues also correlated with earliness. Evidently, several parameters take part in the determination of the bud breaking process and must be taken into account with plant growth regulators. (Duygu)

CHEMICAL AND GENETIC REGULATION OF GROWTH

Chemical and genetic growth regulation has been recognized for decades as being basic to increasing biomass, improving crop yield, and promoting conservation of nonrenewable resources. Judging by the number of participants who commented on ways to use natural and synthetic growth regulators, the development and application of such substances may be the most important strategy for the future.

●When discs of chicory or Jerusalem artichoke tissue are placed for 3 days in water, their weight increases by only about 15%. When similar discs are placed in a solution of any auxin, the weight increases dramatically. With 2,4-D at 10^{-5} M, for example, the increase is about 200%. There is, however, no increase in cell number as a result of treatment--but cell enlargement does occur to a marked extent. The clue to what is happening comes when the cell contents of the untreated and treated tissues are run on a paper chromatogram. It is then clear that the 2,4-D has resulted in hydrolysis of insoluble polysaccharides to soluble sugars (notably glucose and fructose). The release of these soluble sugars into the cell increases the osmotic pressure and water is drawn into the cell.

Studies at Wye College have shown that the 2,4-D treatment in this tissue leads to the production of a highly active and very specific increase which brings about the hydrolysis noted above. Here then is an important example of how an auxin can influence a plant enzyme system. This work encourages us to seek further examples of such an effect in our attempts to put auxin action on a proper biochemical basis.

The other example of growth substance/enzyme relationships, of course, is the gibberellin field where GA affects the amylase activity in the cereal grain. (Wain)

●Following the discovery by Kögl in 1934 that IAA is a plant growth hormone there were rapid developments. New synthetic auxins were discovered, some of which found uses in agriculture--for such purposes as rooting of cuttings, setting fruit in absence of pollination, preventing the preharvest drop of apples, etc. However, the most important development was the use of auxins in selective weed control. This opened up a gigantic market in the agricultural chemicals field, and the use of compounds such as 2,4-D; MCPA; 2,4-DB; and MCPB is the main reason why cereal yields have increased so dramatically since these compounds were introduced.

Now we are interested in how research can be planned to make plant growth regulators even more important in agricultural production. But, in fact, we might be slipping back in this respect. No longer can we boast that our plant growth regulators represent the most important group of selective herbicides on the world market, as they were for many years. They have now lost this pride of place to simazine, atrazine, and other compounds which together are known as the triazines.

Should we not investigate more intensively how our existing and new plant growth regulators can be used to kill unwanted plants (weeds) in the presence of the growing crop? The physiologist has an important role to play here as well as the chemist. (Wain)

● Although synthetic indole, naphthyl, and chlorophenoxy acids were widely tested as root-inducing substances in the 1950s, apart from indole-3-butyric acid (IBA), none of the many compounds tested has found widespread use in horticultural practice, mainly because many of the compounds tested possess halogen substituents which frequently caused harmful secondary effects on the plant cutting. In view of the discovery that phenylacetic acid (PAA) and 4-chloroindole-3-acetic acid (4CL-IAA) are naturally occurring auxin substances, and the demonstration that PAA is equally effective with IAA, and more effective than IBA, in promoting the initiation of lateral root primordia in pea seedlings, the capacity of 4CL-IAA, PAA, and chlorophenylacetic acids to promote the rooting of horticulturally important wood cuttings should be fully investigated. Further, since phenyl compounds appear to be more stable than indole compounds to bacterial breakdown or the conversion within the plant to inactive products, 4CL-IAA and the chlorophenyl acids might show good penetration and sufficient long-term stability (in dusting powders or treatment solutions) to enable them to induce good root initiation in many "difficult to root" wood cuttings without at the same time showing any of the harmful side effects produced by the chlorophenoxy acids. (Wightman)

● I learned many years ago that segments of coleoptiles and other seedlings elongated in test solutions they excreted protons and the solution became acid. But dilute (about 10^{-5} M) solutions of cobalt salts prevent the acidification, and at the same time they promote the elongation. Thus perhaps they force the protons back into the tissue in some way. It is possible, then, that cobalt might prove useful in some of the inhibitions Dr. Wareing discussed (see Chapter 17). (Thimann)

● It is strange that, in an agriculture so dominated by seeds as ours is, we know so little about the filling of the seed. This is an area absolutely central to the possibility of major increases in grain yield.

First, we must ask ourselves why is it that only the flagleaf and the upper part of the stem contribute C_{14} to the grain? In our isolated senescing leaves we find that the movement of amino acids, and to a lesser extent that of carbohydrates, is basipetally polar--much like the movement of auxin, though less rapid. I suggest, therefore, that the movement of photosynthates out of the lower leaves and in the subflag region of the stem is basipetally polar. CCC, by making the internodes shorter, would make the polarized region shorter and so make it possible for some of the products from the senescing lower leaves to reach the ear.

Now, cytokinin prevents the polar movement in the leaf and holds the photosynthate there, and this causes or accompanies the delay of senescence. If we treat the flagleaf with cytokinin we would delay its senescence and so give more time for it to produce photosynthate for the grain. However, this would not be enough, for it would be necessary later on to induce the flagleaf to senesce so as to be sure that all of its photosynthate has moved out into the ear in time for harvesting. We know already from the work on leaf senescence how to delay and how to hasten senescence by simple chemical treatments. Thus, such a dual procedure, first delaying and then hastening senescence, could be an important strategy for the future. (Thimann)

● Delay of senescence in certain crops such as wheat, rice, and some grain legumes should be beneficial, with an estimated 3-5% additional yield potential in wheat for each day delay in senescence. It would be useful to discover the initial molecular event that triggers senescence. Carbon dioxide enrichment delays senescence in grain legumes, presumably by enabling the plant to meet its nitrogen needs by fixation without forcing breakdown of leaf protein. In other cases, as for multiple cropping senescence, enhancers may be desirable. (Hardy)

● See Hardy under ENRICHMENT OF SOIL AND AIR.

● There may well be times when you wish to change the genetic potential midseason with regulators. The following scenario can be envisaged: Farmers in variable rainfall regions are often convinced to plant the lower-yielding drought resistant dwarf wheats. In years when rainfall is higher, there is a large loss in yield. If we could, in these high rainfall years, treat these plants to "make" them into the intermediate size, later-ripening wheats, we would have a large market for a useful regulator. (Gressel)

● A major chemical breakthrough in the genetics of N_2 would be a catalyst that enabled a zero direct energy input oxidation of N_2 with the O_2 in the air at about 25°C. (Hardy)

● In at least some legumes up to 40 or 50% of photosynthate is transferred to the root, with large losses there as respired CO_2.

Is this huge loss of CO_2 necessary, or are roots inefficient, and might genetic or chemical regulation improve this efficiency? The nodule is especially inefficient, using 10-20 K_s CH_2O to fix 1 K_s N_2. (Hardy)

NATURAL HERBICIDES

● Plants have built-in defense mechanisms. One of the most common is allelopathy, defined as mutual harm, and explained by one species or culture of plant inhibiting the growth of another through the production of secondary metabolites as defensive agents in plant-to-plant relationships, usually by chemical means. The phenomenon offers an exciting alternative to the use of chemical herbicides, which are now the most extensively used of all substances for crop production. While most commonly expressed in the survival of desert plant communities, allelopathy has now been observed with at least four economically important crops--cucumbers, asparagus, sorghum, and sudan grass. There are important varietal differences within crops.

One potential application is for allelopathic cover crops to be used as an alternative to chemical herbicides in conservation tillage. Weed-suppressing crop residues could thus reduce the energy inputs into agricultural production and the dependence on synthetic herbicides, help eliminate an environmental hazard, and decrease the number of weak propagules. Characterization of natural plant toxins could lead to the synthesis of analogues with even greater efficiency and safety as herbicides for crop production. Although such developments will not escape regulatory constraints, the exploitation of allelopathic responses in economically important crops stands as one of the most exciting possible strategies for plant regulation and world agriculture. (Wittwer)

● See also Wain under REGULATION OF GROWTH for synthetic herbicides.

TISSUE CULTURE

● "The tissue culture technique is one of the cheapest used in agricultural research. In certain areas and especially for crop improvement it has great potential." (Nitsch) Another of its virtues is that it combines practical genetics and physiological considerations. Surely further investigation needs to be done on a technique which emphasizes rapid transfer of laboratory results to improvements in the field.

● In China the tissue culture technique has been used and developed to speed up work in plant breeding. New varieties of tobacco, rice, and wheat have been selected for high yield and shorter growing cycle. Moreover, they are adapted for the different regions. The main cost of tissue culture is in hand labor, which is usually readily available in developing countries. This technique is also used extensively to cure virus-infected plants by the meristem culture method. In forestry it is also a valuable tool for vegetative propagation of the trees. (Nitsch)

● Recent experiments have shown conclusively that somatic hybrid plants can be produced in combinations where sexual hybridization is not possible. It is difficult to visualize, however, the retention and expression of the complete genomes of both the parents in somatic hybrid plants of completely unrelated species. Judging from the behavior of such hybrid cell lines in animals, it would appear that chromosomes of one parent will be gradually eliminated. Indeed, evidence for this has been provided for soybean and tobacco cell lines. One can thus visualize a plant obtained from the fusion of a legume and a cereal protoplast in which all the cereal chromosomes are retained but only those chromosomes of the legume are present which enable it to associate with Rhizobia. Such an engineered cereal plant, when and if obtained, should have the ability to form a symbiotic association with Rhizobia. For the purpose of illustration, this scenario has been oversimplified, but it does not ignore the many difficult problems involved. If successful, culture of cereal protoplasts can influence selection of specific cell lines, the biology of rhizobial symbiosis, the energy requirements of nitrogen fixation, etc.

It must be emphasized that conventional plant breeding procedures will continue to be the dominant means of crop improvement, and somatic hybridization in time will supplement it only to a limited extent, in particularly difficult--but important--cases. (Vasil)

● In connection with the role of callus, it is suggestive that many cuttings including those of apples will form good callus although they will not root. The formation of callus is a sign that the cells of the cut surface are active, but one often gets the impression that callus and roots are alternatives, in that callus actually inhibits root formation. In Dr. Nitsch's cuttings cytokinins inhibit rooting (Chapter 4), and it has been shown recently that lateral root formation is powerfully inhibited by cytokinins. It may be, therefore, that callus is an active seat of cytokinin synthesis, and this would fit well with Dr. Lenz's finding (Chapter 9) that callus increases the apparent rate of photosynthesis of leaves, for cytokinin opens the stomata. (Thimann)

● The culture of pollen grains or anthers of seed plants to produce haploids may provide new potential for biomass production as an energy resource. Haploids may flower but produce no seed. Senescence is delayed or prolonged indefinitely. The possibilities with woody species should be explored. No photosynthetically fixed energy would be diverted to wasteful seed production. Similarly, continued growth of forage crops for livestock in the absence of seed production would be a boon to enhancement of feed production for ruminant animals. (Wittwer)

● Experiments on associated cultures of plant cells with nitrogen fixing bacteria provide valuable information which can be useful for providing or creating more suitable conditions for ideal natural- or forced-symbiotic associations in nature (see Vasil, Chapter 5). (Vasil)

● A type of highly significant fusion not discussed is the direct and simple transfer of a useful cytoplasm from one species to another without the need of crosses and backcrosses. Workers have recently been able to rapidly transfer cytoplasmic male sterility, an important factor for genetic hybridization, from one species of Nicotiana to another. The trick was to inactivate the nucleus of the male sterile plant by irradiation prior to fusion, thus leaving only the nucleus of the other species active. In a similar manner it might be possible to transfer cytoplasmically inherited herbicide resistance from the wild Brassica campestris to the Brassica crops. (Gressel)

● Though I do not know of any studies done on the use of ethylene in haploid culture, I personally feel that a study on CO_2 concentration in the culture vials might be more promising. Ethylene has been used in vitro culture to induce flowering in short-day plants grown under long days. (Nitsch)

● Generally, tissues and organs develop better in vitro without a solidifying agent that probably physically inhibits uptake of nutrients and sometimes contains inhibiting substances. Therefore, if we could design some supporting apparatus for tissues or organs, the use of a liquid medium is a preferable strategy, particularly when additions are to be given to or samples are to be taken from the medium, or the tissues or organs are to be transferred from one medium to another. (Bruinsma)

TEMPERATURE EFFECTS

● Climate, as related to crop productivity, should be viewed as an economic resource. It is scarce and needs to be allocated for specific crops in specific locations. "Climate fertility" has been suggested as equal in importance to soil fertility in total world agriculture. The most important parameters are temperature, precipitation, and sunlight.

The challenge for the future is to make climate a more useful and less hazardous resource. Climate on a global scale is exacting an enormous toll in reduced crop productivity, potential food production, and instability of supplies. (Wittwer)

● Plant growth regulators are known to modify the response of crops to climate, especially by reducing some of the hazards of low temperature. This is particularly manifested with sugarcane in the semi-tropics. Treatment of sugarcane with gibberellin during winter months has resulted in increased growth and a 10% gain in sugar yield. The use of gibberellin sprayed on forage grasses in early spring to stimulate growth and yield should be further explored. It is likely that if additional fertilizer nitrogen and other nutrients were added, growth and yields could be maintained during later harvests. (Wittwer)

● See Nitsch under BIOMASS.

● Because we know that there is already sufficient genetic and physiological hardiness in many crop plants of the temperate zone to survive extreme cold, provided plants can be acclimated and de-acclimated, we should aim at putting some of the "timidity" of this type of plant into some of our species that are more suited to optimum growth under warm conditions. "Timidity" means the slowness to growth early in spring when the risk of frost is high and air temperatures are warm but soil temperatures are low. Survival in this period is often critical to ultimate yield. Seed dormancy that requires a cold period to permit normal generation or a slow de-acclimation period in native plants or seedlings that overwinter are the natural mechanisms in wild plants to survive this critical period of warm days but frosty nights. (Simpson)

● Certain bulbs and tubers, such as *Ranunculus* and *Leucojum*, commence growth particularly early in spring. Is anything known about the temperature ranges over which the enzymes of these bulbs and tubers are active? Or is it possible that because they represent active tissue rather than dry seeds their enzymes are already in a free or active state? While those in seeds have to be released from bound or precursor forms? In either case this would seem to be a worthwhile area for study. (Thimann)

DROUGHT RESISTANCE

Since drought is one of the chief causes of loss of standing crops, ways must be found to make economically important crops more resistant to drought and to reduce the effects of water stress. There are both chemical and genetic means by which this may be accomplished.

• If the changes in the hormonal balance reported by Karamanos (see Chapter 23) and Simpson (see Chapter 7) are correlated with the variations in plant water potential both in the diurnal and the long-term scale, then it should be relatively easy to provide plant breeders with the so-called "magic box" for selecting genotypes for drought resistance. Instead of using sophisticated and expensive apparatus for the identification of the hormones, simpler instruments, for example the pressure bomb or the diffusion porometer, could provide easy and quick information. The fact that plant water potential was found to be correlated with the diurnal variations in the hormonal balance is a promising perspective. (Karamanos)

• We (and others) have found that cytokinins cause stomatal opening in the dark, but they will maintain stomatal opening in light. In isolated leaves we can thus maintain opening for 5 days continuously in light.

Cytokinins also control the synthesis of polysaccharides from sugar, and cytokinins applied to roots inhibit the growth of laterals.

Thus three of the phenomena described by Lenz (Chapter 9) could be due to cytokinins produced by the forest and transported to the leaves. It would be worthwhile to see if the influence on forests could be initiated by treating the leaves with cytokinin.

Also, it may be that treatment of leaves with stomatal opening substances (cytokinins or other) would have a good effect in keeping up photosynthetic rates, particularly in plants whose stomata tend to close during the afternoon. (Thimann)

• Ethylene and water stress--It has been shown that when plants of *Vicia fabia* and other species are subjected to water stress there is a rapid increase in endogenous ethylene by the plant. These ethylene changes appear to be responsible for some of the symptoms of water stress by leaf epinasty, senescence, and abscission and flower and fruit drop. I do not think that we can use ethylene to control water stress, but it may be possible to use inhibitors of ethylene biosynthesis to reduce some of the effects of water stress. (Wareing)

● Membrane-structural changes and permeability will continue to be among the leading problems in plant physiology for at least the next decade. Resistance to all kinds of stress, far more than being a matter of osmoregulation, is probably principally a matter of membrane-properties-mediated permeability. (Bruinsma)

● An interesting question to pursue is whether there is a sufficient amount of water lost via the cuticle to justify looking for chemical ways (i.e., with growth regulators) to modify cuticle composition. (Gressel)

● See also Wittwer under ENRICHMENT OF SOIL AND AIR.

SEEDS

● There are many advantages of seed preconditioning by growth regulator infusion or by osmotic treatment with PEG-6000. These include (a) advancement of germination time, (b) decrease in the spread of germination, (c) alleviation of environmental stress, (d) production of uniform seedlings, (e) invigoration of seeds as measured by increased rate of root and shoot growth, and (f) increase in yield. (a) through (e) have been tested in soybeans, peas, cabbage, brussels sprouts, lettuce, and celery with positive results.

Highly encouraging results have been obtained in field trials conducted on several cultivars of lettuce in combination treatments in which fusicoccin or cotylenin were fused into lettuce seeds via acetone and then pelleted. Time of emergence and percentage emergence in treated seeds were considerably higher than in untreated seeds.

Seeds of brussels sprouts and cabbage conditioned in 25% PEG-6000 in the presence of 0.2% thiram showed both advancement of emergence and increase in percentage emergence. Soybeans and peas osmoconditioned in the presence of thiram and GA_3 showed marked advancement in emergence time. The major advantage of osmotic treatment with PEG-6000 is that conditioned seeds perform well at suboptimal temperatures such as 5-10°C. This should allow planting of conditioned seeds early in the spring when the soil is moist and cold, and result in increased vegetative growth, a factor of considerable importance in improving yield in such seeds as soybeans. This is particularly true in regions having short growing seasons.

--Many seed protectants can be added to the PEG solution during conditioning at 15°C to control seed-borne and soil-borne pathogens.

--Osmoconditioning of vegetable and flower seeds advances germination time. Thus, it should be possible to increase turnover of flowers and vegetables, especially in glass houses.

--By infusing growth regulators such as fusicoccin and cotylenin into seeds such as lettuce prior to and during osmoconditioning, it should be possible to induce both low temperature and high temperature tolerance.

--By incorporating growth regulators such as a combination of GA, cytokinin, and ethephon during osmotic treatment, it is possible to prevent the induction of secondary dormancy both in the soil and during the osmotic treatment as determined by subsequent germination. Thus it should be possible to spray fields with the appropriate growth regulator combinations to prevent the induction of secondary dormancy in these seeds. (Khan)

● Recent studies reveal that the presence of such gases as O_2, CO_2, and C_2H_4 in the ambient atmosphere, in at least low concentrations, are necessary for the efficient working of exogenous growth regulators such as kinetin plus GA in lettuce seeds. This is especially true under stress conditions (i.e., suboptimal temperatures). Conversely, a combination of all these gases seems to improve germination of lettuce seeds at suboptimal levels of exogenous hormones. Thus by increasing the levels of appropriate gases or growth regulators under various conditions, it should be possible to increase the performance of seeds in the soil. (Khan)

● Several species of Rhizobium, e.g., R. japonicum, have been used to coat seeds of legumes to improve seed and plant performance. The fungi are mixed with lime which is then coated onto the seeds. (Khan)

● One of the greatest potential disseminators of weed seed is open irrigation channels, especially where they are earthen. It would be very interesting to make weed seed counts on the filters used in some trickle irrigation systems which are fed by channel water to assess how much weed seed is disseminated in the unfiltered water used in furrow irrigation. (Gressel)

OTHER SUGGESTIONS

The following are several suggestions which do not fit neatly under any of the above rubrics. They are nevertheless worthy of consideration, especially since they are, in the main, manipulations of existing technology.

- Possibilities for parthenocarpy in olives must be taken into consideration as a strategy. Olive is a very important crop in all the Mediterranean countries, and approximately 40% of the fruit consists of a hard seed that is unused. Therefore, different types of growth regulators should be tried and a way found to obtain parthenocarpic fruits. It will then be possible to get a 40% increase in the edible part of the olive fruit, which will help a great deal in increasing the total yield. (Vardar)

- Dr. Lenz (see Chapter 9) stated that if a fruit tree yielded many fruits, the average size of the fruits tended to be smaller than if the tree had set few fruits. Could we somehow manipulate the control processes in operation so that when numerous fruits are set assimilates would be diverted into the fruits to render them larger? This could be done at the expense of deploying assimilates to leaves, stems, and roots, although the long-term needs of the tree to remain vigorous would have to be satisfied. (Baxter)

- The suggestion of using C_4 plants that are weeds as crop plants in saline conditions because they are generally halophytes might not be the optimum way to reclaim land that has become saline through poor agronomic practice. If C_4 plants generally have a requirement for sodium, whereas C_3 plants do not, then C_4 plants may merely cause more sodium to accumulate in the top layers of the soil unless the plants are physically removed. Even grazing would return plant debris and urine to the surfaces. Would it not be better, for the purposes of reclaiming salty soils, to use C_3 plants, which would avoid sodium uptake? Leaching by rain could still move salts downward and there might be a chance to reclaim the soil for normal cropping rather than perpetuate the saline conditions by using only halophytes. (Simpson)

- The yields from peasant cassava fields are often pitifully low, and the two main reasons for this are: (1) Virus infection, and (2) No fertilizers used.

It was shown by laying down demonstration plots adjoining peasant holdings in Nigeria that, by using virus-free stocks and a proper fertilizer program, yields of 24 tons of cassava per acre could be obtained, whereas the peasant farmers were only getting 2 tons per acre on the same soil. (Wain)

- Plant growth regulators could be used to induce plant tolerance to insects and diseases. For example, use plant growth regulators to inhibit new growth of cotton in late season to control pinkworm in California and Arizona. (Ku)

- Chemical and physical methods to prevent crop loss during harvesting, handling, shipping, and storage may be an interesting topic for discussion. Vegetable and fruit losses due to postharvest mishandling may be as high as 5% of the crop. Loss of grain during storage is estimated at about 6%. Controlled-atmosphere and CO_2 storage for apples is one well-known technology being used today to prevent these losses. (Ku)

- Modern plant tissue culture techniques can be of much value and use in practical agriculture. Unfortunately, there has been no close collaboration or coordination of such research with the work of plant breeders, microbiologists, soil scientists, etc. Such collaboration will hasten the translation of laboratory successes into actual practice in the field. (Vasil)

- It has been shown that the flowering stimulus or influence increases in amount in a graft host. Thus it behaves like a virus or a plasmid, and it seems as if this must limit its chemical nature to that of a nucleic acid. This agrees with the observation that it is not transferred in extracts and does not diffuse across a tissue discontinuity, yet it is transmissible across a graft, i.e., in living tissue. I wonder if we should not pay more attention to this aspect. (Thimann)

Numerous suggestions have been made as to how we can extend currently available technology and develop new techniques to increase crop yield. Needless to say, no one of these proposed strategies will solve the problems of world agriculture. What will be required is careful consideration of many ideas of this sort.

LIST OF PARTICIPANTS

Acikgöz, N.	Agriculture Faculty, Ege University, Izmir, Turkey
Agaoglu, S.	Faculty of Agriculture, University of Ankara, Ankara, Turkey
Andersen, A. Skytt	Department of Plant Physiology, Royal Veterinarian & Agricultural University, Thorvaldsensvej, DK 1871, Copenhagen V, Denmark
Bagni, N.	Institute of Botany, University of Bologna, via Irnerio, 40126, Bologna, Italy
Baxter, R.	Shell Biosciences Laboratory, PBCD, Broad Oak Road, Sittingbourne, Kent, United Kingdom
Bayraktar, K.	Faculty of Agriculture, Ege University, Izmir, Turkey
Bennink, G. J. H.	Matthijs Tinxgracht 10, 1135WX Edam, The Netherlands
Bopp, M.	Botanisches Institut der Universität, Im Neuenheimer Feld 360, D-6900 Heidelberg, Federal Republic of Germany
Bozcuk, N.	Department of Botany, Hacettepe University, Ankara, Turkey
Bozcuk, S.	Department of Botany, Hacettepe University, Ankara, Turkey
Bruinsma, J.	Agricultural University, Arboretumlaan 2, Wageningen, The Netherlands
de Silva, W. H.	c/o Dr. R. Maag Ltd. Chemical Works, 8157 Dielsdorf, Switzerland
Duygu, E.	Department of Botany, University of Ankara, Ankara, Turkey
Ercoskun, T.	Department of Botany, University of Ankara, Ankara, Turkey
Eris, A.	Faculty of Agriculture, University of Ankara, Ankara, Turkey
Gökceoglü, M.	Department of Botany, Ege University, Izmir, Turkey
Görk, G.	Department of Botany, Ege University, Izmir, Turkey
Gressel, J.	Department of Plant Genetics, Weizmann Institute of Science, Rehovot, Israel
Güven, A.	Department of Botany, Ege University, Izmir, Turkey
Hardy, R. W. F.	Central Research and Development, E. I. du Pont de Nemours & Company, Wilmington, Delaware, 19898, U.S.A.
Hugill, J. A. C.	World Sugar Research Organization Ltd., 58 Jermyn Street, London SW1, United Kingdom

Istar, A.	Agriculture Faculty, Atatürk University, Erzurum, Turkey
Jennings, J. V.	Dunlop Ltd. Bio-Activities, 22 Northways Parade (College Crescent), Swiss Cottage, London, NW3 5EM, United Kingdom
Jones, R. L.	Department of Botany, University of California, Berkeley, California, 97420, U.S.A.
Jung, J.	BASF - Versuchsstation, D-6703 Limburgerhof, Postfach 220, Federal Republic of Germany
Kacar, B.	Faculty of Agriculture, University of Ankara, Ankara, Turkey
Karamanos, A. J.	Department of Plant Physiology, Agricultural College of Athens, Votanikos, Athens (T.301), Greece
Karanov, E.	c/o Acad. C. Daskalov, Bulgarian Academy of Science, UI 7, No. 1, Sofia, Bulgaria
Kaska, N.	Department of Pomology, Faculty of Agriculture, Cukurova University, Adana, Turkey
Khan, A. A.	New York State Agricultural Experiment Station, Cornell University, Geneva, New York, 14456, U.S.A.
Kisman, I.	Department of Pomology, Ege University, Izmir, Turkey
Köksal, G.	Nuclear Center, Cekmece, Istanbul, Turkey
Ku, H. S.	Diamond Shamrock Corporation, P.O. Box 348, Painesville, Ohio, 44077, U.S.A.
Kutlu, M.	Faculty of Medicine, Ege University, Izmir, Turkey
Kutlu, Y. Z.	Regional Agriculture Research Institute, P.O. Box 9, Menemen, Turkey
Laetsch, W. M.	Department of Botany, University of California, Berkeley, California, 94702, U.S.A.
Lenz, F.	Institute für Obstbau und Gemüsebau der Universität Bonn, Auf den Hügel 6, 53 Bonn, Federal Republic of Germany
MacConnell, J. T.	Glasgow College of Technology, Cowcaddens Red, Glasgow, G4 OBA, Scotland, United Kingdom
Malagamba, P.	Regional Agriculture Research Institute, P.O. Box 9, Menemen, Turkey
Mert, H. H.	Department of Botany, Ege University, Izmir, Turkey
Nitsch, C.	CNRS, Génétique et Physiologié du Développement des Plantes, 91190 Gif-sur-Yvette, France
Peterson, L. W.	Shell Development Company, P.O. Box 4248, Modesto, California, 95352, U.S.A.

Polar, E.	Isotope Center, Ege University, Izmir, Turkey
Powell, L. E.	Department of Pomology, Cornell University, Ithaca, New York, 14853, U.S.A.
Raman, D.	Tate & Lyle, Ltd. Group Research and Development, P.O. Box 68, Reading, Berkshire, RG6 2BX, United Kingdom
Rufener, J.	c/o CIBA-GEIGY, C-H Stein-Sächingen, Switzerland
Sagsöz, S.	Agriculture Faculty, Atatürk University, Erzurum, Turkey
Scott, T. K.	Department of Botany 010-A, University of North Carolina, Chapel Hill, North Carolina, 27514, U.S.A.
Schulke, G.	c/o Sandoz A.S., CH-4108 Witterswil/SO, Switzerland
Secer, M.	Isotope Center, Ege University, Izmir, Turkey
Secmen, Ö.	Department of Botany, Ege University, Izmir, Turkey
Shahbaghi, S.	College of Agriculture, Rezaiveh, Iran
Sharif, M.	Government of Pakistan Agricultural Research Council, L-13, Al-Markaz, F-7/2, P.O. Box 1031, Islamabad, Pakistan
Shen-Miller, J.	National Science Foundation, 1800 G Street, N.W., Washington, D.C., 20550, U.S.A.
Simpson, G. M.	Crop Science Department, University of Saskatchewan, Saskatoon, Saskatchewan, Canada
Szczepanski, C. von	Shering AG, Agrochemical Research, Postfach 65 03 11, D-1000 Berlin 65, Federal Republic of Germany
Tanrisever, A.	Agriculture Faculty, Ege University, Izmir, Turkey
Tekinel, O.	Faculty of Agriculture, Department of Agricultural Economics & Cultural Technology, Cukurova University, Adana, Turkey
Thimann, K. V.	The Thimann Laboratories, University of California, Santa Cruz, California, 95064, U.S.A.
Vardar, Y.	Yali Cad. Yillar Apt. 468/5, Karsiyaka-Izmir, Turkey
Vasil, I. K.	Department of Botany, University of Florida, Gainesville, Florida, 32611, U.S.A.
Veen, H.	Cent Voor Agrobiol Onderzoek (CABO), Bornsesteeg 65, P.O. Box 14, Wageningen, The Netherlands
Vlitos, A. J.	Tate & Lyle, Ltd. Group Research and Development, P.O. Box 68, Reading RG6 2BX, United Kingdom

Wain, R. L.	Agricultural Research Council, Wye College, Ashford, Kent TN25 5AH, United Kingdom
Wareing, P.	Department of Botany & Microbiology, The University of Wales, Aberystwyth, SY23 3DA Wales, United Kingdom
Wightman, F.	Department of Biology, Carleton University, Ottawa, Canada K1S 5B6
Wittwer, S. H.	Agricultural Experiment Station, Michigan State University, East Lansing, Michigan, 48824, U.S.A.
Yalcin, I.	Department of Botany, University of Ankara, Ankara, Turkey

AUTHOR INDEX

Numbers underlined indicate the page on which references are given in full.

PLANT NAME INDEX

SUBJECT INDEX